COMPLETE NURSE'S GUIDE

TO DIABETES CARE

SECOND EDITION

COMPLETE NURSE'S GUIDE

TO DIABETES CARE

SECOND EDITION

Belinda P. Childs, ARNP, MN, CDE, BC-ADM, Editor
Marjorie Cypress, PHD, MSN, RN, C-ANP, CDE, Editor
Geralyn Spollett, MSN, C-ANP, CDE, Editor

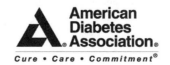

American Diabetes Association

Cure • Care • Commitment®

Director, Book Publishing, Robert Anthony; *Managing Editor*, Abe Ogden; *Acquisitions Editor, Professional Books*, Victor Van Beuren; *Editor*, Aime Ballard-Wood; *Production Manager*, Melissa Sprott; *Composition*, Aptara, Inc.; *Cover Design*, Koncept, Inc.; *Printer*, Transcontinental Printing.

Printed in Canada
1 3 5 7 9 10 8 6 4 2

The suggestions and information contained in this publication are generally consistent with the *Clinical Practice Recommendations* and other policies of the American Diabetes Association, but they do not represent the policy or position of the Association or any of its boards or committees. Reasonable steps have been taken to ensure the accuracy of the information presented. However, the American Diabetes Association cannot ensure the safety or efficacy of any product or service described in this publication. Individuals are advised to consult a physician or other appropriate health care professional before undertaking any diet or exercise program or taking any medication referred to in this publication. Professionals must use and apply their own professional judgment, experience, and training and should not rely solely on the information contained in this publication before prescribing any diet, exercise, or medication. The American Diabetes Association—its officers, directors, employees, volunteers, and members—assumes no responsibility or liability for personal or other injury, loss, or damage that may result from the suggestions or information in this publication.

♾ The paper in this publication meets the requirements of the ANSI Standard Z39.48-1992 (permanence of paper).

ADA titles may be purchased for business or promotional use or for special sales. To purchase more than 50 copies of this book at a discount, or for custom editions of this book with your logo, contact the American Diabetes Association at the address below, at booksales@diabetes.org, or by calling 703-299-2046.

American Diabetes Association
1701 North Beauregard Street
Alexandria, Virginia 22311

DOI: 10.2337/9781580403252

Library of Congress Cataloging-in-Publication Data

Complete nurse's guide to diabetes care / Belinda P. Childs, editor ; Marjorie Cypress, Geralyn Spollett, associate editor[s]. -- 2nd ed.
  p. ; cm.
 Includes bibliographical references and index.
 ISBN 978-1-58040-325-2 (alk. paper)
 1. Diabetes--Nursing. I. Childs, Belinda. II. Cypress, Marjorie. III. Spollett, Geralyn. IV. American Diabetes Association.
 [DNLM: 1. Diabetes Mellitus--nursing. WY 155 C737 2009]
 RC660.C515 2009
 616.4'620231--dc22
                              2009011302

Contents

DISEASES AND TREATMENTS THAT AFFECT DIABETES

DIABETES CARE IN COMMUNITY SETTINGS

Preface

Diabetes is a devastating disease that has become a worldwide epidemic. The prevalence of type 1 diabetes has remained steady, whereas the incidence of type 2 diabetes is growing at epidemic proportions. Currently, 23.6 million Americans have diabetes, 7.8% of the population. There are 17.9 million known to have the disease and 5.7 million are undiagnosed (1). This is an increase from 18 million with known diabetes, 6.3% of the population, in 2003. A recent paper in *Diabetes Care* suggests that >40% of people ≥20 years of age have hyperglycemic conditions and that the prevalence is higher in minority populations (2).

Individuals with pre-diabetes may be able to prevent the development of full-blown diabetes, as was shown in the Diabetes Prevention Program, by increasing activity and decreasing weight. This epidemic in pre-diabetes is being driven by our sedentary lifestyles and increasing rates of obesity. Today, even our children are developing type 2 diabetes at an alarming rate. One in three children will develop diabetes in his or her lifetime.

Uncontrolled diabetes is the leading cause of cardiovascular disease, kidney disease, amputation, and blindness and occurs more often in Latinos, Native Americans, and African Americans. It costs $174 billion annually, up from $134 billion in 2005 (3).

On a positive note, there have been great strides in diabetes care in just the past 5 years. New medications, strategies for treatment, and technologies have given us new tools to address diabetes care and its comorbidities. This guide will provide the latest information to help guide your practice.

In the first edition, I introduced you to Denver, my father-in-law, who died from the complications of diabetes at the age of 85. He had been in and out of the hospital and skilled care facilities and had lived at home with my mother-in-law with the support of home health nurses. It was always the nurse who was at the front line of his care, providing direction and support for my mother-in-law as she provided day-to-day care. What I did not tell you, is that not only has this family's experiences with nurses guided my desire to educate nurses and fueled my passion for diabetes, but I also grew up with a favorite aunt who was diagnosed at age 3 in 1939. She died on dialysis with significant retinopathy and neuropathy. My brother was diagnosed with type 1 diabetes in 1978, and a niece, his daughter, was diagnosed in 2006. My niece just had a healthy baby boy. My brother's care and health after 30 years of diabetes has been vastly different from my aunt's, and my hope is my niece will not have to live a lifetime with diabetes.

While my initial passion for diabetes was driven by my family experiences, I have found, like many other nurses, that a specialty in diabetes offers the opportunity to affect patients' lives in a unique and rewarding way. In caring for the person with diabetes, nurses are an integral part of the diabetes team, providing education, counseling, and disease management.

Nurses take care of people with diabetes every day, no matter where they work. Diabetes affects the rate of recovery from all of the other diseases that the individual with diabetes may encounter. Nurses knowledgeable in diabetes care can improve outcomes and reduce complications. Whether in hospitals, outpatient clinics, community health settings, or public health service, nurses have always played an important role in the care of a person with diabetes, and they will continue to be an essential part of the health care team.

Despite the number of diabetes educators, diabetes nurse specialists, and diabetes education programs across the country, they are few compared with the number of individuals with diabetes. To improve outcomes for individuals with diabetes, we believe it is important that all nurses have a good understanding of diabetes care and education. All nurses must be knowledgeable about diabetes, regardless of their setting. The nurse must have information that is up to date and easily accessible when they are providing patient care, and it is my hope that this book will be a valuable resource for nurses in all settings as they care for patients with diabetes. My co-editors, Marjorie Cypress, PhD, C-ANP, CDE, and Geralyn Spollett, MSN, C-ANP, CDE, and I asked many of the leading experts in diabetes to contribute to this book. The majority are nurses, so it is a book for nurses written by nurses. It is our hope that through this effort patients may be diagnosed earlier, care may be improved in all settings, and diabetes may even be prevented by the actions of nurses.

In 1973, the American Association of Diabetes Educators (AADE) was founded (3). This organization provides training and information for the diabetes educator. Their membership includes nurses, dietitians, pharmacists, social workers, psychologists, physicians, exercise specialists, and others interested in diabetes education. This group recognized the need for a specialty certification examination. The National Certification Board for Diabetes Educators (NCBDE) bestows the title of Certified Diabetes Educator (CDE) on those who pass the examination, which has been offered by the NCBDE since 1986 (4). (More information is available in the RESOURCES section of this book.) At present, there are over 16,000 CDEs, and the AADE has ~12,000 members. More than 50% of the members of AADE document a discipline of RN, NP, or CNS.

In 2002, the first diabetes specialty certification through the American Academy for Nurse Credentialing was administered. This certification recognizes nurses, dietitians, and pharmacists with master's degrees who have met the eligibility criteria for advanced practice providers and have passed an exam. The certification is designated as Board Certified–Advanced Diabetes Management (BC-ADM).

Since 1986, the American Diabetes Association (ADA) has recognized diabetes education programs that meet the criteria for recognition (5). In many cases, ADA Recognition is required for insurance and Medicare reimbursement. Over 2,060 programs at 3,308 sites throughout the U.S. are recognized by the ADA.

The Joint Commission Certificate of Distinction for Inpatient Diabetes Care recognizes hospitals that make exceptional efforts to foster improved outcomes across all patient settings. The Joint Commission and the ADA have identified that most successful inpatient diabetes programs possess several critical attributes, including staff education, written blood glucose monitoring protocols, plans for treatment of hypoglycemia and hyperglycemia, tracking of hypoglycemia incidence, patient education on self-management of diabetes, and a diabetes champion or diabetes team within the inpatient setting (4). You may be a member of this team.

Diabetes Spectrum is a journal published by the ADA that translates research into practice for the diabetes care specialist. The readership consists of nurses, dietitians, psychologists, social workers, pharmacists, physician's assistants, nurse practitioners, and physicians.

Many resources are available for patients and professionals alike. This book has an extensive resources section to assist the health care professional and individual with diabetes in gaining the most up-to-date information.

Knowledge is a key to success whether you are a health care professional, a person with diabetes, or a family member of someone with diabetes. The advances in the understanding of diabetes and treatment strategies change almost daily. This is an exciting time to be caring for individuals with diabetes. Science is adding to our knowledge about obesity-related hormones. New hormones such as amylin have been identified and are now available as a treatment. Fat is now being considered an endocrine organ that produces hormones that affect one's ability to regulate food intake. We have new insulins and new insulin delivery systems and today can say the continuous glucose sensor is a reality.

Nursing can be challenging for many reasons, from long working hours and staffing issues to complexity of care. But it can also be one of the highlights of one's life. There is no greater satisfaction than making a difference in a person's life and health outcomes. Advocating for a person with diabetes is a joy. In helping patients accept the challenges before them, guiding someone toward financial support for medication, referring a family to a support group, or providing hope to the child newly diagnosed with diabetes, you make a difference. Consider yourself a coach. You, the nurse, are providing strategies that assist the individual with diabetes live each day to its fullest. It takes all of us to support individuals with diabetes and their families.

This book has been designed and developed to be used as a resource guide. It is organized into sections. These sections are Fundamentals of Diabetes Care, Complications, Diabetes Care and Management, Special Populations, Diseases and Treatments That Affect Diabetes, Diabetes Care in Community Settings, and Resources. Each chapter features helpful Practical Points, implications for nursing practice that are interspersed throughout, and a summary, which is provided at the end.

Thank you for your interest in diabetes. I encourage you to be an enthusiastic coach for the person with diabetes and hope that the *Complete Nurse's Guide to Diabetes Care* will support you in your work and lifelong learning.

BELINDA P. CHILDS, ARNP, MN, CDE, BC-ADM
Editor

REFERENCES

1. Centers for Disease Control and Prevention: National diabetes fact sheet: United States, 2007 [Internet]. Available from http://www.cdc.gov/diabetes/pubs/pdf/ndfs_2007.pdf. Accessed 1 March 2009

2. Cowie CC, Rust KF, Ford ES, Eberhardt MS, Byrd-Holt DD, et al.: Full accounting of diabetes and pre-diabetes in the U.S. population in 1988–1994 and 2005–2006. *Diabetes Care* 32:287–294, 2009

3. American Diabetes Association: Economic costs of diabetes in the U.S. in 2007 [Internet]. http://www.diabetes.org/diabetes-statistics/cost-of-diabetes-in-us.jsp. Accessed 1 March 2009

4. Joint Commission: Inpatient Diabetes Certification [Internet]. Available from http://www.jointcommission.org/CertificationPrograms/Inpatient+Diabetes. Accessed 1 March 2009

5. American Diabetes Association: Standards of medical care for diabetes—2009 (Position Statement). *Diabetes Care* 32 (Suppl. 1):S13–S61, 2009

Current Knowledge on Diabetes

- Type 2 diabetes can be prevented with changes in lifestyle
- The complications of diabetes can be delayed or prevented with
  - Optimal glucose control (glycated hemoglobin A1c <7.0%) and early, aggressive treatments
  - Management of lipids
    - HDL cholesterol >40 mg/dl
    - LDL cholesterol <100 mg/dl (<70 mg/dl for those with diabetes and overt cardiovascular disease)
      - Triglycerides <150 mg/dl
  - Management of blood pressure
    - <130/80 mmHg
- Smoking cessation is imperative
- One aspirin (75–162 mg) daily for those >40 years of age for primary and secondary prevention of cardiovascular disease

These recommendations are taken from the ADA Clinical Practice Recommendations, which are updated annually (5).

About the Editors

Belinda P. Childs, ARNP, MN, CDE, BC-ADM, is a diabetes nurse specialist at Mid-America Diabetes Associates in Wichita, KS. She received her bachelor's and master's degrees in nursing from Wichita State University. She has worked with Drs. Richard and Diana Guthrie for over 30 years. She is the clinic and research coordinator for the practice and provides diabetes care and education for children, adults, and their families. She has authored several book chapters and journal articles and has done numerous presentations. She is a past editor of *Diabetes Spectrum*, a publication of the American Diabetes Association (2001–2005). Lindy is an adjunct faculty member and instructor in the Department of Nursing at Wichita State University. She is a past President, Health Care & Education, of the American Diabetes Association (1996–1997). She is the co-founder and chair of the Parish Nursing Ministry at her church.

Marjorie Cypress, PhD, MSN, RN, C-ANP, CDE, is an adult nurse practitioner with ABQ Health Partners, Department of Endocrinology in Albuquerque, NM. She received her bachelor's degree from C.W. Post College, her MS in nursing from State University of New York at Stony Brook, and her PhD in Nursing at the University of New Mexico. She has worked in diabetes management and in education of patients and health care professionals for 25 years in New York and New Mexico. She has authored articles in professional and patient diabetes journals and has done numerous presentations. In 2004, Marjorie received the Outstanding Educator in Diabetes Award from the American Diabetes Association (ADA) and the Distinguished Service award from the National Certification Board for Diabetes Educators (NCBDE). She is a past chair of the NBCDE, served on the ADA national board of the directors, and is a member of the State of NM, Diabetes Advisory Committee, and president of the New Mexico Leadership Board for ADA.

Geralyn Spollett, MSN, C-ANP, CDE, is an adult nurse practitioner and associate director at the Yale Diabetes Center, affiliated with the Yale School of Medicine and the Yale New Haven Hospital. During her 30-year career as a nurse practitioner and diabetes educator, Geri has worked with Native American, Hispanic, and African American populations to improve diabetes care and delivery systems. She received her BSN from Fairfield University and MSN from Boston College. During her 10 years at the Yale School of Nursing, she taught in Adult/Family Nurse Practitioner Program and the diabetes care concentration, conducted research in type 2 diabetes in African-American women, and lectured nationally and internationally on diabetes management from a nurse practitioner perspective. Geri has served as associate editor for *Diabetes Spectrum* and written for many of the leading nursing- and diabetes-related journals. She is an active member of the American Diabetes Association (ADA), having served on its board of directors and program committees for the ADA Postgraduate Course and Scientific Sessions. She received the ADA Outstanding Educator in Diabetes Award in 2006. Geri has been active on the National Certification Board of Diabetes Educators, chairing multiple committees and serving as the chair of the Board of Directors.

Acknowledgments

We thank all of the authors who contributed to this book. We would also like to thank our colleagues at Mid-America Diabetes Associates, ABQ Health Partners, and Yale University who have supported us in this endeavor. We are especially indebted to the Guthries for their everlasting impact on thousands of diabetes care providers and individuals with diabetes across the U.S. and internationally. They had a vision and believed that their calling was to promote the importance of diabetes self-management and patient and professional education throughout their lives.

The American Diabetes Association (ADA) must be acknowledged for recognizing the need for a comprehensive book dedicated to the role of the nurse in providing care for people with diabetes. A heartfelt thank you goes to the dedicated ADA staff that provided countless hours, enthusiastic energy, and incredible expertise in making this book a reality. In particular, Victor Van Beuren, Abe Ogden, Stephanie Dunbar, and Sue Kirkman, MD, deserve recognition.

We also thank our families for their support and understanding as we live our passion, the care of people with diabetes. Without their love, support, and guidance, we would not have been able to undertake this endeavor.

And finally, we are grateful to those who live with diabetes for all that they have taught us throughout our lifetimes.

Belinda P. Childs, ARNP, MN, CDE, BC-ADM
Marjorie Cypress, PhD, MSN, RN, C-ANP, CDE
Geralyn Spollett, MSN, C-ANP, CDE

FUNDAMENTALS OF
DIABETES CARE

1. Diagnosis and Classification

Marjorie Cypress, PHD, MSN, RN, C-ANP, CDE,
and Jeremy Gleeson, MD, FACP, FACE, CDE

D iabetes is one of the most common diseases that nurses will deal with in their professional lives. It is so widespread it is called an epidemic, and it is a major health problem in the U.S., as well as in the rest of the world. The prevalence of diagnosed diabetes in the U.S. has increased from 5.6 million people in 1980 to 17.9 million in 2007 (1). The World Health Organization estimates that more than 180 million people worldwide have diabetes, and that number is expected to double by the year 2030 (2). For those people over the age of 65 years, 38% of the population suffers from diabetes. It is listed as the 7th leading cause of death and is linked with heart disease, hypertension, blindness, kidney disease, nervous system disease, amputations, and dental disease (3).

Because diabetes is a chronic and progressive disease, diagnosing diabetes early and intervening even before the diagnosis can help improve health and decrease the burden on individuals, families, communities, and society. This chapter will review the current criteria for diagnosing and classifying diabetes.

Diabetes is a group of related conditions characterized by abnormalities in the metabolism of carbohydrates, protein, and fat, resulting in elevated blood glucose levels. Although insulin, a hormone secreted by β-cells in the pancreatic islets, is mainly responsible for controlling blood glucose levels, several other hormones that affect fuel metabolism also have an effect on glucose control. Amylin is one such hormone whose significance has been recently recognized. Diabetes may result from defects in insulin secretion or action or a combination of both factors. Regardless of the underlying cause, the diagnosis of diabetes is straightforward and based on elevation of blood glucose alone.

Chronic hyperglycemia causes damage to blood vessels and is associated with several diabetes complications—most notably damage to the eyes, kidneys, and nerves, as well as other organs. These complications appear to be direct consequences of blood glucose elevation. Importantly, patients with diabetes are also at much higher risk for cardiovascular events, such as heart attack and stroke. Symptoms of diabetes, all caused by elevated blood glucose, include polyuria, polydipsia, weight loss, fatigue, blurred vision, and dry mouth. Many people, usually those with milder elevations in blood glucose, have no symptoms at all or may not recognize them as problems. The diagnosis may therefore first be suspected on routine measurement of blood glucose or on an incidental finding of glucose in the urine. Sometimes diagnosis occurs when there is already evidence of chronic diabetes complications such as vascular disease or neuropathy. The onset of diabetes is generally insidious. Because many patients, especially those with type 2 diabetes, are free of symptoms, they may remain undiagnosed for prolonged periods.

CLASSIFICATION OF DIABETES

There are several distinct classes of diabetes. The most common forms of diabetes are designated type 1, type 2, and gestational. Type 1 diabetes is caused by an absolute deficiency of insulin secretion, whereas type 2 diabetes is caused by a combination of insulin resistance and a relative, progressive decrease in insulin secretion. Approximately 90% of patients with diabetes have type 2 diabetes. Diabetes first diagnosed in pregnancy is designated gestational diabetes mellitus (GDM); most patients with GDM have features in common with type 2 diabetes. Type 1 and type 2 diabetes encompass the vast majority of patients with diabetes. Some patients may have overlapping features of both type 1 and type 2 diabetes. Rarer forms of diabetes occur as a result of genetic defects in β-cell function, pancreatic diseases, various endocrine diseases, and drug-induced diabetes. To avoid patient misclassification, the terms insulin-dependent diabetes mellitus and non-insulin-dependent diabetes mellitus, for type 1 and type 2 diabetes, respectively, are no longer used. Many patients with type 2 diabetes "depend" on insulin for glucose control.

EPIDEMIOLOGY

The incidence of diabetes is increasing at an alarming rate among all races, ethnicities, ages, and weight classes. In the U.S., 7% of the entire population is believed to have diabetes. Among men over the age of 20 years, 10.5% have diabetes, and among women of the same age, 8.8% have diabetes (3). This is believed to be related to the increasing rates of obesity and higher prevalence of sedentary lifestyle among Americans and the rapidly growing high-risk populations of Native Americans, Hispanics/Latinos, African Americans, Asians, and Pacific Islanders. In those under 20 years of age, 1 in 400 has diabetes. Although historically diagnoses of diabetes in children have been almost exclusively of type 1, the incidence of the development of type 2 diabetes in children has increased significantly as a result of increasing obesity. Worldwide there is a significant increase in the prevalence of type 2 diabetes in children and adolescents, particularly among those ethnic groups with high susceptibility to type 2 diabetes. Whereas the actual statistics in the U.S. are not known, there have been reports that as many as 8–45% of children with newly diagnosed diabetes have type 2 diabetes (4,5).

In the U.S., type 2 diabetes is more common in minority populations. From an international perspective, however, an increased risk for type 2 diabetes is seen in many diverse ethnic groups. Typically, type 2 diabetes increases when susceptible populations adopt a westernized lifestyle with increased caloric intake and reduced physical activity.

GDM occurs more frequently in African American, Hispanic/Latino, and Native American populations. Approximately 4% of all pregnancies in the U.S. result in GDM, but the prevalence rate ranges from 1 to 14% depending on the population studied (5). Although GDM is glucose intolerance during pregnancy, 5–10% of women with GDM are discovered to have type 2 diabetes, and women with a history of GDM have a 40–60% chance of developing diabetes over the next 5–10 years (3).

HIGH-RISK ETHNICITIES AND TYPE 2 DIABETES

Non-Hispanic blacks/African Americans. A total of 13.3% of all non-Hispanic blacks ≥20 years of age have diabetes. The risk of type 2 diabetes is 1.8 times that for non-Hispanic whites (3).

Hispanic/Latino Americans. An estimated 9.5% of Hispanics ≥20 years of age have type 2 diabetes. Hispanic/Latino Americans are 1.7 times more likely to have diabetes than non-Hispanic whites. Mexican Americans have a risk for diabetes more than twice that of non-Hispanics, and Puerto Ricans are 1.8 times more likely to have diabetes than non-Hispanic whites (3).

Native Americans/Alaska Natives. Native Americans/Alaska Natives have the highest risk of developing type 2 diabetes (2.3 times that of non-Hispanic whites), and it is estimated that 15.1% of this population ≥20 years of age has type 2 diabetes. Among all Native Americans, Alaska Natives have the least risk (8.2%), whereas Native Americans in the southeastern U.S. (27.8%) and in southern Arizona (27.8%) have the highest risk of developing diabetes (3).

Asians/Native Hawaiians/Pacific Islanders. Although there are no specific percentages regarding the prevalence of diabetes in these populations, it is believed that this group is at least twice as likely to develop type 2 diabetes as non-Hispanic whites (3).

DIAGNOSING DIABETES

The recommended screening and diagnostic test for diabetes (Table 1.1) is to measure fasting plasma glucose (6,7). Individuals suspected of having diabetes and those with high risk factors (Table 1.2), even though asymptomatic, should be tested for diabetes. Adults over the age of 45 years should be screened every 3 years. Screening should occur earlier and potentially more often (every 1–2 years) in patients with any of the following:

- overweight (body mass index [BMI] ≥25 kg/m^2)
- history of GDM or delivery of a baby weighing >9 lb

- history of vascular disease
- first-degree relative with diabetes
- high-risk ethnic group
- previously found to have impaired glucose tolerance or impaired fasting glucose
- signs of insulin resistance, such as acanthosis nigricans, hypertension, dyslipidemia, or polycystic ovary syndrome

Diabetes may also be diagnosed based on an oral glucose tolerance test (OGTT) (Table 1.1). This test is not routinely recommended in clinical practice because evaluating fasting plasma glucose is simpler and more convenient. However, an OGTT will identify some individuals as having diabetes who would not be diagnosed based on fasting glucose alone. A 75-g OGTT is used in nonpregnant individuals, and a 100-g OGTT is most commonly used in the U.S. to screen for GDM (see below). Use of the glycated hemoglobin A1c (A1C) measurement,

Table 1.1 American Diabetes Association Criteria for Diagnosing Diabetes

In nonpregnant adults	Testing for type 2 diabetes in children
Symptoms of diabetes and casual plasma glucose ≥200 mg/dl (≥11.1 mmol/l). Casual is defined as any time of day without regard to time since last meal. The classic symptoms of diabetes include polyuria, polydipsia, and unexplained weight loss. OR Fasting plasma glucose ≥126 mg/dl (≥7 mmol/l). Fasting is defined as no caloric intake for at least 8 h. OR 2-h plasma glucose ≥200 mg/dl (≥11.1 mmol/l) during an OGTT. The test should be performed using a glucose load containing the equivalent of 75 g anhydrous glucose dissolved in water.	Overweight (BMI >85th percentile for age and sex, weight for height >85th percentile, or weight >12–30% over ideal for height) PLUS Any two of the following risk factors: ■ Family history of type 2 diabetes in first- or second-degree relative ■ Race/ethnicity (Native American, African American, Hispanic/Latino, Asian American, Pacific Islander) ■ Signs of insulin resistance or conditions associated with insulin resistance (acanthosis nigricans, hypertension, dyslipidemia, history of small-for-gestational-age birth weight or polycystic ovary syndrome) ■ Maternal history of diabetes or GDM during the child's gestation Age of initiation: age 10 years or at onset of puberty if puberty occurs at an earlier age Frequency: every 3 years Test: fasting plasma glucose preferred

From the American Diabetes Association (8). OGTT, oral glucose tolerance test.
These criteria should be confirmed by repeat testing on a different day. Clinical judgment should be used for diabetes in high-risk patients who do not meet these criteria.

Table 1.2 Risk Factors for Type 2 Diabetes

Age ≥45 years
Overweight (BMI ≥25 kg/m2; may not be correct for all ethnic groups)
Family history of diabetes (e.g., parents or siblings with diabetes)
Habitual physical inactivity
Race/ethnicity (e.g., African Americans, Hispanic Americans, Native Americans, Alaskan Americans, and Pacific Islanders)
Previously identified as having impaired glucose tolerance or impaired fasting glucose
History of GDM or delivery of a baby weighing >9 lb
Hypertension (≥140/90 mmHg in adults)
HDL cholesterol ≤ 35 mg/dl and/or triglyceride level ≥250 mg/dl
Polycystic ovary syndrome
History of vascular disease

From the American Diabetes Association (8).

which is a standard test for monitoring glucose control in patients with diabetes, is not currently recommended for establishing the diagnosis of diabetes. In clinical practice, however, a markedly elevated A1C is virtually diagnostic of diabetes. An expert committee convened in 2008 will likely recommend that A1C become the preferred diagnostic test for diabetes; however, the diagnostic cut points had not been published at the time of this writing (8).

PRE-DIABETES

Individuals who do not meet the criteria for diabetes but who clearly have abnormal glucose levels as evidenced by a fasting plasma glucose >100 mg/dl (>5.6 mmol/l) but <126 mg/dl (<7 mmol/l) (impaired fasting glucose) or an OGTT 2-h postglucose level ≥140 mg/dl (≥7.8 mmol/l) and <200 mg/dl (<11.1 mmol/l) (impaired glucose tolerance) are considered to have pre-diabetes. As suggested by the term "pre-diabetes," these individuals have a very high risk of subsequent diabetes. See Table 1.3 for diagnostic criteria, including pre-diabetes.

Table 1.3 Diagnostic Criteria

Normoglycemia	Pre-Diabetes	Diabetes
FPG 100 mg/dl (5.6 mmol/l) 2-h PG <140 (<7.8 mmol/l)	FPG >100 mg/dl (>5.6 mmol/l) 2-h PG ≥140 mg/dl (≥7.8 mmol/l) and <200 mg/dl (11.1 mmol/l)	FPG ≥126 mg/dl (≥7 mmol/l) 2-h PG ≥200 mg/dl (≥11.1 mmol/l) Symptoms of diabetes and casual plasma glucose concentration (random) ≥200 mg/dl (≥11.1 mmol/l)

FPG, fasting plasma glucose; PG, plasma glucose.

DIAGNOSING GDM

If possible, a patient's risk for GDM should be determined before conception, but certainly at the onset of the diagnosis of pregnancy. Women who are obese or have a prior history of GDM, a family history of diabetes, or glycosuria should have glucose screening done as soon as possible. Other women who are of average risk, older than age 25 years, overweight, or a member of a high-risk ethnic group, or who have a history of poor obstetrical outcomes (e.g., spontaneous abortion, congenital malformation, fetal macrosomia) should be screened for GDM at 24–28 weeks' gestation. Screening for GDM is performed with a glucose challenge or OGTT (Table 1.4). The diagnosis of GDM can be made with either a 100-g OGTT as the initial test or a two-step screening approach that begins with a 50-g glucose challenge, followed by the 100-g OGTT if the postchallenge glucose is >130 mg/dl (>7.2 mmol/l). Using a cutoff of ≥130 mg/dl, this two-step screening approach identifies 90% of women with GDM (6).

It is important to be aware that overt type 2 diabetes may manifest early in pregnancy because of weight gain and the increasing insulin resistance of pregnancy. Abnormal blood glucose levels before the 24- to 28-week period of pregnancy suggest a diagnosis of type 2 diabetes or pre-diabetes as opposed to typical GDM. Regardless, because the diagnosis of GDM is a risk factor for the development of type 2 diabetes, women with abnormal blood glucose levels should be screened for diabetes 6–12 weeks postpartum, using OGTT criteria for individuals

Table 1.4 GDM Diagnosis

Diagnosis of GDM with a 100-g oral glucose load after an overnight fast of at least 8 hours

Time	mg/dl (mmol/l)
Fasting	≥95 (5.3)
1 h	≥180 (10)
2 h	≥155 (8.6)
3 h	≥140 (7.8)

Diagnosis of GDM with a 75-g oral glucose load

Time	mg/dl (mmol/l)
Fasting	≥95 (5.3)
1 h	≥180 (10)
2 h	≥155 (8.6)

From the American Diabetes Association (6). Two or more of the venous plasma concentrations must be met or exceeded for a positive diagnosis. The test should be done in the morning after an overnight fast of at least 8 h and after at least 3 days of unrestricted diet (≥150 g carbohydrate/day) and unlimited physical activity. The person should remain seated and should not smoke throughout the test.

who are not pregnant, and continue to be followed and screened for the development of pre-diabetes or diabetes (8).

PATHOGENESIS OF DIABETES

TYPE 1 DIABETES

The pathogenesis of type 1 diabetes is divided into autoimmune-mediated diabetes and idiopathic diabetes. In autoimmune-mediated diabetes, insulin-producing β-cells are destroyed by an autoimmune-mediated process. Typically, β-cells are totally destroyed, but in some patients, destruction is incomplete, resulting in residual insulin production. The rate of destruction is variable. In children, it is often rapid, whereas in adults, it may take several years. Antibody markers are usually seen. These include islet cell antibodies, insulin autoantibodies, and antibodies to glutamic acid decarboxylase (GAD), among others. Antibodies that are present early in the course of diabetes may subsequently become undetectable. There are well-recognized associations with several genes in the HLA (human leukocyte antigen) loci, including both predisposing and protective genes. Patients with type 1 diabetes have increased incidences of other autoimmune diseases, including Hashimoto's thyroiditis, Graves' disease, pernicious anemia, vitiligo, celiac disease, and Addison's disease. In type 1 diabetes, deficiency of the β-cell hormone amylin occurs along with insulin deficiency. This hormone has important effects on glucose disposal after eating.

There is a less common form of type 1 diabetes known as idiopathic diabetes, in which there is no evidence of autoimmune disease and immune markers are absent. This appears to be inherited, but the cause is unknown. Idiopathic diabetes is more common in those of African or Asian ethnic origin and is characterized by episodic ketoacidosis and varying degrees of insulin deficiency. The need for insulin replacement is intermittent—it may come and go.

TYPE 2 DIABETES

The pathogenesis of type 2 diabetes is complex. Type 2 diabetes develops progressively, with the pathogenic abnormalities already present in the phase of pre-diabetes. Virtually all individuals with type 2 have insulin resistance combined with varying degrees of insulin deficiency. Typically, this is a relative, not absolute, insulin deficiency. Early in the course of type 2 diabetes, insulin secretion may be increased in relation to that in individuals without diabetes; however, it is always deficient in terms of the amount required to overcome the insulin resistance. Later in the course of type 2 diabetes, insulin deficiency is often more pronounced.

The progressive decline in β-cell function over several years, regardless of type of therapy, was demonstrated in the U.K. Prospective Diabetes Study (UKPDS) (9), wherein the ability to maintain A1C levels continued to decrease markedly throughout the 9 years of follow-up, even when the researchers controlled for lifestyle issues such as diet, physical activity, and medication. Notably, in the UKPDS, insulin resistance did not change, suggesting that decreasing β-cell function is responsible for diabetes progression. This progression of insulin deficiency is reflected in the treatment required by those with type 2 diabetes. Many individuals with type 2 diabetes require multiple oral medications and will go on to require insulin therapy either in combination with oral agents or as monotherapy.

Type 2 diabetes shows a strong familial tendency. There are likely to be multiple genes involved, but none has been clearly identified. Obesity and sedentary lifestyle are major risk factors for development of type 2 diabetes. Obesity, particularly abdominal obesity, increases insulin resistance and the risk for type 2 diabetes. Genetic factors, i.e., those unrelated to obesity, also contribute to insulin resistance. Clearly though, many obese individuals do not develop type 2 diabetes. They presumably have adequate β-cell function to produce sufficient insulin to overcome the insulin resistance. Even with insulin resistance, diabetes will usually not develop unless there is a concomitant defect in β-cell function resulting in a deficiency of insulin secretion. Weight loss in overweight individuals with diabetes improves insulin resistance but usually does not fully restore insulin sensitivity.

GDM

Diabetes that is first recognized in pregnancy is classified as GDM, although most patients with GDM share pathogenic features in common with type 2 diabetes. The insulin resistance of pregnancy leads to hyperglycemia in susceptible women that often resolves after delivery but may recur in subsequent pregnancies. Screening on the first prenatal visit should include assessment for high-risk ethnic group, personal history of impaired glucose tolerance or fasting glucose, family history of diabetes, previous history of GDM, and obesity (6). Consistent with this pathogenesis, women who have had GDM are at increased risk of developing diabetes later in life and should be screened for the subsequent development of diabetes throughout their lives. Any form of diabetes, including type 1 diabetes, can be first recognized in pregnancy and would be technically included in the definition of GDM (6).

OTHER CAUSES OF DIABETES

Diabetes may be seen in diseases of the exocrine pancreas, such as cystic fibrosis. Various endocrine diseases, such as Cushing's syndrome, acromegaly, and pheochromocytoma, can cause diabetes. Drug-induced diabetes is an important clinical problem. Corticosteroid drugs are the most frequent cause of hyperglycemia in clinical practice, but numerous other drugs can impair insulin action and precipitate diabetes. Most likely, these drugs are not the sole cause of diabetes but unmask hyperglycemia in individuals already at risk (6). See chapter 28 for additional information.

MATURITY-ONSET DIABETES OF THE YOUNG

Although the genes that underlie type 2 diabetes have not been identified, various genetic defects have been recognized that cause more rare forms of diabetes.

Several genetic defects in β-cell function are known to result in diabetes at an early age. They cause impaired insulin secretion without insulin resistance. At least six specific gene mutations have been identified; they are all inherited in an autosomal-dominant fashion. These rare forms of diabetes have been called maturity-onset diabetes of the young (MODY). Prevalence rates are not well known, but are estimated to be approximately 1% of all diabetes in the U.S. This term, however, should not be applied to the more common type 2 diabetes that, unfortunately, is occurring more frequently in children and adolescents.

CLINICAL FEATURES OF TYPE 1 AND TYPE 2 DIABETES

Most often, type 1 diabetes occurs in children and young adults, but it may occur in individuals of any age. The rate of β-cell destruction varies; it is typically more rapid in younger individuals, who present frequently with severe symptomatic hyperglycemia and sometimes with diabetic ketoacidosis. This suggests severe insulin deficiency. Insulin therapy is required for survival. Those with a slower progression of β-cell destruction may retain some insulin secretion for many years and may present with only modest asymptomatic hyperglycemia. As the disease progresses, they require insulin for survival and are at risk for ketoacidosis. Patients with type 1 diabetes are not typically obese at diagnosis; however, obesity at the time of diagnosis does not exclude a diagnosis of type 1 diabetes.

The clinical presentation of type 2 diabetes is even more variable than that of type 1 diabetes. Because the insulin deficiency is only relative, many of these patients can be treated without insulin, at least initially. Most patients with type 2 diabetes are obese or overweight with increased abdominal adiposity. It is most commonly seen in adults, but is also increasingly being seen in adolescents and children, usually in association with obesity. Symptoms may be mild or nonexistent in many patients with type 2 diabetes. Although diabetic ketoacidosis is characteristically associated with type 1 diabetes, it may be seen in some cases in which patients with type 2 diabetes are under severe physical stress, such as major infection. This is different from the situation in type 1 diabetes, where patients are ketosis prone and may develop ketoacidosis rapidly by simply omitting insulin.

Although it may be easy to distinguish the classic presentation of type 1 diabetes seen in a lean child with weight loss and ketoacidosis and that of type 2 diabetes seen in an obese older adult with no symptoms and mildly elevated glucose levels, other individuals may be difficult to classify in the initial stages of the disease process. Overlap between the two common forms of diabetes does exist. It may not be clear whether a middle-aged adult with onset of fasting hyperglycemia has type 2 diabetes or a slowly evolving form of type 1 diabetes. In addition, an individual with a clear history of type 1 diabetes may subsequently

---

PRACTICAL POINT

Carefully assessing all patients with new-onset hyperglycemia to determine whether they are insulin deficient or insulin resistant is critical for deciding the safest and most effective treatment plan.

Clues to Determining Type of Diabetes

Type 1 Diabetes	Type 2 Diabetes
Usually lean	Usually overweight or obese
May not have a family history	Almost always has a family history
May not be a member of a high-risk ethnic group	Often a member of a high-risk ethnic group
Ketosis prone	Not ketosis prone
Onset slow to rapid (3–4 weeks)	Onset usually slow and progressive
Usually young but can be any age	Usually over age 30 years, but can occur in youth May have history of GDM or delivery of baby >9 lb
	May have associated complications, such as hypertension, atherogenic dyslipidemia, cardiovascular disease, or risk factors
	Markers for insulin resistance

become obese and develop additional features associated with insulin resistance that are common in patients with type 2 diabetes. Some patients who develop diabetes in adulthood and who may initially appear to have type 2 diabetes may have a form of autoimmune diabetes. These individuals are usually leaner than the typical patient with type 2 diabetes. Insulin deficiency may develop more rapidly than in a typical type 2 diabetes patient but more slowly than in a child with type 1 diabetes. Some of these patients may have autoimmune markers such as anti-GAD antibodies, indicating autoimmune β-cell destruction as the cause of their diabetes. The term latent autoimmune diabetes of adulthood (LADA) has been applied to this group. They are frequently misdiagnosed as having type 2 diabetes and may respond to insulin secretagogues for a limited period of time. However, as they become more insulin deficient, the hyperglycemia and symptoms become more pronounced. They may exhibit ketonuria, and insulin is the only appropriate treatment.

The development of type 2 diabetes in children and adolescents is a rapidly increasing clinical problem. These individuals are usually obese and most often belong to ethnic groups with a high incidence of type 2 diabetes. No longer is age of onset a reliable indicator of the type of diabetes present.

SUMMARY

The diagnosis of diabetes is made strictly by blood glucose testing. Therapy is initiated based on the level of blood glucose and the type of diabetes diagnosed.

Nurses in all settings have the opportunity to identify patients who are at risk for diabetes, have pre-diabetes, or have diabetes. Studies indicate that early diagnosis and aggressive therapy will delay and possibly prevent the complications of diabetes. Nurses therefore have the opportunity to counsel, refer, and promote healthy behaviors among individuals with diabetes and pre-diabetes and those at high risk for diabetes.

REFERENCES

1. Centers for Disease Control and Prevention: National diabetest fact sheet: general information and national estimates on diabetes in the US, 2007. Atlanta, GA; US Department of Health and Human Services, Centers for Disease Control and Prevention, 2008

2. World Health Organization: Diabetes Fact Sheet November 2008 [Internet]. Available from http://www.who.int/mediacentre/factsheets/fs312/en/index.html. Accessed 27 January 2009

3. NIDDK: National Diabetes Statistics, 2007 [Internet]. Available from http://www.diabetes.niddk.nih.gov/dm/pubs/statistics/. Accessed 26 January 2009

4. American Diabetes Association: Type 2 diabetes in the young: The evolving epidemic (Consensus Statement). *Diabetes Care* 27:1798–1811, 2004

5. Fagot Campagna A: Emerging type 2 diabetes mellitus in children: epidemiological evidence. *J Pediatr Endocrinol Metab* 13 (Suppl. 6):1395–1402, 2000

6. American Diabetes Association: Diagnosis and classification of diabetes mellitus (Position Statement). *Diabetes Care* 30 (Suppl. 1):S55–S60, 2008

7. American Diabetes Association: Screening for type 2 diabetes (Position Statement). *Diabetes Care* 27 (Suppl. 1):S11–S14, 2004

8. American Diabetes Association: Standards of medical care in diabetes—2009 (Position Statement). *Diabetes Care* 31 (Suppl. 1):S13–S61, 2009

9. UK Prospective Diabetes Study Group: Overview of 6 years' therapy of type II diabetes: a progressive disease. *Diabetes* 44:1249–1258, 1995

Dr. Cypress is an Adult Nurse Practitioner and Certified Diabetes Educator in the Division of Endocrinology at ABQ Health Partners in Albuquerque, NM. Dr. Gleeson is Chair of the Division of Endocrinology and Medical Director of the Diabetes Program at ABQ Health Partners, Albuquerque, NM.

2. Prevention and Risk Reduction

Marjorie Cypress, PHD, MSN, RN, C-ANP, CDE, and
Jeremy Gleeson, MD, FACP, CDE

The 2007 cost of diabetes and its comorbidities was estimated to be $174 billion (1). While the prevalence of diabetes continues to grow, there are believed to be 54 million people in the U.S. over the age of 21 that have pre-diabetes (2). Prevention and risk reduction include not only reducing the risk for developing diabetes, but also preventing the vascular diseases that are associated with diabetes. Preventing diabetes and its complications should be a focus of all health care professionals. Interventions to recognize high-risk individuals and strategies to decrease risk should be considered an essential part of medical and nursing care.

PREVENTING DIABETES

Attempts to prevent type 1 diabetes have been largely unsuccessful. The large, multicenter Diabetes Prevention Trial (3) in type 1 diabetes sought to prevent the development of type 1 diabetes in people at high risk by using low-dose injected, as well as oral, insulin. These interventions proved ineffective.

Several studies that focused on preventing type 2 diabetes had more success (4–7). In the U.S., the Diabetes Prevention Program (7) demonstrated that type 2 diabetes could be either prevented or delayed in a population of people identified to have increased risk of diabetes because of impaired glucose tolerance. This study, a controlled trial conducted in 27 sites in the U.S. and Canada, randomly assigned 3,234 participants ages 25–85 years to an intensive lifestyle intervention consisting of a weight-loss diet and 150 min of exercise a week, a medication intervention group (metformin), or a control group. The results showed that individuals in the lifestyle intervention group, whose sustained average weight loss was ~5% of body weight and exercised averaged >150 min/week, had a 58%

decrease in the risk for developing type 2 diabetes. There was a 31% decrease in the risk for developing type 2 diabetes among individuals in the metformin group. The lifestyle group was most successful in decreasing the risk of developing diabetes in the population >60 years of age. Of note, 45% of the study population was from high-risk minority groups. This and other studies have provided the evidence for preventing type 2 diabetes. Unfortunately, no studies have yet shown that these interventions prevent cardiovascular disease, which is the most significant complication of diabetes.

CARDIOMETABOLIC RISK

Many people with and without type 2 diabetes have a constellation of risk factors that predispose them to diabetes and to cardiovascular disease. These include being overweight or obese (BMI ≥ 25); having hypertension, dyslipidemia (high triglyceride and low HDL cholesterol levels), hyperinsulinemia, insulin resistance, family history, or microalbuminuria; and smoking (Fig. 2.1).

People with diabetes are at risk for chronic microvascular and macrovascular complications; approximately 80% of people with diabetes will develop and may die of cardiovascular disease (8). People with diabetes and no prior history of myocardial infarction have a risk of dying from heart disease that is comparable to those who have had a myocardial infarction but do not have diabetes (9). As a result, the National Cholesterol Education Program (NCEP) lists diabetes as a coronary disease risk factor equivalent in the Adult Treatment Panel guidelines (10).

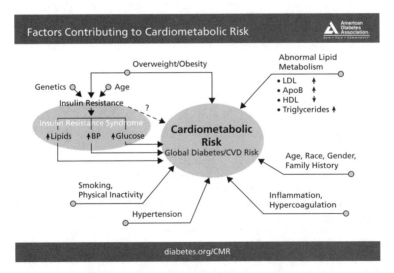

Figure 2.1 Cardiometabolic risk factors. (From the American Diabetes Association. Available at http://professional.diabetes.org/UserFiles/File/ Resources%20for%20Professionals/CMR_Chart.pdf.)

DIABETES AND CARDIOVASCULAR DISEASE PREVENTION STRATEGIES

Prevention strategies can be divided into primary and secondary prevention. In individuals who have already been diagnosed with diabetes, strategies should be aimed at preventing cardiovascular disease and other complications of diabetes. In individuals with pre-diabetes, cardiometabolic risk factors, or a high risk for developing type 2 diabetes, the focus is on preventing the onset of diabetes and treating cardiovascular risk factors (Table 2.1).

IDENTIFYING HIGH-RISK INDIVIDUALS

Adults of any age who are overweight or obese and have additional risk factors should be tested for diabetes or pre-diabetes (11). (See chapter 1 for diagnostic criteria.)

People with obstructive sleep apnea have been found to be 2.5 times more likely to develop type 2 diabetes than people without sleep apnea (12). There is evidence that the intermittent shortage of oxygen in the body from sleep apnea may cause a stress response that can alter glucose metabolism and may play a role in insulin resistance. In addition, sleep apnea has been associated with hypertension and heart failure and may be an independent risk factor for the development

Table 2.1 Recommendations for Preventing or Delaying Diabetes

- Individuals at high risk should be educated about the benefits of modest weight loss and regular physical activity.
  - Medical nutrition therapy: Reduce fat, especially saturated fat (<7% of calories); increase dietary fiber; control calories.
  - Physical activity: Perform 30 min of moderate-intensity exercise or activity a day, 5–7 days a week.
- Screen high-risk individuals with risk factors for pre-diabetes or with diagnosed pre-diabetes (BMI >25 kg/m^2, family history of diabetes, family member with early cardiovascular disease, member of a high-risk ethnic group, history of giving birth to a baby >9 lb, history of impaired glucose tolerance or glycosuria, history of GDM).
  - If normal, re-screen at 3-year intervals or more frequently if indicated.
  - If abnormal, confirm test on another day.
- Counsel all individuals with pre-diabetes on weight loss, if needed, and physical activity. Refer to a dietitian for education and follow-up.
- Assess for other cardiovascular risk factors.
  - Stop smoking.
  - Control blood pressure.
  - Manage lipid levels.
  - Control hyperglycemia.
- Recommend or refer for appropriate treatment, e.g., smoking cessation program, primary care provider for control of hypertension and dyslipidemia, dietitian, CDE, exercise physiologist, community resources, mental health specialist, etc.
- Consider drug therapy (metformin) for diabetes prevention in some individuals, and evaluate whether there is a need for aspirin therapy.

of hypertension. The International Diabetes Federation (IDF) (13) suggests further testing on people who have symptoms of sleep apnea (witnessed apnea, heavy snoring, daytime sleepiness). The treatment includes weight reduction (if overweight), decreased alcohol intake, and use of CPAP (Continuous Positive Airway Pressure). In addition, the IDF recommends that because metabolic diseases, including type 2 diabetes, are very common in patients with sleep apnea, they be screened for these metabolic abnormalities.

Community blood glucose screening is often done at health fairs and shopping malls, but it is difficult to evaluate and is subject to wide variability and inaccuracies. Its cost effectiveness, sensitivity, and specificity have been challenged (14,15), and this type of screening is not recommended. However, community screening in the form of risk factor assessment to identify individuals who have multiple risk factors for developing type 2 diabetes and cardiovascular disease may be beneficial. Community risk factor screening can also provide the opportunity to heighten awareness of diabetes, identify high-risk individuals, refer them for appropriate testing, and promote early intervention or prevention strategies. It is therefore important that screening be conducted by a health professional with specific plans and referrals for people with and without regular medical care who have clear risk factors.

LIFESTYLE INTERVENTIONS

One of the most important lifestyle interventions focuses on healthful eating, maintenance of a desirable body weight, and regular, routine physical activity. Medical nutrition therapy and physical activity are effective in helping people lower their risks for developing diabetes, hypertension, dyslipidemia, and heart disease.

Waist circumference has been seen to be a better predictor of diabetes than BMI (16). Waist circumference is also associated with increased cardiometabolic risk and can be used to monitor an individual's response to diet and exercise when BMI does not change. Men with a waist circumference >40 inches and women with a waist circumference >35 inches are considered to be at high risk for diabetes and cardiovascular disease.

Medical nutrition therapy should focus on decreasing total calories as well as the intake of fat, particularly saturated fat, and increasing the intake of whole grains and dietary fiber. It is important to incorporate individual circumstances, health status, preferences, and cultural and ethnic considerations (17). There is no standard nutrition plan; neither is there an "ADA diet" applicable to all individuals with diabetes. However, making healthy food choices and striving to reach a healthy body weight (BMI 18.5–24.9 kg/m^2) should be the focus of medical nutrition therapy. (See chapter 3 for more on lifestyle interventions.)

Physical activity should be universally encouraged. The Centers for Disease Control and Prevention, the American College of Sports Medicine, and Healthy People 2010 all recommend moderate-intensity physical activity for a minimum of 150 minutes a week, 30 min/day, 5 days a week or vigorous-intensity physical activity for 20 min/day, at least 3 days a week (18). Starting to exercise or increasing physical activity to 20 or 30 min/day may be too difficult a goal initially. Advise sedentary people to begin increasing their physical activity gradually. Walking 10 minutes several times a day may be easier for some people than trying to walk for 30–40 minutes at a time. Exercise can be a variety of activities. It can include such activities as walking instead of driving, playing with children or grandchildren, gardening, cleaning house, playing tennis, biking, or swimming. Assessing individual preferences, physical ability, and safety is important when choosing the type of exercise. Stress the importance of adequate hydration while doing any type of physical activity.

Changing behavior or maintaining healthy behaviors is challenging. People need to be ready to change and to view these lifestyle behaviors as important. Assessment must include readiness to change, how behavior change or health is valued, and one's confidence in the person's ability to be successful.

Because it is well known that lifestyle changes can decrease the risk for developing type 2 diabetes, improve lipids, improve blood pressure, lower weight, and generally decrease risk for cardiovascular events, identifying high-risk individuals and intervening with prevention strategies is of utmost importance (Table 2.1). Screening, counseling, monitoring, and perhaps initiating drug therapy may be indicated.

SMOKING

Smoking is believed to be a risk factor for the development of diabetes (19,20) because it is associated with insulin resistance, increased abdominal fat distribution, dyslipidemia, and hypertension. Cigarette smoking and diabetes markedly increase the risk not only for macrovascular disease but for diabetes-related microvascular disease (21). The risks of smoking may be well known, but it is important that health care providers continue to urge individuals who smoke to stop and to educate people who smoke about the increased risks of cardiovascular disease and other diabetes complications. All smokers should be asked about their readiness to stop smoking and be referred to smoking cessation programs (22). It may be advantageous to combine the medication varenicline or bupropion with a cessation program. In addition, health care providers should advise all individuals with diabetes or risk factors for diabetes and vascular diseases not to start smoking.

HYPERGLYCEMIA

Recommendations for the treatment for people with pre-diabetes (impaired fasting glucose or impaired glucose tolerance) are to normalize glucose levels with lifestyle modification. In those with additional risk factors (Table 2.2), the initial treatment may be lifestyle modification along with metformin (23). In patients with type 2 diabetes, lifestyle modification and metformin treatment are recommended at diagnosis (24). (See chapter 5 on treatment of type 2 diabetes.) Targets for glycemic control are A1C <7% in people with diabetes (70–130 mg/dl preprandial [3.9–7 mmol/l] and <180 mg/dl postprandial [<10 mmol/l]—both capillary blood glucose) and A1C in the normal range (4–6%) for diabetes prevention (11).

HYPERTENSION

The goal for managing hypertension in diabetes is a blood pressure <130/80 mmHg. Lifestyle management is the first intervention. Initial medications include angiotensin converting enzyme (ACE) inhibitors or angiotensin receptor blockers (ARBs), which have been demonstrated to delay the progression to

Table 2.2 Treatment Recommendation for Individuals with IFG, IGT, or Both (23)

Population	Treatment
IFG or IGT	Lifestyle modification (i.e., 5–10% weight loss and moderate-intensity physical activity ~ 30 min/day)
Individuals with IFG and IGT and ANY of the following: ■ <60 years of age ■ BMI ≥35 kg/m² ■ Family history of diabetes in first-degree relative ■ Elevated triglycerides ■ Reduced HDL cholesterol ■ Hypertension ■ A1C >6%	Lifestyle modification (as above) and/or metformin (850 mg, twice a day)

nephropathy (25). Most people will generally require two or more medications to control blood pressure in the target range (11). (See chapter 8 on cardiovascular complications.)

DYSLIPIDEMIA

Fasting lipids should be measured at least annually. Target ranges for lipids in diabetic patients are LDL <100 mg/dl, HDL >50 mg/dl, and triglycerides <150 mg/dl. In those with existing or high risk for cardiovascular disease, targets are lower. A statin is the initial drug of choice for most patients (8,11). (See chapter 8.)

MICROALBUMINURIA

Microalbuminuria is a marker for cardiovascular risk. All individuals with diabetes should be screened annually, starting 5 years after diagnosis of type 1 and upon diagnosis of type 2. Good glycemic control and management of hypertension with ACE inhibitors or ARBs and other drugs as necessary can slow the progression to macroalbuminuria. Blood pressure control has also been shown to decrease cardiovascular events in people with diabetes (26).

ASPIRIN THERAPY

There is evidence that aspirin therapy can reduce the risk of cardiovascular events in individuals with diabetes without a diagnosis of cardiovascular disease and in individuals who have already been diagnosed with cardiovascular disease. The American Diabetes Association recommends aspirin therapy (75–162 mg/day) for primary prevention of cardiovascular events in individuals with diabetes who are over 40 years of age or have additional risk factors

Current ADA Goals

- A1C to <7% in general for nonpregnant adults. In some patients a lower A1C goal, with avoidance of hypoglycemia, may be appropriate.
- Less stringent goals may be appropriate for children; patients with a history of severe hypoglycemia, limited life expectancy, or comorbid conditions; and those with longstanding diabetes who have had difficulty reaching the target A1C despite self-management education, appropriate glucose monitoring, and effective doses of multiple glucose-lowering agents, including insulin.
- Patients with diabetes should be treated to a blood pressure of <130/80 mmHg.
- In people without overt cardiovascular disease, the LDL cholesterol goal is <100 mg/dl (2.6 mmol/l). In people with existing cardiovascular disease, the LDL cholesterol goal is <70 mg/dl (1.8 mmol/l). Triglyceride levels <150 mg/dl (1.7 mmol/l) and HDL cholesterol >40 mg/dl (1.0 mmol/l) in men and >50 mg/dl (1.3 mmol/l) in women are desirable.

From the American Diabetes Association's Standards of Medical Care in Diabetes—2009 (27).

and for secondary prevention in individuals with diabetes and a history of cardiovascular disease, unless contraindicated (27). An alternative to aspirin is clopidogrel, which has been shown to reduce cardiovascular events in individuals with diabetes (11).

ALCOHOL

Carefully assess alcohol consumption and counsel patients on the dangers of excessive alcohol intake. Aside from being high in calories, stimulating appetite, and perhaps being contraindicated with certain medications, excessive alcohol consumption is associated with other social and health problems. It appears that excessive alcohol intake may contribute to the development of diabetes but low to moderate amounts may decrease the risk (17,28). Modest alcohol intake (1–2 drinks/day [one drink is the equivalent of 5 oz of wine, 12 oz of light beer, or 1.5 oz of 80-proof distilled spirits]) may be incorporated into the nutrition plan for individuals who choose to drink.

IMMUNIZATIONS

Individuals with diabetes, especially those with vascular complications, are at high risk for morbidity and mortality associated with influenza and pneumococcal disease. Patient education regarding the need for vaccinations is necessary. Individuals with diabetes who are ≥6 months of age should receive an influenza vaccine every fall. A pneumococcal revaccination is recommended for individuals ≥65 years of age who were previously immunized when they were <65 years of age if the vaccine was administered >5 years ago. Revaccination may also be advised in individuals with diabetes who suffer from renal disease or other immunocompromised states (11).

PERIODIC MEDICAL VISITS

It is often challenging to convince individuals who feel healthy to see their health care providers for routine visits. However, individuals with multiple risk factors need regular evaluation and management. A person with a chronic illness may need to be seen three to four times a year. Health care providers must emphasize the need for regular screening and evaluation not only in these individuals, but in their family members as well. Identification of individuals at high risk for diabetes and cardiovascular disease may be effectively done when patients come in accompanied by a family member who has obvious risk factors. Education regarding the risks of developing type 2 diabetes should be done at that time, and those family members should be referred for further evaluation.

Individual health care beliefs may present a barrier to preventive care if individuals at high risk do not perceive themselves as susceptible to illness. It is the duty of the health care team to be cognizant of the health care beliefs of the individuals they see. The health care team should work together to identify, screen, and diagnose high-risk individuals so that early intervention strategies can be initiated.

SOCIO-ECOLOGICAL PERSPECTIVE

A multifaceted approach is necessary to prevent diabetes, reduce risk, and promote health. It is important that nurses view the individual within the larger context of family, community, and society. This may include cultural traditions, food preferences, access to medical care, social and community support, and resources such as environments conducive to health. These resources may include safe walking trails, access to healthy and fresh produce, healthier choices in vending machines, and physical education in the schools.

A1C may also be reported as an estimated average glucose (eAG) as follows:	
A1C %	eAG (range) in mg/dl
5	97 (76–120)
6	126 (100–152)
7	154 (123–185)
8	183 (147–217)
9	212 (170–249)
10	240 (193–282)
11	269 (217–314)
12	298 (240–347)

From Nathan et al. (30).

SUMMARY

Primary and secondary intervention is essential in the prevention of diabetes and the potential complications of diabetes. Interventions to recognize high-risk individuals and strategies to decrease the risk of diabetes and diabetes-related vascular complications should be considered an essential part of nursing care. Every January, the American Diabetes Association publishes the updated Standards of Medical Care in Diabetes based on the latest research findings. The Standards can be accessed on the Internet at www.diabetes.org.

REFERENCES

1. American Diabetes Association: Economic costs of diabetes in the U.S. in 2007. *Diabetes Care* 31:1–20, 2008

2. Benjamin SM, Valdez R, Geiss LS, Rolka DB, Narayan KMV: Estimated number of adults with prediabetes in the United States in 2000: Opportunities for prevention. *Diabetes Care* 26:645–649, 2003

3. Diabetes Prevention Trial–Type 1 Diabetes Study Group: Effects of insulin in relatives of patients with type 1 diabetes mellitus. *N Engl J Med* 346:1685–1691, 2002

4. Eriksson KF, Lindegarde F: Prevention of type 2 (non insulin dependent) diabetes mellitus by diet and physical exercise: the 6-year Malmo feasibility study. *Diabetologia* 34:891-898, 1991

5. Pan XR, Li GW, Hu YH, Wang JX, Yang WY, et al.: Effects of diet and exercise in preventing NIDDM in people with impaired glucose tolerance: the Da Qing IGT and Diabetes Study. *Diabetes Care* 20:537–544, 1997

6. Tuomilehto J, Lindstrom J, Eriksson JG, Valle TT, Hamalainen H, et al.: Prevention of type 2 diabetes mellitus by changes in lifestyle among subjects with impaired glucose tolerance. *N Engl J Med* 344:1343–1350, 2001

7. Diabetes Prevention Program Research Group: Reduction in the incidence of type 2 diabetes with lifestyle intervention or metformin. *N Engl J Med* 346:393–403, 2002

8. Buse JB, Ginsberg HN, Bakris GL, Clark NG, Costa F, et al.: Primary prevention of cardiovascular diseases in people with diabetes mellitus: A scientific statement from the American Heart Association and the American Diabetes Association. *Diabetes Care* 30:162–172, 2007

9. Haffner SM, Lehto S, Rönnemaa T, Pyörälä K, Laakso M: Mortality from coronary heart disease in subjects with type 2 diabetes and in nondiabetic subjects with and without prior myocardial infarction. *N Engl J Med* 339:229–234, 1998

10. Expert Panel on the Detection, Education, and Treatment of High Blood Cholesterol in Adults: Executive summary of the third report of the National

Cholesterol Education Program (NCEP) Expert Panel on Detection, Education, and Treatment of High Blood Cholesterol in Adults (Adult Treatment Panel III). *JAMA* 285:2486–2497, 2001

11. American Diabetes Association: Clinical Practice Recommendations 2009. *Diabetes Care* 32 (Suppl. 1):S1–S97, 2009

12. Botros NA, Shah N, Mohsenin V, Roux F, Yaggi HK: Obstructive sleep apnea as a risk factor for type II diabetes (Abstract). *Am J Respir Crit Care Med* 175 (Suppl.):A359, 2007

13. Shaw JE, Punjabi NM, Wilding JP, Alberti KM, Zimmet PZ: Sleep disordered breathing and type 2 diabetes: a report from the International Diabetes Federation Task Force on Epidemiology and Prevention. *Diabetes Res Clin Pract* 81:2–12, 2008

14. Bahman P, Tabaei BP, Burke R, Constance A, Hare J, May-Aldrich G, et al.: Community-based screening for diabetes in Michigan. *Diabetes Care* 26:668–670, 2003

15. Rolka DB, Narayan KMV, Thompson TJ, Goldman D, Lindenmayer J, Alich K, Bacall D, Benjamin EM, Lamb B, Stuart DO, Engelgau MM: Performance of recommended screening tests for undiagnosed diabetes and dysglycemia. *Diabetes Care* 24:1899–1903, 2001

16. Waist circumference and cardiometabolic risk: a consensus statement from Shaping America's Health: Association for Weight Management and Obesity Prevention; NAASO, The Obesity Society; the American Society for Nutrition; and the American Diabetes Association. *Diabetes Care* 30:1647–1652, 2007

17. American Diabetes Association: Nutrition principles and recommendations in diabetes (Position Statement). *Diabetes Care* 31 (Suppl. 1):S61–S78, 2008

18. Centers for Disease Control and Prevention: Physical activity recommendations [Internet]. Available at: www.cdc.gov/physicalactivity/everyone/guidelines/adults.html. Accessed 30 March, 2009

19. Foy CG, Bell RA, Farmer DF, Goff DC Jr, Wagenknecht LE: Smoking and incidence of diabetes among U.S. adults: findings from the insulin resistance atherosclerosis study. *Diabetes Care* 28:2501–2507, 2005

20. Wannamethee SG, Shaper AG, Perry IJ: Smoking as a modifiable risk factor for type 2 diabetes in middle-aged men. *Diabetes Care*. 2001;24:1590–1595.

21. De Cosmo S, Lamacchia O, Rauseo A, Viti R, Gesualdo L, et al.: Cigarette smoking is associated with low glomerular filtration rate in male patients with type 2 diabetes. *Diabetes Care* 29:2467–2470, 2006

22. American Diabetes Association: Smoking and diabetes (Position Statement). *Diabetes Care* 27 (Suppl. 1):S74-S75, 2004

23. American Diabetes Association: Impaired fasting glucose and impaired glucose tolerance: implications for care. *Diabetes Care* 30:753–759, 2007

24. Nathan DM, Buse JB, Davidson MB, Ferrannini E, Holman RR, et al.: Medical management of hyperglycemia in type 2 diabetes: a consensus algorithm for the initiation and adjustment of therapy: a consensus statement from the American Diabetes Association and the European Association for the Study of Diabetes. *Diabetes Care* 31:1–11, 2008

25. Arauz-Pacheco C, Parrott MA, Raskin P: The treatment of hypertension in adult patients with diabetes. *Diabetes Care* 25:134–147, 2002

26. Heart Outcomes Prevention Evaluation Study Investigators: Effects of ramipril on cardiovascular and microvascular outcomes in people with diabetes mellitus: results of the HOPE study and MICRO-HOPE substudy. *Lancet* 355:253–259, 2000

27. American Diabetes Association: Standards of medical care in diabetes—2009. *Diabetes Care* 32 (Suppl. 1):S13–S61, 2009

28. Athyros VG, Liberopoulos EN, Mikhailidis DP, Papageorgiou AA, Ganotakis ES, et al.: Association of drinking pattern and alcohol beverage type with the prevalence of metabolic syndrome, diabetes, coronary heart disease, stroke, and peripheral arterial disease in a Mediterranean cohort. *Angiology* 58:689–697, 2008

29. American Diabetes Association: Influenza and pneumococcal immunization in diabetes (Position Statement). *Diabetes Care* 27 (Suppl. 1):S111–S113, 2004

28. Nathan DM, Kuenen J, Borg R, Zheng H, Schoenfeld D, et al.: Translating the A1C assay into estimated average glucose values. *Diabetes Care* 31:1473–1478, 2008

Dr. Cypress is an Adult Nurse Practitioner and Certified Diabetes Educator in the Division of Endocrinology at ABQ Health Partners in Albuquerque, NM. Dr. Gleeson is Chair of the Division of Endocrinology and Medical Director of the Diabetes Program at ABQ Health Partners, Albuquerque, NM.

3. Healthy Lifestyle Changes: Food and Physical Activity

Anne Daly, MS, RD, BC-ADM, CDE

TWIN EPIDEMICS: DIABETES AND OBESITY

Recent evidence demonstrates the unfolding of a diabetes epidemic in the U.S. According to the Centers for Disease Control and Prevention, diabetes now affects nearly 21 million Americans—or 7% of the U.S. population—and more than 6 million of those people do not know they have diabetes (1). This number represents an additional 2.6 million people with diabetes since 2002. Another 54 million people are estimated to have pre-diabetes, a condition that increases the risk of developing type 2 diabetes, as well as heart disease and stroke. Of particular concern is that in the last two decades, type 2 diabetes (formerly known as adult-onset diabetes) has been reported among U.S. children and adolescents with increasing frequency (1,2). Simultaneously, since the mid-1970s, the prevalence of overweight and obesity has increased sharply for both adults and children (2,3). This increasing incidence of obesity and low levels of physical activity are thought to be major contributors to the diabetes epidemic, bolstered by the growth of population groups with high incidences of type 2 diabetes and the aging of the American population.

How do we address these epidemics? Recent evidence has shown that people with pre-diabetes can successfully prevent or delay the onset of diabetes by losing 5–7% of their body weight. This can be accomplished through 30 min or more of moderate physical activity most days of the week and a low-calorie, low-fat eating plan, rich in whole grains, fruits, and vegetables. Most important, supporting people with diabetes in achieving lifestyle-related goals and maintaining healthy lifestyles requires the coordinated effort of a team that includes physicians, nurses, registered dietitians (RDs), and diabetes educators. Living a healthy lifestyle is like swimming upstream against a powerful daily tide of environmental and commercial messages to "Eat more. It's OK."

ROLE OF LIFESTYLE CHANGES IN DIABETES PREVENTION

Strong evidence suggests that lifestyle changes, especially healthy eating and physical activity, are beneficial for people with impaired glucose tolerance, or pre-diabetes, and insulin resistance. A recent large systematic review summarized the evidence from worldwide clinical trials for the effectiveness of formal lifestyle interventions to prevent or delay the development of type 2 diabetes (4). Pooled estimates from 12 trials showed that lifestyle interventions reduce the risk of developing diabetes by 49% compared with standard treatment alone. Lifestyle interventions generally consisted of specific meal plans/diets and regular physical activity.

The greatest and most compelling evidence for the risk-reducing benefits of lifestyle modification in the U.S. comes from the Diabetes Prevention Program (DPP). The DPP was the first randomized trial to compare lifestyle and a pharmacological intervention with placebo (5). The DPP randomly assigned 3,234 overweight or obese pre-diabetic adults (mean age 51 years) from 27 medical centers to one of three conditions: an intensive, structured lifestyle modification group; a medication (metformin) group; or a control group using standard lifestyle advice plus placebo. Recruitment efforts aimed to ensure that more than half the participants were from the ethnic groups in the U.S. with the highest risk of developing diabetes, which include African Americans, Native Americans, Hispanics/Latinos, Asians, and Pacific Islanders, and in the end, participants from these groups made up 45% of the study population. The goal of the intensive lifestyle modification group was to lose 7% of their starting body weight. Results showed that at average follow-up of 2.8 years, the lifestyle intervention reduced the incidence of diabetes by 58% in all participants (71% for adults over age 60 years) and by 31% in those assigned to metformin as compared with the incidence in the control group. Weight loss was the predominant predictor of reduction in diabetes incidence, with a 16% reduction in risk per every 1 kg of weight lost (6). However, those who achieved exercise goals, but not weight loss goals, also experienced some reduction in diabetes risk (44%). Changes in physical activity and diet, primarily reduced calories from fat, predicted weight loss, and weight loss in turn was associated with reduced diabetes risk.

Education and concerted support from a health care team were key elements of the DPP. Within the first 24 weeks, participants in the intensive lifestyle intervention group attended 16 group sessions in which a structured core curriculum was used. After the core curriculum was delivered, participants met with their case managers monthly. Participants in the standard treatment group received written information and one 20- to 30-min individual session with a case manager. Participants in the standard treatment group were encouraged to follow the food pyramid and the equivalent of the National Cholesterol Education Program (Step 1) diet.

The DPP results are consistent with earlier reports of the Finnish Diabetes Prevention Study, a smaller study that involved a single ethnic group (6). In that study, the intervention group received detailed and individualized counseling aimed at reducing weight, reducing total intake of fat and saturated fat, and increasing fiber, along with personal guidance on increasing physical activity. This counseling was provided in seven sessions with a nutritionist during the first year and one session every 3 months during the study. The control group received general oral and written information about diet (a two-page leaflet) and physical activity at annual visits. The incidence of diabetes in the intervention group was reduced by 58%, a rate identical to the U.S. study.

The success of these lifestyle intervention programs depends upon the implementation of structured lifestyle change programs. Although pessimism is commonly expressed with regard to the challenge of inducing lifestyle change in overweight and sedentary people, recent lifestyle intervention trials demonstrate that this pessimism is unwarranted. The conclusions of these major studies are remarkably consistent, and the clinical implications are clear: type 2 diabetes is not inevitable, individuals at high risk to develop diabetes can be identified, and with early lifestyle intervention, diabetes can be delayed, if not prevented (5,6). Interventions to reduce diabetes risk in overweight or obese individuals should target weight reduction (7,8). Currently, a large National Institutes of Health–sponsored clinical trial designed to determine if long-term weight loss in people with diabetes will improve glycemia and prevent cardiovascular events is under way. One-year results showed impressive improvements in glucose control and cardiovascular risk factors (9).

Recent evidence (10) calculates the national burden of diabetes to be in excess of $174 billion, resulting in higher insurance premiums paid by employees and employers, reduced earnings through productivity loss, and reduced overall quality of life for people with diabetes and their families and friends. Thus, an effort to prevent and/or delay diabetes is worthwhile. Policymakers and health care systems must develop low-cost ways to promote physical activity and weight loss. Evidence is strong that the DPP lifestyle intervention is cost-effective as delivered in the DPP trial (11,12). Evidence indicates this lifestyle intervention can be effectively delivered in a group format (13), rather than the one-to-one format used in the DPP. This significantly reduces the cost of the program, thus increasing its cost effectiveness. In most clinical settings, weight management is not considered a primary intervention for the prevention or treatment of type 2 diabetes. However, the DPP clearly demonstrated that early referral to a structured lifestyle change program to prevent the development of diabetes in those who are deemed at high risk is essential. Other clinical trials, including the U.K. Prospective Diabetes Study (UKPDS), have demonstrated that nutrition therapy is most effective in the initial phases of type 2 diabetes, when insulin resistance is likely to be the greatest (14).

ROLE OF DIABETES NUTRITIONAL CARE IN LIFESTYLE CHANGE

Over the past decade, along with changes in the medications used for treating diabetes have come changes in medical nutrition therapy (MNT) and behavior-change strategies. Gone are the days when the primary nutrition messages for people with diabetes were to limit sugar intake and follow a "diabetic diet" with a specified calorie level. Before 1994, American Diabetes Association (ADA) nutrition recommendations attempted to define ideal macronutrient percentages for a diabetes nutrition prescription. Although individualization was a basic principle, it had to be done within the confines of the nutrition prescription.

Now, instead of a rigid nutrition prescription, MNT is based on an assessment of lifestyle changes that would assist the person with diabetes in achieving and maintaining clinical goals, but it is focused on changes the person with diabetes is able and willing to make (15). Studies have shown that a positive approach—focusing on "to do" behaviors rather than "not to do" behaviors—is more effective in producing improved clinical outcomes (16) and weight loss (17). Table 3.1 illustrates the paradigm shift that has occurred in nutrition therapy.

THE PROCESS OF MNT

MNT is the service provided by an RD that, when implemented properly, consists of a four-step nutritional care process (18):

1. Nutrition assessment
2. Nutrition diagnosis
3. Nutrition intervention
4. Nutrition monitoring and evaluation

MNT is effective in diabetes management (19,20). Evidence from randomized controlled trials, observational studies, and meta-analyses has shown that MNT improves metabolic outcomes such as blood glucose and glycated hemoglobin A1c (A1C) in people with diabetes (Table 3.2).

Dietitians have found it helpful to prioritize nutrition advice based on the nutrition assessment. Patients often choose small, gradual changes in lifestyle, and it is essential that lifestyle goals be changes that the patient is willing and likely to be able to make. Initially, choosing just one or two primary behavior-change areas is suggested so as not to overwhelm the patient. Focusing on specific "how to" steps is helpful for successful behavior change (see also "What Can I Eat?" a patient booklet available from the ADA at 1-800-DIABETES). Providing the patients with a written copy of the goals is recommended.

Once an assessment has been completed, the RD will determine the nutrition diagnosis, which includes the presence of, risk of, or potential for developing a nutritional deficit that can be addressed by nutrition therapy. Nutrition interventions are specific actions to remedy the nutrition diagnosis and can include clinical and behavioral goals agreed upon with the patient, as well as specific nutrition intervention strategies. These might include selecting a meal-planning strategy and suggesting a specific education resource for the patient to use. No single strategy or method can be recommended because a variety of methods have been tested and demonstrated to facilitate attainment of nutrition goals. During initial phases of education (survival education), simplified resources, such as the Food Guide Pyramid, that can illustrate basic nutrition guidelines are recommended. There are basic diabetes nutrition messages that are associated with improved outcomes:

Eat similar amounts of carbohydrate throughout the day each day, and distribute the carbohydrate fairly evenly throughout the day. To control blood glucose levels, the first priority is to eat consistent amounts of carbohydrate at meals

Table 3.1 Outdated Versus Updated Diabetes Nutrition Recommendations

Outdated	Updated
MNT was a calculated ADA diet with calculated calories and percentages of carbohydrate, protein, and fat. Pre-calculated diets were distributed.	There is no one diet for all people with diabetes. Dietitians work collaboratively with each patient to individualize a "prescription" based on assessment, therapy goals, and meal planning approaches that meet the patient's needs. The use of diet sheets or a one-time "diet instruction" is rarely effective to change eating habits. Lifestyle changes that result in positive clinical outcomes require education and counseling in both nutrition and physical activity with support over time.
Weight loss was prioritized below glucose control.	Weight loss is recommended for all overweight and obese individuals who have or are at risk for diabetes.
Ideal body weight (per Metropolitan Life Insurance) was the goal.	Even modest weight loss (5–7% of starting body weight) can improve glucose, lipids, and insulin resistance. Participation in a structured and intensive maintenance program improves long-term weight maintenance.
Sugars and sweets are forbidden because they are rapidly digested and absorbed and cause blood glucose levels to go higher than do starches.	Evidence from many clinical studies has demonstrated that sugars do not increase glycemia more than isocaloric amounts of starch.
Protein is recommended because it slows the absorption of carbohydrates and prevents hypoglycemia.	Ingested protein does not slow the absorption of carbohydrate, nor does adding protein prevent or assist in the treatment of hypoglycemia.
"When diet and exercise fail, add medications." The implication: No need to pay attention to lifestyle.	Diet doesn't fail, the pancreas does. Type 2 diabetes is a progressive disease. MNT should continue to be an essential part of the treatment plan. Patients can "eat their way through" any medications they are given.

and to eat at similar times of day. Carbohydrate is the primary predictor of post-prandial blood glucose levels because carbohydrate in foods raises blood glucose levels fastest and the most after eating. This does not mean foods containing carbohydrate should be eliminated, but simply that their consumption should be controlled and consistent. Foods that contain carbohydrate are among the healthiest foods—starches, whole grains, fruits, vegetables, and milk. An adult typically needs between three and five carbohydrate servings (starches, fruits, milk, or yogurt) per

Table 3.2 Lessons Learned from Nutritional Outcomes Research

- Nutrition therapy does not fail. It is essential for optimal diabetes management. The β-cells of the pancreas fail.
- In the U.K. Prospective Diabetes Study (UKPDS), intensive nutrition therapy provided by dietitians decreased A1C levels by ~2%.
- Other studies have shown that nutrition therapy provided by RDs lowers A1C by 1–2% and fasting plasma glucose levels by 50–100 mg/dl (2.8–5.6 mmol/l).
- The UKPDS revealed that type 2 diabetes is a progressive disorder, and therapy—medication(s) combined with nutrition therapy—needs to be intensified over time.
- The focus of lifestyle interventions should be on improving blood glucose control, lipids, blood pressure, and weight.
- Teach patients which foods contain carbohydrate, emphasize portion sizes, and specify the number of servings for meals and snacks.
- Shape eating behaviors to include generous amounts of fruits and vegetables (at least 5 1-cup servings total/day), low-fat dairy products (3 servings), and whole-grain products (3 servings).
- Encourage 30 min of physical activity on most days of the week.
- Monitor blood glucose, lipids, blood pressure, and weight to determine effectiveness of therapy.

meal. One serving is equal to 15 g carbohydrate. Nonstarchy vegetables contain smaller amounts of carbohydrate and are encouraged because they provide good nutrition and volume. Distribution of carbohydrate foods is difficult for many patients, especially those who skip breakfast. When a person with diabetes eats only one or two meals per day or drinks large volumes of regular soda or fruit juice, simply changing to three spaced meals and using calorie-free beverages can improve blood glucose significantly.

Practice portion control. In our "super-sized" world, adjusting portions to reasonable sizes is essential for optimal glucose and weight control. Encourage people

PRACTICAL POINT

It is important when developing behavioral goals with patients that the goals be attainable and very specific regarding the type, frequency, and duration of the behavior. For example:

- "I will decrease the number of fast food meals I eat to one a week for the next 2 months."
- "I will walk 20 min, 5 days a week, for the next month."
- "I will increase the amount of green vegetables I eat to at least two servings a day for the next month."
- "I will replace lard with canola oil in my cooking for the next 3 months."

Be sure to follow up with patients to evaluate their progress toward meeting their goals or to help them identify barriers and develop new goals.

to continue to eat the foods they enjoy, but to eat smaller portions. An RD can help people with diabetes learn what portions are appropriate for them. Eating smaller portions is a first step. However, substituting high-fiber, low-fat foods is a necessary strategy to keep people satisfied and at the same time reduce total fat and calorie intake. Asking patients to fill their plates only once without going back for seconds can lower caloric intake and blood glucose levels.

Skim the fats. Fat is loaded with calories, and all fats (except omega-3s) may be associated with insulin resistance. A reduction in fat helps with weight loss and maintenance and improves lipid levels. Fat is found in salad dressing, margarine, oil, chips, fried foods, and more. Saturated fat is found in meats, whole milk, other full-fat dairy foods, butter, and coconut, palm, and hydrogenated oils. Trans fats are found in processed foods and baked goods, shortening, and some fast food items, such as french fries. Trans fats are now listed on food labels, making it easier to identify the foods that contain them. As noted above, trying to eat less of the same high-fat foods does not work; helping patients learn to eat more of the low-fat foods is a more successful way to achieve reduced calorie intake and heart-healthy eating, without reducing the amount of food at a meal. Increasing fruits and vegetables to at least seven servings total per day is an excellent way to add volume to meals but decrease calorie and dietary fat intake at the same time. This is an example of how using a positive approach, focusing on "to do" behaviors rather than "not to do" behaviors, can be effective. In essence, eating more fruits and vegetables becomes a backdoor way of decreasing fat.

Engage in adequate physical activity. Ideally, patients should accumulate a total of 30 min of physical activity most days of the week, according to the American Diabetes Association Standards of Medical Care in Diabetes, as well as the Surgeon General's report on physical activity and health (21,22). Being active helps improve blood glucose levels, lowers risk of mortality, and improves insulin sensitivity. It may also improve other common metabolic abnormalities of insulin resistance, including hypertension, hyperlipidemia, and atherosclerosis. Encourage patients to identify activities they can enjoy safely and can realistically include in their schedule. In the case of children and adolescents, encourage a reduction in time spent doing sedentary activities, including computer and TV time.

Get to or stay at a healthy weight. Encourage patients to maintain a healthy weight. Overweight patients who lose as little as 10 lb can have significant improvements in blood glucose, blood pressure, and lipids and can also decrease insulin resistance. This message is one of the most helpful that patients can hear. Discuss what reasonable body weight and weight loss goals would be for each individual's situation. An RD will often recommend that a patient record food intake along with blood glucose levels, which often helps reduce caloric intake and promote weight loss.

Subsequently, more complex MNT approaches, such as calorie or carbohydrate counting, *Choose Your Foods: Exchange Lists for Diabetes* (23), insulin adjustments using insulin-to-carbohydrate ratios, or even medically supervised very-low-calorie diets, may be appropriate. Offering a variety of nutrition interventions provides greater flexibility and choices to the person with diabetes and is especially useful for individuals who have been discouraged or frustrated by previous nutrition instruction methods. Although ideally the approach that best meets the individual needs of the client is chosen, the choice of a food plan is also influ-

Table 3.3 Toolbox Approaches to Structured Lifestyle Changes to Promote Weight Loss and Problem Solving

- Increase frequency of contact with health care provider
- Review self-monitoring skills (e.g., records of food, activity, weight, blood glucose levels, medications)
- Change self-monitoring approach, if needed
- Provide recipes
- Assign calorie goal or lower fat/calorie goal
- Refer to RD for structured meal plans
- Involve significant other(s)
- Conduct small group visits
- Schedule meeting with behavioral therapist
- Use meal replacements for one to two meals per day
- Try calorie/fat-controlled frozen entrees
- Recommend RD-led grocery store visit
- Borrow self-help materials
- Provide motivational strategy/incentive/contract
- Refer to a dietitian, fitness club, etc., for additional coaching

enced by the RD's experience with different strategies. This means the RD needs a toolbox of approaches for supporting patients in structured lifestyle change to promote weight loss (Table 3.3), with close monitoring of outcomes to determine whether goals are being met. These approaches are used in multicenter clinical trials and have been found to be effective.

Many printed resources are available to support nutrition interventions. The ADA and American Dietetic Association continuously update their numerous co-published diabetes meal planning resources, which are designed to reflect the most recent ADA nutrition recommendations (15), updated nutrient composition data, consumer trends, and feedback from educators (24). These resources include the following titles:

- *What Can I Eat? The Diabetes Guide to Healthy Food Choices* (English and Spanish)
- *Choose Your Foods: Plan Your Meals* (English and Spanish)
- *Eating Healthy with Diabetes: Easy Reading Guide*
- *Choose Your Foods: Exchange Lists for Diabetes* (English and Spanish)
- *Choose Your Foods: Exchange Lists for Weight Management*

These publications can be ordered from the ADA at 1-800-DIABETES or http://store.diabetes.org. In addition, ADA's website features an online nutritional tool, MyFoodAdvisor (http://www.diabetes.org/food-nutrition-lifestyle/nutrition/my-food-advisor.jsp), that provides an interactive resource for patients.

THE GLYCEMIC INDEX

The glycemic index (GI) was developed to compare the postprandial responses to constant amounts of various carbohydrate-containing foods (25). The GI of a food is the increase above fasting in the blood glucose area over 2 h after ingestion of a constant amount of that food (usually a 50-g carbohydrate portion) divided by the response to a reference food (usually white bread or glucose). The glycemic loads of foods, meals, and diets are calculated by multiplying the GIs of the constituent foods by the amounts of carbohydrate in each food and then totaling the values for all foods.

The use of diets with a low GI in the management of diabetes is controversial, with contrasting recommendations around the world. Findings of randomized controlled trials have been mixed; some studies have shown statistically significant improvements, whereas others have not (26). The variability in responses to specific carbohydrate-containing food is a concern (27). As a result, the issue of the GI has been fraught with controversy and has polarized the opinion of leading experts.

After reviewing the evidence in 2007, the ADA again concluded that the total amount of available carbohydrate is more important than the source (starch or sugar) or type (low or high GI), and although low-GI foods may reduce postprandial hyperglycemia, there was not sufficient evidence to recommend use of low-GI diets as a primary strategy in food/meal planning (15). Rather, the use of GI is raised as an additional technique beyond considering the total amount of carbohydrate alone (28). Primary nutrition interventions documented to have the greatest impact on metabolic outcomes should be selected as follows:

- In the case of type 1 diabetes, adjusting insulin based on the carbohydrate content of the meal would appear to be a better primary strategy than trying to follow a low-GI diet (28).
- For type 2 diabetes, primary nutrition interventions should focus on behavioral strategies such as reduced calorie intake, modest weight loss, and basic carbohydrate counting. These strategies have been demonstrated to produce better outcomes than a low-GI diet approach. For instance, using a moderate-carbohydrate approach reduced A1C by ~20%, compared with 7.4% from a low-GI diet (28). Information on glycemic responses of foods can perhaps best be used for fine-tuning glycemic control.

HIGH-FAT, HIGH-PROTEIN, LOW-CARBOHYDRATE DIETS

The optimal macronutrient distribution of weight loss diets has not been established (15). While low-fat diets have traditionally been promoted for weight loss, two randomized controlled trials found that subjects on low-carbohydrate diets lost more weight at 6 months than subjects on low-fat diets (29,30). Another study of overweight women randomized to one of four diets showed significantly more weight loss at 12 months with the Atkins low-carbohydrate diet than with the higher-carbohydrate diets (31). However, at 1 year, the difference in weight loss between the low-carbohydrate and low-fat diets was not significant, and weight loss was only modest with both diets. Further research is needed to determine the long-term efficacy and safety of low-carbohydrate diets (32). The recommended dietary allowance (RDA) for digestible carbohydrate is 130 g/day and is based on providing adequate glucose to fuel the central nervous system without reliance on glucose production from ingested protein or fat (33). Although brain fuel needs can be met on lower-carbohydrate diets, long-term metabolic effects of very-low-carbohydrate diets are unclear, and such diets eliminate many foods that are important sources of energy, fiber, vitamins, and minerals and are important in dietary palatability (33).

It is true that high-protein, low-carbohydrate eating plans produce substantial initial weight loss-partly because of fluid loss and partly because people end up eating fewer calories because of the limited choices and the effect of ketones to decrease appetite. However, these eating plans do not appear effective for long-term weight maintenance (34). If a patient chooses to follow a low-carbohydrate diet, lipid profile, renal function, and protein intake (if nephropathy is present) should be monitored, and glucose-targeted medication should be adjusted as necessary (15).

ROLE OF PHYSICAL ACTIVITY IN RISK FACTOR REDUCTION

The possible benefits of physical activity for patients with and at risk for type 2 diabetes are substantial. Several long-term studies have demonstrated a consistent beneficial effect of regular physical activity on carbohydrate metabolism and insulin sensitivity. Improvements in A1C are most marked in patients with mild type 2 diabetes and in individuals who are likely to be the most insulin resistant (35).

Multiple epidemiological studies have shown an inverse relationship between physical activity and the risk of coronary heart disease (CHD). Sedentary individuals have almost twice the risk of CHD as those performing high-intensity activity. However, the optimal level of activity for preventing CHD is unclear. In some studies, the reduction in risk from increased levels of activity appeared to be linear up to a certain level, above which there was no further benefit; in others, the effect was restricted to the highest categories of total energy expenditure (36).

Physical activity decreases cardiovascular risk through a number of mechanisms:

- decreased blood pressure
- increased HDL cholesterol level
- decreased triglyceride level
- reduced weight
- increased fibrinolysis in response to thrombotic stimuli
- increased insulin sensitivity and potentially improved blood glucose levels
- reduced susceptibility to serious ventricular arrhythmias
- associated behavioral changes, e.g., smoking cessation, healthier eating, stress reduction
- psychological benefits, e.g., decreased depression and anxiety

Aerobic activity benefits the cardiovascular system by decreasing heart rate and increasing stroke volume at rest and during physical activity and increasing cardiac output. Physical activity of moderate intensity is usually recommended for people with known coronary artery disease (CAD) in the absence of ischemia or significant arrhythmias. Physical activity of moderate intensity is also generally recommended for the person with hypertension. This level of activity can be targeted to 60–80% of maximum heart rate, which corresponds to 50–75% of maximum oxygen consumption. High-intensity activity should be minimized because it can cause a significant rise in blood pressure.

Physical activity reduces blood pressure by 5–10 mmHg in some people, and its effects are usually noted within 10 weeks of training. Before starting a physical activity program, people with hypertension require adequate blood pressure control because physical activity causes acute increases in systolic pressure and this increase can be exaggerated in diabetes. The blood pressure response to physical activity should be monitored initially, and adjustments in therapy should be made accordingly.

Before increasing usual patterns of physical activity or beginning an exercise program, the person with diabetes should undergo a detailed medical evaluation with appropriate diagnostic studies. He or she may require an exercise stress test (see below). Physical activity should be performed on most days of the week or at least four times per week, with each session lasting between 30 and 60 min. Physical activity at regular intervals has been noted to decrease the risk of myocardial infarction. Sedentary individuals experience a higher relative risk of myocardial infarction after an episode of heavy exertion compared with individuals who engage in physical activity five or more times per week.

In addition to cardiovascular disease, sedentary lifestyles are closely associated with obesity. Physical activity is a potent physiological stimulus of lipolysis, which results in the release of free fatty acids from triglycerides stored in fat for use as an energy source by muscle. Therefore, physical activity increases energy expenditure, which results in a negative calorie balance, adding potential for weight loss to occur. Although physical activity alone may produce a 2–3% reduction in BMI, it is more effective when used as an adjunct to MNT (37). Multiple studies have shown that once weight loss has been accomplished, physical activity is the primary predictor of weight maintenance (38). Without increasing physical activity, weight loss is often temporary.

GETTING STARTED WITH PHYSICAL ACTIVITY

Walking is the most commonly prescribed activity and the most likely to be successful because of both safety and accessibility. Almost anyone can participate in brisk walking, and when a pedometer is used, the individual has feedback about the number of steps or miles walked. Monitoring physical activity data is useful for shaping this behavior in small, simple steps. Individuals might begin by walking for 5–10 min 3 days/week and gradually increase duration, frequency, and intensity of walking to the target level. The DPP intervention included 150 min/week of medium-intensity activity, equivalent to brisk walking (1 mile/15–20 minutes). Proponents of counting steps advocate establishing a baseline, working up to 4,000 steps per day, and increasing to 10,000 steps daily over a 6-month period. The National Weight Control Registry, a group of successful weight maintainers, reports participants engage in an average of 2,800 calories of physical activity per week (39).

Getting started with a physical activity program is not easy, and keeping one going can be even more difficult. The use of written goal-oriented plans is associated with success. Other factors that promote increased physical activity are

- doing some activity daily
- doing some activity before noon
- having a home option, e.g., treadmill, neighborhood walking route
- using multiple, short bouts of exercise (10–20 min at a time)
- doing multiple types of activities
- follow-up with a case manager/coach

EVALUATION BEFORE RECOMMENDING PHYSICAL ACTIVITY

Past ADA guidelines have suggested that patients with diabetes and multiple cardiovascular risk factors be assessed for CAD before beginning a program of physical activity. However, because the area of CAD screening remains unclear, ADA now recommends that providers use clinical judgment and encourage high-risk patients to start with short periods of low-intensity activity and increase the intensity and duration gradually over time (21). In addition, patients with diabetes should be evaluated for conditions such as uncontrolled hypertension, severe neuropathy, and advanced retinopathy that might contraindicate certain types of activity or predispose them to injury.

Little is known about the cardiovascular risk or risk reduction of physical activity training in individuals with type 1 diabetes because most research is conducted in people with type 2 diabetes. Until additional information is available, anyone with the onset of type 1 diabetes in childhood or adolescence who is over the age of 35 years or who has had diabetes for >15 years should be considered a high-risk patient.

ROLE RESPONSIBILITIES

Because of the complexity of nutrition issues, both the ADA (15) and the Institute of Medicine (40) recommend that an RD who is knowledgeable and skilled in MNT play the lead role in providing MNT. However, it is essential that all team members, including physicians and nurses, be knowledgeable about MNT and support its implementation. Table 3.4 lists nurse and other health care professional and dietitian responsibilities related to MNT.

SUMMARY

The evidence for more aggressive treatment of diabetes using nutrition and physical activity is growing. To best meet the challenge and manage the diabetes epidemic in the U.S., all health care professionals must accept expanding role responsibilities. To effectively help people with diabetes achieve behavior change, it is important to recognize the person with diabetes as the most important person on the health care team. Nurses should encourage small, gradual changes in just one or two behaviors and emphasize the "to do" behaviors rather than the "not to do" behaviors. These strategies are associated with improved behavioral and clinical outcomes. Teaching strategies that help the person become his or her own

Table 3.4 Nurse and RD Responsibilities Related to MNT

Nurse's responsibilities
1. Refer patient to an RD for MNT.
2. Provide referral data: diabetes treatment regimen, laboratory values for A1C, glucose values, cholesterol fractions, blood pressure, and presence of microalbuminuria; medical goals for patient care; medical history; medications that affect MNT; and clearance for physical activity.
3. Collaborate with the patient to establish medical treatment goals.
4. Provide and reinforce basic nutrition messages.
5. Reinforce the importance of working with an RD on nutrition self-management.

RD's responsibilities

1. Obtain referral data and treatment goals before the initial nutrition intervention.
2. Obtain and assess information about patient's eating habits, activity, self-monitoring of blood glucose levels, cultural and ethnic background, psychosocial and economic issues, and support system(s).
3. Assess patient's knowledge, age, skill level, readiness to change, and goals.
4. In partnership with the patient, select and implement appropriate nutrition prescription and use appropriate teaching tools to provide education on food, meal planning, and self-management.
5. Evaluate the effectiveness of MNT based on treatment targets and adjust MNT as needed.
6. Make recommendations to the nurse based on the outcomes of nutrition interventions and communicate progress/outcomes of nutrition interventions; communicate progress/outcomes to all team members.
7. Plan for follow-up and ongoing education.

manager of behavior change are likely to result in the most lasting change. The nurse should be knowledgeable about community resources to refer the patient for additional nutritional services such as diabetes self-management programs and dietitians.

REFERENCES

1. Centers for Disease Control and Prevention: National Diabetes Fact Sheet, United States, 2005 [Internet]. Available from http://www.cdc.gov/diabetes/pubs/pdf/ndfs_2005.pdf. Accessed 29 January 2009

2. Mokdad AH, Bowman BA, Ford ED, Vinicor F, Marks JS, Koplan JP: The continuing epidemics of obesity and diabetes in the United States. *JAMA* 286:1195–1200, 2001

3. Alberti G, Zimmet P, Shaw J, Bloomgarden Z, Kaufman F, Silink M: Type 2 diabetes in the young: the evolving epidemic: the International Diabetes Federation Consensus Workshop (Consensus Statement). *Diabetes Care* 27:1798–1811, 2004

4. Gilies CL, Abrams KR, Lambert PC, Cooper NJ, Sutton AJ, et al.: Pharmacologic and lifestyle interventions to prevent or delay type 2 diabetes in people

with impaired glucose tolerance: a systematic review and meta analysis. *BMJ* doi:10.1136/bmj.39063.689375.55 (published 19 January 2007)

5. Diabetes Prevention Program Research Group: Reduction in the incidence of type 2 diabetes with lifestyle intervention or metformin. *N Engl J Med* 346:393–401, 2002

6. Finnish Diabetes Prevention Study Group: Prevention of type 2 diabetes mellitus by changes in lifestyle among subjects with impaired glucose tolerance. *N Engl J Med* 344:1343–1350, 2001

7. Hamman RF, Wing RR, Edelstein SL, Lachin JM, Bray GA, et al.: Effect of weight loss with lifestyle intervention on risk of diabetes. *Diabetes Care* 12:1426–1434, 2004

8. Anderson JW, Kendall C, Jenkins DJ: Importance of weight management in type 2 diabetes: review with meta-analyses of clinical studies. *J Am Coll Nutr* 22:331–339, 2003

9. Look AHEAD Research Group, Pi-Sunyer X, Blackburn G, Brancati FL, Bray GA, et al.: Reduction in weight and cardiovascular disease risk factors in individuals with type 2 diabetes: one-year results of the look AHEAD trial. *Diabetes Care* 30:1374–1383, 2007

10. American Diabetes Association: Economics costs of Diabetes in the U.S. in 2007. *Diabetes Care* 31:596–615, 2008 (published erratum 31:1271, 2008)

11. Herman WH, Hoerger TJ, Brandle M, Hicks K, Sorenson S, et al.: The cost-effectiveness of strategies to prevent type 2 diabetes. *Ann Intern Med* 142:1–28, 2005

12. The Diabetes Prevention Program Research Group: Costs associated with the primary prevention of type 2 diabetes mellitus in the Diabetes Prevention Program. *Diabetes Care* 26:36–47, 2003

13. Mayer-Davis EJ, D'Antonio AM, Smith SM, Kirkner G, Martin SL, et al: Pounds Off With Empowerment (POWER): a clinical trial of weight management strategies for Black and White adults with diabetes who live in medically underserved rural communities. *American Journal of Public Health* 94:1736–1742, 2004

14. Franz M, Green-Pastors J, Warshaw H, Daly A: Does diet fail? *Clinical Diabetes* 18:162–168, 2000

15. American Diabetes Association: Nutrition recommendations and interventions for diabetes (Position Statement). *Diabetes Care* 31:S61–S78, 2008

16. Nicholson AS, Sklar M, Barnard ND, Gore S, Sullivan R, Browning S: Toward improved management of NIDDM: a randomized, controlled, pilot intervention using a low fat, vegetarian diet. *Prev Med* 29:87–91, 1999

17. Epstein LH, Gordy CC, Raynor HA, Beddome M, Kilanowski CK, Paluch R: Increasing fruit and vegetable intake and decreasing fat and sugar intake in families at risk for childhood obesity. *Obes Res* 9:171–178, 2001

18. American Dietetic Association: *International Dietetics and Nutrition Terminology (IDNT) Reference Manual.* Chicago, American Dietetic Association, 2008

19. Pastors JG, Warshaw H, Daly A, Franz M, Kulkarni K: The evidence for the effectiveness of medical nutrition therapy in diabetes management. *Diabetes Care* 25:608–613, 2002

20. Pastors JG, Franz M, Warshaw H, Daly A, Arnold M: How effective is medical nutrition therapy in diabetes care? *J Am Diet Assoc* 103:827–831, 2003

21. American Diabetes Association: Standards of Medical Care in Diabetes—2009. *Diabetes Care* 31 (Suppl. 1):S13–S61, 2008

22. U.S. Department of Health and Human Services, Centers for Disease Control and Prevention, National Center for Chronic Disease Prevention and Health Promotion: *Physical Activity and Health: A Report of the Surgeon General.* Atlanta, GA, Centers for Disease Control and Prevention, 1996

23. American Diabetes Association and The American Dietetic Association: *Choose Your Foods: Exchange Lists for Diabetes.* Alexandria, VA, American Diabetes Association, 2007

24. Wheeler M, Daly A, Franz M, Geil P, Holzmeister LA, et al.: *Choose Your Foods: Exchange Lists for Diabetes*, sixth edition, 2008: description and guidelines for use. *J Am Diet Assoc* 108:883–888, 2008

25. Jenkins DJ, Wolever TM, Taylor RH, Barker H, Fielden H, et al.: Glycemic index of foods: a physiological basis for carbohydrate exchange. *Am J Clin Nutr* 34:362–366, 1981

26. Sheard NF, Clark NG, Brand-Miller JC, Franz MJ, Pi-Sunyer FX, et al.: Dietary carbohydrate (amount and type) in prevention and management of diabetes. *Diabetes Care* 27:2266–2271, 2004

27. Wylie-Rosett J, Segal-Isaacson CJ, Segal-Isaacson A: Carbohydrates and increases in obesity: does the type of carbohydrate make a difference? *Obes Res* 12 (Suppl. 2):124S–129S, 2004

28. Franz M: The glycemic index: not the most effective nutrition therapy intervention (Editorial). *Diabetes Care* 26:2466–2468, 2003

29. Foster GD, Wyatt HR, Hill JO, McGuckin BG, Brill C, et al.: A randomized trial of a low carbohydrate diet for obesity. *N Eng J Med* 348:2082–2090, 2003

30. Stern L, Iqbal J, Seshadri P, Chicano KL, Daily DA, McGrory J, Williams J, Gracely EJ, Samaha FF: The effects of low-carbohydrate versus conventional weight loss diets in severely obese adults: one-year follow-up of a randomized trial. *Ann Intern Med* 140:778–785, 2004

31. Gardner C, Kiazand A, Alhassan S, Soowon K, Stafford R, et al.: Comparison of the Atkins, zone, Ornish and LEARN diets for change in weight and related risk factors among overweight and premenopausal women. *JAMA* 297:969–977, 2007

32. Klein S, Sheard NF, Pi-Sunyer X, Daly A, Wylie-Rosett J, et al.: Weight management through lifestyle modification for the prevention and management of type 2 diabetes: rationale and strategies: a statement of the American Diabetes Association, the North American Association for the Study of Obesity, and the American Society for Clinical Nutrition. *Diabetes Care* 27:2067–2073, 2004

33. Institute of Medicine: *Dietary Reference Intakes: Energy, Carbohydrate, Fiber, Fat, Fatty Acids, Cholesterol, Protein and Amino Acids.* Washington, DC, National Academies Press, 2002

34. Friedman MR, King J, Kennedy E: Popular diets: a scientific review. *Obes Res* 9 (Suppl. 1):1S–40S, 2001

35. American Diabetes Association: Physical activity/exercise and type 2 diabetes (Position Statement). *Diabetes Care* 29 :1433–1438, 2006

36. Wannamethee SG, Shaper AG: Physical activity in the prevention of cardio-vascular disease: an epidemiological perspective. *Sports Med* 31:101–114, 2001

37. Pi-Sunyer FX, Becker DM, Bouchard C, et al.: NHLBI Obesity Education Initiative Expert Panel on the Identification, Evaluation, and Treatment of Overweight and Obesity in Adults. *Obes Res* 6 (Suppl. 2):51S–209S, 1998

38. The Diabetes Prevention Program Research Group: Achieving weight and activity goals among Diabetes Prevention Program lifestyle participants. *Obes Res* 12:1426–1434, 2004

39. McGuire MT, Wing RR, Klem ML, Seagle HM, Hill JO: Long-term maintenance of weight loss: do people who lose weight through various weight loss methods use different behaviors to maintain their weight? *Int J Obes* 22: 572–577, 1998

40. Institute of Medicine: *The Role of Nutrition in Maintaining Health in the Nation's Elderly: Evaluating Coverage of Nutrition Services for the Medicare Population.* Washington, DC, National Academies Press, 2000, p. 118–131

Ms. Daly is the Director of Nutrition and Diabetes Education and a co-founder of the Springfield Diabetes and Endocrine Center, Springfield, IL.

4. Treatment Strategies for Type 1 Diabetes

Belinda P. Childs, ARNP, MN, CDE, BC-ADM, and
Davida Kruger, ANP, MSN, BC-ADM

Type 1 diabetes is a complex, multihormonal disease. Insulin has been the primary treatment for type 1 diabetes. However, to successfully manage type 1 diabetes, individuals must integrate several diabetes treatment components into their lifestyle, including insulin action times, food intake, and physical activity. The individual with type 1 diabetes and the health care provider must share an understanding of the disease process and available treatment strategies and collaborate in determining the best treatment choices.

EPIDEMIOLOGY

The incidence of type 1 diabetes in the U.S. in people <20 years of age is estimated at 19 in 100,000 per year. In adults, type 1 diabetes accounts for 5–10% of all diagnosed cases of diabetes. It is estimated that around 700,000 people have type 1 diabetes. The risk for type 1 diabetes is higher for whites than for African Americans or Hispanics/Latinos (1).

Autoimmune type 1 diabetes has multiple genetic predispositions and is also related to poorly defined environmental factors. People with type 1 diabetes are prone to other autoimmune disorders, such as Graves' disease, Hashimoto's thyroiditis, Addison's disease, vitiligo, pernicious anemia, and celiac disease. Evidence also supports an increased risk for multiple sclerosis in those with type 1 diabetes.

The genes that confer susceptibility for type 1 diabetes are located in the HLA (human leukocyte antigen) region of chromosome 6. Genetically susceptible individuals who also have autoantibodies to islet cell antigens, insulin, and GAD (glutamic acid decarboxylase) are at greatest risk of developing type 1 diabetes (2). Tests are available to identify those at risk, but lacking a way to prevent type 1 diabetes, testing is not typically done. Many individuals were screened as part of the Diabetes Prevention Trial–Type 1, which attempted unsuccessfully to prevent type 1 diabetes with insulin therapy in those at risk. The follow-up study is called the TrialNet Natural History Study. Information can be obtained online at http://www.diabetestrialnet.org.

PATHOPHYSIOLOGY

Type 1 diabetes occurs most frequently in children and young adults but may be diagnosed at any age, even in the eighth and ninth decade. As stated in chapter 1, there are two types of type 1 diabetes: immune-mediated and idiopathic, the former being much more common. The etiology of type 1 diabetes remains unclear, but the key is insulin deficiency due to the failure of the β-cell to produce adequate insulin to control blood glucose levels. Type 1 diabetes has been referred to in the past as insulin-dependent diabetes and juvenile-onset diabetes.

Other hormones involved in glucose regulation include glucagon, somatostatin, and amylin (Fig. 4.1). Glucagon, produced by the α-cells in the islets of Langerhans in the pancreas, plays a major role in sustaining plasma glucose production. Glucagon maintains the basal blood glucose within a normal range during fasting. In the nondiabetic milieu, if the glucose level falls below normal, glucagon is released; this in turn triggers the release of hepatic glucose from the liver (glycogenolysis). The blood glucose level returns to normal. This glucose release is not needed after a meal. Normally, glucagon is suppressed by the effect of insulin on the liver, and glucagon is almost totally suppressed after a meal. In diabetes, there is an inadequate suppression of postprandial glucagon (hyperglucagonemia), resulting in increased hepatic glucose production (gluconeogenesis). Exogenous insulin is unable to restore normal postprandial insulin concentrations in the portal vein or suppress the postprandial glucagon secretion. This results in an abnormal glucagon-to-insulin ratio, the release of hepatic glucose and, ultimately, hyperglycemia (3). Somatostatin, which is produced by the δ-cells in the islets of Langerhans, also plays a role in the regulation of insulin and glucagon release.

Amylin (discovered in 1987) is the most recently identified regulatory hormone and is co-secreted by the β-cells with insulin. It appears to play a role in postprandial glucose regulation by reducing excess glucagon in the postprandial period and regulating gastric emptying from the stomach to the small intestines. Amylin also appears to have an effect on satiety.

Glucose homeostasis is complex. In addition to the above-mentioned hormones, several "incretin" hormones also play a role in postprandial glucagon and insulin secretion, as well as gastric emptying. Currently identified incretin hormones are glucagon-like peptide-1 (GLP-1) and gastric inhibitory polypeptide (GIP) (3).

DIAGNOSIS

Although the symptoms of type 1 diabetes (Table 4.1) can arise suddenly, the disease is now considered to have an insidious onset. In the past, most patients newly diagnosed with type 1 diabetes were hospitalized with ketoacidosis. Today, however, most are identified by symptoms and early glucose testing before becoming ill.

THE IMPORTANCE OF OPTIMAL GLUCOSE CONTROL

The findings of the Diabetes Control and Complications Trial (DCCT) left no doubt that glucose control reduces the likelihood of developing the microvascular complications of diabetes (4). Data from the DCCT show that the risk of the development of microvascular complications decreases as hemoglobin A1c (A1C)

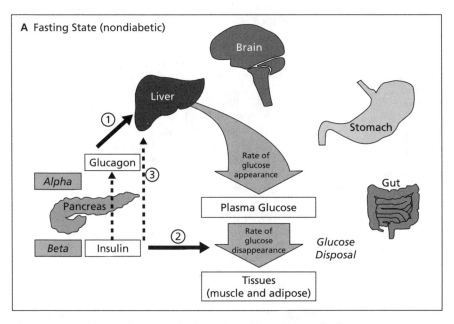

Figure 4.1 Glucose homeostasis: role of insulin and glucagon. *A:* For nondiabetic individuals in the fasting state, plasma glucose is derived from glycogenolysis under the direction of glucagon (1). Basal levels of insulin control glucose disposal (2). Insulin's role in suppressing gluconeogenesis and glycogenolysis is minimal because of low insulin secretion in the fasting state (3). *B:* For individuals with diabetes in the fasting state, plasma glucose is derived from glycogenolysis and gluconeogenesis (1) under the direction of glucagon (2). Exogenous insulin (3) influences the rate of peripheral glucose disappearance (4) and, because of its deficiency in the portal circulation, does not properly regulate the degree to which hepatic gluconeogenesis and glycogenolysis occur. From Aronoff et al. (3).

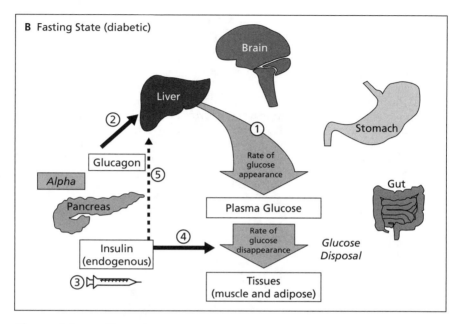

B Fasting State (diabetic)

Figure 4.1 *continued.*

nears the normal level. Any lowering of A1C and blood glucose level decreases the risk of developing microvascular complications.

A cohort of 1,349 patients who participated in the DCCT has been followed since the completion of the DCCT. This follow-up study, Epidemiology of Diabetes Interventions and Complications (EDIC), has demonstrated a beneficial effect of optimal glucose control 7–8 years after the DCCT's completion. Those who had near-normal glycemia during the DCCT continue to have less albumin excretion and reduced incidence of hypertension compared with the less well-controlled group, regardless

Table 4.1 Symptoms of Type 1 Diabetes

Polyuria—increased urination
Polyphagia—increased appetite
Polydipsia—increased thirst
Unexplained weight loss
In children, bedwetting
Yeast infections
Flushed skin
Fruity breath
Severe abdominal pain
Nausea and/or vomiting
Lethargy

of their current glucose control (5). Additionally, they have been found to have reduced rates of myocardial infarction, stroke, and cardiovascular death (6).

BASAL-BOLUS INSULIN THERAPY

In individuals without diabetes or impaired glucose tolerance, nature carefully controls blood glucose levels within a very narrow range. This is accomplished by the continuous secretion of a small amount of insulin, termed basal insulin, at a relatively constant level, i.e., it never "peaks." Superimposed on the basal insulin is a bolus of insulin that the body secretes with each feeding. Figure 4.2 shows normal physiology.

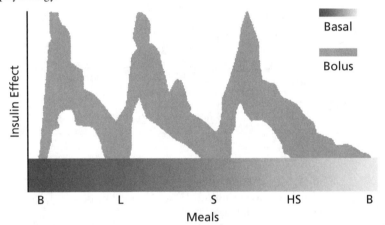

Figure 4.2 Physiologic insulin secretion. B, breakfast; L, lunch; S, supper; HS, bedtime.

It is possible to closely mimic the pattern of basal and bolus insulin using exogenous insulin. One option is to use a continuous subcutaneous insulin infusion (CSII) pump, which can be programmed to release basal insulin at chosen rates, plus bolus insulin controlled by the pump wearer (see chapter 24 for further information on CSII). Multiple daily injections using a long-acting (peakless or nearly peakless) insulin analog plus a rapid-acting insulin analog to cover meals also allow physiological basal-bolus insulin therapy. To maximize the advantages of these approaches, it is important that both patient and provider understand not only the basal-bolus concept but also the action times of the various insulins (Table 4.2).

INSULIN TIMING AND ACTION

There are four general categories of insulin based on action times:

- rapid acting: insulins lispro, aspart, and glulisine, which are genetically engineered insulin analogs
- short acting: regular soluble insulin

Table 4.2 Insulin Action Times

	Onset (h)	Peak (h)	Effective duration (h)
Rapid acting			
Insulin lispro (analog)*	0.25–0.5	0.5–2.5	≤5
Insulin aspart (analog)*	<0.20	1–3	3–5
Insulin glulisine (analog)	<0.2–0.5	1–3	3–4
Short acting			
Regular (soluble)	0.5–1	2–3	3–6
Intermediate acting			
NPH (isophane)	2–4	4–10	10–16
Long acting			
Detemir	2+	4–6	
Insulin glargine (analog)	2–4	Nearly peakless	20–24
Combinations			
50% NPH, 50% regular	0.5–1	Dual	10–16
70% NPH, 30% regular	0.5–1	Dual	10–16
70% NPA, 30% aspart	<0.25	Dual	10–16
75% NPL, 25% lispro	<0.25	Dual	10–16

*Per manufacturers' data; other data indicate equivalent pharmacodynamic effect (Plank J, Wutte A, Brunner G, Siebenhofer A, Semlitsch B, et al.: Direct comparison of insulin aspart and insulin lispro in patients with type 1 diabetes. *Diabetes Care* 25:2053–2057, 2002).

- intermediate acting: NPH, an isophane insulin
- long acting: insulin glargine and insulin detemir, genetically engineered analogs

Table 4.2 summarizes the action profiles, i.e., the time to onset, time to peak action, and duration of action, of these preparations. The values shown are for human insulin. Porcine insulin is still available, but most patients use genetically engineered human insulin.

For most individuals with type 1 diabetes, a basal-bolus approach to management is the best choice. The basal insulin reduces hepatic glucose production, keeping it in equilibrium with the use of basal glucose by the brain and other tissue. After meals, bolus (prandial) insulin secretion stimulates glucose use and storage while inhibiting hepatic glucose output, thereby limiting the meal-related glucose excursion. Individuals with type 1 diabetes lack both basal and bolus insulin production. The basal-bolus approach allows for the most flexible lifestyle.

One basal-bolus strategy is to use glargine/detemir as the basal insulin and insulin lispro/aspart/glulisine as the bolus insulin (Fig. 4.3). Usually, 40–60% of the total daily insulin dose is for basal needs and the remaining would go to the bolus doses, divided based on meal content and composition. Glargine/detemir can be given at any time of day but should be given at a consistent time of day, e.g., in the morning or at bedtime. Alternatively, NPH in two or three doses per day can be used to provide basal needs.

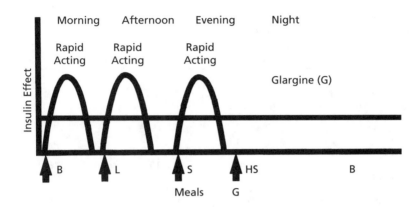

Figure 4.3 Representation of idealized insulin effect provided by three daily injections of rapid-acting insulin with an evening injection of insulin glargine. B, breakfast; L, lunch; S, supper; HS, bedtime.

Insulin mixtures are also available. Premixed insulins do not allow as much flexibility in eating and physical activity times and are usually not the best choice in type 1 diabetes. Carefully instruct patients about the onset of action of insulin and time of administration. Premixed 70/30 NPH/regular should be taken 30 min before eating, whereas a 70/30 NPA/aspart or 75/25 NPL/lispro dose is administered with the meal.

Education and caution to ensure accurate dosing are needed when patients are asked to mix insulins themselves. The rule is to draw the clear insulin, e.g., regular, lispro, aspart, or glulisine, before the cloudy insulin, e.g., NPH. The dose should be given within 2–10 min of mixing. The exceptions are glargine and detemir, which cannot be mixed with any other insulin or drawn into a syringe that contained any other insulin. Also, glargine should be administered immediately after being drawn into a syringe (7), unlike NPH, which can be stored in syringes and refrigerated for up to 30 days (8). If glargine, detemir, or any other clear insulin has particles or has become cloudy, a new vial or pen should be used and the contaminated vial/pen discarded.

STARTING INSULIN

Starting doses of insulin are best calculated based on body weight. The initial dose is usually 0.5–1.5 units/kg body wt/day. The starting dose is determined within this range by the degree of ketosis with which the patient presents, not the blood glucose level. Most individuals with type 1 diabetes have some level

> **PRACTICAL POINT**
>
> Although insulin does not have to be refrigerated, it should not exceed 86°F.

of ketosis and may have initially been treated with intravenous insulin and rehy-drated (see chapter 7). Others may be identified early in the disease process and simply need insulin replacement, which will mean a lower starting dose.

Children and adolescents with newly diagnosed type 1 diabetes usually have some degree of ketosis or acidosis and thus are very insulin deficient and require high doses of insulin. Children also have a higher metabolic rate than adults and therefore a higher clearance rate of drugs, e.g., insulin. Growth hormones can cause elevated blood glucose levels. Children require higher doses of most insulins, as well as other medications, than do adults. Children and adolescents who develop diabetic ketoacidosis (DKA) are usually treated with low-dose intravenous insulin.

When a patient is stable and ready for subcutaneous insulin, start with a dose of 1–2 units/kg body wt/day, reserving the lower doses for patients who have hyperglycemia and little or no ketosis and the highest dose for patients who have or have had DKA. Children should be fed to satiety (usually 40–60 kcal/kg body wt/day) to replenish their lost stores of body nutrients and given enough insulin to control blood glucose levels and restore anabolism to regain lost weight.

Insulin is divided between a rapid-acting insulin, which is administered with meals, and a longer-acting insulin, such as glargine/detemir, usually administered at bedtime. About 40–60% of the total daily insulin requirement should be given as glargine/detemir and the remaining given as aspart/lispro/glulisine. Mealtime aspart/lispro/glulisine is dosed according to meal size, except that the largest dose per calorie/carbohydrate is normally given with breakfast because of the large amount of growth hormone secreted in the early hours of the night in growing children. In children, especially toddlers, aspart/lispro/glulisine can be given after the meal and the dose adjusted by how much the child has actually eaten.

Regimens using a split mix of NPH and lispro or aspart can be used in patients with type 1 diabetes (Fig. 4.4). Approximately 50–60% would be given as a

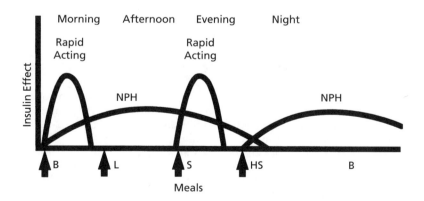

Figure 4.4 Representation of a split mix of NPH and rapid-acting insulin at breakfast, rapid-acting insulin at the evening meal, and NPH at bed-time. B, breakfast; L, lunch; S, supper; HS, bedtime. From Bode (Ed.) (2).

breakfast dose of mixed insulin NPH/lispro; 15–20% would be given as a supper dose of regular, lispro, aspart, or glulisine at the evening meal; and 15–20% as NPH at 10:00 p.m. As noted, it is important to eat meals as the insulin is peaking. Snacks are likely necessary during midmorning and midafternoon and at bedtime. It will be important during the adjustment phase to monitor 3:00 a.m. blood glucose levels to prevent nocturnal hypoglycemia.

INTRODUCTION OF ANALOG AMYLIN

If an individual is insulin deficient, he or she is amylin deficient. The purpose of pramlintide, the synthetic form of amylin, is to reduce postprandial hyperglycemia. It also has been shown to enhance satiety, which leads to the potential for weight loss. The primary side effects are nausea and hypoglycemia. Nausea is the most common side effect with the use of pramlintide. Starting pramlintide at a low dose and gradually increasing the dose helps to minimize nausea. Nausea is typically transient and goes away over time.

Pramlintide is used with insulin and has been associated with insulin-induced hypoglycemia. Lowering the insulin dose when pramlintide is initiated has shown to minimize hypoglycemia.

Individuals must be willing to test their blood glucose levels frequently as they begin pramlintide to minimize the risk of insulin-induced hypoglycemia. Because of the action of pramlintide, the prandial insulin dose needs to be reduced by 30–50%. Some practitioners begin therapy by advising patients to take the pramlintide immediately before the meal and the insulin at the end of the meal so that the individual can adjust the rapid-acting insulin dose if he or she achieves satiety early in the meal. Nausea is also minimized if the individual stops eating when satiety is achieved.

Pramlintide is given as an injection using a Symlin pen, which is available in two sizes, either 60 μg or 120 μg. The 60-μg pen has four doses available: 15 μg, 30 μg, 45 μg, and 60 μg. The 120 μg pen has two doses available: 60 μg and 120 μg.

SELF-MONITORING OF BLOOD GLUCOSE

Self-monitoring of blood glucose (SMBG) is essential to diabetes control, regardless of the treatment strategies. Pattern management is the method of choice for making any insulin dose adjustments but is essential when using basal-bolus insulin therapy with rapid- and long-acting insulin.

Use of a sliding scale is not an effective way to adjust insulin doses. In the past, patients were commonly told to monitor their blood glucose levels before meals and at bedtime. This was done so that insulin could be adjusted on a sliding scale or algorithm according to the blood glucose level at the time. Regardless of the insulin tactics used, this method is retrospective. The calculated change corrects a previous error, which may then overlap another insulin dose and cause hypoglycemia later. This is particularly true when longer-acting insulins are used. Many sliding scales are based on a set of standing orders for all patients regardless of weight or insulin sensitivity.

For example, using a sliding scale with a patient taking mixed regular and NPH insulins could potentially cause significant afternoon hypoglycemia. The morning NPH insulin may be working well, but adding extra regular insulin at noon because the prelunch blood glucose level is high will result in an overlap with the duration of the NPH and may cause afternoon hypoglycemia. The next logical action would be to decrease the evening insulin dose because the presupper blood glucose level is low, which will result in a high bedtime blood glucose level. As is evident, this becomes a vicious cycle. In contrast, the pattern management approach is proactive.

USING SMBG FOR PATTERN MANAGEMENT

With pattern management, blood glucose level is checked at fasting and 2 h postprandially. If the values are >200 mg/dl (11.1 mmol/l) or ketones are present in the urine, supplements or a correction dose can be given immediately. Unless the blood glucose is very high, it is better to observe a 2- to 3-day pattern and then make a change based on the pattern. Correction doses may be given based on the premeal blood glucose as long as it is noted.

Changes in insulin doses are then made according to the type of insulin involved. The fasting blood glucose level is a reflection of the glargine/detemir or bedtime NPH insulin, and if it is too high or too low over a 2- to 3-day period, the glargine/detemir/NPH dose should be adjusted accordingly. Of note, the change should be within 10–20% of the existing dose. If a percentage of the existing dose is used as the adjustment guide, the individual's insulin sensitivity and weight have been taken into consideration. One size does not fit all in insulin management or adjustment.

The blood glucose level after breakfast is used to adjust the prebreakfast rapid-acting insulin dose, the level after lunch is used to adjust the lunchtime insulin dose, and the level after the evening meal is used to adjust the premeal insulin dose. Again, changes are made every 2–3 days in 10–20% increments until the measured values are in the target range agreed to by the patient and/or family.

The American Diabetes Association (ADA) goals of therapy are fasting plasma glucose 70–130 mg/dl (3.9–7.2 mmol/l), postprandial plasma glucose at the highest peak <180 mg/dl (<10.0 mmol/l), and A1C <7% (9). For preschool children, the elderly, and other special situations, these targets may be slightly higher.

Glucose monitoring is an important tool for the individual with diabetes to use for daily adjustment, pattern management, and review with the provider during office visits. Optimal pattern management uses several days of SMBG records, whether handwritten or downloaded from the meter. (Cables and software for downloading meter data are available for most glucose meters.) Downloading meter data offers the individual the opportunity to self-manage blood glucose levels without keeping a log book. Downloaded records may also be appreciated by the provider. However, written records with detailed journaling of factors such as specific food, emotions, and physical activity help the individual with diabetes learn problem-solving skills. Downloaded meter information will require supplemental information about the individual's food plan, medication, activity, and treatment of hypoglycemia so that adjustments in medication, meals, or activity can be based on accurate information. Also, for downloaded information to be useful, it should be downloaded regularly, e.g., weekly. If the meter is only downloaded at the health care provider's office, the individual with diabetes is missing the opportunity to make regular adjustments to his or her meal plan, exercise, and medication.

CORRECTING HYPERGLYCEMIA

Correctional doses of insulin can be given, but care should be taken to avoid overtreating with insulin. If one overtreats hyperglycemia with too much or too frequent insulin, one increases the risk of hypoglycemia. The resultant hypoglycemia may then be overtreated with food, which could result in hyperglycemia and insulin being supplemented again. This is referred to as the sliding-scale effect. The level of hyperglycemia at which a patient corrects may vary between individuals and should be decided by the patient and provider. Extreme caution should be used if using a correction bolus with split-mixed insulin.

For patients who are on intermediate- or long-acting insulin, there is no single value in adjusting it to correct for a high premeal glucose level. In this case, 10% of the total insulin dose may be supplemented as rapid-acting insulin. Another method is to use the rule of 1,700 (Table 4.3). This method involves dividing the total daily dose of insulin, including rapid- and long-acting insulins, into 1,700 (10,11). In this way, the patient with diabetes can determine by approximately how many milligrams 1 unit of insulin will lower the blood glucose. Correction doses should be used cautiously. Food and activity can also be adjusted to alter blood glucose.

CORRECTING HYPOGLYCEMIA

With basal-bolus insulin therapy, the 15 g/15 min rule becomes important. This rule suggests that to treat hypoglycemia, the individual with diabetes should take 15 g glucose, wait 15 min, recheck, and if necessary, retreat with an additional 15 g glucose. In the past, we often taught individuals with diabetes to follow up treatment with a complex carbohydrate/protein snack. However, this may not be necessary. It will depend on the time of day in which the hypoglycemia occurs. If the reaction occurs during the peak of the NPH action, an additional snack may be required to prevent recurrent hypoglycemia (see also chapter 7).

Patients converting from a regimen in which frequent and/or prolonged hypoglycemia existed may find that elevated blood glucose levels will occur after treatment if low blood glucose levels are treated the same way as in their previous

Table 4.3 Calculating Correction or Insulin Sensitivity Factors

1,700 Rule

Determine total daily dose of insulin: Insulin dose is 11 units of aspart before each meal and 35 units of NPH at bedtime. Total daily dose = 68 units.

Divide daily dose into 1,700: Total daily dose = 68 units divided into 1,700 = 25. Thus, 1 unit of aspart will drop blood glucose about 25 mg/dl.

If blood glucose is 200 mg/dl (11.1 mmol/l) before the evening meal, and target blood glucose is 100 mg/dl, 200 − 100 = correction needed for 100 mg/dl.

Using the correction factor, give an extra 4 units aspart to decrease blood glucose to 100 mg/dl (55.6 mmol/l).

regimen. This will be particularly true if these patients eat a high-calorie/high-fat food such as chocolate, in which case they might experience blood glucose levels ≥300 mg/dl (16.6 mmol/l). Assumptions might be made that the high glucose levels that followed the low glucose levels are due to the Somogyi effect, but they are most likely related to the type of treatment or the overtreatment of low blood glucose. The Somogyi phenomenon has been defined as a counterregulatory effect in response to hypoglycemia in which the liver releases glucose. The result is high blood glucose. This is seen sometimes after extreme exercise. However, there is debate as to whether this phenomenon exists. If it does exist, it occurs infrequently.

FOOD PLAN CONSIDERATIONS

Using the basal-bolus regimen provides greater flexibility in lifestyle and schedule for patients with diabetes. Rapid-acting insulin can be adjusted based on the carbohydrate consumption at any given time. Snacks may not be required, as is often the case with the split-mix regimens. However, snacks may be eaten, if desired, without compromising glucose control if carbohydrates are counted and supplemented with insulin. This is a benefit for many children and adults who have been frustrated by a strict eating schedule that required that they eat even when they were not hungry, such as at bedtime. A general guideline is that additional insulin is not needed if the snack contains <120 calories or <20 g carbohydrate, but any food containing >120 calories or >20 g carbohydrate may require additional insulin (12).

The key to achieving the greater flexibility in meal timing and portions afforded by basal-bolus therapy is learning to count carbohydrate intake and match insulin doses appropriately. This can be taught in the course of medical nutrition therapy delivered by a registered dietitian or diabetes educator (see chapter 3). Often, the first step in learning carbohydrate counting is eating consistent amounts of carbohydrates and calories. Advanced carbohydrate counting includes determining the individual's insulin-to-carbohydrate ratios and insulin sensitivity factor and learning how to appropriately use these factors. Total calories should be counted to prevent weight gain, especially after puberty. The ability to be flexible with the timing and quantity of meals has had a major impact on glucose control as well as the ability to control weight.

> **PRACTICAL POINT**
>
> Reviewing a patient's food history in correlation with the blood glucose values is critical to the success of any glucose management strategy, but it becomes essential in basal-bolus therapy.

EXERCISE CONSIDERATIONS

Typically, exercise lowers blood glucose levels. The individual with diabetes will need to either increase caloric intake or decrease insulin with additional physical activity. With a basal-bolus regimen, the patient may lower either the basal or the bolus insulin. If the exercise is anticipated and occurs within 3 h of the rapid-acting dose, the patient can decrease the premeal dose or ingest more calories/

carbohydrates. SMBG to detect postexercise hypoglycemia is needed for up to 36 h after the activity (13). The intermediate- or long-acting dose can be decreased if a prolonged activity, such as an active vacation, or intense physical activity, such as skiing or yard work, is planned. The keys are to individualize the plan and to carefully monitor blood glucose.

INSULIN/PRAMLINTIDE STORAGE AND ADMINISTRATION

Typically, insulins and pramlintide do not need to be refrigerated, but they should not be exposed to extremes in temperature. These products have varying durations of stability once opened and used unrefrigerated. The stability varies from 14 to 30 days depending on the product and whether it is in a vial or pen. Marking the vial, syringe, or pen with the date it should be discarded ensures use before expiration.

Patients should be alert to unexpected changes in blood glucose levels. Unexplained increases should prompt a patient to verify that her insulin is not outdated, has not been exposed to direct sunlight or excessive heat (>86°F for most, >96°F for aspart), and has not been frozen (7).

Insulins that are in suspension (cloudy) should be gently rolled a minimum of 20 times before use. This should be done with consistency because some of the variable absorption of the suspended insulin is related to inconsistent mixing of the suspension. Drawing up a dose and then laying the syringe down before injection requires that the filled syringe be remixed by gentle rolling before administration.

Manufacturers of disposable syringes and pen needles recommend that these devices only be used once. The small gauge needles do not withstand multiple uses without "fraying." Viewed under the microscope, a needle used just two or three times begins to look like a rope unraveling. Another potential issue, which arises with reuse of syringes or needles, is the inability to guarantee sterility. Most insulin preparations have bacteriostatic additives that inhibit the growth of bacteria commonly found on the skin. Nevertheless, syringe/needle reuse may carry an increased risk of infection for some individuals. Patients with poor personal hygiene, acute concurrent illness, open wounds on the hands, or decreased resistance to infection for any reason should not reuse a syringe or pen needle.

Appropriate candidate for pramlintide therapy

- Adherent with current insulin regimen
- Consistent SMBG
- Elevated postprandial glucose levels
- A1C <9%
- No recent history of recurrent severe hypoglycemia requiring assistance
- No hypoglycemia unawareness
- No current diagnosis of gastroparesis
- Not a pediatric patient
- Not pregnant or planning a pregnancy
- Has a diabetes team/provider familiar with intensive insulin management

Pramlintide (Symlin) Initiation Guidelines for Type 1 Diabetes

- Start with 15 µg
  - Immediately before major meal/snack
  - Reduce mealtime insulin by 30–50%
  - Self-monitoring blood glucose
    - Anticipate higher values during initiation period
    - Evaluate long-acting insulin and insulin timing
  - If no significant nausea for 3–7 days, advance Symlin
- Advance in 15-µg increments every 3–7 days as tolerated to maximum of 60 µg (10 units)
  - If nausea occurs and persists, reduce to previous dose
  - Adjust insulin doses to optimize control
    - Consider insulin action, timing, amount

From Childs BP, Kesty NC, Klein E, Rubin R, Wick A: Considering pramlintide therapy for postprandial blood glucose control. *Diabetes Spectr* 20:108–114, 2007; Kruger D, Martin C, Sadler C: New insights into glucose regulation. *Diabetes Educ* 32:221–228, 2006; and Kruger D, Gloster M: Pramlintide for the treatment of insulin-requiring diabetes mellitus: rationale and review of clinical data. *Drugs* 64:1419–1432, 2004.

Some patients find it practical to reuse syringes/needles. If needle reuse is planned, the needle must be recapped after each use. Certainly, a needle should be discarded if it is noticeably dull or deformed or if it has come into contact with any surface other than skin. With just one injection, tips of the newer, smaller (30- and 31-gauge) needles can become bent into a hook form that can lacerate tissue or break off, leaving needle fragments in the skin. The medical consequences of this are unknown, but it may increase lipodystrophy or have other adverse effects. In addition to the dulling of the fine needle after puncturing the bottle and the skin, lubrication is lost and the next injection can be painful. Advise patients who are reusing needles to inspect injection sites for redness or swelling and to consult their health care provider before initiating the practice and if signs of skin inflammation are detected.

Insulin may be injected into the subcutaneous tissue of the upper arm or the anterior and lateral aspects of the thigh, buttocks, and abdomen (with the exception of a circle within a 2-inch radius around the navel). Pramlintide may be injected into the abdomen or upper thigh in the same way insulin would be administered. Intramuscular injection is not recommended for routine insulin injections, although it may be given under some circumstances, e.g., DKA or dehydration, because the rate of absorption is faster. Exercise increases the rate of absorption from injection sites, particularly of NPH and Regular formulations, probably by increasing blood flow to the skin and perhaps also by local actions.

Site selection should take into consideration the variable absorption between sites. Rotating within one area (e.g., rotating injections systematically around the abdomen), rather than rotating to a different area with each injection, decreases

Insulin Injection Tips

- Select a site that has no lipohypertrophy or scar tissue.
- Use the same anatomical region for selected injections, e.g., all morning shots in the abdomen, evening meal injection in the arm, bedtime injection in the thigh.
- Use insulin that is at room temperature.
- Make sure no air bubbles remain in the syringe before injection.
- Day-to-day use of topical alcohol is not required. If used, wait until alcohol has evaporated completely before injection.
- Keep muscles in the injection area relaxed, not tense, when injecting.
- Penetrate the skin quickly.
- Do not change the needle's direction during insertion or withdrawal.
- Count to 5 to ensure that all insulin is delivered through a small-gauge needle; count to 10 if using an insulin pen.
- Do not wipe the needle with alcohol. Recap carefully.

Insulin Pen Tips

- Screw on the pen needle until it is snug, not tight.
- Prime before every injection with 1–2 units to make sure the needle is not clogged and insulin is coming out the tip of the needle.
- Use a pen needle that is long enough to go into the subcutaneous tissue. Thin people and children may be able to use the 5-mm "mini" length, while heavier people may need to use the ½-inch to 12-mm length to achieve improved insulin absorption.
- Continue to hold the dose knob down while counting to 10 to assure that all the insulin is delivered.
- Release the pinch before removing the needle to allow the insulin to "depot" and not be as likely to come back out on the skin.
- If bruising occurs or if a drop of blood is noted at the injection site hold pressure over the injection site for about 10 seconds to help clot the small blood vessel. Do not rub.
- Dispose of pen needles in sharps containers or according to local guidelines.
- Dispose of empty plastic pens in the trash.

variability in insulin absorption from day to day. However, glargine and detemir are reported to have consistent absorption regardless of injection site.

Rotation of the injection site is also important to prevent lipohypertrophy or lipoatrophy. Lipohypertrophy is a buildup of fat at the injection site. Lipoatrophy is a loss of fat that causes dimpling of the tissue at injection sites. Hypertrophy and atrophy can occur with overuse of an injection site. Some patients are more prone to lipohypertrophy and lipoatrophy. Both were more common with insulins from animals and are less common with the new insulin preparations. Areas of hypertrophy usually lead to slower inconsistent absorption. Autoimmunity to the insulin may play a role in the development of lipohypertrophies and lipoatrophies. If a patient has hypertrophied injection sites, precautions should be taken to prevent hypoglycemia when insulin is injected into a new site because a dramatic decrease in insulin requirements and hypoglycemia may be seen. In addition, unexplained hypoglycemia may occur if insulin is consistently injected into a hypertrophied area.

INSULIN DELIVERY SYSTEMS

Insulin delivery methods include syringes, pens, injectors, and insulin pumps. It is vital that both health care providers and individuals with diabetes understand the options available for achieving optimal glucose control.

INSULIN PENS

Not only are insulin pens convenient, but individuals are more likely to deliver accurate doses with insulin pens. Patients may be able to see the numbers on the dial or screen better than on a syringe and may be able to manipulate a dialing mechanism more easily than a syringe plunger. Also, when beginning insulin, an anxious patient is often less threatened by an insulin pen than by a needle, syringe, and vial. The smaller volume of insulin that needs to be carried around, compared with a vial and syringe, means that there is less exposure of the insulin to the temperature fluctuations and elements of daily living. The cartridges and pre-filled pens hold 300 units each. Insulin pens are available with replaceable cartridges or as disposable pens. Note the following three important patient education points:

- The needles should be removed after each use.
- The user should "prime every time" to assure that insulin is at the tip of the needle and to make sure that there is no air in the cartridge.
- The needle should remain in the skin for the count of 10 to ensure that all the insulin has been delivered before the needle is removed.

The pen needle should be removed from the pen immediately after an injection is complete. The needle provides an opening into the sterile chamber, permitting an entry for bacteria and/or leakage of insulin. In the case of cloudy suspension, the concentration may be altered by leakage of fluid when insulin is not fully suspended.

OTHER INSULIN DELIVERY DEVICES

PRACTICAL POINT
Long-lasting basal insulins should be given within about an hour of the same time every day for best consistency.

Needleless air injectors are available, but they are costly and frequently not covered by insurance. Many people with type 1 diabetes, from children to elders, use CSII with an insulin pump. Learning to use an insulin pump successfully requires a program of user education and frequent support from the health care team (see chapter 24). Another option is the use of an injection

Future Treatments

Only continued research will reveal the prevention and cure for type 1 diabetes. Although pancreas transplantations are sometimes an option, they are usually performed only if the individual with diabetes also needs a kidney, and there are not enough donor organs to treat everyone with type 1 diabetes. The pancreas is difficult to transplant, and 10–20% of transplants fail within the first year. In addition, there are risks associated with the need for antirejection medications (14,15).

Islet transplantations are another potential cure under investigation. A multicenter clinical trial is finding that up to 50% of transplant recipients remain free of the need for exogenous insulin for 1 year after receiving islet cells. Major obstacles are islet cell rejection, a limited supply of islets, and the risk of long-term use of antirejection medications (16).

Investigations of other new therapies center on amylin (pramlintide), a neuroendocrine hormone regulator of insulin action that is co-secreted with insulin, as well as incretin hormones from the gut that regulate glucose; new insulin analogs; stem cell advances; and new insulin delivery systems, such as a portable, possibly implanted, closed-loop insulin delivery system that would both sense glucose levels and release appropriate amounts of insulin.

port, such as the I-Port. For individuals who are giving multiple injections, the port prevents the need to use multiple sites a day. Like an insulin pump needle, the port site is to be changed every 3 days.

SUMMARY

Near-physiological glucose control is achievable in type 1 diabetes with a motivated individual and a knowledgeable health care team. An insulin regimen can be crafted to match each individual's lifestyle. The person with diabetes must understand insulin action times and his or her individualized response to insulin. The effects of the food plan, physical activity, and emotions can be evaluated with regular monitoring of blood glucose levels. The ability to optimally manage hyperglycemia and hypoglycemia empowers people to be independent. To achieve optimal glucose control requires that the individual become active in self-managing his or her disease and that the health care team provide coaching and support.

REFERENCES

1. National Institute of Diabetes and Digestive and Kidney Diseases, National Diabetes Information Clearinghouse: National Diabetes Statistics, 2007, Prevalence of Diagnosed and Undiagnosed Diabetes among People Aged 20 Years or Older, United States, 2007 [Internet]. Available at http://diabetes.

niddk.nih.gov/dm/pubs/statistics/#i_youngpeople. Accessed 30 January 2009

2. Bode BW (Ed.): Medical Management of Type 1 Diabetes. 4th ed. Alexandria, VA, American Diabetes Association, 2004

3. Aronoff SL, Berkowitz K, Shreiner B, Want L: Glucose metabolism and regulation: beyond insulin and glucagon. *Diabetes Spectrum* 17:183–190, 2004

4. Diabetes Control and Complications Trial Research Group: The effect of intensive treatment of diabetes on the development and progression of long-term complications in insulin dependent diabetes mellitus. *N Engl J Med* 329:977–986, 1993

5. DCCT/EDIC Writing Group: Sustained effect of intensive treatment of type 1 diabetes mellitus on development and progression of diabetic nephropathy. *JAMA* 290:2159–2167, 2003

6. The DCCT/EDIC Study Research Group: Intensive diabetes treatment and cardiovascular disease in patients with type 1 diabetes. *N Engl J Med* 353:2643–2653, 2005

7. Grajower MM, Fraser CG, Holcombe ML, Daugherty ML, Harris WC, et al.: How long should insulin be used once a vial is opened? (Editorial). *Diabetes Care* 26:2665–2669, 2003

8. American Diabetes Association: Insulin administration (Position Statement). *Diabetes Care* 27 (Suppl. 1):106–109, 2004

9. American Diabetes Association: Standards of medical care in diabetes—2009 (Position Statement). *Diabetes Care* 32 (Suppl. 1):S13–S61, 2009

10. Warshaw HS, Kulkarni K: *Complete Guide to Carbohydrate Counting*. Alexandria, VA, American Diabetes Association, 2001, p. 148–149

11. Hinnen DH, Guthrie DW, Childs BP, Friesen J, Rhiley D, Guthrie RA: Pattern management of blood glucose. In *A Core Curriculum for Diabetes Education: Diabetes Management Therapies*. Franz M, Ed. Chicago, IL, American Association of Diabetes Educators, 2003, p. 220–221

12. Guthrie RA, Childs BP, Guthrie DW: *Rapid and Long Acting Insulin Analogs: Strategies for Patient Use*. Monograph. 2nd ed. Wichita, KS, Quontum Press, 2004

13. American Diabetes Association: Physical activity/exercise and diabetes (Position Statement). *Diabetes Care* 27 (Suppl. 1):S58–S62, 2004

14. National Institute of Diabetes and Digestive and Kidney Diseases, National Diabetes Information Clearinghouse: Pancreatic islet transplantation [Internet]. Available from http://diabetes.niddk.nih.gov/dm/pubs/pancreaticislet/index.htm. Accessed 30 January 2009

15. American Diabetes Association: Pancreas transplantation [Internet]. Available from http://www.diabetes.org/type-1-diabetes/pancreas-transplants.jsp. Accessed 30 January 2009

16. American Diabetes Association: Islet transplantation [Internet]. Available from http://www.diabetes.org/type-1-diabetes/islet-transplants.jsp. Accessed 30 January 2009

Ms. Childs is a Diabetes Nurse Specialist at Mid-America Diabetes Associates, Wichita, KS. Ms. Kruger is a Certified Nurse Practitioner at Henry Ford Health Systems, Detroit, MI.

5. Treatment Strategies for Type 2 Diabetes

Andrea Zaldivar, MS, ANP-BC, CDE, and
Jane Jeffrie Seley, MPH, MSN, GNP, CDE

T he majority of diabetic patients encountered over the course of a nursing career will have type 2 diabetes. Type 2 diabetes affects 90–95% of all people with diabetes. Because hyperglycemia develops slowly over time, many people are asymptomatic and may have had type 2 diabetes for up to 7–12 years before diagnosis. Because of this prolonged period of unknown hyperglycemia, there may already be diabetes complications (1,2). Type 2 diabetes is most common in obese individuals who are at least 45 years of age, but because of the increasing rate of obesity, we now see type 2 diabetes in children as young as age 10 years (3,4). The public health ramifications of a formerly adult disease affecting children and adolescents remain to be seen. Whether a nurse chooses to work with adults or children, he or she should become familiar and comfortable with the early identification and management of type 2 diabetes.

If glucose is to be used or stored efficiently in the body, the pancreas must secrete sufficient insulin and it must be used properly by the body. In type 2 diabetes, this altered process represents two main defects. People with type 2 diabetes have insufficient insulin production; however, the deficiency is relative because some insulin is still produced in the pancreas (5). In addition to insulin deficiency, the predominant problem is increased insulin resistance in the muscle, adipose cells, and liver (6). In individuals with type 2 diabetes, overproduction of glucose by the liver appears to coexist (6) with decreased insulin secretion and increased insulin resistance. A good strategy to use when treating patients with type 2 diabetes is to select medications that address these defects.

Research in the past several years has revealed other factors in the pathophysiology of type 2 diabetes. Glucagon-like peptide-1 (GLP-1) and gastric inhibitory polypeptide (GIP), which are secreted in the gut (incretin hormones), and amylin (a neuroendocrine hormone), which is secreted in the β-cells of the pancreas all appear to have an impact on glucose homeostasis. Research into these hormones has led to the development of new drugs. GLP-1 receptor agonists and dipeptidyl peptidase (DPP)-IV inhibitors stimulate insulin secretion while inhibiting glucagon, thus lowering blood glucose (7). Amylin regulates glucose metabolism in the stomach and liver by delaying glucose transport in the postprandial state (8). Many of these newer drugs have an added benefit of producing satiety and possibly weight loss in some patients.

The American Diabetes Association Standards of Medical Care in Diabetes (1) recommend the use of metformin as initial therapy in type 2 diabetes and even in some patients with pre-diabetes. This recommendation directs the health professional to initiate treatment of the insulin resistance first and insulin deficiency second.

TREATING INSULIN DEFICIENCY

Health care professionals who treat people with diabetes today are fortunate to have a large list of oral medications to assist in treating the insulin deficiency found in type 2 diabetes.

SULFONYLUREAS

A class of long-acting insulin secretagogues known as sulfonylureas has been in existence since the 1950s and is sometimes the first choice for pharmacological treatment of type 2 diabetes (Table 5.1). Sulfonylureas, which stimulate the β-cells in the pancreas to produce more insulin, appear to work quickly in reducing blood glucose levels.

Table 5.1 Medications That Increase Insulin Secretion

Sulfonylureas stimulate insulin secretion in the pancreatic β-cells.

Second generation:
Glyburide/DiaBeta, Micronase, Glynase Prestabs (1.25–10 mg), Glipizide/Glucotrol, Glucotrol XL (2.5–20 mg), Glimepiride/Amaryl (1–4 mg)

Notes:
- Taken before meals
- Hypoglycemia is the most common side effect
- Contraindicated during pregnancy or in people allergic to sulfa

Meglitinides stimulate insulin production in the pancreatic β-cells (shorter acting than sulfonylureas).

Repaglinide/Prandin (0.5–16 mg), Nateglinide/Starlix (60–120 mg × 3 days)

Notes:
- Taken just before meals and omitted if a meal is missed
- Hypoglycemia is the most common side effect
- Can be titrated according to meal size
- Contraindicated during pregnancy

> ### PRACTICAL POINT
>
> By definition, a person who has type 2 diabetes has insulin resistance. When recommending meal planning, physical activity, and medications, treatment strategies should address both the insulin resistance and the insulin deficiency.

When sulfonylureas were first introduced, health care providers were often disappointed with the unpredictable way in which they stimulated the β-cells to secrete insulin. The first generation of sulfonylureas often encouraged insulin secretion when insulin was not needed, resulting in hypoglycemia. Fortunately, most of the newer, or second-generation, sulfonylureas cause less hypoglycemia (except glyburide) than their predecessors because they are shorter-acting (6). Weight gain and hypoglycemia continue to be potential side effects of this class of medication (9).

The U.K. Prospective Diabetes Study (UKPDS) documented a progressive decline in β-cell function in individuals with type 2 diabetes, commencing years before the actual diagnosis of diabetes and continuing throughout the person's life, regardless of mode of treatment (10). For sulfonylureas to be effective, they require functioning β-cells; therefore, they are most useful in the earlier stages of type 2 diabetes. Over time, sulfonylureas become less effective, and other medication will be needed to achieve glycemic targets.

MEGLITINIDES

Meglitinides are short-acting insulin secretagogues that are taken just before a meal (Table 5.1). Meglitinides are more sensitive than sulfonylureas to being activated in the presence of hyperglycemia or a meal. For this reason, meglitinides appear to produce less hypoglycemia. Meglitinides should be taken immediately before a meal and omitted if the meal is skipped. This group of medications works well in individuals with unpredictable eating patterns because the dose can be varied according to the size of the meal or not taken if the meal is missed. At the same time, because meglitinides are taken before every meal, they may not be the best choice for patients who have trouble remembering to take their medications. Meglitinides, like sulfonylureas, are not recommended for use during pregnancy (11).

TREATING INSULIN RESISTANCE

Early in the progression of the disease, a person with type 2 diabetes experiences resistance to insulin in the liver as well as in the adipose and muscle cells (6). When insulin resistance is present, more insulin is required to lower glucose levels. Initially, an individual may be able to adequately compensate and produce sufficient insulin to meet the body's metabolic needs. He or she may experience a period of increased insulin production or "hyperinsulinemia" before having overt diabetes.

Although the exact mechanism is unknown, hyperinsulinemia is associated with macrovascular risk factors, including dyslipidemia and hypertension (6). Whether referred to as the metabolic syndrome, dysmetabolic syndrome, syndrome X, or the insulin resistance syndrome, the characteristics of hypertension, dyslipidemia, and central obesity put the individual with type 2 diabetes at higher risk for developing cardiovascular disease (6). The UKPDS highlighted the need to tightly control hypertension in individuals with type 2 diabetes to decrease the occurrence of cardiovascular events. This study further showed that control of blood pressure might require the use of multiple medications (10).

Insulin resistance in the liver, muscle, and adipose cells appears long before type 2 diabetes (12). Eventually the pancreas cannot keep up with the increased demands of extra insulin to compensate for the insulin resistance, and glucose control becomes challenged. Insulin resistance can be decreased through weight loss, physical activity, and the use of insulin sensitizers, such as biguanides and thiazolidinediones (9,13).

Medications that treat insulin resistance act primarily on the liver (biguanides) or in the muscle and adipose cells (thiazolidinediones) (Table 5.2). Because of their abilities to target insulin resistance in two different areas, biguanides and thiazolidinediones can be taken together to produce a greater effect (11).

BIGUANIDES

Biguanides, of which metformin is only one, work to control diabetes by decreasing glucose production in the liver (particularly during the night), thus lowering fasting blood glucose levels. Biguanides also lower peripheral insulin resistance, although to a lesser extent. Lactic acidosis, though rare, is a potential risk of this category of medication. Any individuals who are predisposed to lactic acidosis, such as binge drinkers, those with New York Heart Association (NYHA) class III or IV heart failure, and people with impaired renal function (creatinine 1.5 mg/dl in men and 1.4 mg/dl in women), should not take biguanides. Caution should be taken in the elderly, with kidney function evaluated and closely monitored. The common side effect seen with biguanides is gastrointestinal complaints, especially if the dosage is too quickly advanced when initiated or initiated at too high a dose. This side effect is lessened when the medication is taken with food and/or gradually titrated or when an extended-release formulation is used. Many patients report a decrease in appetite and subsequent modest weight loss when taking biguanides (9).

THIAZOLIDINEDIONES

Thiazolidinediones decrease insulin resistance primarily in muscle and adipose cells. Their glucose-lowering effect is not based on stimulating insulin production; therefore, these agents do not produce hypoglycemia when used as monotherapy. Thiazolidinediones have also been shown to have both lipid-lowering and antihypertensive effects (6). The main side effects associated with thiazolidinediones are weight gain and edema. Patients should be observed for signs and symptoms of heart failure. Thiazolidinediones are not recommended for use in patients with NYHA class III or IV heart failure (9). Newer black-box warnings caution that thiazolidinediones can cause or worsen heart failure and should not be used if the patient is symptomatic for heart failure (11). Rosiglitazone has been associated with an increased risk of myocardial infarction and is not recommended for use with insulin or nitrates (14,15). Pioglitazone, however, was not found to have any sig-

---

Table 5.2 Medications That Reduce Insulin Resistance

Biguanides suppress glucose production in the liver and decrease insulin resistance.

Metformin/Glucophage, Glucophage XR, Fortamet/Riomet (500–1,000 mg)

Notes:
Taken with meals
- Gastrointestinal complaints are the most common side effect
- Should be stopped the day of any procedure using iodinated contrast media or major surgical procedures and restarted 48 h later if renal function has been confirmed to be adequate and stable
- Contraindicated
  - during pregnancy
  - in renal disease (serum creatinine ≥1.5 mg/dl in men and ≥1.4 mg/dl in women, or abnormal creatinine clearance)
  - in liver dysfunction
  - in congestive heart failure
  - with history of alcohol abuse
  - in acute or chronic metabolic acidosis
- If age >80 years, confirm normal renal function with creatinine clearance test before initiating therapy and monitor closely

Thiazolidinediones decrease insulin resistance in adipose and muscle cells.

Pioglitazone/Actos (15–45 mg), Rosiglitazone/Avandia (4–8 mg)

Notes:
- Usually taken once daily with the first meal (rosiglitazone may be given once or twice daily)
- Weight gain and fluid retention are the most common side effects
- Contraindicated during pregnancy
- Use with caution in liver disease; liver function tests should be done before initiating therapy and according to the prescriber's discretion (the authors recommend quarterly for the first year), and then annually
- Contraindicated in patients with NYHA class III and IV cardiac status; observe patients for signs and symptoms of heart failure, especially increased shortness of breath, edema, and weight gain
- Possible additional beneficial effect of pioglitazone on cardiovascular disease

---

See also "Oral Agents" in RESOURCES.

nificant effects (when compared with placebo) on cardiovascular outcomes (included all-cause mortality, nonfatal and silen myocardial infaction, stroke, major leg amputation, acute coronary syndrome, coronary artery bypass graft or percutaneous coronary intervention, and leg revascularization) after 3 years of follow-up (16). The most recent ADA guidelines for medical management of type 2 diabetes do not recommend using rosiglitazone, particularly since there is more beneficial data on using pioglitazone (17). Liver toxicity was a concern with an earlier medication in this class. The newer thiazolidinediones do not seem to produce this side effect, but should be used with caution when liver disease is present. Liver function tests should be done before initiating therapy and according to the prescriber's discretion. If any elevation is present at baseline, more frequent testing is prudent.

INSULIN THERAPY IN TYPE 2 DIABETES

Because type 2 diabetes is chronic and progressive, β-cell function is decreased by at least 50% at diagnosis and by 75% 6 years later (18). β-Cell function may also be impaired temporarily in the case of severe hyperglycemia known as glucose toxicity (6). In either case, insulin therapy should be considered whenever optimal glucose control, i.e., glycated hemoglobin A1c (A1C) <7%, cannot be reached to decrease the risk of long-term microvascular complications (18). The decision to initiate insulin therapy should be made based on glycemic control, not patient and provider readiness. Whenever insulin is mentioned, it is not uncommon for patients to plead for more time to eat better, exercise more, and improve their glycemic control. It should be stressed that the initiation of insulin is not intended to punish patients for not taking care of themselves; rather, it is simply necessary to achieve glycemic control. Insulin is a natural hormone that, when deficient, requires replacement. Many patients express a fear of weight gain and hypoglycemia while on insulin.

Weight gain as a result of initiating insulin therapy is a valid concern for the patient with type 2 diabetes and his or her health care provider. As glycemic control improves, glycosuria decreases and calories once wasted by the body are now stored as fat. Intermittent overinsulinization may result in hypoglycemia that leads to hunger and an increase in caloric consumption (19). Weight gain can be minimized with attention to carbohydrate counting and increased physical activity as insulin therapy is advanced. Concurrent use of metformin along with insulin therapy has also been shown to minimize weight gain (20, 21). If still effective, sulfonylureas combined with insulin can lower the insulin dose by 25–50% with less weight gain (19). In two separate studies, bedtime administration of NPH instead of daytime NPH and use of insulin glargine instead of NPH yielded less weight gain (19). Levemir has also been associated with little or no weight gain (22).

Many patients verbalize a fear of the actual act of injecting the insulin and of the increased risk of hypoglycemia with insulin therapy. In reality, the rates of severe hypoglycemia in type 2 diabetes are low. The Kumamoto study (23), for example, showed an average A1C of 7.1% for the tightly controlled group and the same rate of mild hypoglycemia as that of the conventional therapy group, which had a mean A1C of 9.4%. Nurses can be influential in helping patients understand the benefits of insulin therapy and the ease of use and increased accuracy of new delivery devices such as insulin pens (19,24). Patient education regarding the signs, symptoms, and especially prevention of hypoglycemia can help allay fears. In addition, showing patients an insulin syringe or pen and short pen needle and asking them to try an injection usually is met with surprise at how tiny the needle actually is and how little pain is experienced.

The initiation of insulin therapy is often delayed because of both patient

> **PRACTICAL POINT**
>
> Insulin therapy should never be used as a threat. The natural progression of the disease tells us that most people with type 2 diabetes will need insulin eventually, regardless of previous therapies. It does not indicate that the patient failed.

and provider resistance. Health care providers often bargain with patients and place insulin initiation on the backburner because insulin self-care education involves considerable time and effort in a busy practice setting where there may not be any skilled personnel available. Insulin is often used as a threat to patients rather than a valuable tool. The reality is that the longer a person lives with type 2 diabetes, the fewer functioning β-cells they have, and the need for insulin becomes inevitable over time (6). We must prepare patients for this by talking about insulin in a positive way.

The rationale for starting insulin for a patient with type 2 diabetes is initially different from that in the case of type 1 diabetes. This is because the pancreas in type 2 diabetes patients may still be able to "help" by producing some insulin. The current philosophy is to use a simple and easy-to-follow regimen, keeping the oral agents the same and adding a single injection of insulin once daily at a convenient time, such as in the morning or at bedtime (23). The current options include a long-acting basal insulin, such as glargine or detemir, an intermediate-acting insulin, such as NPH, or a premixed insulin, such as 70/30 or 75/25 (6). Glargine can be given either in the morning or at bedtime, depending on patient preference. Although the single injection of NPH is often given at bedtime, it could also be given before breakfast or before supper depending on the patient's lifestyle or preferences and the insulin chosen. The premixed insulins are best given before meals, such as before breakfast and before supper. Because of insulin resistance, insulin dose requirements in type 2 diabetes are often much higher than in type 1 diabetes (19). The important thing to remember is that there is no one treatment regimen for all patients but rather individualized regimens should be designed or tailored to a patient's particular needs and abilities.

As type 2 diabetes progresses, more intensive insulin regimens will be needed to achieve the same glycemic goals (insulin treatment is more fully covered in chapter 4). Basal-bolus regimens such as those used in type 1 diabetes will help patients reach glycemic targets when other therapies no longer can because of the progression of type 2 diabetes (19). The use of exogenous insulin administered in a way that mimics normal physiology will help reduce the chance of long-term complications (23). Once insulin therapy is agreed upon, it is important that the patient receive extensive patient education beyond lifestyle interventions, including education in

- proper storage and administration of insulin
- site selection and rotation
- time-action profile(s) of insulin
- disposal and reuse of syringes and pen needles
- hypoglycemia treatment and prevention
- blood glucose monitoring targets
- sick-day management

In addition, the patient should be followed closely and taught to adjust the insulin, if possible, as needed to achieve optimal glycemic control. If the patient is not able to learn how to adjust insulin doses, a plan should be made for regular phone, fax, or e-mail contact with a health professional to evaluate blood glucose levels and discuss treatment changes. The patient expects improvement with insulin therapy, and it is up to the provider to facilitate success by both optimizing therapy and encouraging patient self-management.

Table 5.3 Medications That Reduce Glucose Absorption

α-Glucosidase inhibitors decrease carbohydrate absorption in the gastrointestinal tract.

Acarbose/Precose (25–100 mg), Miglitol/Glyset (25–100 mg); 3 times/day

Notes:
- Taken with the first bite of each main meal
- Flatulence and gastrointestinal complaints are the most common side effects
- Contraindicated
  - during pregnancy
  - during breast-feeding
  - for children
  - in cirrhosis of the liver
- Not recommended in patients with creatinine clearance of <25 ml/min (23) or inflammatory bowel disease

See also "Oral Agents" in RESOURCES.

SLOWING GLUCOSE ABSORPTION

Unlike the other medications used to treat type 2 diabetes that increase insulin production or decrease insulin resistance, α-glucosidase inhibitors work in the intestinal tract to slow glucose absorption (Table 5.3). These medications are usually most effective in the early stages of type 2 diabetes, when postprandial excursions of glucose seem to be the primary issue involved in controlling glucose (6,12), and in patients who ingest large amounts of carbohydrates (6). The most common side effects seen in this class of medication are flatulence and diarrhea. These side effects seem to subside after 3–4 weeks of use (6,9). α-Glucosidase inhibitors do not cause hypoglycemia when used as monotherapies (12). Hypoglycemia can occur when these agents are used in combination with other diabetes medications that can cause hypoglycemia, such as insulin secretagogues or insulin. Because α-glucosidase inhibitors slow down the digestion of carbohydrates into glucose, glucose tablets should be used to effectively treat hypoglycemia (12).

AMYLIN MIMETICS, INCRETIN MIMETICS, DPP INHIBITORS

These agents work by suppressing glucagon secretion, slowing gastric emptying, and increasing satiety. Some, such as the incretin mimetic exenatide, also work by increasing glucose-dependent synthesis and secretion of insulin by the β-cells in the pancreas. (See Table 5.4.)

PRAMLINTIDE

Pramlintide, a synthetic form of amylin, is an injectable medication that can be useful in optimizing glycemic control in patients taking insulin. Pramlintide works

Table 5.4 Medications That Have Several Actions

Pramlintide/Symlin slows gastric emptying, suppresses glucagon secretion, and promotes satiety.
Injectable: 30–120 μg before meals, depending upon whether used in type 1 or type 2 diabetes

Notes:
- Take immediately prior to meals (may need to decrease preprandial insulin by 50%).
- Do not mix with insulin (in same syringe).
- Do not take pre-meal if meal is < 250 calories or < 30 Grams of carbohydrates, or a skipped meal.
- Titration should be done slowly and carefully.
- Nausea is the most common side effect.
- Severe hypoglycemia is a risk when used along with insulin.
- Contraindicated
  - during pregnancy
  - in gastroparesis or other serious gastrointestinal problem
  - in presence of hypoglycemia unawareness
  - if A1C >9% (21)

Exenatide/Byetta slows gastric emptying, suppresses glucagon secretion, promotes satiety, and increases insulin secretion in response to meals.
Injectable: 5–10 μg twice daily

Notes:
- Inject no more than 60 min before meals (two largest meals of the day).
- Can cause hypoglycemia if used with insulin, sulfonylurea, or meglitinide.
- Most common side effect is nausea.
- Pancreatitis has been noted post-marketing.
- Store unused pen in refrigerator; open pen keep <77°F; use pen only for 30 days.
- Contraindicated
  - during pregnancy
  - in type 1 diabetes
  - in end-stage renal disease
  - in the presence of gastroparesis or other serious gastrointestinal problem
  - if A1C >9%
  - in pancreatitis (27)

Sitagliptin/Januvia is a DPP-IV inhibitor that decreases glucagon secretion and increases insulin secretion and release.
Oral medication: 25, 50, or 100-mg once daily

Notes:
- Can cause hypoglycemia if used with sulfonylurea.
- Can be used with metformin (precautions are those associated with metformin).
- Generally weight stable.
- Contraindicated
  - in type 1 diabetes
  - during pregnancy
  - if hypersensitivity to drug (angioedema)
  - caution in renal insufficiency (37)

together with insulin to reduce postprandial hyperglycemia by suppressing glucagon secretion, slowing gastric emptying, and increasing satiety, thereby decreasing food intake. Pramlintide is particularly useful in patients who are on basal-bolus insulin therapy and are still unable to achieve optimal postprandial blood glucose levels. Pramlintide can be used in both type 1 and insulin-treated type 2 diabetes (11,25).

EXENATIDE

Exenatide lowers postprandial blood glucose by increasing insulin secretion by β-cells, lowering glucagon levels (without disturbing the glucagon response to hypoglycemia), suppressing appetite, and slowing gastric emptying. One of the benefits of exenatide is often weight loss. Exenatide is given twice daily as a 5- to 10-μg subcutaneous injection. The most common side effect is nausea, which frequently subsides with use. It is very important that patients be educated to eat within 60 min of injecting the medication. If they do not plan to eat, the exenatide dose should be omitted. Exenatide is contraindicated in patients with type 1 diabetes because functioning β-cells are required for the medication to enhance insulin secretion. It is also contraindicated in patients with end-stage renal disease or any major gastrointestinal disease. Exenatide can be used in conjunction with metformin, thiazolidinediones, and/or sulfonylureas (26,27).

DPP INHIBITORS

Sitagliptin, a DPP-IV inhibitor, is an oral agent that works by blocking DPP-IV and thus prolonging the availability of GLP-1 and GIP, the hormones that stimulate insulin secretion, inhibit gastric emptying, and inhibit insulin secretion. Sitagliptin can be used as monotherapy or taken in conjunction with metformin, sulfonylureas, or thiazolidinediones. Unlike injectable incretins (exenatide), sitagliptin is not associated with weight loss. Kidney function should be assessed and dosage reductions made for renal insufficiency. This drug is not recommended for use in type 1 diabetes or in ketoacidosis. Sitagliptin is taken once daily. Possible side effects include upper respiratory infection, nasopharyngitis, and headache (11).

ENCOURAGING WEIGHT LOSS

It is no coincidence that both diabetes and obesity are on the rise in the U.S. According to a study published in the *Journal of the American Medical Association* (28), obesity rose from 19.8 to 20.9% of adults in the U.S. in the same year (2000–2001) that diagnosed diabetes rose from 7.3 to 7.9%. A strong correlation was found between overweight or obesity and diabetes in all races, ages, educational levels, and smoking levels and in both sexes (28). Although being overweight is associated with insulin resistance, not all overweight people develop type 2 diabetes. Therefore, other factors besides obesity must be present to facilitate the onset of diabetes (29).

On a more positive note, even a modest weight loss in overweight adults significantly reduces the risk of developing diabetes. In one study, there was a 33%

> ### PRACTICAL POINT
>
> When addressing weight loss, work closely with a dietitian to set mutually acceptable and attainable goals. Treatment of hyperglycemia may cause weight gain as there is a decrease in loss of calories from glycosuria. A possible first goal can be not to gain any weight between visits.

lower risk of an individual developing diabetes for every kilogram lost per year over a 10-year period (24). In addition, in three randomized control trials in China, Finland, and the U.S., the incidence of type 2 diabetes in people who were at high risk for developing diabetes was reduced by up to 58% with lifestyle interventions that included modest weight loss (30–32).

Weight loss and regular physical activity are primary treatment strategies in type 2 diabetes. Over time, they can lead to a reduced need for medication as well as improved glycemic control. It is important for nurses to place the same emphasis on meal planning and physical activity as on pharmacological interventions. Newer agents such as exenatide and pramlintide may be helpful to patients who have difficulty controlling portion sizes, since they have the potential to produce satiety and decrease food intake. Some patients have achieved significant weight loss on these medications.

A simple strategy that can be used to promote weight loss is to assist individuals in recognizing the antecedents and consequences to overeating and their actual eating behaviors. An example would be asking a patient to examine how skipping a meal could promote overeating at the end of the day and then asking them to evaluate how they feel when they overeat (take note that skipping meals cannot be done if the patient is taking certain medications). Providers should tailor behavior changes accordingly (33). These lifestyle changes can help patients achieve the glycemic targets that will reduce their risk of serious complications. Sensible weight loss takes time and perseverance. Many patients get frustrated and need ongoing guidance and support. Emphasizing even the smallest improvement in weight, especially if it correlates with a decrease in A1C level, helps keep patients encouraged and motivated. Referral to a dietitian and/or certified diabetes educator for medical nutrition therapy will be beneficial for the individual with type 2 diabetes.

TREATING TYPE 2 DIABETES

As type 2 diabetes progresses and β-cell function decreases or insulin resistance increases, medical treatment must be advanced (34). Most people with type 2 diabetes will require more than one medication over time, with each targeting a different organ and defect. Figure 5.1 shows a consensus algorithm for the treatment of type 2 diabetes recently developed by the American Diabetes Association and the European Association for the Study of Diabetes (17). Coupled with the comorbidities associated with increased insulin resistance, such as hypertension and dyslipidemia (23), this often translates into an individual with type 2 diabetes taking a large number of medications daily (i.e., polypharmacy, see chapter 23).

Tier 1: Well-validated core therapies

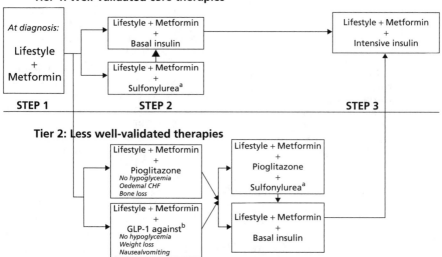

Tier 2: Less well-validated therapies

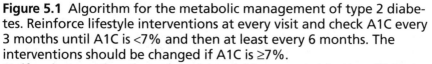

Figure 5.1 Algorithm for the metabolic management of type 2 diabetes. Reinforce lifestyle interventions at every visit and check A1C every 3 months until A1C is <7% and then at least every 6 months. The interventions should be changed if A1C is ≥7%.
aSulfonylureas other than glyburide or chlorpropamide; binsufficient clinical use to be confident regarding safety.

> **PRACTICAL POINT**
>
> As medications are being added or changed, remember to reinforce treatment goals with patients, stressing their relationship to avoiding diabetes-related complications.

The use of polypharmacy in patients with type 2 diabetes creates several challenges for the nurse. First, the nurse must be diligent in learning the action, side effects, and drug-to-drug interactions of each medication and how to optimize benefits so that he or she can educate the patient. Second, the nurse must find creative ways such as the use of pillboxes or reminder cues to assist the patient in adhering to complex medication regimens. Nurses must also be cognizant of the overall cost of taking multiple medications daily and assist patients with social services and pharmaceutical indigent care program referrals when needed.

Effective communication between the patient and health care provider is crucial if patients are to execute complex treatment recommendations. At least 14% of the nation's population speaks a language other than English at home (35). Adhering to complex medication regimens may be especially difficult when a nurse attempts to assist a patient whose primary language is not English. Nurses

<table>
<tr><td>

PRACTICAL POINT

To facilitate adherence to treatment recommendations, make sure patients can describe how they should be taking their medications and what they should do if they have questions about their medications before they leave your facility.

</td></tr>
</table>

must be proactive in developing strategies to deal with the needs of culturally diverse populations. The use of bicultural/bilingual staff, use of internal language banks, and language skills training may assist nurses in facilitating communication between themselves and diverse patients (36).

Nurses should offer additional emotional and practical support to the individual with type 2 diabetes who must begin insulin therapy. Many of these patients need assistance in accepting this inevitable step in the progression of their disease and the reality that it is not their fault. Individuals with type 2 diabetes need information about the targets for glycemic control and the relationship between control and risk of complications. Avoiding diabetes-related complications is an important goal for both the nurse and the patient.

SUMMARY

Type 2 diabetes is a complex, progressive disease associated with numerous comorbidities including hyperlipidemia, hypertension, obesity, and depression. Because of the progressive nature of the disease, not the failure of the patient or health care provider, most patients will need insulin in their lifetime. The nurse will play an important role in assisting patients in understanding the nature of their disease, including the necessity of medications to treat insulin resistance, insulin deficiency, and other defects of type 2 diabetes as well as the importance of healthy lifestyle behaviors.

<table>
<tr><td>

TYPE 2 DIABETES SYMLIN INITIATION

- Start 60 micrograms
  - Immediately before major meal/snack.
  - Reduce mealtime insulin 50%.
  - Self-monitoring blood glucose
    - Anticipate higher values during initiation period.
    - Evaluate long-acting insulin and insulin timing.
  - If no significant nausea for 3–7 days, advance Symlin.

- Advance to 120 μg
  - If nausea occurs and persists, reduce to 60 μg.
  - Adjust insulin doses to optimize control.
    - Consider insulin action, timing, amount.
    - Evaluate food/activity.

</td></tr>
</table>

REFERENCES

1. American Diabetes Association: Standards of medical care in diabetes—2009. *Diabetes Care* 32 (Suppl.1):S13–S61, 2009

2. U.S. Preventive Services Task Force: Screening for type 2 diabetes mellitus in adults: U. S. Preventive Services Task Force (Recommendation Statement). *Ann Intern Med* 148:846–854, 2008)

3. Mayer-Davis E: Type 2 diabetes in youth: epidemiology and current research toward prevention and treatment. *J Am Diet Assoc* 108 (Suppl.1):s45–s51, 2008

4. Liese AD, D'Agostino RB Jr, Hamman RF, Kilgo PD, Lawrence JM, et al.: The burden of diabetes mellitus among US youth: prevalence estimates from SEARCH for Diabetes in Youth Study. *Pediatrics* 118:1510–1518, 2006

5. Stumvoll M, Goldstein B, van Haeften T: Type 2 diabetes: principles of pathogenesis and therapy. *Lancet* 365:1333–1346, 2005

6. Beaser RS: *Joslin Diabetes Deskbook: A Guide for Primary Care Providers.* 2nd ed. Philadelphia, Lippincott Williams and Wilkins, 2007

7. Goldberg RB, Holman R, Drucker DJ: Clinical decisions: management of type 2 diabetes. *N Engl J Med* 358:293–297, 2008

8. Riddle MC, Drucker DJ: Emerging therapies mimicking the effects of amylin and glucagon-like peptide 1. *Diabetes Care* 29:435–449, 2006

9. Fonseca VA, Kulkarni K: Management of type 2 diabetes: oral agents, insulin and injectables. *J Am Diet Assoc* 108 (Suppl.1):s29–s33, 2008

10. UK Prospective Diabetes Study Group: Intensive blood-glucose control with sulfonylureas or insulin compared with conventional treatment and risk of complications in patients with type 2 diabetes (UKPDS 33). *Lancet* 352:837–853, 1998

11. *Physicians' Desk Reference.* 62nd ed. Montvale, NJ, Medical Economics, 2008

12. Reaven G: Metabolic syndrome: pathophysiology and implications for management of cardiovascular disease. *Circulation* 106:286–288, 2002

13. Franz MJ, Kulkarni K, Polonsky WK, Yearbough P, Zamudio V (Eds.): *A Core Curriculum for Diabetes Educators.* 4th ed. Chicago, American Association of Diabetes Educators, 2003

14. Nissen SE, Wolski K: Effect of rosiglitazone on the risk of myocardial infarction and death from cardiovascular causes. *N Engl J Med* 356:2457–2471, 2007

15. Singh S, Loke YK, Furberg CD: Long-term risk of cardiovascular events with rosiglitazone: a meta-analysis. *JAMA* 298:1189–1195, 2007

16. Dormandy JA, Carbonnel B, Eckland DJA, et al.: Secondary prevention of macrovascular events in patients with type 2 diabetes in the PROactive (PROspective pioglitAzone Clinical Trial in macrovascular Events): a randomized controlled trial. *Lancet* 366:1279–1289, 2005

17. Nathan DM, Buse JB, Davidson MB, Ferrannini E, Holman RR, et al.: Medical management of hyperglycemia in type 2 diabetes: a consensus algorithm for the initiation and adjustment of therapy. *Diabetes Care* 31:1–11, 2008

18. Dewitt DE, Dugdale DC: Using new insulin strategies in the outpatient treatment of diabetes. *JAMA* 289:2265–2269, 2003

19. DeWitt DE, Hirsh IB: Outpatient insulin therapy in type 1 and type 2 diabetes mellitus. *JAMA* 289:2254–2264, 2003

20. Riddle M: Combined therapy with insulin plus oral agents: is there any advantage? An argument in favor. *Diabetes Care* 31:S125–S130, 2008

21. Holman RR, Thorne KI, Farmer AJ, Davies MJ, Keenan JF, et al.: Addition of biphasic, prandial or basal insulin to oral therapy in type 2 diabetes. *N Engl J Med* 357:1716–1730, 2007

22. Home P, Kurtzhals P: Insulin detemir: from concept to clinical experience. *Expert Opin Pharmacother* 7:325–343, 2006

23. White JR: Clarifying the role of insulin in type 2 management. *Clinical Diabetes* 21:14–21, 2003

24. Rubin R, Peyrot M: Factors affecting use of insulin pens by patients with type 2 diabetes. *Diabetes Care* 31:430–432, 2008

25. Amylin Pharmaceuticals: Symlin package insert. 2008

26. Peters A, Miller D: New insights: clinical pearls for using incretin mimetics in type 2 diabetes. *Diabetes Educator* 33 (Suppl. 1), 14S–19S, 2007

27. Eli Lilly: Byetta package insert. 2008

28. Mokdad AH, Ford ES, Bowman BA, Dietz WH, Vinicor F, et al.: Prevalence of obesity, diabetes, and obesity-related health risk factors, 2001. *JAMA* 289:76–79, 2003

29. Romao I, Roth J: Genetic and environmental interactions in obesity and type 2 diabetes. *J Am Diet Assoc* 108 (Suppl. 1):S24–S28, 2008

30. Diabetes Prevention Program Research Group: Impact of intensive lifestyle and metformin therapy on cardiovascular disease risk factors in the Diabetes Prevention Program. *Diabetes Care* 28:888–894, 2005

31. Tuomilehto J, Lindstrom J, Eriksson JG, Valle TT, Hamalainen H, et al.: Prevention of type 2 diabetes mellitus by changes in lifestyle among subjects with impaired glucose tolerance. *N Engl J Med* 344:1343–1350, 2001

32. Pan XR, Li GW, Hu YH, Wang JX, Yang WY, et al.: Effects of diet and exercise in preventing NIDDM in people with impaired glucose tolerance: the Da Qing IGT and Diabetes Study. *Diabetes Care* 20:537–544, 1997

33. Wylie-Rosett J, Swencionis C, Caban A, Friedler A, Schiffer N: *The Complete Weight Loss Workbook: Proven Techniques for Controlling Weight-Related Problems.* 2nd ed. Alexandria, VA, American Diabetes Association, 2007

34. Robertson C: Physiological insulin replacement in type 2 diabetes. *Diabetes Educator* 32:423–432, 2006

35. Shin H, Bruno R: *Language Use and English-Speaking Ability, 2000.* Census 2000 Brief. Washington, DC, U.S. Department of Commerce Economics and Statistics Administration, U.S. Census Bureau (Pub. C2KBR-29), 2003

36. National Alliance for Hispanic Health: *A Primer for Cultural Proficiency: Towards Quality Health for Hispanics.* Washington, DC, Estella Press, 2001

37. Merck: Januvia package insert. 2007

Ms. Zaldivar is the Director, Geriatrics and Diabetes, Lighthouse International, New York, NY. Ms. Seley is a Diabetes Nurse Practitioner at New York Presbyterian/Weill Cornell Medical Center, New York, NY.

6. Evolution of Self-Management Practices

Deborah Hinnen, ANP, BC-ADM, CDE, FAAN, and
Richard A. Guthrie, MD, FACE

Problem solving, detecting patterns, and making proactive changes in the food plan, physical activity, or medication protocol are the essence of diabetes self-management (1). These are advanced skills for people with diabetes. First, the basic self-care skills for diabetes management must be mastered, including glucose monitoring, insulin injection and/or oral medication dosing and timing, hypoglycemia prevention and treatment, daily schedule delineation, basic meal planning, and knowing when to call the practitioner. As a facet of continuous, lifelong outpatient diabetes education, all nurses working with people with diabetes can teach, reinforce, and verify these daily care activities.

Self-management of diabetes requires that people have essential information in order to make changes to their treatment regimen to achieve optimal control of diabetes. Technological advances have been significant over the past two decades in both glucose monitoring and insulin delivery systems. Self-monitoring of blood glucose (SMBG) was introduced in the late 1970s, replacing the retrospective urine glucose testing methods previously used. The benefits of frequent blood glucose monitoring were seen in the Diabetes Control and Complications Trial, which verified that glucose control could be achieved with intensive management.

The newest type of monitoring, continuous glucose monitoring (CGM) is an exciting technology that is becoming more widely used. CGM uses a sensor that monitors interstitial tissue glucose on a continuous basis, allowing patients to make various adjustments to improve their glucose control. Unfortunately, current reimbursement is minimal, contributing to the modest usage of the technology. The ultimate goal of diabetes management for insulin-requiring people is to be able to continuously collect glucose data and feed that into an insulin delivery system, creating a closed loop. Until closed-loop technology is perfected, the process of analyzing logbooks or downloading data and using computer software

---

PRACTICAL POINT

Adult learners learn best by experiential learning. Learning a skill such as glucose monitoring is a hands-on activity that must include a return demonstration to verify the patient's ability to obtain accurate results.

---

to evaluate glucose values is necessary to make sense of all those glucose measurements.

GLUCOSE MONITORING

Glucose monitoring puts patients in the role of self-manager. It is probably the most important part of being able to problem solve and manage diabetes on a daily basis. It provides feedback on changes in food intake, physical activity, medications, and daily living. SMBG allows patients to make changes in their everyday regimens and gives them immediate information about how different factors affect their glycemic control.

Blood glucose monitoring is primarily done with a blood glucose meter. The choice of a blood glucose meter should be based on several factors.

MATCHING METER TO PATIENT

Here are the facts on today's glucose meters:

- All meters are essentially accurate if the manufacturer's instructions are followed.
- All newer meters are plasma referenced, which makes them comparable to the hospital and practitioner's office results.
- Today's meters require a minimal amount of blood.
- Most meters have a capillary "sipping" action, therefore drawing in a precise amount of blood.
- Most meters range in size from a deck of cards to a Pop-Tart.
- Meters have varying degrees of memory (10–3,000 data points).
- Most meters provide results in <5 seconds.
- Most meters have some internal technology or computer software to assist with analyzing and summarizing the data.
- All major manufacturers have comparably priced test strips.
- It is more difficult to obtain sample meters for patients than in the past. Sample test strips are rarely available.

Given these facts, consider the following when helping a patient choose a meter:

- Does the patient have insurance to obtain strips and supplies?
  - If not, refer him or her to a social worker or to local resources for purchasing strips at a reduced rate.
  - Consider a generic-labeled meter and test strips and less frequent but carefully staggered testing times.
- Does the insurance company have a preferred meter on formulary?
  - If yes, then that is the meter to recommend.
  - If there are no meter formulary restrictions, consider employment, lifestyle, and patient preference. For instance, people who are frequent

computer users, piano players, guitar players, etc., may prefer alternate site testing (forearm, abdomen, or thigh).
- Does the patient have good vision and dexterity?
  - If not, consider a meter with strips in a drum or disc to reduce the need to open cans or foil wrappers.
  - Techno-savvy people may want a meter with extended memory, data storage, and data management capabilities. Seniors or those who want something simpler may want a meter that has fewer steps and a larger screen.

KEY METER SKILLS TO TEACH

- If the patient has never performed a capillary blood glucose test, do a test with a drop of control solution on the patient's finger so the patient can see how simple it is to perform the test. This also verifies that the strips are good.
- Help the patient get an adequate-sized blood sample.
  - Washing hands in warm soapy water cleanses the skin and helps dilate the capillaries, making it easier to obtain the drop of blood. There is no need to use alcohol to clean the skin; alcohol only dries the skin and causes stinging if a puncture is done while the alcohol is wet.
  - If using an alternate site like the arm, rubbing may increase circulation to the site.
  - Select a finger that does not have calluses.
  - Ask the patient to hang the hand in a dependent position for 30–60 seconds and shake it (as if shaking down a thermometer) or snap the fingers to increase blood flow.
  - After the puncture, gently milk (rather than squeeze) the finger, from the base of the finger to the finger tip
  - If not enough blood is obtained, adjust the lancing device depth (bigger number = deeper penetration).
- Return demonstration will help identify mistakes.
- Provide the toll-free customer service number (normally found on the back of the meter or on the packaging) for assistance with such tasks as setting the date and time or changing the code.
- If an inpatient, encourage self-management by having the patient perform his or her own blood glucose test on his or her own meter when it is the routine testing time. Patients can measure their blood glucose levels and compare those values with results obtained from the laboratory. The values should be within 10–15% of each other.
- Teach patients to carefully dispose of test strips and lancets in a container, not the trash.
- Disposal guidelines may vary from state to state. Find out what precautions need to be taken in your state.
- During an office visit, have the patient do a reading. Even those with long-standing diabetes my have technical issues.

Table 6.1 Common User Errors and Corrective Actions

Error	Correction
Not enough blood	Use deeper penetration of lancet.
Blood not adequately filling the test strip chamber	Make sure blood touches strip and is held there until strip chamber is filled. May require more blood.
Meter not calibrated to current strips	Teach patients to calibrate strips every time they open a new vial or box of strips.
Ruined strips, strips that have been out of the container for too long, out of date, or mail order strips that got too hot or cold	Open a new box or vial of strips. Teach patients not to store strips out of the container.
Not using control solution to check test strips or using control solutions that are too old	Teach patients to use control solution to ensure the strips are reading accurately. Date control solution when opened and discard after 90 days (even if date on box is current).

COMMON USER ERRORS AND CORRECTIVE ACTIONS

For common user errors and the ways to prevent or correct them, see Table 6.1.

MOTIVATING RELUCTANT TESTERS

- Experiment with blood glucose testing before and after certain foods, e.g., a glass of orange juice at breakfast, a meal with dessert, a fast-food meal (hamburger, fries, and soft drink).
- Many patients have symptoms that are nonspecific and describe it as "feeling funny." Tell patients to test when they feel "funny" to see if the symptoms are attributable to their blood glucose levels. Sometimes those feelings can be a sign of something other than diabetes (e.g., heart problems, hypertension, etc.). It is difficult to discern hypoglycemia from a myocardial infarction in people with diabetes. If a patient has low blood glucose with chest pain or other symptoms, and those symptoms are relieved with treatment for the hypoglycemia, the symptoms are likely those of hypoglycemia. However, it is important to teach patients how to respond to symptoms that are not resolved by treatment for hypoglycemia. It is often reassuring for patients to be able to attribute those "funny feelings" to a glucose value.
- Ask a patient to speak at a diabetes support group meeting where he or she can show new patients how to keep a logbook and lead a discussion of pattern recognition and problem solving.

- Negotiate with someone else at home to do the testing for 1 week.
- Negotiate the testing frequency based on what the patient is willing/able to do.
- Negotiate weekly data review with the patient by fax, phone, or e-mail.

GLUCOSE MONITORING SCHEDULES

Patients who use insulin are often asked to test three or more times per day: fasting/premeal and 2 h after each meal, and between 2:00 and 3:00 a.m. The American Diabetes Association (ADA) recommendations state that postprandial testing may be appropriate to achieve postprandial glucose targets, but that "the frequency and timing of SMBG should be dictated by the particular needs and goals of the patients" (2). In patients with type 2 diabetes who are not being treated with insulin, some regimen of SMBG may correlate with a reduction in glycated hemoglobin A1c (A1C); however, other factors, such as diet and exercise counseling or other pharmacological intervention, make it difficult to assess the contribution of SMBG alone (3–5).

Pre- and postprandial testing allows the calculation of glycemic excursions. Glycemic variability research suggests that the excursion, or variable "swing in glucose," triggers reactive oxidative stress, which has been implicated in both micro- and macrovascular complications of diabetes (6). When glycemic goals are reached in type 2 diabetes, testing may be less frequent (four times per day, 3–4 days per week). People who count their carbohydrate intake and determine their insulin dose using insulin-to-carbohydrate ratios will test before meals to determine how much insulin to take for the meal. Women who are pregnant and people using insulin pumps are asked to test every day, four to six times per day.

People using oral agents may test less often after reaching glycemic goals. There is little literature that guides home blood glucose testing schedules or frequency in those who use oral medications for their diabetes. If the person is insured by Medicare, 100 test strips for a 3-month period are covered. This dictates testing frequency to a great degree. If people choose to test their glucose level daily either fasting or fasting and at 4:00 p.m., they will miss postprandial glucose excursions. Therefore, alternating days and times during the day to provide a more complete glucose pattern would be a better use of testing supplies. Testing four times per day, 2 days per week is consequently the recommendation for many people on oral agents (1,7,8). Some practitioners recommend testing two times per day, 4 days per week. Individualization is the key to successful testing. For instance:

- All patients need more blood glucose tests during illness, medication changes, dietary changes, and stress (1).
- During acute illness, premeal or hourly testing is needed to determine the need for and specific dose of any supplemental rapid-acting insulin.
- Asymptomatic hypoglycemia, i.e., hypoglycemia unawareness, requires more frequent and regular testing on a daily basis, particularly at peak insulin times and before driving, as a precaution for identifying low blood glucose levels.
- Pregnancy requires frequent SMBG, e.g., five to seven times per day, every day to make the adjustments needed to optimize blood glucose control.

OTHER MEASURES OF GLUCOSE CONTROL

A1C

The gold standard in overall diabetes control is the A1C level. This measure of control provides an average (or weighted mean) of the blood glucose level over the past 2–3 months. The glycation process, in which glucose attaches to the hemoglobin molecule, is irreversible and linear, with higher glucose levels causing increased glycation, thus higher A1C values. Therefore, A1C provides a picture of the average blood glucose level during the 120-day lifespan of the hemoglobin molecule.

A Case in Problem Solving: John

John is a 57-year-old man who has had type 2 diabetes for 5 years. He works as a manager at Wal-Mart and has no known complications. John is taking the following diabetes medications:

■ Morning: 10 mg glipizide, 1,000 mg metformin
■ Evening: 10 mg glipizide, 1,000 mg metformin

His food plan consists of 1,800 calories.

	Monday	Wednesday	Saturday
Glucose values (mg/dl)			
Fasting	187	199	203
2 h after breakfast	139	144	148
Before lunch			
2 h after lunch	152	133	121
Before dinner			
2 h after dinner	128	146	138

Changes in schedule/routine
Diet
Insulin/medication
Reactions
Activity

Problem: High fasting blood glucose levels

Possible cause: Inadequate medication in evening or at bedtime to prevent excessive hepatic glucose release

Options:

■ Assure John that the high fasting glucose levels are likely not because he ate too much at dinner or during the evening. Explain that food that is eaten is used or stored in 4–5 h. Explain how the liver releases excessive glucose in the early morning hours if adequate insulin is not available.
■ Consider adding exenatide (Byetta) or bedtime NPH or a glargine/detemir insulin dose (initiate bedtime basal dose at 10% of total body weight).
■ Consider adding a third oral agent.

A Case in Problem Solving: Mary Jane

Mary Jane is a 40-year-old woman who has had type 1 diabetes for 18 years. She works in a call center. Mary Jane has mild peripheral neuropathy in both feet, with no visual changes. Recently, she began a daily four-injection regimen to improve her glucose control.

- Breakfast: 12 units insulin lispro
- Lunch: 10 units insulin lispro
- Dinner: 14 units insulin lispro
- Bedtime: 40 units insulin glargine

Her food plan consists of 1,600 calories (three meals and one snack) with an additional 2 units insulin lispro for each additional carbohydrate choice (15 g) eaten (1:7 insulin-to-carbohydrate ratio).

	Wednesday	Friday	Sunday
Glucose values (mg/dl)			
Fasting	100	110	103
2 h after breakfast	315	292	248
Before lunch			
2 h after lunch	269	233	149
Before dinner			
2 h after dinner	144	136	137
Changes in schedule/routine			
Food	donut	O.J., toast	Pancakes
Insulin/medications			
Reactions			
Activity			Walk after lunch

Problem: Pattern of high blood glucose levels after breakfast on 3 days and lunch on 2 days

Possible causes:

- Too much carbohydrate at breakfast/lunch for the current insulin dose
- Too many calories for breakfast
- Not enough insulin before breakfast/lunch
- Insulin-to-carbohydrate ratio is incorrect, needs to be recalculated
- Not counting carbohydrate correctly
- Not using insulin-to-carbohydrate ratio

Options: Consider changing something in routine before the high tests:

- Decrease total carbohydrate at breakfast/lunch.
- Change the composition of breakfast (i.e., add protein and fat to carbohydrate).
- Decrease total calories at breakfast/lunch.
- Increase the dose of insulin lispro before breakfast/lunch, e.g., by 10%.
- Increase the insulin-to-carbohydrate ratio at breakfast, e.g., 1:6 (2.5 units insulin lispro per carbohydrate serving).
- Include exercise after breakfast; it was effective on Sunday after lunch.

The ADA has effectively promoted a standardization process for this test (9). High-performance liquid chromatography and immunoassay methods are now commonly used to measure A1C. The normal range is 4–6%. With consistency from hospital, clinic, and physician laboratories, this test and the anticipated normal ranges allow practitioners to speak a common language in regard to diabetes control.

ESTIMATED AVERAGE GLUCOSE

The correlation of average glucose to the longer-term measure of glycated hemoglobin has been determined through a large study using CGM and SMBG in people with type 1, type 2, or no diabetes (10).

Many pharmaceutical companies and the ADA on its website provide teaching materials, charts, and calculators to explain the relationship of a normal A1C value of 6% to a correlated average glucose of 126 mg/dl (7 mmol/l) for the past 2–3 months. As the A1C value goes up 1 percentage point, the glucose averages go up ~28.7 mg/dl (1.6 mmol/l). Consequently, an A1C of 7% equals an average glucose of 154 mg/dl (8.6 mmol/l). See Table 6.2.

The ADA's Standards of Medical Care in Diabetes (2) recommend an A1C goal <7% (corresponding to average blood glucose values of <154 mg/dl [8.6 mmol/l]). Testing should be done every 3 months until glycemic goals are reached and then every 6 months. The recommendation to take action if the value is >7% is critical to the prevention of long-term complications of diabetes.

According to the ADA, the A1C goals should be individualized based on duration of diabetes, pregnancy status, age, comorbid conditions, hypoglycemia unawareness, and other individual patient considerations. More stringent glycemic goals may be appropriate in some individuals if this can be achieved without risk of hypoglycemia. Conversely, less stringent goals than <7% maybe appropriate for patients with limited life expectancy, advanced microvascular complications, or cardiovascular disease or those with a history of severe hypoglycemia (2).

Table 6.2 Estimated Average Glucose (eAG)

	mg/dl[*]	mmol/l[†]
A1C (%)		
5	97 (76–120)	5.4 (4.2–6.7)
6	126 (100–152)	7.0 (5.5–8.5)
7	154 (123–185)	8.6 (6.8–10.3)
8	183 (147–217)	10.2 (8.1–12.1)
9	212 (170–249)	11.8 (9.4–13.9)
10	240 (193–282)	13.4 (10.7–15.7)
11	269 (217–314)	14.9 (12.0–17.5)
12	298 (240–347)	16.5 (13.3–19.3)

Data in parentheses are 95% CIs. [*]Linear regression eAG (mg/dl) = 28.7 x A1C – 46.7. [†]Linear regression eAG(mmol/l) = 1.59 x A1C – 2.59. From Nathan et al. (10).

Glycemic variability suggests that managing A1C alone may not be enough to prevent long-term complications of diabetes. Glycemic extremes trigger reactive oxidative stress, which initiates a cascade of events that lead to micro- and macrovascular damage. Postprandial variability is associated with a decrease in carotid intima-media thickness, which is a clinical marker for atherosclerosis (6,11).

Analyzing glucose records to determine and minimize glycemic variability is gaining importance. Many of the download printouts from the meters and the CGM systems are reporting more statistics than just averages and number of tests per time period. Evaluating glycemic variability can be accomplished by reviewing such summary data from glucose meter and sensor downloads as

1. Mean blood glucose: This represents an average during a specific time period, e.g., average of fasting glucoses, average after breakfast glucose values.
2. Standard deviation: This is an indicator of extremes of glucose levels. It is a representation of the highest and lowest blood glucose levels in a time period or of the total number of glucose tests. If mean glucose is near the goal, clinicians suggest that two times standard deviation should be less than the mean. For example, if the average glucose is 139 mg and the standard deviation is 45, then two times the standard deviation ($45 \times 2 = 90$) is less that the mean ($90 < 139$).
3. Median: The median is the middle point of the distribution of values: half of the values are above and half are below that point.
4. MAGE: MAGE stands for the mean amplitude of glycemic excursion, or the area under the curve. This method evaluates how high the glucose level is and long it has been above target.

Additional information available may include the low blood glucose index, high blood glucose index, or average daily risk range.

FRUCTOSAMINE: GLYCATED ALBUMIN

The glycation of serum albumin is a process similar to the glycation of hemoglobin. The result, however, provides a glucose average of the past 10 days. Conceptually, this would be valuable for medication adjustment. Fructosamine would be especially useful in situations when short-term measurements are needed, such as in pregnant women, elderly patients, or patients unable to do SMBG. Fructosamine may also be very helpful in patients with hemoglobinopathies, where the A1C may not be accurate.

Normal ranges vary with the different methods used. This test is not as standardized as the A1C. The lack of standardization of the testing procedure has limited the use of this measure.

KETONE TESTING

Ketone testing provides an important indicator of fat metabolism and free fatty acid conversion in the liver. In the face of hyperglycemia, this is an indication of insulin insufficiency and alternate fuel availability. The ketone bodies are weak acids: acetone, acetoacetic acid, and β-hydroxybutyric acid. The accumulation of these acids decreases the pH and eventually leads to diabetic ketoacidosis (DKA). Therefore, it is important to test for ketones when glucose levels are elevated and especially during illness.

Ketones can be tested by a urine dipstick or plasma testing for β-hydroxybutyric acid with the Precision Xtra (Abbott) glucose meters. Urine ketone testing is done by dipping a ketone test strip into a urine sample and comparing it with the color chart in the appropriate time period advised by the manufacturer.

Ketones are rarely present in patients with type 2 diabetes because these patients still have endogenous insulin production, unless there is weight loss due to inadequate calorie intake. However, on sick days, counterregulatory hormones and catecholamines may trigger ketosis in patients with type 2 diabetes as well as in those with type 1 diabetes (see also "Be Prepared: Sick Day Management," a patient handout in resources). Therefore, all people with diabetes need to test for ketones when they are ill. In pregnant women, ketones and hyperglycemia (DKA specifically) during the first trimester are incompatible with fetal viability. Later in the pregnancy, positive ketones are usually an indication of a hypocaloric situation called starvation ketosis. This can often be rectified with the addition of a bedtime snack containing carbohydrate.

Indications for ketone testing:

- when blood glucose levels exceed 250–300 mg/dl (13.9–16.6 mmol/l), especially in patients with type 1 diabetes
- during illness
- when fasting, during pregnancy
- if glucose levels exceed 150 mg/dl (8.3 mmol/l) during pregnancy

PROBLEM SOLVING AND SELF-MANAGEMENT

CONCEPTS OF PATTERN MANAGEMENT

Pattern management is a comprehensive approach to blood glucose management that includes all aspects of current diabetes therapy (1,12–15). Although this approach is typically identified with intensive or flexible insulin therapy, pattern management should also include changes in nonpharmacological therapies, i.e., nutrition therapy and physical activity, and combinations of oral agents to improve glycemic control.

Elements of pattern management include:

- The motivation on the part of the person with diabetes to be an active participant in care
- Individualized blood glucose goals negotiated by the person with diabetes and diabetes care team
- Frequent SMBG or CGM recorded in a logbook or with software, to provide data for making adjustments
- A food plan to follow, starting with eating consistent amounts of calories/carbohydrates as a basic skill. An advanced skill would be to determine insulin-to-carbohydrate ratios (developed by measuring the usual amount

of insulin needed to cover varying amounts of carbohydrate), which are used for adjusting insulin dose based on carbohydrate intake (16)

■ Multiple injections of insulin, insulin pump therapy, or combinations of oral agent(s)/insulin
■ Self-adjustments, based on blood glucose monitoring data, food intake, physical activity, and medication(s) to achieve glycemic goals
■ Frequent interaction between individuals with diabetes and the diabetes care team, using telephone, fax, and e-mail to discuss glucose values between visits
■ Comprehensive self-management training, including:
  • Coverage of the education content areas identified by the National Standards for Diabetes Self-Management Education (17)
  • The relationship of glucose levels, food, activity, and medications
  • Prevention of hypoglycemia or hyperglycemia
  • Sick-day management
  • Purpose, strategies, and value of pattern management for intensive therapy to achieve blood glucose goals
  • Empowerment of the patient through education for decision making and problem solving, goal setting, and long-term motivation
  • An understanding of the personal belief systems related to the value of health and intensive diabetes management
  • Access to diabetes and health-related supplies
  • Support systems to provide emotional and clinical management support
  • Diabetes care team with on-call clinical support
  • Ongoing education, such as support groups offered via the ADA, hospital, or education center (18,19)

STRATEGIES FOR PATTERN MANAGEMENT

Pattern management involves reviewing several days of glucose records and making adjustments in diabetes treatment based on trends, rather than reacting to a single high or low blood glucose reading. Adding supplemental or sliding-scale insulin at the time of the elevated glucose level solves the problem only for that particular point in time but does not prevent the problem from occurring again (20–22). Effective pattern management takes into account all variables that affect blood glucose levels—including food, physical activity, stress, and illness—not just insulin or other medication adjustments (1).

The patient must have a food plan that he or she can consistently follow. The number of calories and/or carbohydrate servings is determined by the person with diabetes in consultation with a dietitian. To determine patterns, food intake, physical activity, and timing and doses of insulin or other medications must be as consistent as possible. This helps prevent blood glucose fluctuations that can mask true patterns.

In individuals using insulin, if blood glucose levels are out of goal range, consider whether

■ the individual prefers to change calorie/carbohydrate intake, change physical activity, or make adjustments in insulin or other medications. Although it is easier to make insulin or other medication adjustments, weight management must be a consideration. Increasing insulin to cover extra food or carbohydrates will anabolically store total calories and potentially increase weight.

■ the individual is on enough insulin, too much insulin, or the wrong insulin regimen (23–25).

In individuals with type 2 diabetes, if blood glucose levels are out of goal range, consider whether the individual

■ has a food plan that he or she is able to follow.
■ requires a change in medication dose.
■ requires the addition of other diabetes medications (26).
■ requires the addition of evening insulin.
■ requires a change to a comprehensive insulin-only regimen.

The first step in pattern management is to identify blood glucose trends in relation to glucose goals. The individual with diabetes needs to provide multiple data points at critical times for evaluation and problem solving and to collect sufficient data to evaluate whether goals are being met. Ideally, this means monitoring four to seven times a day, but adequate data can be obtained by testing four times a day, 2 or 3 days per week or testing two times per day, at alternating times, for 1 or 2 weeks. Food records with the number of calories and carbohydrate servings compared with blood glucose readings can then be analyzed once or twice a week.

When looking for patterns, read down the columns of blood glucose records to review all of the readings at the same time of day, e.g., fasting. A sample blood glucose record is provided in Table 6.3. Three high readings at the same time each day show a pattern of high blood glucose levels. Several low readings at the same time show a pattern of low blood glucose levels. If blood glucose readings are high at a specific time for 3–5 days, that is a pattern. Potential causes for the elevated levels should be examined so that the problem can be corrected. Causes of high blood glucose levels can be any of the following:

■ Eating too much carbohydrate or more calories than usual.
■ Doing less physical activity than usual.

6.3 Sample Blood Glucose Log

	Fasting blood glucose (mg/dl)	After breakfast (mg/dl)	After lunch (mg/dl)	After supper (mg/dl)
Monday	106	198	84	112
Tuesday	159	210	178	191
Wednesday	141	188	—	113
Thursday	139	222	132	233

- Taking too little insulin, missing an insulin dose, or having problems with the dose, type, or combination of oral medications.
- Using expired or improperly stored insulin or not taking oral agents as prescribed.
- Experiencing emotional or physical stress, including illness.
- Having a rebound response from the liver releasing excessive amounts of glucose from glycogen as a result of hypoglycemia.
- Overtreating hypoglycemia.

If blood glucose levels are low for several days at the same time, potential causes should be examined. Low blood glucose levels are usually corrected before high levels. Untreated hypoglycemia can cause a rebound glucose response, induced by the counterregulatory hormone glucagon, with hyperglycemia to occur later. Causes of low blood glucose levels can be any of the following:

- Eating too little carbohydrate or less than usual, i.e., too few calories.
- Doing more physical activity than usual.
- Taking too much insulin or oral medication.
- Taking a hot bath/shower for an extended period of time.

QUESTIONS TO ASK WHEN EVALUATING BLOOD GLUCOSE VALUES

- Is there a pattern when evaluating 3–5 days of blood glucose readings?
- Does something happen at the same time every day, such as an insulin reaction, high glucose after breakfast, etc.?
- Are there blood glucose readings representing all "times" of the day?
- Are there blood glucose readings reflecting the "peak" times of each medication (insulins and/or oral agents)?
- Are there after-meal glucose values that represent peak glucose values?
- Are there "other notes" or "changes" to account for observed patterns, such as meal times, carbohydrate or calorie variances, exercise changes, unusual hours of work or school, stress, illness, etc.?
- Is prevention of weight gain or weight loss important for the patient? If so, consideration must be given to trying to reduce the use of hypoglycemic medications (i.e., insulin or insulin secretagogues), especially if low blood glucose levels are occurring routinely.
- Does the patient have a history of weight gain? Is the weight gain the result of overtreatment of frequent episodes of hypoglycemia?
- Does the patient have a history of weight loss? Is the weight loss caused by poor glycemic control (1)?

INTERPRETING BLOOD GLUCOSE READINGS FOR PEOPLE TAKING INSULIN

Knowing what the glucose level means based on when the test was performed is critical to effective decision making.

■ Premeal glucose measurements are needed to monitor basal (or background) insulin dose(s) (e.g., NPH, glargine, or detemir). If fasting or pre-dinner readings are out of the target range, consider adjusting basal insulin doses. Premeal testing may also be used to determine if a supplemental/correction insulin dose is needed to add or subtract from the bolus dose.

■ Two-hour postprandial glucose readings are needed to titrate rapid-acting insulin (e.g., lispro, aspart, glulisine) for mealtime injections. If the difference in premeal and postprandial glucose readings is more than 40–50mg mg/dl (2.2 mmol/l), consider adjusting the mealtime rapid-acting insulin by 10% (27).

■ Two-hour postprandial readings are also used to evaluate the effectiveness of incretins (exenatide, sitagliptin, thiazolidinediones, glimepiride, glipizide, glyburide, repaglinide, nateglinide, α-glucosidase inhibitors, and other glucose-lowering agents). Two-hour postprandial glucose testing is helpful in patients with type 2 diabetes when evaluating the effect of meals and certain foods on blood glucose levels (26).

■ Elevated fasting glucose levels require 3:00 a.m. testing and recording at least once or twice a week to determine the cause. High fasting glucose levels can be caused by any of the following:
  • Overnight hypoglycemia that triggers the liver to release glucose (Somogyi or rebound effect)
  • Normal hormonal changes that trigger the liver to release excessive glucose in the early morning (dawn phenomenon)
  • Insufficient basal or background insulin
  • In youth, growth hormone secreted at night during growth spurts
  • Excessive hepatic glucose release in type 2 diabetes

INTERPRETING CGM DATA

Individuals with diabetes who are using CGM and providers alike will find that they will need to change how they "think" when evaluating CGM data. This is still an evolving science. Individuals have real-time data to evaluate continuously and can make decisions on the spot, but they must remember that there is a 2- to 3-min lag time between the interstitial glucose and the capillary glucose (28). A blood glucose of 70 mg/dl by the sensor may be 55 mg/dl by a capillary glucose. New treatment targets for the patient may need to be set with guidance from the provider. Alarms should be set at higher than usual targets, e.g., not at 55 mg/dl but at 70 mg/dl or 80 mg/dl to alert the individual that there is a falling glucose. This allows the individual to be proactive rather than reactive. Learning to respond to trends rather than responding to a single number will be important.

Since it is real-time data, it is easy to treat the current blood glucose but not take time to evaluate the patterns that may evolve day to day. One of the most valuable tools is the event markers an individual can use to record information about meals, insulin doses, and other events. The individual can then look for patterns based on these events. Potential changes may include timing of the bolus doses, amount of the bolus doses, amount of the basal insulin, and changes in the insulin-to-glucose correction dose (29). It is important that patients be able to use the software program that comes with their CGM system to analyze the data. The software allows patients and providers to evaluate the glucose information continuously, hourly, in time blocks, by meals, by days of the week, by weekend, or by weekday. Individual time blocks can be set by the provider with the patient or by the patient herself. Any number of days—up to 60 on some programs—can be "overlaid" and the trend identified. The median and the standard deviation for various times may be more important than an average.

LIFESTYLE ISSUES

Self-management is central to integrating successful glycemic control with flexibility of lifestyle. Two common issues illustrate how this is done.

TRAVELING

Travel is not the cumbersome experience it once was for people with diabetes. However, security issues have changed in recent years. People with diabetes must familiarize themselves with the Federal Aviation Administration (FAA) guidelines. The information is summarized on the ADA web site at www.diabetes.org.

- It is recommended that all medications have the pharmacy label. The pharmacy label is typically applied to an insulin box, so advise individuals to save boxes, even from insulin pens.
- Meters, pumps, and supplies can go through the security check without damage to the equipment.
- On overseas flights, patients may order special meals, but airlines should be notified well in advance or during the purchase of tickets. Snacks are not always available on domestic flights. It is advisable to carry extra snacks when flying.
- All supplies (medication, testing supplies, items to treat hypoglycemia, and snacks) should be in a carry-on bag, not packed in checked luggage, so that temperature-sensitive supplies are protected and supplies are at hand.
- Documentation from a practitioner explaining that the person has diabetes and must carry various medications and supplies is not required by the FAA because of the increased risk of forgery. However, some customs agents accept such letters.
- Education on travel outside of the country should include arranging emergency medical contacts.
- Instructions on acquiring medication if the traveler has his or her carry-on bag stolen should include going to the emergency room or pharmacy in that country. Insulin may be a different concentration, i.e., U40 (40 units/cc) or U80 (80 units/cc) rather than U100 (100 units/cc). However, the person can obtain that country's "meal/bolus" insulin and "basal" insulin and syringes to match. A unit of insulin is an international measure, but the dilution of the insulin will be variable. If the person needs 10 units of insulin lispro for lunch, he or she will need 10 units of regular (or other available rapid insulin) in U80 or U40 strength, drawn up in the appropriate U80 or U40 syringe. The amount will look different because of the dilution of the insulin.

- In the past, crossing time zones has been the greatest challenge for insulin users. The use of insulin glargine or detemir has made this much less difficult. Keep the injection time for glargine/detemir on the same schedule as in the patient's original time zone. Other meal insulins may change to match the meal times of the new destination. People using insulin pumps may need to adjust the timing of their nighttime basal rates based on when they sleep in the new time zone. However, flexibility in meal times continues to be a strength for those using pumps.
- Keeping supplies from getting too hot is another consideration whether flying or driving. Travel kits with cool gel packs are available from pharmacies for a reasonable cost. Insulated lunch bags are also useful for moderating temperatures.
- Traveling always requires that snacks and glucose for treating hypoglycemia be available and within reach at all times. Temperature control for supplies is a concern. People should not leave their emergency snacks or medication in the car when they go into a restaurant for lunch.
- Traveling to high altitudes may affect meter readings and reduce appetite. If skiing or hiking, the insulin dose may need to be reduced because of increased activity and lower caloric intake. Snacks and glucose should be carried in a pocket or backpack.

DRINKING ALCOHOL

The literature is confusing regarding the benefits and risks of alcohol intake. For some, drinking alcohol may be harmful, particularly if they are taking certain medications. However, if the person with diabetes chooses to drink, the key is to understand the physiology and make informed decisions.

- Alcohol is detoxified in the liver, where the glycogen reserves are stored and normally released in case of hypoglycemia. At the time alcohol is consumed, glucose values will likely rise because of the carbohydrate in the beer, wine, or mixed drinks. However, the later and more dangerous effect of alcohol is a hypoglycemic effect. This hypoglycemic effect may take place anywhere from 10 to 20 h after drinking. If the person has had enough to drink and becomes hypoglycemic during the night while sleeping, the liver may not be able to release glycogen reserves to protect and correct the low blood glucose. This situation is potentially fatal.
- Drug interactions are known to occur with several oral agents.
  1. Sulfonylureas (especially the older drug chlorpropamide) may cause an Antabuse, or disulfiram, reaction when the person drinks. This will be evident by flushing and nausea.
  2. Binge drinking (defined by the ADA as five or more drinks on one occasion) while on metformin can increase lactate levels, potentially leading to lactic acidosis, and may be fatal. Flu-like symptoms may be a confusing side effect that can also occur with intoxication.
- For the person who chooses to drink, the key is moderation.
  1. If the person is in optimal glycemic control, the ADA guidelines for alcohol intake suggest a maximum of one to two drinks per day.

2. Alcohol should be consumed with food.
3. Alcohol calories should be calculated into the total daily intake.
4. Even if blood glucose values are elevated, the bedtime snack should not be skipped.

SUMMARY

Monitoring-based self-management is the standard of diabetes care. The technology, medications, and education available to people with diabetes and providers have vastly improved. These pieces of the puzzle, when put together in an organized fashion, create a picture of flexibility and optimal glycemic control that is clearer now than ever before. The elusive nature of diabetes care and glycemic control has been replaced with a sharper image—a clearly focused, detailed picture of diabetes management that is patient driven. Nurses can help patients take ownership in this intensive management approach. Commitment to long-term self-care, together with education on diabetes care rationale and goals, empowers the patient to set personal short- and long-term goals and to seek help with obstacles, including the challenge of maintaining long-term motivation.

REFERENCES

1. Hinnen D, Childs B, Guthrie D, Guthrie RA, Martin S: Overcoming clinical inertia with pattern management. In *The Art and Science of Diabetes Education: A Reference Book for Health Professionals*. Mensing C, Ed. Chicago, American Association of Diabetes Educators, 2006

2. American Diabetes Association: Standards of medical care in diabetes—2009 (Position Statement). *Diabetes Care* 32 (Suppl. 1):S13–S61, 2009

3. Welschen LM, Bloemendal E, Nijpels G, Dekker JM, Heine RJ, et al.: Self-monitoring of blood glucose in patients with type 2 diabetes who are not using insulin: a systematic review. *Diabetes Care* 28:1510–1517, 2005

4. Farmer A, Wade A, Goyder E, Yudkin P, French D, Craven A, et al.: Impact of self monitoring of blood glucose in the management of patients with non-insulin treated diabetes: open parallel group randomised trial. *BMJ* 335:132, 2007

5. O'Kane MJ, Bunting B, Copeland M, Coates VE: Efficacy of self monitoring of blood glucose in patients with newly diagnosed type 2 diabetes (ESMON study): randomised controlled trial. *BMJ* 336:1174–1177, 2008

6. Monnier L, Mas E, Ginet C, Michel F, Villon L, Cristol J-P, Colette C: Activation of oxidative stress by acute glucose fluctuations compared with sustained chronic hyperglycemia in patients with type 2 diabetes. *JAMA* 295:1681–1687, 2006

7. Guthrie DW, Guthrie RA (Eds.): *Nursing Management of Diabetes Mellitus.* 5th ed. New York, Springer, 2002

8. American Association of Clinical Endocrinologists/American College of Endocrinology Diabetes Recommendations Implementation Writing Committee: ACE/AACE Consensus Conference on the Implementation of Outpatient Management of Diabetes Mellitus: Consensus Conference Recommendations. *Endocr Pract* 12 (Suppl. 1):6–12, 2006

9. American Diabetes Association: Tests of glycemia in diabetes (Position Statement). *Diabetes Care* 27 (Suppl. 1):S91–S93, 2004

10. Nathan DM, Kuenen J, Borg R, Zheng H, Schoenfeld D, Heine R: Translating the A1C assay into estimated average glucose values. *Diabetes Care* 31:1473–1478, 2008

11. Esposito K, Giugliano D, Nappo F, Marfella R, for the Campanian Postprandial Hyperglycemia Study Group: Regression of carotid atherosclerosis by control of postprandial hyperglycemia in type 2 diabetes mellitus. *Circulation* 110:214–219, 2004

12. Davidson J, Reader D, Rickheim O: *Blood Glucose Patterns: A Guide to Achieving Targets.* Minneapolis, MN, International Diabetes Center Park Nicollet Institute, 2003

13. Pearson J, Bergenstal R: Fine-tuning control: pattern management versus supplementation: pattern management: an essential component of effective insulin management. *Diabetes Spectrum* 14:75–78, 2001

14. Nathan DM, Buse JB, Davidson MB, et al.: Management of hyperglycemia in type 2 diabetes: a consensus algorithm for the initiation and adjustment of therapy. *Diabetes Care* 29:1963–1972, 2006

15. Lorenzi G: Implementation of diabetes education. In *The Art and Science of Diabetes Education: A Reference Book for Health Professionals.* Mensing C, Ed. Chicago, American Association of Diabetes Educators, 2006, p.

16. American Dietetic Association, American Diabetes Association: *Advanced Carbohydrate Counting.* Chicago, IL, American Dietetic Association; Alexandria, VA, American Diabetes Association, 2003

17. American Diabetes Association: National standards for diabetes self-management education (Position Statement). *Diabetes Care* 27 (Suppl. 1):S143–S150, 2008

18. Pieber TR, Brunner GA, Schnedl WJ, Schattenberg S, Kaufmann P, Krejs GJ: Evaluation of a structured outpatient group education program for intensive insulin therapy. *Diabetes Care* 18:625–630, 1995

19. Hirsch IB, Farkas-Hirsch R: Sliding scale or sliding scare: it's all sliding nonsense. *Diabetes Spectrum* 14:79–81, 2001

20. Shagan BP: Does anyone here know how to make insulin work backwards? Why sliding-scale insulin coverage doesn't work. *Pract Diabetol* 9:1–4, 1990

21. Sawin CT: Action without benefit: the sliding scale of insulin use. *Arch Intern Med* 157:489–491, 1997

22. Guthrie RA, Childs B, Guthrie D: *Rapid and Long Acting Insulin Analogs: Strategies for Patient Use.* Monograph. 2nd Ed. Wichita, KS, Quontum Press, 2004

23. Hirsch IB, Bergenstal RM, Parkin CG, et al.: A real-world approach to insulin therapy in primary care practice. *Clinical Diabetes* 23:78–86, 2005

24. Brunelle BL, Llewelyn J, Anderson JH, Gale EA: Meta-analysis of the effect of insulin lispro on severe hypoglycemia in patients with type 1 diabetes. *Diabetes Care* 21:1726–1731, 1998

25. Childs BP, Guthrie RA, Carr M, McDaniel J, Rhiley D: Incorporating new diabetes oral agents into clinical practice. *Diabetes Spectrum* 9:266–268, 1996

26. Bolli G: Clinical strategies for controlling peaks and valleys: type 1 diabetes. *Int J Clin Pract* 120 (Suppl.):65–74, 2002

27. Brownlee M, Hirsch I: Glycemic variability: hemoglobin A1C-independent risk factor for diabetic complications. *JAMA* 295:1707–1708, 2006

28. Buckingham B, Block J, Willson DM: Continuous glucose monitoring. *Curr Opin Endocrinol Diabetes* 12:273–279, 2005

29. Hirsch IB, Armstrong D, Bergenstal RM, Buckingham B, Childs BP, Clarke WL, Peters A, Wolpert H: Clinical application of emerging sensor technologies in diabetes management: consensus guidelines for continuous glucose monitoring (CGM). *Diabetes Tech Ther* 10:232–246, 2008, doi:10.1089/dia.2008.0016

Ms. Hinnen is a Diabetes Clinical Nurse Specialist at Mid-America Diabetes Associates, Wichita, KS. She coordinates a multidisciplinary team that provides education and care for an American Diabetes Association–recognized program. Dr. Guthrie is the Medical Director at Mid-America Diabetes Associates, Wichita, KS.

COMPLICATIONS

7. Acute Complications of Diabetes

Irl B. Hirsch, MD

D iabetic ketoacidosis (DKA), hyperosmolar hyperglycemic syndrome (HHS), and hypoglycemia are the most common acute complications of diabetes. To prevent significant mortality and morbidity, it is important for the health care provider and the individual with diabetes to identify the symptoms and institute appropriate treatment promptly.

DKA AND HHS

EPIDEMIOLOGY

Despite the fact that insulin was first used clinically over 80 years ago, hyperglycemic crisis continues to be a major public health problem. DKA has an incidence rate of four to eight cases per 1,000 patients with diabetes (1,2), and it appears that hospitalizations for DKA are increasing in the U.S. (3). Currently, DKA accounts for 4–9% of all hospitalizations of people with diabetes. HHS, on the other hand, is more difficult to quantify but is thought to comprise <1% of all hospitalizations of people with diabetes (4).

The cost of treating DKA is staggering. In the state of Rhode Island, it was estimated that the cost of DKA in 1983 was $225 million (2). More recently, the American Diabetes Association (ADA) estimated the cost of DKA to be approximately $1 billion each year (5). Even more alarming is that DKA is responsible for $1 out of every $4 spent on direct medical care for adult patients with type 1 diabetes in the U.S. The mortality rates are <5% for DKA in experienced centers and ~11% for HHS, and the rates increase with age and comorbidities (5). Deaths associated with either of these conditions are more often due to the underlying precipitating factor than to the metabolic crisis itself.

PATHOPHYSIOLOGY

DKA consists of the triad of hyperglycemia, ketonemia, and acidemia. The ADA classifies DKA by level of acidemia and level of stupor. Although infection is usually thought of as the most likely precipitating factor, omission of insulin is actually the most common etiology in both the U.S. and Europe. This omission may occur from the inability to obtain the insulin for financial reasons, as part of an eating disorder, or as part of some other type of psychological disease process.

Up to 20% of cases of DKA or HHS may present without a previous diagnosis of diabetes. HHS, more often a disease of the elderly, can be caused by acute illness or drug therapy. The former would most commonly include an infection, such as pneumonia or sepsis; a vascular event, such as a myocardial infarction or cerebrovascular accident; or acute pancreatitis. The latter includes agents such as glucocorticoids, diazoxide, diuretics, and β-blockers. In both DKA and HSS, the fundamental defect is a decrease in the net effective concentration of insulin coupled with a massive elevation of the counterregulatory hormones (glucagon, cortisol, growth hormone, and epinephrine). In DKA, the insulin deficiency is either absolute or relative in relation to the counterregulatory hormones that overwhelm the body's ability to suppress lipolysis. In HHS, there is a residual amount of insulin that suppresses ketosis but cannot control hyperglycemia. This leads to severe dehydration and impaired renal function that eventually leads to even more severe hyperglycemia. For this reason, hyperglycemia is more profound in HHS than in DKA.

At both the molecular and cellular levels, there has been a substantial improvement in our understanding of both of these conditions during the past 30 years. As is the case with chronic vascular complications of diabetes, we now appreciate that these two conditions are proinflammatory states generating oxidative stress. Despite this understanding, what has not changed is that many of these hyperglycemic crises are preventable and that prevention is the fundamental goal.

ASSESSMENT AND CLINICAL PRESENTATION

DKA and HHS are both medical emergencies that require a brief but directed assessment. Key issues that require special assessment include 1) airway patency, 2) mental status, 3) cardiovascular and renal status, 4) possible source of infection, and 5) state of hydration. Although there are many similarities in the presentation of DKA and HHS, there are some subtle differences. Table 7.1 presents the similarities and differences. DKA usually presents quickly, often over the span of 24 h, whereas HHS usually presents over several days because the level of consciousness often decreases in a less acute manner. DKA is also more often associated with nausea, vomiting, and abdominal pain. The classic rapid deep breaths observed with acidosis (Kussmaul breathing) are not generally seen with HHS. The fruity breath associated with DKA is a result of acetone loss through the lungs. Patients with HHS are more often hyperosmolar than those with DKA; thus, obtundation and coma are more common in this group. Another important detail for those with HHS is that even though infection is a common precipitating event, fever is rare, even with sepsis, because of skin vasodilation related to the dehydration and volume depletion.

Table 7.1 Comparison of DKA and HHS

	DKA	HHS
Features		
Age of patient	Usually <40 years	Usually >60 years
Duration of symptoms	Usually <2 days	Usually >5 days
Glucose level	Usually <600 mg/dl (<33 mmol/l)	Usually >800 mg/dl (>44 mmol/l)
Sodium concentration	Likely normal or low	Likely normal or high
Potassium concentration	High, normal, or low	High, normal, or low
Bicarbonate concentration	Low	Normal
Ketone bodies	Present	Usually absent
pH	Low, <7.3	Normal
Serum osmolality	Usually <350 mOsm/kg	Usually >350 mOsm/kg
Cerebral edema	Often subclinical	Rare
Assessment		
Skin	Flushed: dry, warm	Pallor: moist, cool
Breath	Fruity, acetone	Normal
Vital signs	Blood pressure decreased, pulse increased	Blood pressure decreased, pulse increased, afebrile
Gastrointestinal	Severe abdominal pain, nausea, vomiting	Mild abdominal pain, nausea, vomiting
Mental status	Lethargic	Lethargic
Prognosis	<5% mortality	~11% mortality

In a patient with known diabetes, a presumptive diagnosis can usually be made quickly by a capillary glucose measurement and a urine dipstick. Because patients with DKA may present to the outpatient clinic, these tests are relatively easy to obtain, but for the obtunded individual in an emergency room, a urinary catheter is often required. Nevertheless, for definitive diagnosis, laboratory studies will be needed.

LABS AND TESTS

For either of the hyperglycemic emergencies, it is necessary to send stat labs for plasma glucose, electrolytes, urea nitrogen, creatinine, complete blood count (with differential), serum acetone, and arterial blood gas. The severity of the DKA is determined by the degree of acidemia and mental status: pH <7.24 and a stuporous level of consciousness is considered "moderate" DKA, whereas pH <7.00 with coma is considered "severe." Many mild cases of DKA, especially when there are no abnormalities in mental status, can be managed in an outpatient setting or after volume repletion in an emergency room.

Note that a person can have DKA without substantial hyperglycemia. Euglycemic DKA is defined as DKA in an individual with plasma glucose level <300 mg/dl (<16.6 mmol/l). This condition most often occurs when volume depletion is not severe but there is absolute insulin deficiency, as in type 1 diabetes.

The initial urinalysis may need to be interpreted with caution. Urine (and for that matter, serum) ketones are evaluated by the nitroprusside reaction, which is a semiquantitative test for acetoacetate and acetone but not for β-hydroxybutyrate, the main keto acid of DKA (6). Therefore, laboratory assessment often underestimates the severity of the DKA. A recent study suggested serum β-hydroxybutyrate may be a better test for DKA than the traditional bicarbonate level, which is much less specific (7).

> **PRACTICAL POINT**
>
> Euglycemic DKA can be seen in surgical patients with type 1 diabetes when adequate intravenous fluids are given to prevent dehydration but insulin is either withheld or administered in doses too low to prevent ketosis.

With the initial blood draw, if there is no obvious etiology, it is reasonable to draw blood for blood cultures. Obviously, if another etiology becomes apparent, the cultures can be canceled. Similarly, a urine culture should be obtained with the initial laboratory assessment.

While the electrolytes are being analyzed, an electrocardiogram should be obtained, especially for adults. First, a myocardial infarction can precipitate DKA or HHS. In children, an electrocardiogram can give important clues to hypokalemia or hyperkalemia. Second, if there are abnormalities with the T-waves, suggesting abnormalities in potassium homeostasis, a telemetry device needs to be placed immediately because hypokalemia from the treatment of these emergencies is a common cause of mortality.

When evaluating laboratory data, it is important to understand two key formulas. Perhaps the most important is the anion gap, defined as the serum sodium – (chloride + bicarbonate). Usually, the anion gap is calculated as part of the electrolyte measurement; if not, the clinician needs to perform the calculation. In modern assays, the normal anion gap is 7–9 mEq/l. An elevated anion gap confirms an unmeasured anion. Although this may include β-hydroxybutyrate (and acetoacetate), the differential diagnosis for an anion gap acidosis includes lactic acidosis, uremic acidosis, salicylate intoxication, rhabdomyolysis, and ethylene glycol intoxication. There are numerous different acid-base disturbances that need to be diagnosed because both metabolic alkalosis and primary respiratory diseases causing hypoventilation or hyperventilation may also present with DKA. Furthermore, a non–anion gap acidosis can be seen in DKA, as can a mixed–anion gap and hyperchloremic acidosis.

The other important formula that needs to be calculated is the total serum osmolality. This is calculated as:

$$2 \times [\text{serum sodium (mEq/l)}] + [\text{glucose (mg/dl)}/18] + [\text{blood urea nitrogen (mg/dl)}/2.8]$$

The normal range for this measurement is 290 ± 5 mOsm/kg. The diagnosis of HHS can be made with a serum osmolality >330 mOsm/kg, usually with a blood glucose level >600 mg/dl and the absence of significant ketonemia.

Several other issues related to laboratory assessment should be considered. The first is that serum creatinine may be falsely elevated because of acetoacetate interfering with the assay. After treatment, the creatinine level will usually return to normal or at least to the baseline level. Next, high amylase levels need to be interpreted cautiously in the initial evaluation of DKA because these may be the result of extrapancreatic secretion. A leukocytosis with very high white blood cell counts is common and does not necessarily reflect an infectious process. Again, with therapy for DKA, the white blood cell count will normalize, but if it remains high after successful treatment, investigation for an occult infection should be considered.

Hyperglycemia will result in a falsely low sodium level because of the movement of water from the intracellular to the extracellular space in the presence of hyperglycemia. To calculate the corrected serum sodium level in the context of hyperglycemia, add 1.6 mEq/l to every 100 mg/dl above 180 mg/dl. If severe hyponatremia is still present after this calculation, other etiologies of hyponatremia need to be considered. Most patients with HHS present with profound hypernatremia, indicative of a severe free-water deficit. When the serum sodium is corrected for the hyperglycemia in these patients, the corrected sodium level is often >170 mEq/l.

Special attention needs to be paid to serum potassium levels. First, despite massive kaliuresis from hyperglycemia and often further potassium losses from vomiting, serum potassium levels are usually normal or even high. The reason for this is that insulin deficiency, acidemia, and hyperosmolarity all result in potassium moving from the cell into the blood. Clinicians should not be misled; potassium levels can drop quickly, leading to life-threatening arrhythmias as fluids and insulin are replaced. For this reason, potassium replacement is a key component of the therapy of DKA and HHS and is the reason many of these patients, especially older patients with possible coronary artery disease at risk for arrhythmias, need to be monitored with telemetry.

TREATMENTS

Nursing plays a vital role in the therapy for acute hyperglycemic episodes. Appropriate monitoring is the first important component of therapy. This is best addressed with a complete flow sheet that includes both physical examination findings (e.g., blood pressure, heart rate) and laboratory results (e.g., glucose, bicarbonate, potassium, phosphate). The flow sheet should also include aspects of therapy, e.g., rate and type of fluid, insulin and potassium rates, bicarbonate and phosphate rates. Table 7.2 presents an example of a flow sheet for tracking DKA therapy. Table 7.3 presents key treatment tips.

One of the most controversial areas in the treatment of hyperglycemic crisis has been the rate and type of fluids that should be infused. Initially, this should be determined by the volume status of the patient. Supine hypotension signifies an ~20% decrease in extracellular fluid, whereas orthostatic hypotension confirms a 15–20% reduction in extracellular volume. An orthostatic increase in pulse without a change in blood pressure suggests a 10% reduction in extracellular volume. For all of these situations, there is now agreement that the first fluid infused should be 0.9% normal saline, administered as quickly as possible over the first hour, followed by 500–1,000 ml/h for the next 2 h of either 0.9% normal saline or 0.45% normal saline, depending on the degree of hydration and the serum sodium

Table 7.2 Suggested DKA/HHS Flowsheet

DATE: HOUR:	ER													
Weight (daily)														
Mental Status*														
Temperature														
Pulse														
Respiration/Depth**														
Blood Pressure														
Serum Glucose (mg/dl)														
Serum Ketones														
Urine Ketones														
ELECTROLYTES														
Serum Na+ (mEq/l)														
Serum K+ (mEq/l)														
Serum Cl- (mEq/l)														
Serum HCO3- (mEq/l)														
Serum BUN (mg/dl)														
Effective Osmolality														
2[measured Na (mEq/l)]														
+ Glucose (mg/dl)/18														
Anion Gap														
A.B.G.														
pH Venous (V) Arterial (A)														
pO2														
pCO2														
O2 SAT														
INSULIN														
Units Past Hour														
Route														
INTAKE FLUID/METABOLITES														
0.45% NaCl (ml) past hour														
0.9% NaCl (ml) past hour														
5% Dextrose (ml) past hour														
KCL (mEq) past hour														
PO4 (mmol/l) past hour														
Other (e.g., HCO3-)														
OUTPUT														
Urine (ml)														
Other														

*A-ALERT D-DROWSY   S-STUPOROUS   C-COMATOSE
**D-DEEP S-SHALLOW   N-NORMAL

From ABA (8).

Table 7.3 Acute Complication Treatment Tips and Precautions

Establish diagnosis; if known to have diabetes and unable to test glucose, assume hypoglycemia and give intravenous glucose or glucagon.

If triage call, vomiting present, or hyperglycemia, request urine ketone measurement.

Treat the volume depletion first.

Insulin should not be replaced until the potassium level is known.

HHS/DKA usually requires intensive care monitoring for at least 12 h.

Monitor and replace potassium to prevent life-threatening arrhythmias.

Cerebral edema is a risk with too rapid correction of blood glucose.

Consider a major vascular incident in the elderly as etiology for hyperglycemic crisis.

level. Even with severe dehydration and hypernatremia, 0.9% normal saline is hypotonic compared with the extracellular fluid. Some authors advocate hypotonic saline (0.45% normal saline) from the outset if the effective serum osmolality [calculated as 2 × measured sodium (mEq/l) + glucose (mg/dl)/18] is >320. Others, including this author, prefer the initial use of 0.9% saline for the first hour, followed by 0.45% saline unless volume losses are severe and hypotension is not corrected after the first liter of fluid.

Dextrose (5%) should be added to the solution when blood glucose reaches 250 mg/dl (13.9 mmol/l) in DKA or 300 mg/dl (16.6 mmol/l) in HHS. There are two main reasons for this. First, it allows continued insulin administration to control ketogenesis in DKA. Furthermore, particularly in children, too rapid a decrease in blood glucose can result in cerebral edema. Another important point is that once blood pressure is stabilized and glucose levels decrease to the point that osmotic diuresis is not leading to further water and electrolyte losses, urine volumes will also decrease, allowing a decrease in intravenous fluids. This is critical in young children and older adults, who are at a greater risk of overhydration. The excess of free water from overhydration can also result in cerebral edema. The exact fluid rate will vary depending on the clinical situation, but will generally range from 4 to 14 ml/kg/h. Although there are large variations, the average duration of time that intravenous hydration will be required is ~48 h.

Perhaps the most important point about the use of insulin therapy in either DKA or HHS is that electrolyte levels need to be confirmed before starting an intravenous insulin infusion. In the rare patient who presents with hypokalemia, insulin therapy needs to be postponed until the potassium levels are corrected. Although controversial, most authorities begin the insulin infusion (all human regular insulin) with an intravenous bolus of 0.1–0.15 units/kg, followed by 0.1 units/kg/h. Some endocrinologists will use intramuscular insulin at 7–10 units, except when hypotension is present, in which case only the intravenous route can ensure appropriate absorption. Occasionally, insulin resistance will require much larger doses of insulin than the starting rates noted above. However, even very low doses of insulin will inhibit lipolysis and ketogenesis. When the blood glucose level reaches 250–300 mg/dl (13.3–16.3 mmol/l), the insulin infusion rate can be decreased and the intravenous dextrose added. In general, it is appropriate to measure blood glucose every hour in these patients. The electrolytes can be measured less frequently. The blood glucose should decrease at a rate of 50–70 mg/dl/h. If blood glucose is not improving, other etiologies should be investigated, such as patient's volume status not being corrected or an error in the insulin infusion mixture.

In general, these patients may have a 500 to 700 mEq/l potassium deficit when they present. Intravenous fluids will increase renal plasma flow, whereas intravenous insulin will result in a movement of potassium from extracellular to intracellular areas. These two events will lead to a profound decrease in serum potassium levels shortly after the treatment of a hyperglycemic emergency. When hypokalemia is present at the onset, potassium levels should be replaced at least to a level of 3.3 mEq/l before insulin is started. These patients should also be monitored with telemetry. In general, potassium replacement should not exceed 40 mEq the first hour and then 20–30 mEq/h after that. Because potassium chloride in addition to the saline used will usually result in hyperchloremia, many authors recommend replacing some of the potassium as either potassium phosphate or potassium acetate. However, there are no studies examining a change of outcomes with these alternative potassium solutions.

Bicarbonate use is also a controversial topic in the treatment of DKA. There is little reason to consider adding bicarbonate for most of those with DKA because acidemia will improve as bicarbonate is generated by the liver while the ketogenesis is reversed by insulin therapy. In children, it is suggested that bicarbonate will result in more profound altered consciousness and headache (9,10). Clearly, the addition of bicarbonate will lead to more profound hypokalemia. It is for this reason that some authors feel the only indication for the use of bicarbonate therapy is life-threatening hyperkalemia. However, there are now controlled trials examining the use of bicarbonate therapy in severe acidemia (pH 6.9–7.1) (11). The results of these small trials showed no beneficial or adverse effects from the bicarbonate therapy. The ADA suggests bicarbonate therapy for those patients who present with severe acidemia (pH < 6.9) because of the potential for severe vascular effects (5). The solution should never be given as a bolus, but rather infused as 1 ampoule (50 mmol) into another solution, such as a liter of 0.45% normal saline.

As with potassium, initial levels of serum phosphate are often normal or increased despite a total-body deficit. Insulin therapy will result in a shift of phosphate into the cell, often resulting in hypophosphatemia during the treatment of DKA and HHS. However, in the rare situation of the serum phosphate dropping below 1 mg/dl, complications from hypophosphatemia are unusual. Furthermore, controlled trials have not demonstrated a benefit from routine use of phosphate therapy in the treatment of DKA (12,13). Current recommendations are to replace phosphate if levels drop below 1.0 mg/dl (5). This can be accomplished by adding 20–30 mEq/l of potassium phosphate to the intravenous solution over 2–3 h. The most important complication of phosphate replacement is hypocalcemia, so serum calcium levels need to be monitored during the time period.

Protocols for management of DKA and HHS are presented in Figures 7.1 and 7.2. These protocols are taken from the ADA position statement on hyperglycemic crisis in patients with diabetes (8).

Unlike HHS, mild DKA can be managed on an outpatient basis. Patients are encouraged to call their providers when moderate or high urine ketones or

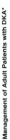

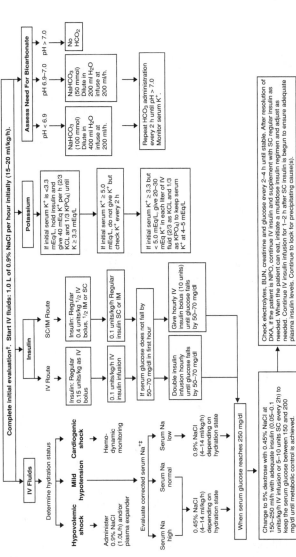

Figure 7.1 Protocol for the management of adult patients with DKA. *DKA diagnostic criteria: blood glucose >250 mg/dl, arterial pH <7.3, bicarbonate <15 mEq/l, and moderate ketonuria or ketonemia. Normal ranges vary by lab; check local lab normal ranges for all electrolytes. †After history and physical examination, obtain arterial blood gases, complete blood count with differential, urinalysis, blood glucose, blood urea nitrogen (BUN), electrolytes, chemistry profile, and creatinine levels *stat* as well as an electrocardiogram. Obtain chest X-ray and cultures as needed. ‡Serum Na should be corrected for hyperglycemia (for each 100 mg/dl glucose >100 mg/dl, add 1.6 mEq to sodium value for corrected serum sodium value). IM, intramuscular; IV, intravenous; SC subcutaneous. *From* American Diabetes Association: Hyperglycemic crises in diabetes (Position Statement). *Diabetes Care* 27 (Suppl. 1):S94–S102, 2004.

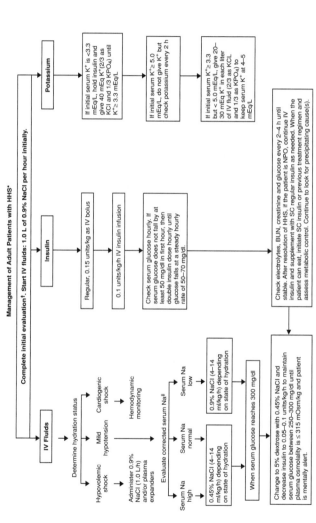

Figure 7.2 Protocol for the management of adult patients with HHS. *Diagnostic criteria: blood glucose >600 mg/dl, arterial pH <7.3, bicarbonate <15 mEq/l, mild ketonuria or ketonemia and effective serum osmolality >320 mOsm/kg H_2O. This protocol is for patients admitted with mental status change or severe dehydration who require admission to an intensive care unit. For less severe cases, see text for management guidelines. Normal ranges vary by lab; check local lab normal ranges for all electrolytes. Effective serum osmolality calculation: 2[measured Na (mEq/l)] + glucose (mg/dl)/18.†After history and physical examination, obtain arterial blood gases, complete blood count with differential, urinalysis, plasma glucose, blood urea nitrogen (BUN), electrolytes, chemistry profile, and creatinine levels *stat* as well as an electrocardiogram. Obtain chest X-ray and cultures as needed. ‡Serum Na should be corrected for hyperglycemia (for each 100 mg/dl glucose >100 mg/dl, add 1.6 mEq to sodium value for corrected serum value). IV, intravenous; SC subcutaneous. *From* American Diabetes Association: Hyperglycemic crises in diabetes (Position Statement). *Diabetes Care 27* (Suppl. 1):S94–S102, 2004.

unmanageable high blood glucose levels are noted. Early replacement of insulin using frequent doses of insulin lispro, insulin aspart, or intramuscular regular insulin (0.1 units/kg) every 2–3 h plus good hydration will allow the individual to decrease the blood glucose levels and restore hydration. Using sports drinks will assist in correcting the electrolyte imbalance. Sugared liquids will be required to prevent a rapid glucose drop from the supplemental insulin. Management principles follow the guidelines for hospital care. If the blood glucose does not decrease within 3–5 h or vomiting occurs, then the individual needs to be treated at the hospital. Antiemetics are not recommended because vomiting may be the symptom that guides whether the metabolic acidosis is being corrected.

EDUCATIONAL/BEHAVIORAL CONSIDERATIONS

The most important area for educational consideration is determining how DKA and HHS can be prevented. Because a large percentage of these patients develop these life-threatening emergencies because of insulin omission, factors leading to this need to be explored and attempts need to be made to correct the situation. The patient who returns with a hyperglycemic crisis on a frequent basis must be assessed for underlying causes. These patients (previously termed brittle) often return in crisis because of some other major problem that could be related to a severe psychological stress, an eating disorder, or even major financial troubles that make obtaining insulin difficult. Alternatively, some patients with frequent hospitalizations have waited too long to ask for assistance during a pump malfunction or systemic infection. If the etiology is related to a psychological problem, the patient will require special attention. A referral to a mental health specialist would be appropriate for the vast majority of these patients.

Education of the individual with diabetes and family is essential. See Table 7.4 for educational tips. Referral to appropriate resources should occur to prevent the next episode.

> **PRACTICAL POINT**
>
> Education is the key to the prevention of the acute complications of diabetes: hypoglycemia and hyperglycemia. Nurses should review with patients their strategies for treating high and low blood glucose levels and potential precipitating causes. Reinforce good practices.

HYPOGLYCEMIA

EPIDEMIOLOGY

Hypoglycemia, defined as a blood glucose level <50–60 mg/dl (<2.8–3.3 mmol/l) is common in type 1 diabetes. It is estimated that most people with type 1 diabetes have at least two symptomatic episodes each week, meaning that they may have thousands of episodes over the course of a lifetime (14). Severe hypoglycemia, defined as requiring the assistance of another person, may occur in many at

Table 7.4 Patient Education Tips

Problem	Key Education Points
Insulin omission	Access to care, including insulin supply Poor storage of insulin, old insulin
Failed sick-day management	Access to ketone monitoring supplies Recognition of symptoms of DKA, HHS, and hypoglycemia Understanding of action needed if ketones present Access to glucose-containing fluids Understanding of when to treat Importance of continuing insulin, even with illness Guidelines for when to call the health care provider/emergency medical services Guidelines, if appropriate, for insulin supplementation during illness
Frequent DKA	Referral to mental health professional

least once yearly. It is estimated that 2–4% of deaths in patients with type 1 diabetes occur because of hypoglycemia (15). Iatrogenic (as a result of treatment) hypoglycemia is much less common in type 2 diabetes. Estimates vary, but severe hypoglycemia appears to occur at a fraction of the rate seen in type 1 diabetes (5). Hypoglycemic death from sulfonylureas has been documented.

PATHOPHYSIOLOGY

Normally, as glucose levels decline, both glucagon and epinephrine levels respond as a protective mechanism against hypoglycemia. In nondiabetic individuals, the glycemic threshold for this counterregulatory response is between 65 and 70 mg/dl (3.6 and 3.9 mmol/l), but this shifts to higher levels in individuals with suboptimally controlled diabetes and lower levels in diabetic individuals with near-normal A1C levels. The glucagon and epinephrine response will result in an increase of hepatic glucose output in addition to a suppression of glycogenesis. Furthermore, the elevated epinephrine levels will result in the autonomic symptoms frequently seen with hypoglycemia: tremor, palpitations, and anxiety. Common signs include elevated heart rate, pallor, and elevated systolic blood pressure. A cold sweat and hunger appear to be cholinergic (not related to epinephrine). Eventually, if oral or parenteral glucose is not provided, neuroglycopenic symptoms will occur, e.g., nausea, diplopia, confusion, seizures, and even coma may result from profound hypoglycemia. These neuroglycopenic symptoms occur after the autonomic symptoms.

The mechanisms for hypoglycemia and hypoglycemia unawareness are better understood in type 1 than in type 2 diabetes. In the former, as endogenous insulin secretion declines, the normal glucagon response to hypoglycemia diminishes to the point that the patient's only initial response is epinephrine secretion. Furthermore, the brain adapts to antecedent hypoglycemia so that the epinephrine response to hypoglycemia is shifted to a lower plasma glucose level.

A severely reduced epinephrine response can be seen in the absence of classic autonomic dysfunction, leading to hypoglycemia unawareness. However, the presence of autonomic neuropathy typically diminishes the epinephrine response, leading to an even higher risk of severe hypoglycemia.

For individuals with type 2 diabetes, the frequency of severe hypoglycemia is similar to that in individuals with type 1 diabetes when matched for duration of insulin therapy. Given the progressive nature of insulin deficiency in type 2 diabetes, clinical hypoglycemia becomes a greater problem as endogenous insulin secretion declines. Table 7.5 lists risk factors for the development of hypoglycemia.

Alcohol consumption is a common etiology of hypoglycemia. Alcohol can inhibit gluconeogenesis, especially in a starved state, placing an insulin-requiring patient at high risk for iatrogenic hypoglycemia. Indeed, even individuals without diabetes can develop hypoglycemia from alcohol. In the fed state, alcohol may actually increase hepatic glucose production, thus making alcohol ingestion quite risky because it may be quite difficult to predict the glycemic effects at any given time. To further complicate matters, the type of alcohol ingested may alter the glucose. For example, a sweet liqueur may raise the glucose, whereas a dry wine may lower it, depending on the fed state of the individual. Given this wide variability, alcohol can be dangerous and should be ingested in moderation. Furthermore, frequent blood glucose testing should be performed to help guide treatment, especially as it relates to the prevention of hypoglycemia because typical symptoms may be altered.

Table 7.5 Risk Factors for Hypoglycemia

Risk Factors	Possible Causes
Insulin excess	Too much insulin, insulin secretagogue, or insulin sensitizer; taken at the wrong time or wrong type
Decreased exogenous glucose	Missed meal or snack; not enough food Overnight fast
Decrease in endogenous glucose production	Alcohol
Increased glucose utilization	Too much exercise or activity without enough food
Increased insulin sensitivity	Late after exercise Improved fitness Weight loss Use of an insulin sensitizer Middle of the night
Decreased insulin clearance	Renal failure
Compromised glucose counterregulation	Insulin deficiency, history of severe hypoglycemia, aggressive therapy and glucose goals, lower A1C

LABS AND TEST

Usually, very little needs to be done for the diagnosis of insulin- or sulfonylurea-induced hypoglycemia. In a symptomatic patient, a capillary blood glucose level will confirm the diagnosis. Those with hypoglycemia unawareness need to perform more frequent self-monitoring of blood glucose in an attempt to avoid severe hypoglycemia. Often, these patients are found to be hypoglycemic on routine blood checks even though they may not have any symptoms.

TREATMENT

Most episodes of symptomatic and asymptomatic (found by checking blood glucose) hypoglycemia can be treated with the ingestion of oral carbohydrate. This carbohydrate may be in the form of glucose tablets, juice, milk, or crackers. The vast majority of these cases can be treated with 15–20 g carbohydrate. This step can be repeated in 15–20 min if the symptoms have not improved or the blood glucose level has not increased. The most common mistake made by patients is to overtreat the hypoglycemic episode because of insatiable hunger, failure of the symptoms to resolve immediately, and/or fear of a continuing drop in glucose levels. All too often this results in posthypoglycemic hyperglycemia because additional insulin is not injected for the extra food ingested.

Treating Severe Hypoglycemia

Parenteral therapy is required when the patient is unable to take carbohydrate orally. Crushed glucose tablets or gel should not be placed in the mouth or rubbed onto the buccal mucosa of a person who is not able to swallow. Glucagon or intravenous glucose is the only remedy. Subcutaneous or intramuscular glucagon is often used by family members in patients with type 1 diabetes. Glucagon is less helpful for individuals with type 2 diabetes because it stimulates insulin secretion as well as glycogenolysis. After glucagon administration, the patient will often experience nausea, vomiting, and headache.

When possible, intravenous glucose is the preferred treatment for severe hypoglycemia. The usual treatment is 10–25 g of 50% dextrose administered over 1–3 min. Blood glucose level should be checked after completion of the administration. Doses are variable, based on the weight of the individual, the type of diabetes, and the cause of the hypoglycemia. A continuous glucose infusion of 10% dextrose may be needed because the glucose bolus is transient. In patients who are unable to ingest oral carbohydrates or those with sulfonylurea-induced hypoglycemia, the hypoglycemia may be prolonged.

A patient who has been treated for hypoglycemia with glucagon or intravenous glucose should be provided oral carbohydrates as soon as he or she is able to eat.

HYPOGLYCEMIA UNAWARENESS

Hypoglycemia unawareness is defined as the loss of the epinephrine-mediated warning symptoms of hypoglycemia. Hypoglycemia unawareness is associated with hypoglycemia frequency. The more hypoglycemia a patient experiences, the lower the threshold for symptoms. Fortunately, clinical trials have shown that this type of hypoglycemia unawareness may be reversed by strict avoidance of hypoglycemia. Most clinicians advise individuals with hypoglycemia unawareness to measure their glucose before driving. Until the technology for glucose sensors improves, it would seem prudent for these individuals to measure their blood glucose when driving more frequently if the trip is during a time of suspected glycemic reduction, e.g., after exercise or 1–2 h after injecting a rapid-acting analog (Table 7.6).

EDUCATIONAL/BEHAVIORAL CONSIDERATIONS

All patients at risk for iatrogenic hypoglycemia need to learn typical symptoms and treatment. These patients would include individuals prescribed sulfonylureas, insulin secretagogues, and insulin. Aspects that require review include strategies for prompt oral treatment and avoidance of overtreatment. Family members of individuals with type 1 diabetes need training in the use of subcutaneous or intramuscular glucagon.

Patients who develop a severe fear of hypoglycemia (usually after one or more episodes of severe hypoglycemia) require special attention. Families can also become extremely fearful. The provider needs to appreciate that this fear can be overwhelming and that individuals may intentionally maintain extremely high blood glucose levels because of this fear. Often, they require psychological counseling. Slowly lowering glycemic targets over time can be an effective method to address this fear and return to glycemic goals.

Table 7.6 Reduction and Treatment of Hypoglycemia Unawareness

Goal	Actions
Increase symptoms of hypoglycemia	Rigorous avoidance of hypoglycemia Increased glucose monitoring Increase glucose targets for at least 3 weeks
Assist patient in identifying nonclassic symptoms	Possible: Blurred vision, numbness in limbs or lips, nausea, many others Encourage documentation in symptom log Log should include exercise, food, insulin timing Use log to identify atypical symptoms and patterns
Secure assistance at work, school, and home	Identification and training of family, friends, and coworkers to give glucagon and/or know when to call emergency medical services

SUMMARY

Prevention is the key to effective management of the acute complications of diabetes. These complications are costly, not only in the expenditure of health care dollars, but also in the decrease in the quality of life for people with diabetes.

Specific protocols, order sets, treatment algorithms, and clinical pathways should be developed and implemented to guide the best practices in the hospital (see chapter 31). Nurses should take a leadership role in developing and implementing these clinical pathways. Monitoring of the patient with DKA and HHS by the nurse will be crucial. Preventing future episodes of DKA or HHS will depend on patient and family/caregiver education. Managing mild DKA and hypoglycemia at home will require a patient and family who are well educated. The nurse should take every opportunity to assess the patientís and family's knowledge levels and ability to prevent and treat hyperglycemia and hypoglycemia.

REFERENCES

1. Johnson DD, Palumbo PJ, Chu C: Diabetic ketoacidosis in a community-based population. *Mayo Clin Proc* 55:83–88, 1980

2. Faich GA, Fishbein HA, Ellis SE: The epidemiology of diabetic acidosis: a population-based study. *Am J Epidemiol* 117:551–558, 1983

3. Centers for Disease Control and Prevention, Division of Diabetes Translation: *Diabetes Surveillance, 1001.* Washington, DC, U.S. Govt. Printing Office, 1992, p. 635–1150

4. Fishbein HA, Palmubo PJ: Acute metabolic complications in diabetes. In *Diabetes in America.* 2nd ed. Harris MI, Cowie CC, Stern MP, Boyko EJ, Reiber GE, Bennett PH, Eds. Washington, DC, U.S. Govt. Printing Office, 1995, p. 283–291 (NIH publ. no. 95-1468)

5. Kitabchi AE, Umpierrez GE, Murphy MB, Kreisberg RA: Hyperglycemic crisis in adult patients with diabetes: a consensus statement from the American Diabetes Association. *Diabetes Care* 29:2739–2748, 2006

6. Stephens JM, Sulway MJ, Watkins PJ: Relationship of blood acetoacetate and β-hydroxybutyrate in diabetes. *Diabetes* 20:485–489, 1971

7. Shekikh-Ali M, Karon BS, Basu A, Kudva YC, Muller LA, et al.: Can serum β-hydroxybutyrate be used to diagnose diabetic ketoacidosis? *Diabetes Care* 31:643–647, 2008

8. American Diabetes Association: Hyperglycemic crises in diabetes (Position Statement). *Diabetes Care* 27 (Suppl. 1):S94–S102, 2004

9. Glaser NS, Wooten-Gorges SL, Marcin JP, Buonocore MH, Dicarlo J, Neely EK, Barnes P, Bottomly J, Kuppermann N: Mechanism of cerebral edema in children with diabetic ketoacidosis. *J Pediar* 145:149–150, 2004

10. Glaser NS, Wooten-Gorges SL, Buonocore MH, Marcin JP, Rewers A, Strain J, Dicarlo J, Neely EK, Barnes P, Kuppermann N: Frequency of subclinical cerebral edema in children with diabetic ketoacidosis. Pediatr Diabetes 7:75–80, 2006

11. Morris LR: Bicarbonate therapy in severe diabetic ketoacidosis. *Ann Intern Med*; 105:836–840, 1986

12. Fisher JN: A randomized study of phosphate therapy in the treatment of diabetic ketoacidosis. *J Clin Endocrinol Metab* 57:177–180, 1983

13. Barsotti MM: Potassium phosphate and potassium chloride in the treatment of diabetic ketoacidosis. *Diabetes Care* 3:569, 1980

14. Cryer PE: Hypoglycemia: the limiting factor in the glycaemic management of type I and type II diabetes. *Diabetologia* 45:937–948, 2002

15. Laing SP, Swerdlow AJ, Slater SD, Botha JL, Burden AC, Waugh NR, et al.: The British Diabetic Association Cohort Study. II. Cause-specific mortality in patients with insulin-treated diabetes mellitus. *Diabet Med* 26:466–471, 1999

Dr. Hirsch is a Medical Doctor, Diabetes Care Center, at the University of Washington Medical Center, Seattle, WA.

8. Cardiovascular Complications

Deborah A. Chyun, RN, MSN, PHD, FAHA, and
Lawrence H. Young, MD, FACC, FAHA

PATHOPHYSIOLOGY

Cardiovascular disease (CVD), which includes stroke, peripheral vascular disease, hypertension, angina, myocardial infarction (MI), heart failure, and sudden cardiac death, is the leading cause of death in patients with type 1 or type 2 diabetes. Patients with diabetes are two to three times more likely to develop CVD than people without diabetes, and women with diabetes are at especially high risk (1). Hypertension, which is present in ~40–60% of patients with type 2 diabetes, plays a major role in the development of stroke, MI, and heart failure.

The pathophysiology of CVD in individuals with diabetes is complex, and the development of atherosclerotic coronary artery disease (CAD), the focus of this chapter, involves the interaction of many factors, including hypertension, dyslipidemia, impaired endothelial function, inflammation, central adiposity, and hemostatic abnormalities involving platelet function, thrombosis, and fibrinolysis. Although the direct role of hyperglycemia remains controversial, hyperglycemia has an important role in the development of microvascular complications that contribute to adverse outcomes, as well as to lipid and coagulation abnormalities that directly influence the development and progression of CAD. In patients with diabetes, CAD is generally more widespread, with stenosis in a greater number of vessels, along with more obstructive lesions within each vessel. Diffuse disease involving long segments and/or the distal aspects of the artery may be present, thereby limiting the usefulness of either percutaneous or surgical revascularization. Therefore, multiple risk factors must be controlled for successful prevention and management of CAD.

CLINICAL PRESENTATION

In the early stages of CAD, minor atherosclerosis may lead to plaque buildup. Plaque rupture may subsequently lead to acute coronary syndromes, such as unstable angina and acute MI. More advanced atherosclerosis significantly narrows the vessel lumen and restricts blood flow, leading to myocardial ischemia during exercise or emotional stress. Myocardial ischemia sometimes results in angina or dyspnea, but some patients with diabetes may be asymptomatic. The first manifestation of CVD in these individuals may be acute MI, heart failure, or sudden cardiac death. Although as many as one in five individuals with type 2 diabetes may have completely asymptomatic or "silent" ischemia (2), CVD also occurs in patients who have symptomatic ischemia with angina. The mechanisms responsible for asymptomatic CAD in patients with diabetes may include cardiac autonomic neuropathy (3,4), and abnormalities in cardiac autonomic function may also serve as a risk marker in individuals with underlying asymptomatic myocardial ischemia (2). The clinical presentation of CVD is outlined in Table 8.1.

PREVENTION

As the understanding of the pathophysiological mechanisms responsible for CVD in individuals with diabetes continues to evolve, it has become apparent that type 2 diabetes and CVD share many common antecedents. The most effective way of preventing CVD in patients is to prevent diabetes in the first place. Although it is critical that the primary prevention of CVD in all patients with diabetes become a top priority, because CVD may already be established when the person is diagnosed with diabetes, identification of underlying CVD and limiting its progression are additional goals. There is some discrepancy in treatment goals among published clinical practice guidelines, particularly for blood pressure and lipids, as well as for levels at which medications should be started. Yet, no matter how lenient the goal, it is clear that the goals for cardiac risk factors or for blood glucose are not being achieved in most patients with diabetes. Goals and strategies for multifactorial risk reduction are presented in Table 8.2 (5–10).

There recently has been controversy over the benefit of intensive therapy with the goal of normalizing glycemic control in patients with established diabetes. The ACCORD (Action to Control Cardiovascular Risk in Diabetes) Study evaluated patients with type 2 diabetes who underwent intensive lowering of their glycated hemoglobin A1c (A1C) to <6%, the normal level for nondiabetic individuals. The results at 3.5 years of follow-up showed an increase in mortality, without significant reduction of nonfatal MI or stroke, when compared to standard therapy with a goal of 7.0–7.9% (11). This finding raised safety concerns that led the National Heart, Lung, and Blood Institute of the National Institutes of Health to stop the study 18 months earlier than planned (11).

No one medication or combination of medications has been cited as the specific cause for the increased number of deaths in the intensive therapy group. However, many participants were taking three to five oral agents plus insulin (11).

Table 8.1 Clinical Presentation of CVD

Stable angina
- Transient symptoms usually brought on by activity and relieved by rest or nitroglycerin: pressure, squeezing, fullness, or pain in center of chest lasting more than a few minutes; pain or discomfort in one or both arms, back, neck, jaw, or stomach; feeling out of breath with or before the chest discomfort
- In absence of anginal symptoms, "anginal equivalents": excessive fatigue, dyspnea, breaking out into a cold sweat, nausea, or lightheadedness
- Diagnostic: transient ST-segment depression on exercise electrocardiogram, regional contractile abnormalities on exercise echocardiogram, or stress-induced myocardial perfusion imaging

Acute coronary syndromes
- Symptoms: as with stable angina, but change in pattern with increased frequency, severity, and duration, lasting more than a few minutes and not relieved by rest or nitroglycerin
- Signs: cool, clammy skin; increased or irregular heart rate; decreased blood pressure; restlessness; altered mental status
- Diagnostic: ST-segment elevation or depression, significant Q-waves, deep T-wave inversions, left bundle branch block, ventricular arrhythmias or heart block on electrocardiogram; elevation of serum cardiac markers; echocardiogram, myocardial perfusion imaging, and angiogram may be ordered

Heart failure
- Symptoms: swelling in feet, ankles, and legs (edema); difficulty breathing, shortness of breath, dyspnea on exertion, orthopnea, paroxysmal nocturnal dyspnea; weight gain; weakness or dizziness
- Signs: elevated heart rate and blood pressure; S3, S4, cardiac murmurs; crackles on lung examination; jugular venous distention and abdominojugular reflux
- Diagnostic: chest X-ray consistent with heart failure or pulmonary edema; echocardiogram, myocardial perfusion imaging, and angiogram may be ordered

Stroke
- Symptoms: sudden numbness or weakness in face, arm, hand, or leg, especially on one side of body; sudden inability to see out of one eye or to one side; sudden confusion, trouble understanding or speaking; sudden trouble walking, dizziness, or loss of balance or coordination; sudden, severe headache without known cause
- Signs: depends on site involved but may include restlessness, lethargy, altered mental status, hemiplegia, or hemiparesis
- Diagnostic: computed tomographic scans, magnetic resonance imaging, carotid or transcranial ultrasound, cerebral angiography, lumbar puncture

---

The ACCORD findings raise the possibility of harm when A1C is lowered to a normal level, but further research is needed to validate these findings. The American Diabetes Association (ADA), American Heart Association (AHA), and American College of Cardiology (ACC) have co-authored a statement (12) affirming that the control of risk factors remains paramount, specifically, controlling blood pressure, reducing lipid levels with statin drugs, prescribing aspirin, and reemphasizing lifestyle modifications. To reduce microvascular and neuropathic sequelae in both type 1 and type 2 diabetic patients, an A1C of 7% is the goal (12). To affect macrovascular sequelae in those with early type 1 or type 2 diabetes, and A1C of <7% is also a reasonable goal (12).

Table 8.2 Goals and Strategies for Prevention of CVD in Patients with Diabetes

Blood pressure <130/80 mmHg (6,10,14)

- Measure at each visit; if ≥130/80 mmHg, confirm on second day
- Lifestyle modification (weight control, physical activity, limit sodium and alcohol intake) before initiation of medication if blood pressure <140/90 mmHg
- Angiotensin-converting enzyme (ACE) inhibitor or angiotensin receptor blocker considered first-line therapy for renal-protective effect

LDL cholesterol <100 mg/dl (5,6,9,14,17)

- Tested annually or every 2 years if low risk
- Suggested daily intake: carbohydrates, 50–70%; protein, 15–20%; total fat, 25–35%; saturated fat <7–10%; up to 10% polyunsaturated and 20% monounsaturated; cholesterol <200–300 mg; fiber 20–30 g/day
- Regular physical activity
- Weight and glycemic control
- Medication if LDL ≥135 mg/dl; optional (fibric acid derivative or niacin) if HDL is <40 mg/dl and LDL is 100–129 mg/dl (unless known CAD)
- HMG-CoA reductase inhibitors (statins) preferred as first-line therapy; fibrate with statin if triglycerides elevated

Regular physical activity three to four times per week for 30 min (7,14)

- Routinely assess physical activity and exercise status

- Encourage increase in daily activities and moderate aerobic regimen such as brisk walking
- Individualization of exercise prescription and caution with peripheral or cardiac autonomic neuropathy or proliferative retinopathy
- Patient education regarding symptoms of angina and MI

Maintain BMI 21–25 kg/m² and waist circumference <102 cm (40.2 in) in men and <88 cm (34.7 in) in women (14)

- Measured at each visit
- Weight control
- Regular physical activity

Complete smoking cessation (8,14)

- Assess smoking status
- Provide counseling, problem solving, or coping skills training and pharmacotherapy

Aspirin therapy (6,14)

- Consider enteric-coated aspirin, 75–162 mg/day, if age >40 years with one or more additional CAD risk factors
- Initiate in presence of CAD

A1C <7% (6)

- Tested two to three times annually if meeting goal; four times annually if above goal or therapy changed
- Medical nutrition therapy
- Weight control
- Regular physical activity
- Self-monitoring of blood glucose
- Education in self-management and problem solving

The importance of blood pressure control in diabetic patients was demonstrated in the U.K. Prospective Diabetes Study (13). ADA goals call for reduction of blood pressure to <130/80 mmHg (6), and other guidelines call for reducing blood pressure even further (10). Therapeutic lifestyle approaches should be initiated when blood pressure levels are between 130/80 and 139/89 mmHg (6,14). For blood pressure ≥140 mmHg systolic or ≥90 mmHg diastolic, antihypertensive

Table 8.3 Lifestyle Modifications to Manage Hypertension

Modification	Recommendation	Approximate Systolic Blood Pressure Reduction
Weight reduction	Maintain normal body weight	5–20 mmHg/10-kg weight loss
Adopt DASH eating plan	Consume a diet rich in fruits and vegetables and low-fat dairy products with a reduced content of saturated and total fat	8–14 mmHg
Dietary sodium restriction	No more than 2,400 mg/day	2–8 mmHg
Physical activity	Regular aerobic activity such as brisk walking at least 30 min/day most days of the week	4–9 mmHg
Moderation of alcohol consumption	Limit to no more than two drinks per day for men, one for women	2–4 mmHg

From Hinnen et al. (18). DASH, National Heart, Lung, and Blood Institute's Dietary Approaches to Stop Hypertension.

medications are usually instituted in addition to therapeutic lifestyle interventions (Table 8.3).

The major lipid abnormalities associated with insulin resistance and type 2 diabetes include reduced HDL cholesterol and increased triglyceride levels (15). Oxidized, small, dense LDL cholesterol particles are also atherogenic in patients with diabetes, even though LDL cholesterol is not specifically elevated in diabetes (16). The ADA recommends LDL cholesterol levels <100 mg/dl and calls for initiation of statin therapy—in addition to lifestyle modification—in all diabetic patients with overt CVD and in those >40 years of age without CVD but with one or more other CVD risk factors, regardless of baseline lipid levels (6). Goals for HDL and triglyceride levels vary (6,9,14). LDL lowering to <70 mg/dl has been recommended for very-high-risk patients, such as those with established CVD and diabetes (17).

Physical inactivity and obesity play major roles in the development of type 2 diabetes and CVD. Regular physical activity, structured exercise, and dietary modifications have beneficial effects on glycemic control, lipids, weight, and blood pressure. Table 8.4 illustrates the approximate and cumulative LDL cholesterol reduction achieved by dietary modification (10).

Individualized exercise recommendations are required in patients with peripheral vascular disease or cardiac autonomic neuropathy, severe retinopathy, or known CAD (7). Because of the possibility of unrecognized CAD, individuals with type 2 diabetes should generally engage in moderate-intensity exercise regimens. Sedentary individuals should always initiate exercise programs at a low level and gradually increase the intensity of exercise. All patients should be educated about

Table 8.4 Approximate and Cumulative LDL Cholesterol Reduction Achievable by Dietary Modification

Dietary Component	Dietary Change	Approximate LDL Cholesterol Reduction
Major		
Saturated fat	<7% of calories	8–10%
Dietary cholesterol	<200 mg/day	3–5%
Weight reduction	Lose 10 lb	5–8%
Other LDL-lowering options		
Soluble fiber	5–10 g/day	3–5%
Plant sterol/stanol esters	2 g/day	6–15%
Cumulative estimate 20–30%		

From Kruger et al. (19).

the typical and atypical symptoms of myocardial ischemia and instructed to report these symptoms to their care provider if they occur. Prior ADA guidelines suggested that before recommending a program of physical activity, the provider should assess patients with multiple cardiovascular risk factors for CAD. However, the area of screening asymptomatic diabetic patients for CAD remains unclear, and routine screening is not recommended (6). Providers are advised to use clinical judgment (6).

Current recommendations for the use of aspirin call for initiation of low-dose therapy in the presence of known CVD, and aspirin therapy should be considered in individuals with diabetes who are at high risk (6). These individuals include people over the age of 40 years; current smokers; individuals with a family history of CVD; or those with hypertension, obesity, micro- or macroalbuminuria, or elevated lipid levels. Many individuals with diabetes continue to smoke, and complete smoking cessation should be the goal (8). Although glucose control is more strongly linked with microvascular complications of diabetes than with macrovascular disease, optimal glucose control is important to the control of lipid levels and may have an impact on cardiac events.

Recent studies have shown improved mortality and morbidity with optimal glucose control during acute treatment of MI. The Diabetes Mellitus, Insulin Glucose Infusion in Acute Myocardial Infarction (DIGAMI) study demonstrated that intensive insulin treatment improved survival at 1 year and at 3.4-year follow-up (20). The intensive treatment of diabetes, with patient self-monitoring of blood glucose levels to target A1C concentrations <7%, is supported by both the ADA and the AHA (14).

> **PRACTICAL POINT**
>
> Lowering LDL to <70 mg/dl, along with a lowering of the threshold for drug treatment to 100 mg/dl, have been recommended for very-high-risk patients, such as those with established CVD and diabetes.

TREATMENT

NONSURGICAL INTERVENTION

Once the diagnosis of CAD is made, aggressive treatment of dyslipidemia and hypertension, prevention of thrombosis with aspirin, and treatment with medications to reduce myocardial ischemia become even more essential, following the same principles outlined above (Table 8.2). Specific medications for CVD management in patients with diabetes, along with precautions to observe in this population, are outlined in Table 8.5.

The diagnosis of heart failure presents additional challenges. Treatment of heart failure in patients with diabetes should focus not only on the management of heart failure, but also on coexistent hypertension, CAD, and renal disease, as well as glucose control. Guidelines for the overall management of heart failure, based on class I evidence (evidence and/or general agreement that the procedure or treatment is useful and effective) and the four stages of heart failure, are shown in Table 8.6 (22). Stage A includes individuals at high risk of developing heart failure; stage B includes individuals with left ventricular dysfunction but without symptoms; and stage C includes individuals with left ventricular dysfunction with either current or prior symptoms. Refractory, end-stage heart failure is considered stage D.

Blood pressure should be lowered to <130/80 mmHg, and in most patients, even more aggressive lowering of blood pressure is indicated to reduce afterload and reverse left ventricular hypertrophy when present (13). Treatment of heart failure with ACE inhibitors improves clinical outcome, with less frequent hospitalizations for heart failure and fewer deaths (23). ACE inhibitors have an additional benefit in diabetes because of their proven renal-protective effect (24,25), even in high-risk patients without heart failure or known low ejection fractions (26,27). Although there is often reluctance to treat diabetes patients with β-blockers, they clearly benefit from such treatment after MI (28,29). The β-blocker carvedilol improves ventricular function and survival in patients with chronic heart failure and depressed left ventricular function (30). Diuretics also may have an important role in the treatment of advanced symptomatic heart failure (stage C) (31).

PRACTICAL POINTS

Aspirin should be considered in individuals with diabetes who are at high risk (6). These individuals include people aged >40 years; current smokers; individuals with a family history of CVD; or those with hypertension, obesity, micro- or macroalbuminuria, or abnormal lipid levels.

Smoking cessation assistance is available online at the American Cancer Society's web site at http://www.cancer.org/docroot/PED/PED_10_3x_Find_Support.asp.

Table 8.5 Cardiac Medications in Patients with Diabetes

Angiotensin-Converting Enzyme (ACE) Inhibitors
- Contraindications: angioedema, severe cough, bilateral renal artery stenosis, anuric renal failure, significant hyperkalemia, hypotension, shock
- Monitor renal function and potassium levels.

β-Blockers
- Caution: assess for worsening of glycemic and lipid control.
- Contraindications: bradycardia, second- or third-degree arteriovenous block, hypotension, moderate or severe heart failure, active wheezing
- Assess risk of masking hypoglycemia in patients requiring insulin.
- If used in the presence of bronchospastic disease, active heart failure, and conduction system disease, assess for deterioration.
- Initiate slowly and avoid abrupt withdrawal.

Calcium-Channel Blockers
- Diltiazem and verapamil are contraindicated in patients who have heart failure with systolic dysfunction; amlodipine and felodipine may be used to treat angina in patients with heart failure.
- Caution: heart failure, left ventricular dysfunction, arteriovenous block, sinus node dysfunction

Digoxin
- Contraindications: sinus node dysfunction or arteriovenous block
- Potential interactions with many medications
- Monitor renal function and electrolytes (hypokalemia and hypomagnesia).

Diuretics
- Aldosterone antagonist; spironolactone useful, particularly in patients with heart failure, but caution in patients with renal insufficiency because of possible hyperkalemia

Lipid-Lowering Agents
- HMG-CoA reductase inhibitors (statins) contraindicated with acute liver disease, heavy alcohol intake, or significant elevations in liver function tests (LFTs); monitor LFTs and closely monitor patients with hepatic dysfunction; assess for myalgias and potential myopathy with creatine phosphokinase (CPK) measurement, especially when used in combination with fibrates.

Nitrates
- Use with caution in patients with autonomic neuropathy.
- Avoid nitrate tolerance by dosing with 8- to 12-h nitrate-free period.
- Caution in setting of acute MI with presence of hypotension or right ventricular infarction

Platelet Inhibitors and Anticoagulants
- Monitor for bleeding with anticoagulants.
- Maintain partial thromboplastin time (aPTT) (heparin) and prothrombin time.
- International Normalized Ratio (PT/INR) (warfarin).
- Provide patient education regarding possible medication and dietary interactions with warfarin.
- In patients allergic to or unable to take aspirin, use clopidrel.

See also "Antihypertensive Medications" and "Lipid-Lowering Medications" in RESOURCES.

Table 8.6 Recommendations for Treating Heart Failure

- Achieve adequate blood pressure and lipid control.
- Counsel avoidance of smoking, alcohol, and illicit drugs.
- Use ACE inhibitors.
  - Add β-blockers in stage B and prior MI and in all of stage C, once compensated, unless contraindicated.
- Control ventricular rate in atrial fibrillation.
- Treat thyroid disorders.
- Evaluate and treat signs and symptoms
  - Periodic if stage A and regularly if in other stages
  - In stage B and higher, consider valve replacement or repair for hemodynamically significant stenoses/regurgitation.
  - In stage C and higher
    - diuretics if evidence of fluid retention
    - digitalis unless contraindicated
    - withdrawal of drugs known to adversely affect clinical status
  - In stage D
    - meticulous treatment of fluid retention
    - referral for heart failure program and cardiac transplantation

Generally, calcium-channel blockers should not be used in the treatment of heart failure in individuals with diabetes. Metformin and thiazolidinediones (TZDs) are not recommended in patients with moderate-to-severe heart failure because of the risk of lactic acidosis (metformin) and worsening of heart failure (TZDs). Since these medications are still used in patients with diabetes and heart failure, careful monitoring for these complications is necessary. In addition, with TZDs, lower doses should be used in the presence of known heart disease, and slow increases in dosage are advocated (32).

Increasing evidence suggests that individuals with diabetes have an increased risk for heart failure that is independent of the atherosclerosis. In patients with diabetes who are unresponsive to medical therapy, consideration should be given to cardiac transplantation. Transplant rejection is a relatively rare occurrence in the current era of immunosuppressive therapy (33). However, patients requiring insulin are at higher risk for poor outcomes at transplantation. Higher doses of insulin and other adjuvant hypoglycemic agents are usually required during the early post-transplantation phase, when high doses of corticosteroids are used.

In the setting of acute coronary syndromes, which include unstable angina and acute MI, early and appropriate management is critical to limit myocardial damage and prevent complications. MI may occur without the warning of prior angina, and patients may have atypical symptoms that delay them seeking medical attention and thus gaining the benefits of timely reperfusion. Although early coronary reperfusion, aspirin, β-blockers, ACE inhibitors, lipid-lowering agents, and coronary revascularization have dramatically improved the survival of patients with diabetes and MI, those patients with known CVD and diabetes-related microvascular complications still have a higher risk of complications than nondiabetic patients, both during and after hospitalization (Table 8.7) (34-38).

Patients with diabetes presenting with ST-segment elevation, indicative of MI, who are within 12 h of the onset of symptoms, should be considered for

Table 8.7 Complications to Assess and Prevent in Patients with Diabetes and CAD

After acute MI
- Heart failure
- Cardiogenic shock
- Postinfarction angina
- Heart block
- Atrial arrhythmias
- Renal insufficiency
- Recurrent MI and heart failure after discharge

After percutaneous interventions
- MI
- Renal failure
- Stroke

- Retroperitoneal bleeding, femoral hematoma, femoral or iliac artery dissection or occlusion, pseudoaneurysm formation
- Restenosis, MI, and need for repeat revascularization

After coronary artery bypass surgery
- MI
- Renal failure
- Stroke
- Sternal wound infection
- Recurrent angina and heart failure

primary angioplasty with stent placement, particularly when there is evidence of heart failure or hemodynamic instability, where the establishment of secure vessel patency may be critical. At times, additional surgical revascularization is necessary, particularly when significant residual CAD is present with recurrent angina or inducible ischemia (39). In centers where primary angioplasty is not available, thrombolytic therapy should be administered unless there is a contraindication due to bleeding risk. Following revascularization, hemostatic abnormalities in individuals with diabetes remain problematic. Therefore, subsequent antithrombotic treatment to prevent reocclusion is an important part of follow-up care. Adjuvant antithrombotic treatment with glycoprotein IIb/IIIa inhibitors is often administered when intracoronary stents are placed during ST-segment elevation MI in patients with diabetes. In addition, during the acute MI period, aggressive control of blood glucose may improve both short- and long-term outcomes (40,41). After MI, aggressive management of cardiac risk factors is warranted (Table 8.2).

Unstable angina and non–ST-segment MI are part of the spectrum of acute coronary syndromes that leave the individual with diabetes at an increased risk for adverse outcomes (42), including death, progression to ST-segment elevation MI, and subsequent readmission for unstable angina (43). Patients with unstable angina and diabetes have more extensive CAD, involving a greater number and longer segments of vessels, sometimes including the left main coronary artery. Some of these patients may have had prior coronary artery bypass graft (CABG), and patients presenting with imminent closure of diseased saphenous vein grafts pose particular challenges.

Cardiac autonomic neuropathy may further complicate management of patients with diabetes because of the associated increased heart rate and a decreased awareness of ischemic symptoms. The initial therapy of acute coronary syndromes includes the administration of β-blockers, aspirin, heparin, clopidrel or glycoprotein IIb/IIIa inhibitors, and nitrates. Those patients at significant risk for subsequent cardiac events, such as those with marked or widespread resting ST-segment depression, prior MI, decreased left ventricular function, or heart failure, may undergo early coronary angiography and revascularization. A noninvasive approach with further risk stratification based on stress echocardiography or myocardial perfusion imaging may be preferable in lower-risk patients and those with major comorbidity who are at high risk for the invasive approach.

PERCUTANEOUS OR SURGICAL REVASCULARIZATION

The decision to use percutaneous coronary intervention (PCI) or surgical revascularization depends on a number of factors, including the suitability of the target vessels as well as the overall risk status of the patient. PCI is usually implemented for single-vessel disease, and the use of drug-eluting intracoronary stents has improved PCI outcomes by reducing the rate of restenosis. Multivessel disease in patients with diabetes often requires CABG. Although many patients with diabetes safely undergo CABG, older age and the presence of other diabetes-related complications (particularly nephropathy) place the individual at higher risk of poorer operative outcomes. Complications associated with both procedures, which should be assessed, are outlined in Table 8.7.

Strategies for optimizing risk factor control after either PCI or surgical revascularization should be intensified in the population with type 2 diabetes. As with primary prevention in individuals free of CVD and secondary prevention in those with established CVD, there is a critical need for ongoing, intensive, multifactorial risk factor management after PCI or surgical revascularization (Table 8.2).

SUMMARY

Nurses need to have an understanding of the pathophysiology of CVD in individuals with diabetes, along with the clinical presentation of the various manifestations of CVD. Nurses play a particularly important role in coaching those with diabetes regarding the prevention and treatment of CVD. Nurses need to provide education regarding the goals of treatment.

REFERENCES

1. Kannel WB, McGee DL: Diabetes and cardiovascular risk factors: The Framingham Study. *Circulation* 59:8–13, 1979

2. Wackers FJT, Young LH, Inzucchi SE, Chyun DA, Davey JA, et al.: Detection of silent myocardial ischemia in asymptomatic diabetic subjects: the DIAD study. *Diabetes Care* 27:1954–1961, 2004

3. Vinik AI, Mitchell BD, Maser RE, Freeman R: Diabetic autonomic neuropathy. *Diabetes Care* 26:1553–1579, 2003

4. Maser RE, Vinik AI, Mitchell BD, Freeman R: The association between cardiovascular autonomic neuropathy and mortality in individuals with diabetes. *Diabetes Care* 26:1895–1901, 2003

5. American Diabetes Association: Nutrition principles and recommendations in diabetes (Position Statement). *Diabetes Care* 27 (Suppl. 1):S36–S46, 2004

6. American Diabetes Association: Standards of medical care in diabetes—2009. *Diabetes Care* 32 (Suppl. 1):S13–S61, 2009

7. American Diabetes Association: Physical activity/exercise and diabetes (Position Statement). *Diabetes Care* 27 (Suppl. 1):S58–S62, 2004

8. American Diabetes Association: Smoking and diabetes (Position Statement). *Diabetes Care* 27 (Suppl. 1):S74–S75, 2004

9. National Cholesterol Education Program (NCEP): *Third Report of the NCEP Expert Panel on Detection, Evaluation and Treatment of High Blood Cholesterol in Adults (Adult Treatment Panel III)*. Bethesda, MD, National Heart, Lung, and Blood Institute, National Institutes of Health, 2001, p. 1–28

10. Chobanian AV, Bakris GL, Black HR, Cushman WC, Green LA, et al.: The seventh report of the Joint National Committee on Prevention, Detection, Evaluation and Treatment of High Blood Pressure. *JAMA* 289:1560–1572, 2003

11. Writing Committee of the Action to Control Cardiovascular Risk in Diabetes (ACCORD) Study Group: Effects of intensive glucose lowering in type 2 diabetes. *N Engl J Med* 358:2545–2559, 2008

12. Skyler JS, Bergenstal R, Bonow RO, Buse J, Deedwania P, et al.: Intensive glycemic control and the prevention of cardiovascular events: implications of the ACCORD, ADVANCE, and VA diabetes trials: a position statement of the American Diabetes Association and a scientific statement of the American College of Cardiology Foundation and the American Heart Association. *Diabetes Care* 32:187–192, 2009

13. UK Prospective Diabetes Study Group: Tight blood pressure control and risk of macrovascular and microvascular complications in type 2 diabetes: UKPDS 38. *Br Med J* 317:703–713, 1998

14. Grundy SM, Benjamin IJ, Burke GL, Chait A, Eckel RH, et al.: Diabetes and cardiovascular disease: a statement for healthcare professionals from the American Heart Association. *Circulation* 100:1134–1146, 1999

15. Stern MP, Haffner SM: Dyslipidemia in type 2 diabetes. *Diabetes Care* 14:1144–1159, 1991

16. Reaven GM, Chen YD, Jeppesen J, Maheux P, Krauss RM: Insulin resistance and hyperinsulinemia in individuals with small, dense low density lipoprotein particles. *J Clin Invest* 92:141–146, 1993

17. Buse JB, Ginsberg HN, Bakris GL, Clark NG, Costa F, et al.: primary prevention of cardiovascular diseases in people with diabetes mellitus: a scientific

statement from the American Heart Association and the American Diabetes Association. *Diabetes Care* 30: 162–172, 2007

18. Hinnen D, Childs BP, Maryniuk M, Vu J: Pharmaceutical treatment of hypertension and dyslipidemia in people with diabetes: an educator's perspective. Part 1. Hypertension. *Diabetes Spectrum* 17:60–64, 2004

19. Kruger DF, Cypress M, Maryniuk, Childs BP, Tieking J: Pharmaceutical treatment of hyperglycemia and dyslipidemia in people with diabetes: an educator's perspective. Part 2. Dyslipidemia. *Diabetes Spectrum* 17:73–77, 2004

20. Malmberg K: Prospective randomised study on intensive insulin treatment on long term survival after acute myocardial infarction in patients with diabetes mellitus: DIGAMI (Diabetes Mellitus, Insulin Glucose Infusion in Acute Myocardial Infarction) Study Group. *Br Med J* 314:1512–1515, 1997

21. American College of Cardiology/American Heart Association Task Force on Practice Guidelines: ACC/AHA guidelines for the evaluation and management of chronic heart failure in the adult (Executive Summary). *Circulation* 104:2996–3007, 2001

22. Shekelle PG, Rich MW, Morton SC, Atkinson CS, Tu W, et al.: Efficacy of angiotensin-converting enzyme inhibitors and beta-blockers in the management of left ventricular systolic dysfunction according to race, gender, and diabetic status: a meta-analysis of major clinical trials. *J Am Coll Cardiol* 41:1529–1538, 2003

23. Lewis EJ, Hunsicker LG, Bain RP, Rohde RD: The effect of angiotensin-converting-enzyme inhibition on diabetic nephropathy: the Collaborative Study Group. *N Engl J Med* 329:1456–1462, 1993

24. Maschio G, Alberti D, Janin G, Locatelli F, Mann JF, Motolese M, et al.: Effect of the angiotensin-converting-enzyme inhibitor benazepril on the progression of chronic renal insufficiency: the Angiotensin-Converting-Enzyme Inhibition in Progressive Renal Insufficiency Study Group. *N Engl J Med* 334:939–945, 1996

25. Heart Outcomes Prevention Evaluation Study Investigators: Effects of an angiotensin-converting enzyme inhibitor, ramipril, on cardiovascular events in high-risk patients. *N Engl J Med* 342:145–153, 2000

26. Heart Outcomes Prevention Evaluation (HOPE) Study Investigators: Effects of ramipril on cardiovascular and microvascular outcomes in people with diabetes mellitus: results of the HOPE study and MICRO-HOPE substudy. *Lancet* 355:253–259, 2000

27. Kjekshus J, Gilpin E, Blackey A, Henning H, Ross J Jr: Diabetic patients and beta-blockers after acute myocardial infarction. *Eur Heart J* 11:43–50, 1990

28. Viscoli CM, Horwitz RI, Singer BH: Beta-blockers after myocardial infarction: influence of first-year clinical course on long-term effectiveness. *Ann Intern Med* 118:99–105, 1993

29. Bristow MR, Gilbert EM, Abraham WT, Adams KF, Fowler MB, et al.: Carvedilol produces dose-related improvements in left ventricular function and

survival in subjects with chronic heart failure: MOCHA Investigators. *Circulation* 94:2807–2816, 1996

30. Pitt B, Perez A: Spironolactone in patients with heart failure. *N Engl J Med* 342:132–136, 2000

31. Masoudi FA, Wang Y, Inzucchi SE, Setaro JF, Havranek EP, et al.: Metformin and thiazolidinedione use in Medicare patients with heart failure. *JAMA* 290:81–85, 2003

32. Grundy SM, Cleeman JI, Merz CN, Brewer HB Jr, Clark LT, et al.: Implications of recent clinical trials for the National Cholesterol Education Program Adult Treatment Panel III guidelines. *Circulation* 110:227–239, 2004

33. Nesto RW, LeWinter M, Bell D, Bonow RO, Semenkovich CF, et al.: Thiazolidinedione use, fluid retention, and congestive heart failure. *Diabetes Care* 27:256–623, 2004

34. Behar S, Boyko V, Reicher-Reiss H, Goldbourt U: Ten-year survival after acute myocardial infarction: comparison of patients with and without diabetes. *Am Heart J* 133:290–296, 1997

35. Granger CB, Califf RM, Young S, Candela R, Samaha J, et al.: Outcome of patients with diabetes mellitus and acute myocardial infarction treated with thrombolytic agents. *J Am Coll Cardiol* 21:920–925, 1993

36. Barbash GI, White HD, Modan M, Van de Werf F: Significance of diabetes mellitus in patients with acute myocardial infarction receiving thrombolytic therapy. *J Am Coll Cardiol* 22:707–713, 1993

37. Chyun DA, Vaccarino V, Murillo J, Young LH, Krumholz HM: Acute myocardial infarction mortality in the elderly with diabetes. *Heart Lung* 31:327–339, 2002

38. Chyun D, Vaccarino V, Murillo J, Young L, Krumholz H: Mortality, heart failure and recurrent myocardial infarction in the elderly with diabetes. *Am J Crit Care* 11:504–519, 2002

39. Hasdai D, Granger CB, Srivatsa SS, Criger DA, Ellis SG, et al.: Diabetes mellitus and outcome after primary coronary angioplasty for acute myocardial infarction: lessons from the GUSTO-IIb Angioplasty Substudy: Global Use of Strategies to Open Occluded Arteries in Acute Coronary Syndromes. *J Am Coll Cardiol* 1502–1512, 2000

40. Malmberg K, Ryden L, Efendic S, Herlitz J, Nicol P, Waldenstrom A, et al.: Randomized trial of insulin-glucose infusion followed by subcutaneous insulin treatment in diabetic patients with acute myocardial infarction (DIGAMI Study): effects on mortality at 1 year. *J Am Coll Cardiol* 26:57–65, 1995

41. Malmberg K, Norhammar A, Wedel H, Ryden L: Glycometabolic state at admission: important risk marker of mortality in conventionally treated patients with diabetes mellitus and acute myocardial infarction. *Circulation* 138:2626–2632, 1999

42. Braunwald E, Antman EM, Beasley JW, Califf RM, Cheitlin MD, et al.: ACC/ AHA guidelines for the management of patients with unstable angina and non-ST-segment elevation myocardial infarction: executive summary and recommendations: a report of the American College of Cardiology/ American Heart Association Task Force on Practice Guidelines (Committee on the Management of Patients with Unstable Angina). *Circulation* 102:1193–1209, 2000

43. Malmberg K, Yusuf S, Gerstein HC, Brown J, Zhao F, et al.: Impact of diabetes on long-term prognosis in patients with unstable angina and non-Q-wave myocardial infarction: results of the OASIS (Organization to Assess Strategies for Ischemic Syndromes) Registry. *Circulation* 102:1014–1019, 2000

Dr. Chyun is an Associate Professor and Director of the Adult Advanced Practice Nursing Specialty Program at Yale University School of Nursing, New Haven, CT. Dr. Young is a Professor of Medicine, Section of Cardiovascular Medicine, at Yale University School of Medicine, New Haven, CT.

9. Peripheral Vascular Disease

Linda Haas, PHC, RN, CDE

Peripheral vascular disease is an inclusive term referring to peripheral arterial disease (PAD), vasculitis, venous thrombosis, venous insufficiency, and disorders of the lymphatic system. PAD is obstruction of arterial blood flow, not including the cerebral and coronary blood vessels (1). Because PAD is more common in individuals with diabetes (2), with up to one third of individuals >50 of age with diabetes estimated to have the disorder (3), this chapter focuses on PAD, with some reference to venous disease. The critical importance of PAD in diabetes is evidenced by this disorder being a marker for atherosclerotic disease of other blood vessels, including the coronary arteries (4), and a major risk factor for lower-extremity amputation (5).

EPIDEMIOLOGY

PAD affects ~20% of adults >55 years of age (1), ~12 million people in the U.S. (6). Although there are no hard data on the incidence and prevalence of PAD in diabetes, it is estimated that 20–30% of people with symptomatic PAD have diabetes (7). Thus, there may be ~2.5 million people with diabetes and PAD in the U.S. This figure may underestimate the prevalence of PAD in people with diabetes because PAD in these individuals may be asymptomatic because of sensory peripheral neuropathy.

Risk factors for PAD are cigarette smoking, diabetes, older age, hypertension, dyslipidemia (1), and hyperhomocysteinemia (8). In addition to these general PAD risk factors, risk factors in diabetes patients are age, diabetes duration, African-American or Hispanic ethnicity, peripheral neuropathy (9), and hyperglycemia (10). Risk factors for venous disease are age, immobility, recent surgery, residence in residential care facility, previous hospitalization for deep or superficial vein thrombosis, obesity, and trauma (11).

PATHOPHYSIOLOGY

PAD is an atherosclerotic disease of the lower extremities, with vascular inflammation, altered cellular contents of the vasculature and blood cells, and abnormal hemostatic factors. There are abnormalities of endothelial function and regulation of the vasculature, including loss of normal nitrous oxide function, increased atherosclerotic activity in the smooth muscle cells lining blood vessel walls (7), increased oxidative stress, platelet aggregation, and hypercoagulation (8).

PAD in individuals with diabetes is increased because of vascular inflammation and derangement in cellular components. Elevated levels of C-reactive protein (CRP) are strongly associated with the development of PAD (12). In diabetes and impaired glucose tolerance, CRP levels are abnormally elevated. Not only is CRP a marker for the disease process, but it may also play a causative role in the impairment of fibrinolysis and the regulation of vascular tone (4). Vascular abnormalities may present before diagnosis of diabetes and increase with duration of disease and worsening of glucose control.

Venous disease includes varicose veins, caused by incompetency of venous valves; superficial or deep vein thrombosis; and chronic venous insufficiency. The latter is caused by chronic incompetence of the deep veins (11).

ASSESSMENT AND CLINICAL PRESENTATION

Intermittent claudication is the most common manifestation of PAD. Patients should be asked about cramping pain in their calves, thighs, or buttocks that occurs with activity and is relieved by rest. If venous disease is suspected, patients should be asked about feelings of fullness in their legs, a "bursting" sensation, dull aching, and pruritus. These symptoms are usually worse at the end of the day. Table 9.1 provides guidance for forming assessment questions for peripheral vascular disease.

The feet and lower legs should be examined. In PAD, the lower extremities may demonstrate dependent rubor, with pallor on elevation. Presence or absence of hair (if previously present) should be assessed, as well as the condition of the nails, which may be dystrophic in PAD. The area between the toes (interdigital spaces) should be carefully inspected for cracks, fissures, and infection. Debris between the toes may indicate that patients cannot reach their feet to clean between their toes or are not aware of the importance of this hygienic measure. Table 9.1 delineates assessment and intervention strategies for patients with PAD or venous disease.

TESTS AND VALUES

Pedal pulses may be difficult to feel in many patients, particularly for an inexperienced examiner. In addition, the process of locating them can have many

Table 9.1 Nursing Assessment and Interventions and Patient Self-Management Education for Diabetes Patients with Peripheral Arterial and Venous Disease

PAD	Venous Disease
Ask patient about:	**Ask patient about:**

■ Intermittent claudication (pain in calves when walking, especially uphill, relieved by rest)
■ Pain at rest
  • *Gradual onset*, narrowing of vessels
  • *Sudden onset*, complete occlusion
■ May complain of feet feeling cold
	■ May have no symptoms
	■ Aching discomfort
	■ "Bursting" feeling
	■ Tenderness
	■ Pruritus
	■ Footwear too small
	■ Feet too swollen for usual shoes

Examination **Color** ■ Pale or blue, purple ■ Dependent rubor (redness) ■ Blanching when elevated to 45°	**Examination** **Color** ■ Brownish, reddish ■ Mottled
Skin ■ Cool to touch ■ Shiny, thin ■ Loss of hair on toes, lower legs ■ Thickened ridged toenails ■ Nonhealing, distal wounds or ulcers ■ Gangrenous	**Skin** ■ Warm to touch ■ Dry and scaly ■ Edematous (except for toes) ■ Stasis ulcers on malleolus, lower leg
Pulses ■ Diminished or absent dorsalis and posterior tibialis	**Pulses** ■ Peripheral pulses may be difficult to locate because of edema
Interventions ■ Encourage and support efforts at smoking cessation ■ Encourage and support efforts toward increasing walking	**Interventions** ■ Encourage and support efforts at smoking cessation
Instruct patients to ■ Inspect daily for cracks and sores ■ Prevent/protect from trauma ■ If interdigital spaces macerated, wind lamb's wool loosely between toes ■ Sit with feet supported below heart to reduce pain ■ Not use circular bandages or ace wraps on legs ■ Avoid constriction (tight sock band, garters, rubber bands/garters to hold up socks)	**Instruct patients to** ■ Inspect daily for cracks and sores ■ Prevent/protect from trauma ■ Use support hose ■ Elevate feet above heart for 20 min three times a day ■ Avoid constriction (tight sock band, garters, rubber bands/garters to hold up socks) ■ Elevate feet when sitting. Use recliners, foot stools, boxes ■ Tie shoes loosely or wear shoes with an adjustable toe box, e.g., post-op shoes with Velcro closures

Table 9.2 Interpretation of ABI

Ratio	Interpretation
0.91–1.3	Normal
0.7–0.9	Mild obstruction
0.4–0.69	Moderate obstruction
<0.4	Severe obstruction
>1.3	Poorly compressible*

*May indicate medial arterial calcification; ABI is less reliable in this situation.

false-positive and false-negative results. Thus, the ankle-brachial index (ABI) is a preferred measure for screening for PAD in the legs and should be measured for all patients with diabetes over age 50 years who have other risk factors for PAD (8). This test involves measuring the systolic blood pressure just above the ankle and over the brachial artery in the arm with a handheld Doppler device. A ratio is calculated from these measures, with the radial blood pressure as the denominator and the ankle value as the numerator. See Table 9.2 for interpretation of the ABI. In patients with longstanding diabetes, ABI may be inaccurate because of noncompressible blood vessels. In these patients, the toe-brachial index should be used (8). If PAD is diagnosed or strongly suspected, patients should have segmental pressures and pulse volume recordings in a vascular laboratory. Some patients may require treadmill testing, during which a >20-mmHg decrease in ankle pressure usually indicates PAD (8). To confirm the diagnosis of venous disease, continuous-wave Doppler, plethysmography, bidirectional ultrasound, duplex ultrasound, or venography are used in the vascular laboratory (11).

TREATMENTS AND INTERVENTIONS

Treatment of PAD has several aspects. All the conventional risk factors for cardiovascular disease should be addressed, including cigarette smoking, hypertension, and dyslipidemia (8). Antiplatelet therapy is indicated, and clopidogrel or cilostazol may be beneficial in patients with diabetes and PAD (1). An antiatherogenic meal plan may also be advantageous (9).

Cigarette smoking is the single most important modifiable risk factor for the development and exacerbation of PAD (8). Tobacco use is associated with increased risk of amputation.

Hypertension is associated with a two- to threefold increase in claudication and contributes to the development of atherosclerosis. Aggressive blood pressure control, achieving a level of <130/80 mmHg in patients with PAD and diabetes, will help reduce cardiovascular risk.

Although no studies have directly examined the effects of lipid lowering in individuals with diabetes and PAD, there is evidence that lipid-lowering therapies decrease the severity of claudication. In the Scandinavian Simvastatin

PRACTICAL POINT
The use of compression stockings can be difficult for patients who live alone and cannot put on the stockings without help. Silk inner toe liners, stockings with zippered sides, and devices to help put on the elastic stockings are especially helpful for these patients.

Survival Study (4S), the reduction of cholesterol level by simvastatin reduced the risk of new or worsening symptoms of intermittent claudication by 38% (13).

Increased physical activity is an important therapeutic modality and can lead to patients' ability to walk longer distances pain free (13). Walking programs have been shown to increase blood flow, improve collateral circulation, lengthen walking distance capability, decrease the oxygen cost of exercise and the heart rate, and improve functional well-being (14,15). Walking programs are usually carried out in the home setting but may be part of a structured program conducted through a cardiac rehabilitation or physical therapy department. Before a patient starts a walking program, the health care provider or cardiac rehabilitation or physical therapy department should determine if such a program will be safe.

Walking programs must be maintained to be effective, and dropout rates are high. Strategies that assist patients in maintaining a walking regimen include doing some of the cardiac rehab program at home (16), receiving semi-weekly phone calls from health care providers, and self-monitoring progress daily (17). In addition, a computerized feedback system, which tracked progress and set goals, has been shown to decrease and delay dropout rates in a walking program (17).

In some patients, endovascular procedures, such as balloon angioplasty and stenting, may be indicated, as may surgical procedures (8).

A major intervention for venous disorders is use of compression stockings, which should have at least 30–40 mmHg of compression and extend at least to the knee, higher if feasible (11). Patients should avoid long periods during which their legs are dependent, prolonged travel without getting up and walking, and hot weather as much as is feasible. In addition, patients should follow a low-sodium diet to decrease fluid retention. Anticoagulation is usually implemented for superficial or deep vein thrombosis.

INFECTIONS

Patients with diabetes and PAD are more likely to develop severe foot infections. When both neuropathy and PAD are present, the foot is at much greater risk for traumatic ulceration, infection, and gangrene. Patient education in preventive foot care measures becomes critically important in reducing amputation risk. Ischemic ulcers typically form at the edges of the foot, including the tips of the toes and the backs of the heels. Footwear for the neuroischemic foot must fit well to avoid the creation of pressure points or shearing force.

Education/Behavioral Considerations for Peripheral Vascular Disease

Problem	Considerations
Patients with PAD have pain associated with walking.	▪ Encourage and assist to implement a walking program. ▪ Identify barriers to program (external barriers are more easily overcome than internal). ▪ Problem solve ways to overcome these barriers. ▪ Identify or assist patients to identify community resources, such as cardiac rehabilitation, YMCA, senior centers, and shopping mall walking programs, because people are more apt to stay with exercise programs if they have social support.
Many people cannot adequately examine their feet because of obesity, decreased vision, and/or decreased flexibility.	▪ Mirrors on handles may facilitate visual inspection of the plantar surfaces of their feet. ▪ Problem solve methods to raise the feet so patients can reach their feet to wash and dry them appropriately. ▪ Long-handled sponges can enable people to clean their feet and long-handled pointed sponges enable cleaning of the interdigital spaces.

In individuals with diabetes and foot infection, the presenting signs and symptoms are often diminished. An impairment of the neuroinflammatory response reduces the early warning signs of infection. Differentiating between the erythema of cellulitis and the rubor of ischemia may be difficult. The redness of ischemia will disappear on elevation, but in cellulitis, the redness remains, irrespective of positioning.

In cases of severe infection, broad-spectrum intravenous antibiotics will be necessary because the infections are frequently polymicrobial. However, antibiotic treatment alone is not enough to treat most infections. Surgical assessment for debridement and drainage, offloading the ulcer, and applying appropriate dressings plays a vital role in the treatment process.

Future Nursing Research

What strategies will facilitate continuance of walking programs and in which populations? What strategies assist patients to wear appropriate footwear?

SUMMARY

PAD is significantly underdiagnosed and undertreated (11). Although careful examination of the lower extremities can identify PAD, a careful nursing assessment, particularly of exercise patterns and barriers, may identify clues, such as leg pain, that indicate PAD. Clues uncovered during a nursing assessment can also generate ideas for strategies to assist patients in implementing and maintaining an exercise program. These clues include, but are not limited to, previous activity/exercise patterns, occasions when walking was pleasurable, support systems such as family, friends, pets, and seniors groups, and interest in walking groups that might give support for initiation and maintenance of a walking program. Because use of support hose is critical in the treatment of venous insufficiency, the patient's ability to put these on should be assessed. If a patient has difficulty putting compression stockings on, a family member can help; if that is not feasible, a sock assister is very helpful.

PAD is a serious complication associated with diabetes and is often asymptomatic. The clinical presentation varies greatly. Some patients will maintain activity, while others will have difficulty performing daily activities. Since patients with diabetes can present with symptoms that can be confused with neuropathy, PAD can be missed. Clinical evaluation that includes diagnostic vascular testing is important to establish the diagnosis. Vascular consultation followed by appropriate treatment is necessary to preserve and protect the affected limb. Foot care education is a main component in the prevention of foot ulcers and infections. Surgery to restore circulation may be necessary to avoid loss of the limb.

REFERENCES

1. Hankey GJ, Norman PE, Eikelboon JW: Medical treatment of peripheral arterial disease. *JAMA* 295:547–533, 2006

2. American Diabetes Association: Economic costs of diabetes in the U.S. in 2002. *Diabetes Care* 26:917–932, 2003

3. Peripheral arterial disease can be a killer. In *NIH Medline Plus*, 2008, p. 19

4. American Diabetes Association: Peripheral arterial disease in people with diabetes (Consensus Statement). *Diabetes Care* 26:3333–3341, 2003

5. Pecoraro RE, Reiber GE, Burgess EM: Pathways to diabetic limb amputation: basis for prevention. *Diabetes Care* 13:513–521, 1990

6. Fine JJ, Hall PAX, Richardson JH: Predictive power of cardiovascular risk factors for detecting peripheral vascular disease. *South Med J* 97:951–954, 2004

7. Hirsch AT, Criqui MH, Treat-Jacobson D, Regensteiner JG, Creager MA, et al.: Peripheral arterial disease: detection, awareness and treatment in primary care. *JAMA* 286:1317–1324, 2001

8. Hirsch AT, Haskal ZJ, Hertzer NR, Bakal CW, Creager MA, et al.: ACC/AHA guidelines for the management of patients with peripheral arterial disease

(lower extremity, renal, mesenteric, and abdominal aortic) (Executive Summary). *J Am Coll Cardiol* 47:1239–1312, 2006

9. Steffen LM, Duprez DA, Boucher JL, Ershow AG, Hirsch AT: Management of peripheral arterial disease. *Diabetes Spectrum* 21:171–176, 2008

10. Adler AI, Stevens RJ, Neil A, Stratton IM, Boulton AJM, Holman RR, Group UKPDS: UKPDS 59: hyperglycemia and other potentially modifiable risk factors for peripheral vascular disease in type 2 diabetes. *Diabetes Care* 25:894–899, 2002

11. Wennberg PW, Rooke TW: Diagnosis and management of diseases of the peripheral arteries and veins. In *Hurst's The Heart*. 11th ed. Fuster V, Alexander RW, O'Rourke RA, Eds. New York, McGraw-Hill, 2004, p. 2361–2379

12. Shammas ND, Eric J.: Evidence-based management of peripheral vascular disease. *Curr Atheroscler Rep* 7:358–363, 2005

13. Milani RV, Lavie CJ: the role of exercise training in peripheral arterial disease. *Vasc Med* 12:351–358, 2007

14. Hiatt WR: Medical treatment of peripheral arterial disease and claudication. *N Engl J Med* 344:1608–1621, 2001

15. Tan KH, De Cossart L, Edwards P: Exercise training and peripheral vascular disease. *Br J Surg* 87:553–562, 2000

16. Carlson JJ, Johnson JA, Franklin BA, VanerLaan RL: Program participation, exercise adherence, cardiovascular outcomes, and program cost of traditional versus modified cardiac rehabilitation. *Am J Cardiol* 86:17–23, 2000

17. King A, Taylor C: Strategies for increasing early adherence to and long-term maintenance of home-based exercise training in healthy middle-aged men and women. *Am J Cardiol* 61:628–632, 1988

Ms. Haas is the Endocrinology Clinical Nurse Specialist at the VA Puget Sound Health Care System, Seattle, WA, and Metabolic Clinical Nurse Advisor to the Office of Nursing Service, Veterans Health Administration, Washington, DC.

10. Ocular Changes with Diabetes

Roger H. Phelps, OD, FAAO, CDE

D iabetic retinopathy is the leading cause of new blindness in Americans ages 20–74 years, and most diabetes-related blindness is preventable (1–3). Nurses can participate in this prevention by

- knowing the range of effects that diabetes has on the eyes
- assessing the patient's glycated hemoglobin A1c (A1C) history, level of retinopathy (if any), and date of last dilated eye examination
- encouraging diabetes self-management knowledge and skills to promote glycemic and blood pressure control

For every 1% lowering of A1C, there is an ~35% risk reduction for the development or progression of retinopathy. Timely detection and treatment of proliferative diabetic retinopathy can reduce the risk of severe visual loss by 50% (4,5).

The American Diabetes Association (1) recommendations on diabetic retinopathy state that

- An ophthalmologist or optometrist who is knowledgeable and experienced in diagnosing the presence of diabetic retinopathy and is aware of its management should perform annual dilated eye examinations of patients with diabetes.
- Patients who have been identified with a specific risk of visual loss should be referred promptly to an ophthalmologist who is knowledgeable and experienced in the management and treatment of diabetic retinopathy, i.e., an ophthalmologist who is experienced in fluorescein angiography, optical coherence tomography, retinal laser treatment, and intraocular injections.

Herein, the term *retinal specialists* will refer to ophthalmologists who have had specific retinal fellowship training beyond their general ophthalmological training. All eye doctors are licensed to do comprehensive dilated eye examinations and are

Ophthalmologic Examination Schedule

Patient group	Recommendation for exam	Minimum routine follow-up
Type 1 diabetes	Within 3–5 years after diagnosis of diabetes once the patient is aged 10 years	Yearly
Type 2 diabetes	At time of diagnosis of diabetes	Yearly
Pregnancy with preexisting diabetes	Prior to conception and during first trimester	Physician discretion, pending results of first trimester exam

responsible for detecting diabetic retinopathy (6). Nurses working with diabetes patients should know which practitioners on referral lists have specific experience with diabetic eye diseases.

TEMPORARY REFRACTIVE CHANGES

Temporary blurry vision can occur any time individuals with diabetes have a major change in their average glycemic control. Either a major increase or a major decrease in A1C can change the osmotic balance between the aqueous and the crystalline lens in the eye. This is usually a temporary change that is reversible with glycemic stabilization. However, it remains important that the patient have a dilated eye examination any time there is a complaint of blurry vision to rule out any serious cause. Most eye doctors will discuss the costs versus benefits of purchasing a pair of glasses for temporary use while driving or reading until the refractive error stabilizes.

LEVELS OF DIABETIC RETINOPATHY

Microvascular disease of the retina is best predicted by the A1C history and duration of diabetes in a patient (5). The continued hyperglycemia of inadequately

PRACTICAL POINT

The nurse should encourage all patients with diabetes to learn how to establish and maintain glycemic control. When working with individuals who are experiencing significant changes in glycemic control, inform the eye doctor of these changes and send a copy of the most recent A1C value. There appears to be no long-term effect of this temporary refractive change.

Eye Anatomical Terms (see Fig. 10.1)

- **Aqueous:** The clear fluid that is constantly produced by the eye. It drains out of the eye in a circular canal near the iris root.
- **Iris:** The diaphragm that forms the pupil, located in the front portion of the eye. The color of the iris is considered the "eye color."
- **Lens:** The crystalline lens is just behind the iris and is responsible for about one-third of the optical power of the eye. It can change focus until about the age of 40 years.
- **Vitreous:** The vitreous body is the clear gel-like body that fills the large posterior portion of the eye. It is bathed in aqueous fluid, as is the entire inside of the eye, and tends to liquefy with increasing age.
- **Retina:** The photosensitive membrane that lines the inside back of the eye and acts like the film in a camera. It is connected to the brain's seeing mechanism through the optic nerve. It is nourished by its own capillary bed as well as by vessels that underlie it.
- **Optic disk:** The opening in the retina where the optic nerves and major retinal vessels enter and exit the back of the eye.
- **Macula:** This small area of the retina is the most sensitive and central part of our vision.

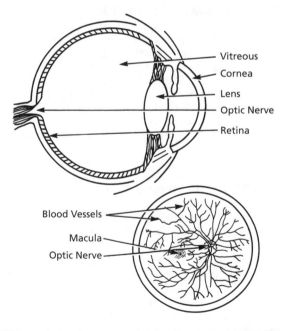

Figure 10.1 Illustration of a normal eye. From Funnell MM, Arnold MS, Lasichack AJ, Barr PA, Eds.: *Type 2 Diabetes: A Curriculum for Patients and Health Professionals.* Alexandria, VA, American Diabetes Association, 2002, p. 347.

controlled diabetes can lead to blindness by the following process. First, high glucose levels damage the capillary walls of the retina, leading to leakage and small blot hemorrhages and microaneurysms. Continued glycemic insult leads to more capillary nonperfusion and the development of intraretinal microvascular abnormalities, venous beading, and the stimulation of chemical factors such as vascular endothelial growth factor. New fragile vessels then grow out from the retina into the vitreous. These leak and bleed easily, forming adhesions between the retina and vitreous, which then lead to traction retinal detachment, vitreous bleeding, and blindness (7).

There are surgical interventions available to stop or slow this process (4), but the best intervention is to optimize glycemic control to keep the retinal capillaries healthy. Often, if the retinopathy is severe, improving glycemic control too quickly can lead to increased retinopathy at first, but after 2–3 years, the benefit of the maintained glycemic control will be realized.

NO DIABETIC RETINOPATHY

This level indicates that no disease is visible on the retina. Although this has been historically uncommon after a long duration of diabetes, it is now becoming more probable with ongoing, consistent glycemic control combined with a timely diagnosis of diabetes.

NONPROLIFERATIVE DIABETIC RETINOPATHY

This level, also called background retinopathy, indicates that there has been some damage to the retinal capillary bed but not to the point that new vessel growth has been stimulated into the vitreous body, which would signify proliferative diabetic retinopathy. These background changes are usually put into three categories: mild, moderate, and severe (or preproliferative) (8).

PRACTICAL POINT

The health of the retinal capillary bed can be best diagnosed by fluorescein angiography and optical coherence tomography. In angiography, a dye is given through an intravenous line, and then carefully timed photographs are taken of the retina to show areas of capillary nonperfusion and leakage. Optical coherence tomography is a newer, noninvasive test that is very sensitive to retinal edema.

Mild nonproliferative diabetic retinopathy. Some scattered small blot hemorrhages and microaneurysms begin to appear on the retina. These can be difficult to see and are easily missed during a nondilated eye examination. There are documented incidences of patients at this mild stage improving their glycemic control and reversing these changes.

Moderate nonproliferative diabetic retinopathy. There is a significant increase in the number of small blot hemorrhages and microaneurysms, with the additional findings of intraretinal microvascular abnormalities or venous beading. This is the point at which the experienced eye doctor will consider a consultation with a retinal specialist.

Severe nonproliferative (preproliferative) diabetic retinopathy. Retinal changes are now becoming a real threat to vision. The retina capillary bed is severely compromised, and more of the retinal findings of the previous moderate stage are present. Chemical mediators, such as vascular endothelial growth factor (VEGF), are now strongly calling out for new vessel growth. The patient should immediately see a retinal specialist for special testing, such as fluorescein angiography and optical coherence tomography, with probable treatment.

PROLIFERATIVE DIABETIC RETINOPATHY

Proliferative diabetic retinopathy indicates that there has been sufficient insult to the vessels that the body has started to try to fix the problem by growing new vessels. However, this "fix" results in more problems for the eye, such as rubeosis iridis, retinal detachment, and vitreous hemorrhage.

Rubeosis iridis. The new vessels most commonly grow from the optic nerve head, but they can also grow elsewhere in the retina and on the iris (called rubeosis iridis). Rubeosis iridis can lead to neovascular glaucoma. A retinal specialist needs to be immediately involved at this stage to minimize the high probability of blindness.

Retinal detachment. The proliferative new vessels are leaky and cause adhesions and tractions that can then pull apart the two layers of the retina, in turn detaching them from the eye wall. If the retina is not surgically reattached, it will deteriorate quickly. Many times, this finding is the first indication of an eye problem in a patient with suboptimally controlled diabetes who has not had an eye examination or routine annual screening. It is not always possible to reattach the retina, and the result is permanent blindness.

Vitreous hemorrhage. A vitreous hemorrhage occurs when the fragile new vessels growing in proliferative diabetic retinopathy break and bleed into the vitreous body. This can be seen as an oily, pink haze or sometimes as a total blockage of vision. Again, this may be the first indication of a diabetes-related eye problem. A retinal specialist usually does a vitrectomy at this point. This surgical procedure removes the jelly-like vitreous material, allowing clear aqueous fluid to fill the eye.

CLINICALLY SIGNIFICANT MACULAR EDEMA

Retinal edema can appear at almost any level of retinopathy and is usually accompanied by some hard exudates. Sometimes these changes can be very subtle and missed by an inexperienced examiner who fails to dilate the pupil. Grid laser treatment, guided by fluorescein angiography and optical coherence tomography needs to be done as soon as possible to minimize the damage caused by the edema to the sensitive macular area. (9)

OTHER RETINAL CHANGES IN THE EYE SOMETIMES ASSOCIATED WITH DIABETES

HYPERTENSIVE RETINOPATHY

High blood pressure combined with weakened retinal capillary beds in suboptimally controlled diabetes can cause a rapid progression in diabetic retinopathy. Hypertensive effects include infarcts in the retinal nerve fiber layer evidenced by cotton wool spots and flame-shaped retinal hemorrhages. These can resolve with better control of blood pressure; however, continued hypertension, even without diabetes, can lead to sight-threatening retinal changes.

Interventions for Diabetic Ocular Complications

- Glycemic control
- Blood pressure control
- Panretinal photocoagulation. A retinal specialist will use a laser to carefully place hundreds of microburns to the peripheral retina. This will decrease the peripheral vision somewhat, but will reduce the demand for new blood vessel growth. This usually dries up the neovascular growth in proliferative diabetic retinopathy, thus preserving the central vision.
- Grid laser treatment. If a fluorescein angiography determines areas of leakages around the macula, a small-grid pattern of microburns will be placed, usually drying up the clinically significant macular edema to prevent further permanent loss to the macular function.
- Subthreshold Diode Laser Micropulse Photocoagulation is being developed as a less destructive alternative laser treatment of the retina for diabetic macular edema.
- Vitrectomy. A retinal specialist, in microsurgery, will remove the vitreous body while carefully protecting the retina from detachment, removing traction membranes.
- Follow-up. Most retinal specialists do not do routine eye care or prescribe low-vision aids, so the optometrist or general ophthalmologist will continue to monitor the patient's visual needs and, if necessary, refer him or her to a low-vision specialist for visual rehabilitation.
- Visual rehabilitation. Similar to physical therapy after a stroke, many patients can learn to adapt to their reduced vision with various new low-vision aids and techniques.
- Many new pharmacological interventions, both oral and injectable, are being studied and show some promise in turning off the chemical mediators in the eye that call out for new blood vessel growth. One such product, an ocular injection of an anti-VEGF pharmaceutical, already has been shown effective and is approved for treatment of the edema associated with wet macular degeneration.

CENTRAL RETINAL VEIN OCCLUSION

Central retinal vein occlusion (CRVO) appears as a hemorrhagic stroke result-ing from an occlusion in the central vein of the eye or a branch of it (BRVO). This problem threatens sight and is more related to the macrovascular changes in diabetes. Cholesterol management together with blood pressure control best prevents it (see chapter 2). Some of the branch occlusions can resolve, but others need laser treatment similar to that in proliferative diabetic retinopathy. Central retinal artery occlusions can happen as well.

AGE-RELATED MACULAR DEGENERATION

Although not specifically associated with diabetes, age-related macular degeneration is the leading cause of legal blindness in senior adults. Injections of pharmaceutical agents that block VEGF have shown remarkable success in maintaining and even restoring vision when given at the beginning signs of macular edema. If a patient with diabetes has already lost vision, special devices, low-vision aids, and proper training can greatly assist the patient in his or her self-management needs, such as in reading blood glucose meters and drawing up insulin.

NONRETINAL CHANGES IN THE EYE SOMETIMES ASSOCIATED WITH DIABETES

DIPLOPIA

A sudden onset of double vision in a patient with diabetes is commonly associ-ated with a complete or partial paresis of cranial nerves III, IV, and VI, which affect the extraocular muscles controlling eye position and movement. Most of these patients can be followed conservatively for 2–3 months, and many times, there is a dramatic recovery. The important exception is when either a third nerve palsy affects the pupil or any palsy lasts >3 months. This situation requires an extensive neuroradiological workup to rule out the possibility of a brain aneurysm or other serious cranial problems.

CATARACTS

Most people who live long enough will benefit from cataract extraction because the lens of their eye becomes less clear in the natural aging process. When the crystalline lens is removed, an artificial lens (intraocular lens) is usu-ally put behind the iris to keep it in proper focus. Although cataracts are more common in individuals with suboptimally controlled diabetes, they are easily detected in routine eye examinations and easily treated when they sufficiently interfere with vision. However, no surgery is without risk, and individuals with diabetes who have a significant amount of retinopathy are at a higher risk of complications during and after the surgery. Many cataract surgeons will request a consultation from a retinal specialist to determine the best time for surgery in these cases.

GLAUCOMA

There are basically three types of glaucoma: primary open-angle glaucoma, primary angle-closure glaucoma, and neovascular glaucoma. All three types are associated with an intraocular pressure that is too high for the health of the optic nerve fibers.

Primary open-angle glaucoma (also known as chronic open-angle glaucoma). It is uncertain whether the diabetic population is at higher risk of developing this most common type of glaucoma. However, the potential for loss of vision is higher in individuals with suboptimally controlled diabetes because of compromised microvascular circulation. Detection and continuous treatment of this condition are important to minimize or prevent vision loss. Almost all routine eye examinations check for glaucoma. Because it is usually asymptomatic, patients are unaware of its presence until much of their peripheral vision is lost. Most patients can be successfully controlled with daily eye drops that lower their eye pressure.

Primary angle-closure glaucoma. Primary angle-closure glaucoma is an ocular emergency and is usually very painful. The cause is an anatomical closure of the drainage canal by the iris. It is also called narrow angle glaucoma. Quick treatment usually prevents any visual loss. Prevention of this condition begins when a narrow drainage angle is discovered during a routine eye examination. The patient would then be referred to an ophthalmologist who has a special laser to open a drainage hole in the iris. This procedure (called YAG iridotomy [neodymium:yttrium aluminum garnet pulsed laser]) can be performed during an office visit, usually permanently prevents closure, and requires no ongoing medication.

Neovascular glaucoma. Neovascular glaucoma is a very serious condition and is associated with suboptimally controlled diabetes. This is a form of proliferative diabetic retinopathy in which new blood vessels form and proliferate along the iris (rubeosis iridis) and into the normal drainage canal of the eye, blocking the normal outflow of the aqueous, causing a painful increase in eye pressure. It is treated in the same way as other proliferative diabetic retinopathy, with panretinal laser photocoagulation and other medical and surgical interventions. Treatment, however, is not always successful in saving vision.

SUMMARY

The nurse can play an important role in reducing the incidence of diabetic retinopathy by providing education in maintaining blood glucose control, helping ensure timely eye examinations, and assisting individuals to achieve better control of blood pressure and lipids. Optimal diabetes control has been shown to prevent or reduce the severity of diabetic retinopathy. Early detection and treatment also decreases the incidence of blindness. Encouragement by the nurse to achieve optimal control and to have annual dilated eye exams is important.

Abbreviations Commonly Used in Ocular Charts and Reports

A1C: Glycated hemoglobin A1c
AMD: Age-related macular degeneration (sometimes ARMD)
BDR: Background diabetic retinopathy (same as NPDR)
CRVO: Central retinal vein occlusion
CSME: Clinically significant (diabetic) macular edema
CW: Cotton wool spots (on retina)
DME: Diabetic macular edema
DR: Diabetic retinopathy
FA: Fluorescein angiography
H/ma: Small-blot hemorrhages and/or microaneurysms
IRMA: Intraretinal microvascular abnormalities
NPDR: Nonproliferative diabetic retinopathy (same as BDR)
NVD: New vessels on the optic disk (this is PDR)
NVE: New vessels elsewhere in the retina (this is PDR)
NVG: Neovascular glaucoma
OCT: Optical coherence tomography
OD: Oculus dexter (right eye)
OS: Oculus sinister (left eye)
OU: Oculus uterque (both eyes)
PACG: Primary angle closure glaucoma
PDR: Proliferative diabetic retinopathy
POAG: Primary (or chronic) open-angle glaucoma
PRP: Panretinal laser photocoagulation
RD: Retinal detachment
RI: Rubeosis iridis (this is PDR)
VEGF: Vascular endothelial growth factor
VB: Venous beading (with retinal veins)
VH: Vitreous hemorrhage

REFERENCES

1. American Diabetes Association: Retinopathy in diabetes (Position Statement). *Diabetes Care* 27 (Suppl. 1):S84–S87, 2004

2. Chous AP: *Diabetic Eye Disease: Lessons from a Diabetic Eye Doctor: How to Avoid Blindness and Get Great Eye Care*. Auburn, WA, Fairwood Press, 2003

3. National Diabetes Education Program web site. Available at http://www.cdc.gov/diabetes/ndep/index.htm. Accessed 8 September 2008

4. American Academy of Ophthalmology (AAO) web site. Available at http://www.aao.org. Accessed 8 September 2008

5. Diabetes Control and Complications Trial Research Group: The relationship of glycemic exposure (HbA1c) to the risk of development and progression of retinopathy in the Diabetes Control and Complications Trial. *Diabetes* 44:968–983, 1995

6. American Optometric Association (AOA) web site. Available at http://www. aoanet.org. Accessed 8 September 2008

7. Aiello LP, Aiello LM, Cavallerano JD: Visual loss. In *Therapy for Diabetes Mellitus and Related Disorders*. 4th ed. Lebovitz HE, Ed. Alexandria, VA, American Diabetes Association, 2004, p. 340–343

8. Aiello LP, Aiello LM, Cavallerano JD: Ocular complications. In *Therapy for Diabetes Mellitus and Related Disorders*. 4th ed. Lebovitz HE, Ed. Alexandria, VA, American Diabetes Association, 2004, p. 344–357

9. Luttrull, JK, Spink CJ: Serial optical coherence tomography of subthreshold diode laser micropulse photocoagulation for diabetic macular edema. *Ophthalmic Surg Lasers Imaging* 37:370–377, 2006

Dr. Phelps has type 1 diabetes, and for many years has taught and lectured locally and internationally on Diabetes and the Eyes. He practices at OjaiEyes Optometry, Ojai, CA.

11. Diabetic Nephropathy and End-Stage Renal Disease

Belinda P. Childs, ARNP, MN, CDE, BC-ADM, and
Kris Ernst, RN, CDE, BSN

EPIDEMIOLOGY OF DIABETIC NEPHROPATHY

Approximately 20 million adults have evidence of chronic kidney disease as determined by a moderately or severely reduced glomerular filtration rate. This represents 7.69% of adults aged 20 and older (1,2). The number of patients with diabetes as the primary cause of end stage renal disease (ESRD) reached 48,157 in 2006. Diabetes accounts for as much as 40% of all new cases of kidney failure (2). This is partly because type 2 diabetes is increasing in prevalence and because people with diabetes now live longer. Minorities are disproportionately affected by kidney disease. African Americans are four times more likely and American Indians six times more likely than non-Hispanic white Americans to develop ESRD (3). In all, 70–80% of people with diabetes never develop ESRD and may live their whole lives without significant renal complications (4).

PATHOGENESIS OF DIABETIC NEPHROPATHY

Studies have suggested that diabetic nephropathy is primarily related to the metabolic changes associated with diabetes.

- Renal changes are initially absent in people with diabetes who have kidney biopsies at diagnosis.
- Renal changes occur in all types of diabetes.
- Renal damage occurs in animal models regardless of whether they have spontaneous or induced diabetes.
- In animal models, reversal of diabetes through intensive insulin therapy or transplantation prevents renal disease and may reverse early histological changes (5).

Natural Course of Renal Disease in Diabetes

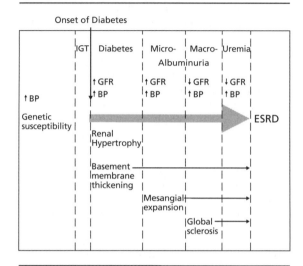

BP, blood pressure; IGT, impaired glucose tolerance; GFR, glomerular filtration rate; ESRD, end-stage renal disease.

Figure 11.1 Natural course of renal disease in diabetes. Adapted from Nelson et al. (6).

The onset of diabetes seems to lead to hemodynamic changes in the renal circulation that lead to increased renal plasma flow, glomerular capillary hyperperfusion, and increased glomerular pressure gradient. These hemodynamic changes are hypothesized to cause functional and structural damage to the glomeruli, which results in defects in glomerular capillary permeability, proteinuria, mesangium changes, and glomerulosclerosis (6). The natural progression of diabetic nephropathy and some of the contributing factors are shown in Fig. 11.1.

RISK FACTORS FOR DIABETIC NEPHROPATHY

Risk factors that contribute to the development of renal disease include duration of diabetes, familial and genetic factors, hypertension, hyperglycemia, plasma prorenin activity, and lipid levels (6). One of the most important risk factors for the development of diabetic nephropathy is duration of diabetes; however, in type 1 diabetes, only 30–50% of patients develop diabetic nephropathy. Therefore, factors other than diabetes itself appear to affect the development of diabetic nephropathy.

FAMILIAL AND GENETIC FACTORS

In patients with type 1 diabetes, if one sibling has diabetes and nephropathy, then it is more likely that another sibling will also have nephropathy. In addition, some studies have found a difference in the distribution of HLA (human leukocyte antigen) markers between those with and without nephropathy in type 1 diabetes. There appears to be familial clustering in patients with type 2 diabetes as well (6).

HYPERTENSION

Hypertension may be a result of nephropathy, but it is also associated with progression and pathogenesis. Both systolic and diastolic hypertension accelerate the progression of diabetic kidney disease. Aggressive management of blood pressure can decrease the rate of fall of the glomerular filtration rate (GFR) (4).

HYPERGLYCEMIA

In the Diabetes Control and Complications Trial (DCCT), intensive therapy focused on attaining a glycated hemoglobin A1c (A1C) level as close to normal range (~7%) as possible reduced the occurrence of microalbuminuria (urinary albumin excretion ≥40 mg/24 h) by 39% and albuminuria (urinary albumin excretion ≥300 mg/24 h) by 54% in the combined cohort (7). Optimal diabetes control in the primary prevention group (those with retinopathy at baseline) in the U.K. Prospective Diabetes Study (UKPDS) demonstrated a reduction in the rate of progression of renal function end points (8).

PRORENIN AND HYPERLIPIDEMIA

Less clear are the roles of prorenin and lipids in the development and progression of nephropathy. Prorenin is the precursor to renin, and an increase in plasma prorenin has been associated with the microvascular complications of diabetes. There are several small studies that have suggested that higher cholesterol level promotes the progression of renal disease.

PREGNANCY

Pregnancy, regardless of whether a woman has diabetes, is associated with a transient rise in GFR and a moderate increase in urinary protein excretion (see chapter 25). Women with preexisting diabetes may experience an increase in proteinuria from the first to third trimester, but this usually returns to normal after delivery. A pregnancy complicated by diabetes does not appear to adversely affect early diabetic renal disease; however, a greater risk of progression may occur in those with hypertension or more severe renal disease (6).

PRACTICAL POINT

A patient with nephropathy may also have diabetic eye disease. The presence of microalbuminuria in all age-groups has been associated with an increased risk for retinopathy. With renal disease, yearly screening for retinal disease becomes essential.

Table 11.1 Strategies to Prevent or Delay the Progression of Diabetic Nephropathy

Primary prevention	Goal: Prevent diabetic nephropathy.
	Optimize glycemic control: A1C <7%
	Blood pressure control: <130/80 mmHg
Secondary prevention	Goal: Prevent or delay the progression from microalbuminuria to overt proteinuria.
	Aggressive control of blood pressure: <120/70 mmHg
	Limit dietary protein: ≤0.8 g/kg body wt/day (10% of daily calories)
	Medical intervention: initiate ACE inhibitor or ARB treatment if increased albumin-to-creatinine ratio
Tertiary prevention	Goal: Prevent or delay the progression of overt diabetic nephropathy and improve clinical outcomes (tertiary care reduces morbidity and mortality by delaying time to dialysis or transplantation).
	Strategies: As above for secondary prevention.

Adapted from ADA (4,9) and DeFronzo (13).

PREVENTION AND TREATMENT

Preventing and delaying the progression of diabetic nephropathy can be achieved with management of the factors known to influence the development and progression of the disease. Table 11.1 contains an outline of treatment approaches divided into primary, secondary, and tertiary prevention strategies.

BLOOD PRESSURE REDUCTION

Hypertension is known to be the single most important factor in the progression of established renal disease. Both systolic and diastolic hypertension accelerate the progression of the disease (5).

According to the American Diabetes Association (ADA) Standards of Medical Care in Diabetes (9), blood pressure should be evaluated at each medical visit. If it is >130/80 mmHg, a second evaluation should be obtained in the near future. The primary goal is to lower blood pressure with lifestyle modifications, such as weight loss (if appropriate), reduction in salt and alcohol intake, and exercise. In 4–6 weeks, if blood pressure has not reached this goal and there are no contraindications for use, then an angiotensin-converting enzyme (ACE) inhibitor or angiotensin receptor blocker (ARB) should be initiated. If initial goals are met and well tolerated, decreasing the blood pressure further may be appropriate. The UKPDS indicated that continuing to lower blood pressure reduced the risk of microvascular complications (8).

In patients with type 1 diabetes, the ADA recommends using ACE or ARB treatment for any microalbuminuria or macroalbuminuria. The current recom-

---

EDUCATION AND SELF-MANAGEMENT

The patient with hypertension should self-monitor their blood pressure. Self-monitoring of blood pressure enhances educational efforts and allows the patient and health care team to work together in detecting, treating, and evaluating the risk for renal complications. Reviewing patients' technique and regularly checking blood pressure monitoring devices can help ensure accurate readings.

---

mendation is to increase the dose of ACE or ARB to reduce or eliminate the microalbuminuria or macroalbuminuria (9).

DIETARY PROTEIN RESTRICTION

Animal studies have shown that reducing dietary protein intake reduces hyperfiltration and intraglomerular pressure and retards the progression of renal disease. Several small human studies have shown a modest reduction in the progression of renal disease using a restriction of 0.8 g/kg body wt/day. The current ADA recommendation is to prescribe the adult Recommended Daily Allowance (RDA) of 0.8–1.0 g/kg body wt/day (~10% of total calories) in the patient with early nephropathy. Because most Americans eat in excess of the recommended amount of protein, portion control that includes weighing and measuring is necessary. It has been suggested that once the GFR begins to fall, it may be helpful to restrict protein intake to 0.8 g/kg/day (10).

Patients using protein-restricted meal plans must be continuously monitored for signs of malnutrition, including weight loss, muscle wasting, weakness, and hypoalbuminemia. In order to consume an adequate number of calories, the patient may need to increase intake of other macronutrients. The additional amount of carbohydrate in this diet can cause blood glucose levels to rise, and insulin and/or oral medications may need to be adjusted. As the renal disease progresses, appetite frequently diminishes, and patients may have to be encouraged to eat adequate calories with enough protein. A dietitian should be consulted for any patient with moderate to severe nephropathy.

DIAGNOSIS AND RENAL FUNCTION TESTS

Diagnostic tests focus on early detection of microalbuminuria. Annual screening for microalbuminuria in type 1 diabetes patients should begin at puberty and/or after 5 years' disease duration. Among people with type 2 diabetes, screening for microalbuminuria should begin at the time of diagnosis. Screening for microalbuminuria can be performed by three methods:

- Measurement of the albumin-to-creatinine ratio in a random spot urine collection
- 24-h urine collection for creatinine and serum creatinine to measure creatinine clearance
- Timed (e.g., 4-h or overnight) collection

Table 11.2 Definitions in Abnormalities in Albumin Excretion

Category	Spot Collection (µg/mg creatinine)
Normal	<30
Microalbuminuria	<30–299
Clinical albuminuria	(≥300 µg/mg)

From ADA (9).

Analysis of the albumin-to-creatinine ratio is the more commonly recommended screening method (4). The other two alternatives (24-h collection and a timed specimen) are rarely used for screening. Normal albumin excretion by spot collection is defined as <30 µg/mg, microalbuminuria is 30–299 µg/mg, and clinical albuminuria is ≥300 µg/mg (Table 11.2). Because of variability in urinary albumin excretion, at least two of three tests performed within a 6-month period should show elevated levels before a patient is designated as having microalbuminuria. Exercise within the preceding 24 h, infection, fever, congestive heart failure, vasculitis, other inflammatory processes (such as acute rheumatoid arthritis), and marked hyperglycemia and hypertension may elevate urinary albumin levels above baseline. If any of these factors were present at the time the urine sample was collected, the test should be repeated. If the albumin screening values are ≥300 µg/mg, then a 24-h urine is ordered to quantify the protein excretion and establish the GFR. In addition, a serum creatinine must be drawn during this time period to determine creatinine clearance, if needed. Creatinine clearance is calculated by comparing the serum creatinine level with the urine creatinine level.

Creatinine clearance was the most widely used direct method of estimating GFR. This value is measured based on a carefully timed urine collection, usually over 24 h. It is critical to note an accurate time frame even if a full 24 h has not passed. A complete sample is imperative. Partial loss of a urine sample or a discrepancy in actual time collected will invalidate the test (10).

Serum creatinine is an indirect measure of GFR. It is now recommended that the serum creatinine be used to estimate GFR and to stage chronic kidney disease. An estimated GFR (eGFR) can also be calculated using the Levey modification of the Cockcroft and Gault method, which uses serum creatinine, patient age, and weight. Online calculators for eGFR can be found at http://www.nkdep.nih.gov/professionals/gfr_calculators/index.htm (4). Most clinical laboratories today report eGFR in addition to serum creatinine.

CHRONIC RENAL DISEASE

Chronic renal disease is defined in two ways (10):

1. Kidney damage for ≥3 months, as defined by structural or functional abnormalities of the kidney, with or without decreased GFR, manifested by either
   a pathological abnormalities or

Table 11.3 Stages of Chronic Kidney Disease

Stage	Description	GFR (ml/min/1.73 m^2)
1	Kidney damage with normal or increased GFR	≥90
2	Kidney damage with mild decrease in GFR	60–89
3	Moderate decrease in GFR	30–59
4	Severe decrease in GFR	15–29
5	Kidney failure	<15 or dialysis

From the National Kidney Foundation (4,18).

     b markers of kidney damage, including abnormalities in the composition of the blood or urine or abnormal imaging tests.

2. GFR <60 ml/min/1.73 m^2 for ≥3 months, with or without kidney damage (10,11).

The stages are shown in Table 11.3.

CLINICAL PRESENTATION AND ASSESSMENT

Individuals are asymptomatic throughout the early stages of diabetic nephropathy. Clinical manifestations of diabetic nephropathy are evident when GFR is 20–35% of normal, and patients become nephrotic with a urinary protein excretion of >4 g/day (12). The clinical management of diabetes with nephrotic syndrome presents a great challenge. The management of blood glucose becomes more difficult as loss of renal function diminishes renal catabolism of insulin. Proteinuria is generally 4–8 g/day, but urinary protein loss can reach 20–30 g/day. Fluid retention is often massive, resulting in weight gain, peripheral edema, congestive heart failure, and pulmonary edema as uremia progresses. Fatigue and shortness of breath result in a reduction of daily activities. Hypertension may become uncontrolled, secondary to fluid volume overload. Uremia becomes evident because of the accumulation of metabolic wastes and toxins.

At equivalent levels of renal failure, patients with diabetes may appear more ill than those without diabetes. Underlying diabetes-induced neurological abnormalities, such as gastroparesis, can exacerbate uremia-induced nausea and vomiting.

A nephrologist should be consulted when GFR is <60 ml/min/1.73 m^2 or if difficulty occurs in the management of hypertension or hyperkalemia (4). Nephrologists should be consulted early in the diagnosis to assure that the patient receives all available preventive measures.

OTHER CONSIDERATIONS IN NEPHROPATHY PROGRESSION

HYPOGLYCEMIA

Patients with renal disease are at higher risk for hypoglycemia because most diabetes medications are metabolized in the kidney. It may be necessary to reduce the dosages of some antihyperglycemic medications and avoid the use of others. Of the oral agents, the sulfonylureas have the greatest risk for inducing and prolonging hypoglycemia. Glimepiride and the meglitinides are least likely to lead to hypoglycemia. Even with these medications, lower dosages will likely be necessary.

The kidneys catabolize one-fourth to one-third of injected insulin. As kidney function declines, exogenous insulin acts longer and in an unpredictable manner (13). Studies have concluded that the kidney can make and release glucose. Based on recent evidence, it would seem that the release of glucose by the kidney might play a role in the regulation of glucose homeostasis. The lack of this production and release may also be a contributing factor in hypoglycemia associated with kidney disease (12,14). Use of insulin analogs, intensive insulin therapy, and hypoglycemia awareness training may all aid in the reduction of severe hypoglycemia in the patient with renal impairment.

PRACTICAL POINT

Patients who present with frequent and unexplained hypoglycemia should have their renal status assessed.

ADDITIONAL COMPLICATIONS

Management and rehabilitation of patients with ESRD are further complicated by the fact that >95% of patients with diabetic nephropathy have some degree of retinopathy, with 50% being blind or having significant vision loss (renal-retinal syndrome). If either renal or retinal disease has been diagnosed, it is important to screen for disease in the other system. Also, microalbuminuria and proteinuria are prognostic indicators of cardiovascular disease in type 2 diabetes.

OTHER THREATS TO THE KIDNEY

Urinary tract infections (UTIs). These are more common in older adults and in those with autonomic neuropathy affecting the bladder. UTIs are often asymptomatic or the patient may complain of unexplained hyperglycemia, incontinence, and vague symptoms, such as fullness in the suprapubic area. It is therefore important that a urinalysis be performed at each clinic visit. If leukocytes or nitrites are present, a urine culture should be obtained. Positive cultures should be treated with an antibiotic. Chronic infections can lead to pyelonephritis. There is debate regarding the importance of asymptomatic bacteremia and the necessity of treatment. Patient education on the symptoms of UTI is important.

Neurogenic bladder. This condition is more common in individuals with diabetes and may predispose individuals to UTIs. Symptoms such as frequent voiding, nocturia, incontinence, and recurrent UTIs may occur sporadically or be considered a result of age or prostatic hypertrophy. If diagnosed, the nurse can teach Credé's manual voiding maneuvers, which should be performed every 8 h. This is often sufficient to prevent the postvoid residual. If not, parasympathetic agents may be tried. If pharmacologic therapy proves unsuccessful, intermittent straight catheterization should be performed two to three times daily.

Dye studies. Intravenous pyelography and other dye studies can be a risk for patients with diabetes, who are at increased risk for acute renal failure after any radiocontrast. Many times, an alternative diagnostic study can be performed. If contrast media are necessary, a minimum amount of dye should be used and adequate hydration with half-normal or normal saline should be ensured prior to the dye study. Serum creatinine tests should be checked daily for 2–3 days after the contrast study (5).

Nephrotoxic drugs. If these drugs (e.g., amphotericin B; aminoglycosides, such as gentamicin; acyclovir; nonsteroidal anti-inflammatory drugs [NSAIDs]) must be used, monitor serum creatinine levels and drug levels and reduce the dosage of the drug administered to patients with impaired renal function. Recommend acetaminophen rather than NSAIDs because these agents reduce prostaglandins and can damage the kidney.

Medication dosages. Because the presence of renal disease can increase the half-life of most medications, new medications should be started at one-half the recommended dosage, and other current medications should be reviewed for possible changes in dosage.

PRACTICAL POINT

In caring for patients with renal disease, consider the following:
- Identify UTIs early and treat aggressively
- Avoid nephrotoxic medications
- Avoid NSAIDs
- Avoid contrast dyes

SPECIAL CONSIDERATIONS IN ESRD

ANEMIA

Anemia caused by ESRD is the result of a decrease in the production of erythropoietin. Because erythropoietin stimulates the production of red blood cells, the anemia often leads to fatigue and decreased activity. The anemia of kidney disease is often managed with regular injections of erythropoietin.

When assessing patients with renal disease and anemia, patient symptoms may not correlate with capillary blood glucose values or with A1C. Thus, it is important to be aware of how anemia can affect tests for glycemic control. With low hemoglobin and low hematocrit levels, some of the commonly used tests are affected and may give inaccurate results. A1C can give a falsely low value. Sometimes, a fructosamine test can be used to assess glycemic control. However, because the fructosamine test is affected by low albumin/protein levels, which are often seen in patients with ESRD, this test may not give an accurate assessment of glycemic control.

Additionally, capillary blood glucose tests can be affected by a low hematocrit level and therefore may also be altered by anemia. Capillary blood glucose results are most accurate when the hematocrit level is between 30 and 50%. However, some glucose meters have a documented accuracy with hematocrit ranges of 25–60% (15). If the patient's symptoms do not correlate with his or her capillary blood glucose levels, the nurse should compare the glucose meter value with a laboratory reference value.

Provided the difficulties concomitant with ESRD and anemia in testing blood glucose values, thorough and careful testing is advised in these patients. Evaluating which meter is less dependent on hematocrit will be important in assisting these patients. If a renal patient is reporting symptoms of hypoglycemia but obtaining normal or high capillary blood glucose levels, it would be prudent to obtain a blood glucose level by the reference laboratory with a simultaneous glucose meter reading.

FLUID VOLUME EXCESS

Fluid volume excess can result from oliguria or anuria. Because of the thirst associated with ESRD, the patient tends to drink in excess and crave sodium, further contributing to the volume excess. The variation in hydration can also affect blood glucose levels. Edema may be a problem associated with the decreased serum osmolality. The nurse needs to assist the patient in identifying ways to relieve this thirst, such as with ice chips, mouth swabs, and sugar-free hard candies as appropriate. These patients are often on fluid restrictions, especially if they have not begun dialysis or are on hemodialysis, so a registered dietitian should be consulted. The nurse should reinforce these fluid restrictions and make it clear that foods that are liquids when at room temperature (e.g., Jell-O, pudding) are also fluids and therefore subject to restriction. In patients who crave sodium, identifying foods that have alternative flavors without sodium, such as lemon, is an option.

Symptoms of electrolyte imbalance include weakness, muscle twitching, nausea, fatigue, headache, and heart palpitations. Other symptoms may include edema, alterations in ECG and chemistry panels, and positional blood pressure changes. Patients need to be cautioned about standing too quickly. This will reduce the potential of falling due to orthostatic hypotension and muscle weakness. Family members may need to be encouraged to support the patient when standing.

DIETARY CHANGES

Protein restriction may be used to prevent the progression of renal disease. But as the disease progresses, patients often experience anorexia, nausea, and vomiting. In addition, foods containing potassium and sodium are often restricted on the renal diet. With the multiple comorbidities of diabetes, it is not uncommon to see a patient trying to manage a meal plan that is low in fat, has consistent carbohydrate content, and is low in potassium and sodium. The challenges this poses can lead to confusion, anger, and feelings of deprivation. Malnutrition can occur because of reduced appetite and dietary restrictions. The nurse should encourage a consultation with a dietitian and make every effort to offer additional food choices if the patient does not eat while in the hospital or in the dialysis unit. During dialysis sessions, dietary restrictions are modified, allowing the patient to enjoy a wider range of foods.

COORDINATION OF CARE

The patient with diabetic nephropathy presents a challenge for nursing. Renal disease itself presents a complex medical program of care. However, when renal disease is coupled with diabetes, the interaction of medical and nursing management issues demands a higher level of nursing care and expertise. Research has demonstrated that excellent diabetes management must be maintained to retard renal deterioration, but with renal disease, diabetes self-management and the patient's ability to achieve glucose goals become increasingly difficult. Foremost, the role of the nurse is to assist the patient in dealing with the complexity of the renal care regimen. A nurse will encounter many of these intricate aspects, including dietary issues and their effects on glucose levels, prevention and treatment of hypoglycemia (including the use of glucagon), issues regarding alterations in activity and increased fatigue associated with anemia and uremia, skin dryness and pruritus, and mental health conditions, such as depression. The patient will be interacting with the health care system at many levels: dietitians, renal and dialysis specialists, diabetes specialists and nurse educators, mental health providers, pharmacists, social workers, etc. As is evident, these many levels of interaction only increase the potential for miscommunication and faulty care coordination. The nurse is the ideal patient advocate to coordinate and facilitate care.

The renal patient has increased physical care needs. Table 11.4 identifies these needs and suggests nursing actions to meet them.

BEHAVIORAL CONSIDERATIONS

Rates of depression, anxiety, and stress may be higher among patients with ESRD than among the general population. These psychological reactions may occur in response to the losses associated with diabetes and renal disease (e.g., loss of physical capacities and loss of control from the complications associated with diabetes). A variety of health care professionals, including mental health professionals, need to be involved in helping patients and families adjust to their losses and to select treatment options. In addition, the involvement of these professionals will make the task of learning a new, often complex treatment regimen more successful (16).

Table 11.4 Physical Care Needs for the Renal Patient with Diabetes

Physical Needs	Nursing Actions
Monitor fluid and electrolyte balance.	1. Weigh patient for fluid retention and measure urinary output/fluid intake. 2. Assess for signs of fluid overload/congestive heart failure. 3. Assess blood pressure and orthostatic changes.
Maintain adequate nutrition status.	1. Evaluate food intake and dietary adherence. 2. Collaborate with the dietitian and provide reinforcement on education regarding potassium and protein restriction. 3. Assess weight changes and alterations in lab values and notify a doctor if necessary. 4. Educate patient in eating smaller, more frequent meals to reduce nausea and maintain blood glucose level.
Maintain skin integrity.	1. Maintain hygiene to prevent infection. 2. Relieve dryness and pruritus by choosing alcohol-free creams and nondrying soaps.
Prevent constipation.	1. Use stool softeners and fiber products. 2. Fluid restrictions and phosphate binders may aggravate constipation. 3. Discourage use of over-the-counter remedies that may cause electrolyte imbalances.
Maintain target glucose levels.	1. Help patient to identify times of the day when hypoglycemia is most likely to occur. 2. Discuss appropriate treatment for hypoglycemia: oral medications and glucagon by injection. 3. Discuss changes in glucose levels with continuous ambulatory peritoneal dialysis fluid changes or before and after dialysis. 4. Encourage patient to keep a glucose log to assist in insulin adjustment decisions.
Encourage safe level of activity.	1. Assess patient's gait, balance, range of motion, muscle strength, and condition of feet. 2. As tolerated, encourage activity to prevent bone demineralization and assist with glucose control.
Increase understanding of complex regimen of care.	1. Help patient to express treatment concerns/fears; refer to mental health professionals as appropriate. 2. Assess treatment schedule to avoid unnecessary fatigue and to better coordinate with diabetes management program. 3. Review alterations in diabetes therapy caused by changes in kidney status.

Adapted from Nettina (17).

Some patients blame themselves when they develop diabetes complications. Scare tactics (e.g., "If you don't control your blood glucose, you will go into kidney failure") are not an effective behavior-change strategy. The fear, anxiety, and stress associated with renal disease may be expressed as anger toward the health care team and reluctance to follow the recommended regimen. Some patients may make comments such as "Why bother?" or "Well, I'm going to have a transplant, so I won't worry about it." It is important that the health care team recognize and validate the patient's feelings in order to ensure that the patient follow the treatment regimen. Avoid giving "pat" answers or responses that can sound patronizing. To assess what feelings and concerns the patient may be experiencing, state the following: "This can be a difficult process for some people, and sometimes they blame themselves. How are you feeling about having a problem with your kidneys?" Allowing the patient to express his or her fears and concerns is the most important intervention.

Support groups and discussion with other individuals and families who have experienced dialysis or transplantation can be an effective intervention for some patients with ESRD. Patients can learn new information, coping skills, and behaviors and adopt positive attitudes from these role models. Having patients and their families available in the clinic setting to meet new patients who are facing a recent diagnosis of renal disease can be very valuable.

CHOOSING A TREATMENT OPTION FOR ESRD

Treatments for ESRD are aimed at replacing the work of the kidneys. Several new treatment options are available for renal replacement therapy. People with diabetes who receive transplants or dialysis experience higher morbidity and mortality than patients without diabetes because of coexisting complications such as coronary artery disease, retinopathy, and neuropathy. Providing education and information on each treatment option allows the patient and family to make an informed choice and enhances the chances of a positive outcome. Benefits and risks of each treatment option should be reviewed with patients and family members for a comparison of options in treating uremia. Direct contact with other patients who are receiving different forms of therapy for ESRD may be valuable in providing education, emotional support, and hope. Supplying list of useful web sites may also be helpful (see RESOURCES).

Dialysis and/or renal transplantation usually occurs earlier in the patient with diabetes than in one who does not have diabetes. Typically, renal replacement therapy will begin when serum creatinine is >6 mg/dl or creatinine clearance is <20 ml/min, but more importantly, it should begin before the development of severe uremic symptoms, such as uremic pericarditis, unresponsive hypertension, muscle deterioration, worsening lethargy, nausea, and vomiting (13).

Planning for treatment should begin early, usually when the serum creatinine level reaches 3 mg/dl (265 μmol/l). Early involvement with a nephrologist, which

---

CANDIDATE SELECTION

Circumstances may be present that limit the patient's choice of treatment. For example, individuals with cardiovascular disease or vascular access problems might be less suitable candidates for hemodialysis. Likewise, individuals unable to tolerate fluid in the peritoneal cavity or those prone to infections would not be appropriate candidates for peritoneal dialysis.

---

is usually recommended when creatinine is 2 mg/dl or GFR is <60 ml/min/1.73 m², is also important to optimize medical therapy as well as help the patient begin the adjustment process. Patients with renal disease will often feel that they are participating in a program in which the goal is to preserve kidney function as long as possible. Late referrals for treatment, which will require hasty decisions regarding type of dialysis or being put on a list for kidney transplantation, frequently result in sentiments of anger and betrayal at the primary care provider for not conveying the seriousness of the kidney disease. If transplantation is under consideration, planning includes tissue typing of family members or other living unrelated donors for possible kidney donation, being placed on a cadaver waiting list, and/or creating vascular access for dialysis.

BEHAVIORAL CONSIDERATIONS WITHIN THE HEALTH CARE TEAM

The health care provider may experience a range of emotions and may need the help of a team member in expressing and dealing with his or her own feelings about what the patient and family are going through and how they are coping.

TREATMENT OPTIONS FOR ESRD

If treatment is not initiated for ESRD, death ensues. Survival is reduced in patients with diabetes compared with those without diabetes. Nearly one-half of all patients with diabetes who begin dialysis die within 2 years. For renal transplant patients with diabetes, the survival rate is much better than that of dialysis-treated patients, primarily because those patients who have kidney or kidney/pancreas transplants have fewer comorbidities.

NO TREATMENT

A patient has the right to choose not to begin dialysis. The patient and family should consider the no-treatment option only after the patient is dialyzed and is not uremic because uremia can affect the mental status. Some patients could be considered incompetent because of uremia. Nurses should encourage the patients and families to discuss the decision not only with their physicians but with clergy, psychologists, social workers, health care teams, and other family members. It is important to evaluate the patient for potentially undiagnosed and/or untreated depression. Planning supportive care (e.g., home care, hospice care) is necessary for the patient who chooses to forgo or discontinue renal replacement therapy.

HEMODIALYSIS

Hemodialysis is the most commonly used kidney-replacement therapy for people with ESRD in the U.S. The use of maintenance hemodialysis requires vascular access, which may be more difficult in the patient with diabetes because of systemic atherosclerosis. A synthetic graft may be used in the patient with diabetes.

Hemodialysis can be performed at a dialysis center or at home. Three types of hemodialysis can occur in the home. Conventional home dialysis is usually done three to four times a week. A new home therapy is now available that is performed five to seven times per week using a newer machine designed for shorter treatments of 2 h each. Nocturnal home hemodialysis consists of a long, slow treatment overnight, usually six nights a week. Training for the individual and the support team/family usually occurs over a 2- to 4-week period (18).

Factors that can alter glucose levels for the patient receiving hemodialysis treatment include the glucose concentration in the dialysate bath, appetite alteration on days with dialysis and days without dialysis, decreased activity on dialysis days, and emotional stress. The following questions are useful in eliciting information regarding causes of blood glucose variability in patients with diabetes who are receiving hemodialysis treatment:

- "Tell me about your glucose pattern on the days you are having dialysis?"
- "Tell me about your pattern on other days?"
- "Tell me when and how much you eat on days you are having dialysis?"
- "What about other days?"
- "Tell me about your activity pattern on days you are having dialysis?"
- "Tell me about your activity pattern on other days?"

Altered hematocrit levels can alter the accuracy of some glucose meters (see "Anemia" above). Sometimes a change in the type of glucose meter used may be warranted to avoid erroneous measurements of blood glucose values. Meter manufacturers provide specifications of hematocrit ranges for their meters. The health care provider should be aware of this potential cause of variability.

PERITONEAL DIALYSIS

Peritoneal dialysis has rapidly grown in popularity because of its advantages of rapid patient training and reduced cardiovascular stress. The use of the mechanical cyclers, called continuous cyclic peritoneal dialysis (CCPD), has simplified the process. Both CCPD and continuous ambulatory peritoneal dialysis carry the risks of peritonitis and gradual decrease in peritoneal surface area. Insulin, antibiotics, and other medications can be added to the dialysate. The amount of insulin required may vary based on the glucose concentration of the dialysate. Typically, regular insulin is added to the dialysate.

Patients requiring insulin can administer regular insulin directly into the dialysate before it is instilled into the peritoneal cavity. This reduces the need for injections because the insulin can be added to the dialysate and represents a more physiological way to deliver insulin because it is continuously absorbed by the hepatic system, much like insulin produced by β-cells.

Factors that can affect glucose regulation for patients on peritoneal dialysis include the concentration of the dialysate solution, method(s) of insulin delivery (e.g., intraperitoneal, subcutaneous, or both), and infection (peritonitis). Carefully written instructions will need to be provided. Self-monitoring of blood glucose is essential. Adjustments in the amount of insulin added to the dialysate should be based on glucose monitoring. A pattern approach should be used. The patient should be encouraged to keep accurate records, noting the glucose concentration of dialysate used, calories/carbohydrates eaten, insulin added to dialysate, and insulin injected. Although regular insulin is preferred in the dialysate, fast-acting insulin can be supplemented for meals and as a correction dose.

KIDNEY TRANSPLANTATION

After kidney transplantation, most individuals with diabetes will require a higher insulin dose because the immunosuppressive medications (i.e., steroids) have a hyperglycemic effect, the newly functioning kidney catabolizes the insulin, and the patient's appetite is often increased with resolution of the uremia due to the effect of the steroids. Patients should be aware that an unexplained and sustained rise in blood glucose may signal a problem with the transplanted kidney. Infection can cause a rise in blood glucose. Prolonged hypoglycemia may signify a reduction in kidney function and a potential rejection episode. If a rejection episode does occur, the medication to prevent the rejection likely will substantially increase blood glucose levels and, consequently, the insulin dose.

SIMULTANEOUS KIDNEY-PANCREAS TRANSPLANTATION

Kidney-pancreas transplantation restores both glucose metabolism and kidney function. Criteria for patient selection vary at each transplant center but typically include the diagnosis of type 1 diabetes, evidence of secondary complications such as moderate or severe neuropathy, metabolic instability, and adequate financial resources/insurance coverage. The complications of kidney-pancreas transplantation are cardiac incompetence, arterial or venous thrombosis, anastomotic leaks and bleeding, and side effects, which include immunosuppression, pancreatitis, and metabolic acidosis related to exocrine pancreatic function.

Renal transplant function is easier to measure than pancreas function. A rise in serum creatinine is a primary indicator of kidney rejection. A decrease in serum amylase or urinary amylase production can signal a jeopardized pancreas. Hyperglycemia occurs late in pancreas rejection. Signs of rejection can be detected earlier in the kidney and treatment can be initiated, thus providing some protection for the pancreas.

SUMMARY

Optimal control of blood glucose and blood pressure are the keys to the prevention of nephropathy. Early detection using the annual albumin-to-creatinine ratio will identify those who are at risk, and aggressive treatment may delay the progression of the disease. The nurse plays a vital role in prevention and detection. If the patient has developed ESRD, it is imperative that the nurse provide support to the patient and family when they are making a decision regarding treatment options.

FUTURE NURSING RESEARCH

Qualitative research is needed to develop a better understanding of how the diagnosis of ESRD affects the individual with diabetes and his or her family. Additional research issues may lie in the area of behavior-changing requirements that are specifically related to the lifestyle modification necessary for adapting to a diagnosis of diabetic nephropathy.

REFERENCES

1. Coresh J, Selvin E, Stevens LA, Manzi J, Kusek JW, et al.: Prevalence of chronic kidney disease in the United States. *JAMA* 298:2038–2047, 2007

2. United States Renal Data System: ESRD incidence and prevalence [Internet], 2007. Available from http://www.usrds.org/2007/pdf/02_incid_prev_07.pdf. Accessed 11 February 2009

3. National Diabetes Information Clearinghouse (NDIC): Complications of diabetes in the United States [Internet]. Available from http://diabetes. niddk.nih.gov/dm/pubs/statistics/index.htm#13. Accessed 22 October 2008

4. American Diabetes Association. Diabetic nephropathy (Position Statement). *Diabetes Care* 27 (Suppl. 1):S79–S83, 2004

5. Bode BW (Ed.): Nephropathy. In *Medical Management of Type 1 Diabetes*. 4th ed. Alexandria, VA, American Diabetes Association, 2004, p. 198–207

6. Nelson RG, Knowler WC, Pettitt DJ, Bennett PH: Kidney disease in diabetes. In *Diabetes in America*. 2nd ed. Bethesda, MD, National Diabetes Data Group, 1995, p. 349–370 (NIH publ. no. 95-1468)

7. Diabetes Control and Complications Trial Research Group: The effect of intensive treatment of diabetes on the development and progression of long-term complications in insulin-dependent diabetes. *N Engl J Med* 329:977–986, 1993

8. UK Prospective Diabetes Study Group: Intensive blood-glucose control with sulfonylureas or insulin compared with conventional treatment and risk of complications in patients with type 2 diabetes (UKPDS 33). *Lancet* 352:837–853, 1998

9. American Diabetes Association: Standards of medical care in diabetes—2009 (Position Statement). *Diabetes Care* 32 (Suppl. 1):S13–S61, 2009

10. Pfeettscher SA: Chronic renal failure and renal transplantation. In *Critical Care Nursing*. Bucher L, Melander S, Eds. Philadelphia, W.B. Saunders, 1999, p. 569–599

11. National Kidney Foundation: K/DOQI clinical practice guidelines for chronic kidney disease: evaluation, classification, and stratification [Internet], 2002. Available from http://www.kidney.org/professionals/kdoqi/guidelines_ckd/toc.htm. Accessed 22 October 2008

12. Gerich JE, Meyer C, Woerle HJ, Stumvoll M: Renal gluconeogenesis: its importance in human glucose homeostasis. *Diabetes Care* 26:382–391, 2001

13. DeFronzo RA: Diabetic nephropathy. In *Therapy for Diabetes Mellitus and Related Disorders*. 4th ed. Lebovitz HG, Ed. Alexandria, VA, American Diabetes Association, 2004, p. 369–397

14. Cryer PE: Hypoglycemic disorders. In *Hypoglycemia: Pathophysiology, Diagnosis, and Treatment*. New York, Oxford, 1997, p. 127–168

15. Tang, Z, Lee TH, Louie RF, Kost GJ: Effects of different hematocrit levels on glucose measurements with handheld meters for point-of-care testing. *Arch Pathol Lab Med* 124:1135–1140, 2000

16. Kleinbeck C: Challenges of diabetes and dialysis. *Diabetes Spectrum* 10:135–141, 1997

17. Nettina SM (Ed.): Renal and urinary disorders: chronic renal failure. In *Lippincott Manual of Nursing Practice*. 6th ed. Philadelphia, Lippincott-Raven, 1996, p. 610–615

18. National Kidney Foundation: Home hemodialysis [Internet]. Available from http://www.kidney.org/atoz/atozItem.cfm?id=74. Accessed 1 October 2008

19. Levey AS, Coresh J, Balk E, Kausz AT, Levin A, et al.: National Kidney Foundation practice guidelines for chronic kidney disease: evaluation, classification, and stratification. *Ann Intern Med* 139:137–147, 2003

Ms. Childs is a Diabetes Nurse Specialist at Mid-America Diabetes Associates, Wichita, KS.

12. Dental Issues in Patients with Diabetes

GERALYN SPOLLETT, MSN, C-ANP, CDE, AND
CHARLES A. CRAPE, DMD

Individuals with diabetes are two to three times more likely than those without the disease to develop dental problems such as caries, periodontal and oral mucosal diseases, and tooth loss. Dental problems can affect glycemic control and may lead to the vascular complications associated with diabetes. Inadequately controlled diabetes can complicate routine dental visits, as well as oral surgery and dental implant procedures. Maintaining appropriate blood glucose levels and following guidelines for good oral hygiene, including regular checkups, can reduce the incidence of dental problems.

PROMOTING DENTAL CARE

Nursing care of patients with diabetes should promote oral hygiene and prevention of dental disease as standard components of continuing diabetes management. Nurses need to emphasize routine dental care not only as a deterrent to tooth loss but also as an important measure in maintaining glycemic control. Patients must understand the integral relationship between dental care and glycemic control, in which a deterioration of one leads to the deterioration of the other.

The Centers for Disease Control and Prevention recommend that patients with diabetes see a dentist every 6 months and more frequently if periodontal disease is present (1). The American Diabetes Association Standards of Medical Care in Diabetes (2) includes an examination of the oral cavity in the initial visit but offers no guidelines for periodic dental examinations.

People with diabetes are less likely than those without diabetes to have had a recent dental examination. In a study by Tomar and Lester (3), subjects who had not seen a dentist in the preceding 12 months cited a lack of perceived need for dental care and an underappreciation of the relationship between oral health and general health. In fact, when compared with other preventive care services (a dilated eye examination and a podiatric examination), dental care visits were the least likely to have occurred.

Inadequate dental care has a strong socioeconomic basis. Patients pay a much larger portion of dental costs out of pocket than they do for most other health care services. Medicare has no provision for dental care, and Medicaid provides only limited coverage in some states. Tomar and Lester (3) found that the disparity in frequency of dental visits among racial, ethnic, and socioeconomic groups was greater than that for any other type of health care visit for subjects with diabetes. Among subjects whose annual household income was more than $50,000, 81.6% had seen a dentist in the preceding 12 months, compared with only 41.2% of those who earned less than $10,000 a year. Similar disparities did not exist for physician visits or foot examinations (3).

COMMON DENTAL PROBLEMS OF INDIVIDUALS WITH DIABETES

Although nursing care for people with diabetes focuses on promoting oral hygiene, nurses must recognize and understand the various dental diseases and conditions commonly found in their patients.

DENTAL CARIES AND GINGIVITIS

Maintaining oral hygiene and preventing dental caries is a necessary component in the overall health of people with diabetes. Tooth decay and loss can compromise the ability to chew nutritious foods such as fruits, vegetables, whole grain or fibrous starches, and meat-based protein. The ingestion of foods that are soft and easy to masticate often causes a sharp rise in glucose levels, affecting diabetes control. Dental treatments such as root canal and bridgework not only are uncomfortable but also require adjustments in food and insulin to maintain glucose control while the dental work is being done. Therefore, emphasis should be placed on the maintenance of excellent oral health and the preservation of tooth integrity.

Topical treatments, such as fluoride applications, fluoride mouth rinses, and salivary substitutes, can help prevent caries and also reduce dry mouth symptoms associated with diabetes.

Gingivitis, or inflammation of the gum tissue, is more prevalent in children and adults with diabetes, despite levels of plaque control similar to those of the general population (4). Patients with diabetes have more decayed and filled tooth surfaces, as well as a higher incidence of root caries, which may be associated with more gingival recession. Often, gingivitis progresses to periodontal disease and subsequent tooth loss. Patients who have partial or total tooth loss

Patient Education Topics for Promoting Oral Health

- Influences of diabetes on oral health
- Achieving glycemic control goals
- Tobacco cessation counseling
- Healthy eating habits
- Oral hygiene measures: routine and between-meal brushing, flossing, using a water pick device
- Topical fluoride applications and dental sealants
- Adjustments in daily diabetes regimen for dental appointments or procedures (e.g., fasting, changes in insulin or diet prior to oral surgery, soft or liquid diet after a procedure)

(edentulism) tend to be older and to have longer duration of disease. They also have higher glycated hemoglobin A1c (A1C) levels and higher rates of microvascular complications, i.e., retinopathy, nephropathy, neuropathy, peripheral arterial disease.

SALIVARY DYSFUNCTION AND XEROSTOMIA

Patients with type 2 diabetes show reduced salivary uptake and excretion (5), and they lack the protective components of saliva that help reduce oral bacteria. During episodes of hyperglycemia, glucose levels in the saliva can increase, providing a medium for bacterial growth. The resulting infection further increases glucose levels, and a vicious cycle of infection and hyperglycemia may ensue.

Xerostomia, or dry mouth, may be related to salivary dysfunction, polydipsia, changes in the salivary basement membranes, or dehydration associated with hyperglycemia. Diuretics, antihistamines, and antidepressants can also affect salivation and aggravate xerostomia.

Patients with xerostomia may experience difficulties in lubricating, masticating, tasting, and swallowing, which can alter nutritional intake and further affect glycemic control. Complications resulting from xerostomia include mucositis, ulcers, and desquamation, as well as opportunistic bacterial, viral, or fungal infections (6). Improvement in glycemic control may alleviate dry mouth and prevent further oral health problems.

ORAL MUCOSAL DISEASES

Oral mucosal diseases occur more frequently in patients with diabetes, perhaps as the result of chronic immunosuppression or acute hyperglycemia. Optimizing glycemic control is the key to prevention and treatment for each of these diseases.

Candidiasis. Fungal infections such as candidiasis are common in individuals with diabetes, particularly smokers with inadequately controlled glucose levels or patients who have dentures or other mouth appliances. Because candidiasis thrives in a warm, moist environment, denture wearers who have diabetes need to remove and clean their dentures daily to maintain healthy gums and oral membranes.

Persistent hyperglycemia can predispose patients to the development of oral candidiasis, which presents as white plaque on the oral mucosa and gums. The area of infection is usually tender and bleeds easily. Medications used to treat this condition are fluconazole and nystatin oral rinse.

Lichen planus. Lichen planus, a chronic mucocutaneous disease, appears to be an immunologically mediated process involving a hypersensitivity reaction at a microscopic level. The lesions associated with lichen planus can contain increased numbers of CD4, CD8, macrophages, dendritic cells, and other immune-regulating cells. Because the corticosteroids and immunomodulating drugs used to treat this condition can lead to hyperglycemia, diabetes therapy must be carefully regulated to reduce glucose levels that can inhibit the healing process.

Angular cheilitis. Angular cheilitis, a lesion that occurs at the outer corners of the mouth, is commonly associated with fungal infections. It is treated with an antifungal cream or an antifungal-steroid preparation applied to the area three to four times a day for 2 weeks. Again, improved glucose levels can help promote healing.

Burning mouth syndrome. Patients with burning mouth syndrome may complain of tongue or mucosal sensations when no lesion is present. Suboptimal glucose control, salivary dysfunction, candidiasis, and neurological abnormalities may all contribute to the syndrome. Treatment may include prescribing salivary substitutes or using benzodiazepine or tricyclic antidepressant therapy to reduce the burning sensation. Patients who decrease their alcohol and caffeine intake may also find relief. Interestingly, burning mouth syndrome has been found in patients with undiagnosed diabetes. When diabetes is diagnosed and glucose control achieved, the symptoms of burning mouth syndrome resolve.

Oral ulcers. Oral ulcers, whether the benign aphthous ulcers or the potentially fatal palatal ulcers, occur more frequently in the diabetic population and must be treated with care. Because individuals with diabetes tend to develop more severe infections, oral ulcers require aggressive management and evaluation by a dental professional.

PERIODONTAL DISEASE

The prevalence of periodontitis in patients with diabetes is 17%, compared with 9% in the nondiabetic population (7). The rate increases dramatically among smokers with diabetes, who are 20 times more likely to develop periodontitis with loss of supporting bone than individuals without diabetes (8). The incidence and severity of periodontal disease increase with inadequate glucose control, age, and duration of disease. Patients with inadequate glycemic control in either type 1 or type 2 diabetes have more interproximal loss of connective tissue attachment and alveolar bone loss than patients with well-controlled diabetes. Many factors contribute to the difficulty in preventing and treating periodontal disease in individuals with diabetes (Table 12.1).

Immune response. Although severe periodontal disease is related to increased plaque or calculus, other mechanisms may also play a role in the development of the disease (9). The presence of diabetes can activate a protective humoral immune response. Smoking and/or the presence of diabetes can alter neutrophil function, lowering the protective response and placing the patient at greater risk for infection. Impairment of the polymorphonuclear leukocyte also leaves the patient with

Table 12.1 Physiological Problems in the Patient with Diabetes That Make Treating Periodontal Disease Difficult

- Increased susceptibility to infection
- Impaired wound-healing ability
- Magnified inflammatory response
- Vascular changes
  - Inhibition of vasodilation
  - Vasoconstriction
  - Accelerated atherosclerosis
  - Focal thrombosis
- Neuropathies from accelerated connective tissue damage
- Gingival changes compromising periodontal integrity

From Hein (7).

a reduced defense against gram-negative microbial infection. Any defect in the function of the polymorphonuclear leukocyte may mean a shift in the balance between destruction and repair in the initiation or progression of periodontal disease (9).

Collagen formation. Hyperglycemia reduces the growth of the fibroblast, an essential element in the building of collagen for the peridontium. A fine balance between destruction and repair of the periodontal tissue already exists; therefore, any element that decreases collagen formation will result in a loss of tissue turnover and will ultimately affect periodontal integrity. Patients with diabetes have an alteration in collagen metabolism and suppressed white blood cell function. Together, these factors increase susceptibility to periodontal infection and reduce healing.

Patients with diabetes may also have an increased level of collagenase, an enzyme that, when activated, can lead to the loss of connective tissue attachment. The decreased formation of collagen and the increased production of collagenase alter the homeostasis within the periodontal tissues (10). This is commonly manifested by "loose teeth," which limit the patient's ability to properly chew food. Once this connective tissue attachment is lost, it cannot be regenerated and usually leads to multiple tooth extractions.

Wound healing and recovery time. Advanced glycosylation end products (AGEs), the result of prolonged hyperglycemia, may alter wound healing and contribute to the severity of periodontal disease. AGEs can change the solubility of collagen and alter its turnover rate. Not only do AGEs bind to phagocytes, initiating an inflammatory response to the bacteria present in the mouth, but they can also activate collagenase. AGEs may also cause a thickening of the basement membrane of blood vessels, which further compromises the wound healing process by inhibiting the activation or exchange of nutrition, oxygen, and various antibodies (10).

Glucose control affects recovery time after treatment of periodontal disease. In one study, patients with well-controlled diabetes had an uneventful recovery, whereas those with inadequately controlled diabetes did well initially but had a more rapid reoccurrence of pockets and a less favorable prognosis (11). Sustaining long-term metabolic control in patients with diabetes is necessary to ensure periodontal health (12). A collaborative effort between dental health providers and the diabetes care team is essential in achieving positive outcomes in periodontal care.

Systemic effects. Periodontal disease has been associated with atherosclerosis and coronary heart disease, particularly in those with diabetes and smokers (13,14). This was also demonstrated in other studies that found that those with severe periodontal disease had 3.2 times greater risk for cardiorenal mortality (15) and for macroalbuminuria and end stage renal disease (16). While more research needs to be done to explore for a causal link, treating the inflammatory nature of periodontal disease may positively influence the severity of diabetes and its complications.

Treatment. In some patients, undiagnosed periodontal disease may disrupt glucose control and increase A1C values. Periodontitis-induced bacteremia may elevate serum proinflammatory cytokines, leading to hyperlipidemia and furthering insulin resistance. Treatment of the dental problem is important to improve glycemic control (17).

PRACTICAL POINT

Advanced periodontitis can present with diffuse gingival inflammation and generalized bleeding of the gum tissue on examination. Patients may complain of "tender gums" that bleed whenever they brush their teeth. This discomfort may lead to increased reluctance to pursue oral hygiene. During treatment for periodontitis, patients must follow specific hygienic measures: use of an automatic toothbrush, interdental cleaning, irrigation with a water pick, and mild abrasive dentifrices (7). Patients with periodontitis will also need more frequent checkups.

Antibiotics, particularly tetracycline and doxycycline, have been prescribed for periodontitis. These drugs seem to reduce the formation of collagenase and/or inhibit the degradation of collagen. They are used with mechanical therapy and may help reduce glucose levels by controlling the infection. Mechanical therapy alone does not completely eliminate periodontal disease when the organisms have invaded connective tissue (7). Chronic gram-negative periodontal infection triggers and sustains systemic inflammation (18).

DENTAL VISITS

To prevent hypoglycemic episodes during the dental examination, the patient must have proper food intake before the appointment. However, some procedures, such as conscious sedation, may require the patient to withhold food for a period of time before or after the procedure (19). In these cases, a reduction in the amount of medication or insulin may be necessary. To avoid hypoglycemia, patients should not schedule the dental appointment during the hours of peak insulin activity or at a usual mealtime. If a hypoglycemic event occurs, the dental procedure should be stopped and 15 g carbohydrate administered. Glucose tabs or gel are often the quickest and easiest form of treatment, and patients should be advised to carry these easy to administer forms of glucose to every dental visit.

Certain dental surgeries should not be done during episodes of severe hyperglycemia because of the higher risk for infection and poor wound healing. One study showed that the risk of infection was linked to higher fasting glucose level (20). Patients with levels <206 mg/dl had no increased risk, whereas patients with glucose levels >230 mg/dl had an 80% risk of developing infection.

MANAGING DENTAL IMPLANTS

Inadequate glycemic control can hinder the success of dental implant procedures. Diabetes-related inhibition of collagen matrix formation and alterations in protein synthesis can affect bone production and repair. Insulin helps modulate normal skeletal growth by stimulating bone matrix synthesis. Through direct and indirect processes, insulin can alter bone turnover rates, decrease the number of osteoblasts and osteoclasts, and reduce osteocalcin. Changes in bone metabolism, association of AGEs with extracellular matrix components, and level of glucose control may influence osseointegration and reduce the percentage of bone-to-implant contact (21).

PRACTICAL POINT

The timing of a patient's dental visit may affect the daily diabetes treatment program. Nurses may need to counsel patients about changes in food or medication schedules as determined by the procedure to be done and the length of recovery. Blood glucose checks should be done before the dental visit and after the procedure, and action should be taken to correct levels outside of the acceptable range for control.

The 1998 National Institutes of Health Consensus Development Conference Statement on Dental Implants (22) underlines the importance of glucose control in patients seeking dental implants. Patients with inadequately controlled diabetes should not be considered candidates for these procedures. A careful preoperative assessment must determine that a patient has no contraindications, but at present there are no established guidelines for selecting candidates for dental implants in the diabetic population. A risk factor analysis for implant loss looks at a variety of issues: type of diabetes, duration of disease, diabetes treatment program, current and previous glycemic control, history of periodontitis, amount of tooth loss, smoking history, and poor wound-healing history.

In the initial evaluation, some dental centers perform a complete blood cell count, fasting glucose, A1C, prothrombin, and partial thromboplastin times. If metabolic control is clinically inadequate, the implant procedure is delayed until glucose levels are within the set parameters. To reduce the risk of infection, a

10-day regimen of a broad-spectrum antibiotic may be prescribed and initiated the day before the procedure (23).

Postoperatively, high circulating levels of glucose reduce wound healing and increase rates of infection, compromising the success of the implant procedure. Strict glucose control and meticulous oral hygiene are vital components of post-procedure care. During this time, patients are encouraged to stop smoking to reduce the risk of implant failure.

SUMMARY

Dental care needs to figure more prominently in the standards for periodic examinations and continuing care of people with diabetes. Just as nurses guide and encourage patients to have routine foot and eye examinations, they must also promote dental checkups as an important component of diabetes management. To help patients make this goal a reality, financial support for dental care must be more readily available to both the general population and individuals with chronic illness. As patient advocates, nurses must help payers to see the importance of dental health in preserving health and function in individuals with diabetes.

REFERENCES

1. Centers for Disease Control and Prevention: *The Prevention and Treatment of Complications of Diabetes, 1991.* Atlanta, GA, U.S. Department of Health and Human Services, Public Health Service, 1991

2. American Diabetes Association: Standards of medical care in diabetes—2009 (Position Statement). *Diabetes Care* 32 (Suppl. 1):S13–S61, 2009

3. Tomar SL, Lester A: Dental and other health care visits among U.S. adults with diabetes. *Diabetes Care* 23:1505–1510, 2000

4. Pinson M, Hoffman WH, Garnick JJ, Litaker MS: Periodontal disease and type 1 diabetes mellitus in children and adolescents. *J Clin Periodontol* 22: 118–123, 1995

5. Kao CH, Tsai SC, Sun SS: Scintigraphic evidence of poor salivary function in type 2 diabetes. *Diabetes Care* 24:952–953, 2001

6. Vernillo AT: Diabetes mellitus: relevance to dental treatment. *Oral Surg Oral Med Oral Pathol Oral Radiol Endod* 91:263–270, 2001

7. Hein C: "Getting it right" in long-term management of chronic periodontitis associated with diabetes, part 1. *Contemporary Oral Hygiene* 3:24–31, 2003

8. Haber J, Wattles J, Crowley M, Mandell R, Joshipura K, Kent RL: Evidence for cigarette smoking as a major risk factor for periodontal disease. *J Periodontol* 64:16–23, 1993

9. Ryan ME, Oana C, Kamer A: The influence of diabetes on the periodontal tissues. *J Am Dent Assoc* 143 (Suppl.):34S–40S, 2003

10. Mattson JS, Cerutis DR: Diabetes mellitus: a review of the literature and dental implications. *Compendium* 22:757–772, 2001

11. Tervonen T, Karjalainen K: Periodontal disease related to diabetics' status: a pilot study of the response to periodontal therapy in type 1 diabetes. *J Clin Periodontol* 24:505–510, 1997

12. Oringer RJ, Research, Science, and Therapy Committee of the American Academy of Periodontology: Modulation of the host response in periodontal therapy. *J Periodontol* 73:460–470, 2002

13. Boehm TK, Scannapieco FA: The epidemiology, consequences and management of periodontal disease in older adults. *J Am Dent Assoc* 138 (Suppl.): 26S–33S, 2007

14. Geismer K, Stoltze K, Sigurd B, Gyntelberg F, Holmstrup P: Periodontal disease and coronary heart disease. *J Periodontol* 77:1547–1554, 2006

15. Saremi A, Nelson RG, Tullock-Reid M, Hanson RL, Sievers ML, et al.: Periodontal disease and mortality in type 2 diabetes. *Diabetes Care* 28:27–32, 2005

16. Shultis WA, Weil EJ, Looker HC, Curtis JM, Shlossman M, et al.: Effect of periodontitis on overt nephropathy and end-stage renal disease in type 2 diabetes. *Diabetes Care* 30:306–311, 2007

17. Iacopino AM: Periodontitis and diabetes interrelationships: role of inflammation. *Ann Periodontol* 6:125–137, 2001

18. Grossi SG: Treatment of periodontal disease and control of diabetes: an assessment of the evidence and need for future research. *Ann Periodontol* 6:138–145, 2001

19. Lalla RV, D'Ambrosio JA: Dental management considerations for the patient with diabetes mellitus. *J Am Dent Assoc* 132:1425–1432, 2001

20. Golden SH, Peart-Vigilance C, Kao WH, Brancati FL: Perioperative glycemic control and the risk of infectious complications in a cohort of adults with diabetes. *Diabetes Care* 22:1408–1414, 1999

21. Fiorellini JP, Nevins ML: Dental implant considerations in the diabetic patient. *Periodontol* 23:73–77, 2000

22. National Institutes of Health: Consensus Development Conference Statement on Dental Implants June 13–15, 1998. *J Dent Educ* 52:824–827, 1998

23. Abdulwassie H, Dhanrajani PJ: Diabetes mellitus and dental implants: a clinical study. *Implant Dentistry* 11:83–85, 2002

Ms. Spollett is an Adult Nurse Practitioner at Yale Diabetes Center, New Haven, CT. Dr. Crape has a private practice in Milford, CT.

13. Dermatological Changes Associated with Diabetes

Geralyn Spollett, MSN, C-ANP, CDE

Just as diabetes interferes with the physiology of the microvasculature of the eye and kidney, it similarly affects the small vessels of the skin, which may lead to skin changes (1). Dyslipidemia and other metabolic changes associated with diabetes can also create dermatological changes. Autoimmune skin diseases such as vitiligo can occur in autoimmune, or type 1, diabetes. In rare cases, medications that are used in the treatment of diabetes can cause adverse skin reactions. In general, how the disruption of normal insulin and glucose metabolism affects the skin is not completely understood (1).

NECROBIOSIS LIPOIDICA DIABETICORUM

Necrobiosis lipoidica diabeticorum (NLD), one of the least common diabetic lesions, has no known etiology (Fig. 13.1). In general, this type of lesion is seen in individuals with diabetes of long duration, but its progression seems to have little to do with glucose control (1). NLD occurs in 0.3–1.6% of individuals with diabetes and is three times more common in women than in men (2). When the lesion occurs in people who do not have diabetes, many of these patients (~90%) go on to develop impaired glucose tolerance or are found to have a family history of diabetes (3). Therefore, screening for diabetes in these individuals is highly recommended.

The NLD lesion progresses through a series of changes, beginning as a shiny, demarcated dusky pink plaque that is slightly elevated. Size varies from 1 to 3 cm to ~25 cm, and over time, it becomes redder and can take on a brownish tinge. As the weeks and months progress, it becomes atrophic, with a thin, shiny, slightly pigmented appearance. The center may have a yellowish tinge, indicating a loss of collagen or severe thinning of the skin, making the subcutaneous fat visible. The lesion may initially present as a series of closely grouped small plaques that coalesce into a larger plaque over time. Usually, the lesions are not painful, but they may be pruritic or tender (4). With thinning, the plaque becomes susceptible to ulceration, and the most minor trauma can cause a rupture. The resulting ulcers are painful and very difficult to heal. Approximately 20% of NLD lesions will resolve spontaneously after 6–12 years (5).

Classically, NLD occurs bilaterally on the pretibial or medial malleolar areas. Lesions can also present on the hands, forearms, abdomen, face, and scalp, but these locations are less often associated with diabetes.

There are no standard guidelines for the treatment of NLD. Middle- to high-potency topical steroids with or without occlusion, intralesional injections of steroids at the active border, and, in some instances, systemic steroids have been used in the treatment of NLD (6). Other treatments such as cyclosporine, psoralen and ultraviolet A light (PUVA), high-dose nicotinamide, clofazimine, pentoxifylline, aspirin, and dipyridamole have been tried with varying rates of success (2). Laser treatment may help reduce bleeding and improve the appearance of the lesion (7). In severe cases, synthetic hydrocolloid dressings have given symptomatic relief. Specialized wound care clinics are best equipped to treat the ulcerated lesions and may use artificial skin substitutes in an attempt to resurface these areas.

GRANULOMA ANNULARE

Although granuloma annulare (GA) is not associated with diabetes, lesion presentation is so similar to NLD that a connection between GA and diabetes has been sought. The initial presentation is small, flesh-colored papule(s) that progress to one larger plaque. The papules may arrange in an annular fashion. The dermal plaques have a ring border and a depressed center. The lesions may be pruritic but are not painful. Histological testing shows collagen degeneration, chronic inflammation, and fibrosis (6). Commonly, lesions appear over the extensor joint areas in children and young adults and may be more generally distributed in middle-aged to older adults. In its more generalized form, plaques are smaller, and hundreds of small lesions may be present. Controversy exists concerning the association of diabetes with this generalized form of GA. At this time, screening for diabetes is recommended for individuals with this form of GA.

Treatment for GA is similar to that for NLD: topical, intralesional, and general steroid use. Other forms of treatment include cryosurgery, ultraviolet-light therapy, and Co2 laser (8). Localized GA remits spontaneously without scarring, but the more generalized version has a longer course with rare spontaneous resolution (2). The duration is variable. It is generally self-limited, and 50% of patients are without lesions within 2 years; however, 40% can experience reoccurrence at the same site (6).

DIABETIC DERMOPATHY

Diabetic dermopathy, also known as shin spots or pigmented pretibial papules, is by far the most common cutaneous manifestation of diabetes (Fig. 13.2). Although it can be present in individuals without diabetes, it is found in as many as 40% of people with diabetes. It occurs more frequently in men aged >50 years (2).

The pigmented shin spots, usually seen on the extensor surfaces of the lower legs, begin as circumscribed round or oval red papules that progress to atrophic hyperpigmented macules. A fine scale over the surface of the macule is sometimes seen. The lesions are usually bilateral but have an asymmetric distribution. They may also appear on the forearms, thighs, and lateral malleoli (2). Histological findings indicate edema of the papillary dermis, thickened superficial blood vessels, extravasation of erythrocytes, and a mild lymphocytic infiltrate (9). Diabetic dermopathy differs from NLD in that the collagen change is much less marked and necrobiosis is absent (10). The lesions of diabetic dermopathy are asymptomatic but may become painful if they ulcerate.

Patients may comment that the lesions occurred after a trauma. Research findings indicate that the blood flow values at dermopathy sites are similar to those found at scar sites. It is possible that the skin scarring seen in dermopathy relates to poor skin perfusion associated with diabetes. However, blood flow studies also indicate that diabetic dermopathy lesions do not represent local ischemia (11).

Although some studies link diabetic dermopathy with the microvascular complications of diabetes, such as nephropathy and retinopathy, other studies have been unable to substantiate these findings. Capillary changes may predispose to shin spots but are not the only cause of this condition (2). Blood glucose control is unrelated to the occurrence or progression of the problem, and there is no effective treatment for these lesions. New lesions appear while old lesions spontaneously heal and leave small scars in their place.

There is no effective treatment. Patients should prevent skin breakdown and infection by using moisturizers and avoiding trauma to the area (8).

DIABETIC BULLAE

Diabetic bullae, also known as bullosis diabeticorum, are a clinically distinct marker for diabetes (Fig. 13.3) often reported in adults with diabetes of long duration and neuropathy. Usually confined to the hands and feet, the blisters occur spontaneously and can be a few millimeters to several centimeters in size.

There are three types of diabetic bullae: *1*) sterile and fluid filled, *2*) hemorrhagic, and *3*) multiple, nonscarring bullae on tanned skin. Of these, only the hemorrhagic type leaves scarring. The bullae resolve spontaneously without treatment in 2–3 weeks but may reoccur in the same or a different anatomical place.

Preventing infection is a major focus in caring for these lesions. Thorough cleaning, topical antibiotics, and clean dressings on a daily basis will reduce the occurrence of infection. The bullae fluid can be aspirated, but the blister roof should be preserved and used as a physiological cover for the wound.

ACANTHOSIS NIGRICANS

Acanthosis nigricans (AN) is characterized by velvety, light brown to black hyperpigmented plaques that appear in the folds of the skin (Fig. 13.4). The thickened skin is most commonly seen around the neck and axillae. Other affected areas include the groin, umbilicus, submammary regions, and hands. It initially presents with hyperpigmentation, which is then followed by a hypertrophy of the epidermis (9).

Although there are eight different forms of AN, the one most commonly seen in diabetes is associated with insulin resistance and obesity. The pathogenesis may be related to insulin-like growth factor receptors on the keratinocytes and dermal fibroblasts, stimulating growth (2). The dark color of these plaques is related to the thickness of the keratin-containing superficial epithelium. AN has been linked to impaired glucose tolerance in younger patients and, as a marker, can serve to alert providers to screen the patient for diabetes. Certain forms of AN are associated with carcinoma (stomach adenocarcinoma) and various endocrinopathies. The sudden appearance of AN after the age of 40 years is an ominous sign. When malignancy is present, the lesion develops suddenly and progresses rapidly. Despite a strong association with diabetes, all AN lesions warrant a workup to rule out underlying causes, the most common of which are pineal tumors, occult malignancies, stomach adenocarcinoma, and drug use (nicotinic acid, estrogen, corticosteroids) (6).

Lesions are usually asymptomatic. Although there is no specific treatment for AN related to diabetes, weight loss and improvement in glucose control, with a lowering of insulin resistance, can improve the condition. Retinoic and salicylic acid may help cosmetic appearance.

DIABETIC THICK SKIN

Diabetic thick skin has been reported in as many as 33% of individuals with diabetes (1) and has been divided into three categories: *1*) scleroderma-like changes of the hand associated with stiff joints and limited mobility, *2*) measurable skin thickness, and *3*) scleredema diabeticorum. The etiology of diabetic thick skin is not fully known. The skin has abnormal collagen accumulation that may be related to hyperglycemic accelerated nonenzymatic glycosylation. A second theory identifies insulin, acting as a growth factor, as causing an overproduction and buildup of collagen.

Tiny pebble-like papules that become confluent appear on the back of the hand, the knuckles, and along the fingernails. Patients may report difficulty completely extending fingers, and slight contractures of the palmar surface (Dupuytren's contracture) may be seen.

Diabetic scleredema (Fig. 13.5) is characterized by diffuse nonpitting induration of the skin with loss of skin markings over the upper back, neck, and shoulders (2). It can extend to the face, arms, chest, and abdomen. The condition is usually asymptomatic, but the lack of skin flexibility may cause neck and back discomfort. Scleredema occurs in 2.5–14% of individuals with type 2 diabetes.

Improved glucose control and use of potent topical and intralesional steroids, penicillamine, intralesional insulin, bath PUVA, low-dose methotrexate, prostaglandin E1, and pentoxifylline have had limited therapeutic success in the treatment of scleredema (2).

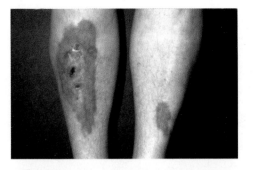

Figure 13.1 Necrobiosis lipoidica diabeticorum. Yellow tinge at the center of the lesion is caused by a lack of collagen.

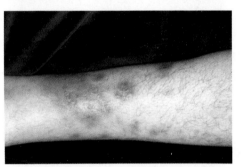

Figure 13.2 Diabetic dermopathy. The most common dermatologic lesion, usually seen in the lower extremities.

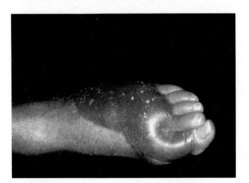

Figure 13.3 Diabetic bullae. Large fluid-filled sacs usually found on the hands are a marker for diabetes.

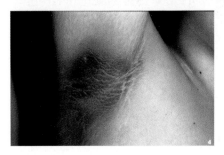

Figure 13.4 Acanthosis nigricans. The dark, velvety appearance of this condition is usually seen in the skinfolds of the neck and axillae.

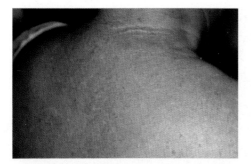

Figure 13.5 Diabetic scleredema. The thickened, nonpitting skin of this condition can affect the flexibility of the upper back, shoulders, and neck.

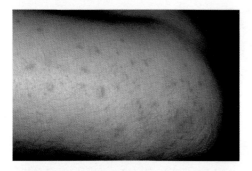

Figure 13.6 Xanthomas. This condition can result from elevated cholesterol, particularly hypertriglyceridemia. Note the pearly color of the lesions.

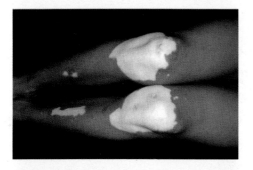

Figure 13.7 Vitiligo. Usually associated with autoimmune type 1 diabetes, loss of skin pigment accounts for the white color of this lesion.

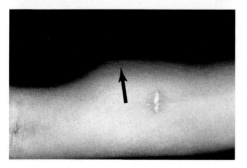

Figure 13.8 Lipohypertrophy. Usually appears in an area of repeated insulin injections.

XANTHOMA

Xanthomas usually appear as a consequence of hyperlipidemia, particularly hyper-triglyceridemia associated with diabetes (Fig. 13.6). Triglyceride levels are often >800 mg/dl and may exceed 1,500 or 2,000 mg/dl (1). Cutaneous xanthomas are a result of an extracellular deposition of lipid in the form of cholesterol or triglyc-erides in the dermis or subcutaneous fat (4). Biopsy of the xanthomas will show lipid-laden macrophages in the mid-dermis. The eruptive lesions develop sud-denly over the extensor surfaces of the arms, legs, and buttocks, originally as red papules but subsequently changing to yellow. The lesion may remain as scattered individual papules or may cluster and form a "rosette."

Diabetes and lipid control play key roles in the resolution of the lesions. If the patient is insulin depleted, as in diabetic ketoacidosis, a rapid correction of glucose levels will lead to a faster resolution of the lesions. However, if the problem is based on chronically elevated triglycerides, once correction of lipid chemistry is achieved, it may take several weeks before the lesions fully respond.

VITILIGO

Vitiligo, an absence of melanocytes that causes hypopigmentation of the skin, can be seen in patients with autoimmune diseases such as type 1 diabetes, Addison's disease, Hashimoto's thyroiditis, and pernicious anemia (Fig. 13.7). The lympho-cytes attack the melanocytes, resulting in chalk-white lesions on the skin that are commonly found over extensor joints such as the elbow and knuckles and around orifices such as the mouth and eye. Although vitiligo can occur in children as well as adults and is found in 0.2–1.0% of the general population, it appears in ~5% of individuals with diabetes (1).

Most patients continue to see new patches of vitiligo throughout their lives. It is not symptomatic but can be disfiguring in darker-skinned people. There is no cor-rective treatment, but some benefit has been seen with potent topical steroid use.

SKIN INFECTION

Skin infections in patients with well-controlled diabetes occur at the same rate and severity as in the general population. However, those with suboptimal gly-cemic control have more frequent infections that are more severe and difficult to resolve. Approximately 20–50% of those with type 2 diabetes experience a skin infection (3). Elevated glucose levels cause numerous immunological dys-functions that make the patient more vulnerable to infection and impede the healing process. With hyperglycemia, leukocytes are not able to move through the thickened capillary wall as effectively, phagocytic action is reduced, and chemotaxis is delayed, allowing an infection to worsen. Neuropathy and periph-eral vascular disease can mask the symptoms of the infection, permitting it to advance unchecked. The presence of the infection further elevates glucose lev-els, contributing to the cycle of hyperglycemia and lengthening the recovery process.

Staphylococcal and fungal infections, particularly of the lower extremities, develop more often in patients with diabetes and are more resistant to therapy. For some patients, the skin infections become chronic problems, promoting skin breakdown and placing them at risk for more severe secondary infections.

Candida infections of the vagina, anogenital area, submammary regions, and axillae tend to be recurrent and occur most frequently in obese patients with type 2 diabetes. In men, the folds of the foreskin and coronal rim of the penis are sites for balanitis and phimosis. Difficult to keep clean and dry, these skinfold areas provide the ideal warm, moist environment for dermatophyte growth. The location of the infection makes applying topical antibacterial or antifungal creams an arduous task, and patients may not complete the full course of therapy, allowing some of the infective agent to persist.

Candidiasis can affect the interdigital web spaces of the hands with eroded patches and inflammatory papules. Frequent hand washing or jobs in which the hands are continually moist predispose to the infection. This condition is called interdigitalis blastomycetia (8).

If the patient suspects an infection, the health care provider should be notified immediately so that treatment can begin as soon as possible. In the individual with inadequately controlled diabetes, the course of therapy may be longer than in the general population, and the patient must understand that to eradicate the infection, the therapy must be used consistently and the course of medication or topical treatment completed.

Skin infections that involve the lower extremities can have severe consequences. Foot ulcers are a leading causative factor in amputations (9). The podiatric emergency and preventive foot care guidelines are discussed in chapter 15. The importance of these guidelines in preventing foot infection or injuries that lead to infection cannot be overemphasized.

PRACTICAL POINT

Prevention of skin infections begins with good personal hygiene, i.e., inspecting and washing areas at highest risk for bacterial or fungal growth. The patient may need assistance from a family member or may need to find creative solutions for accessing hard-to-reach areas, such as using a long-handled sponge to wash and a handheld hair dryer (set to low) to dry the area or a squirt bottle with warm water to help cleanse the anogenital area.

PRACTICAL POINT

Since many patients with neuropathy have impaired sensation, education regarding skin care must emphasize the need to assess the area for changes in color or temperature or the presence of swelling or discharge.

> ## PRACTICAL POINT
>
> When caring for a patient with diabetes, it is important to remember that in areas of reduced blood flow such as the feet, systemic antibiotics used to treat skin infections have difficulty permeating the tissue and their effectiveness is reduced, necessitating a longer time frame for treatment.

INSULIN ALLERGIES AND SKIN MANIFESTATIONS

Although rare, cutaneous reactions to insulin have been reported, usually as raised, warm, itchy nodules forming at the injection site that appear 15 min to 2 h postinjection. With the production of purified and recombinant insulins, the incidence of insulin allergy has been reduced. In some instances, the skin reaction is not to the insulin itself but to the latex of the vial stopper, the alcohol or cleanser used to prepare the injection site, or an intradermal rather than a subcutaneous injection.

True insulin allergy with systemic response such as urticaria or anaphylaxis is rare. Treatment involves a desensitization program that is generally carried out under medical observation.

Use of purified and recombinant insulin has reduced the occurrence of lipoatrophy, a hollowing of the skin at the injection site. More common is the problem of lipohypertrophy in areas of repeated insulin injections (Fig. 13.8). These large fatty-like deposits in the subcutaneous tissue can be disfiguring but are not physically painful. In fact, patients may continue to inject into the area because the sensation of administering the insulin is blunted. However, the continued use of a hypertrophied area may reduce insulin absorption and interfere with glucose control. Ceasing insulin injections at the hypertrophied site allows the skin to return to its normal state. Hypertrophy is avoided by rotating injection sites within anatomical areas and carefully observing the skin's reaction to injections.

Of the oral agents currently on the market, sulfonylureas are most likely to cause dermatological side effects. The sulfa component of the drug can produce an allergic reaction that usually presents as an uncomfortable "measles-like" maculopapular rash. The most common offenders are the first-generation sulfonylureas, such as tolbutamide and chlorpropamide, medications that are rarely used. Occasionally, glyburide, a second-generation drug, has caused urticaria, photosensitivity, erythema, and pruritus; these symptoms disappear with drug discontinuation. Sensitivity to a sulfonylurea may indicate that the patient will react adversely to other sulfa medications. Caution should be used in prescribing any sulfa-containing medication.

SUMMARY

Preventive skin care education that centers on improved hygiene and early assessment and intervention for any suspected skin condition is a key component of nursing care. Many of the lesions associated with diabetes, such as NLD and diabetic bullae, have no prescribed protocol for treatment. The various trials of different forms of treatment, the consistent daily attention that the care of these lesions requires, and the long duration of the self-care process can be a heavy burden for the patient. Supportive nursing care and education enable the patient to understand the condition and be alert for any signs or symptoms of secondary infection.

In other skin conditions, such as xanthomas and injection-site hypertrophy, addressing and treating the underlying cause is an essential component of care. For xanthomas, improved glucose control and lipid management must be achieved for resolution of the lesions to occur. In hypertrophy, patient education regarding insulin injection site rotation and its importance in both skin care and glucose control is central to the plan of care.

In AN, the nurse must realize that not all cases are related to diabetes and that sudden appearance and rapid progression of the lesion may indicate a life-threatening medical condition. Noting changes in size and texture of AN lesions and documenting them provides vital information for future assessment and analysis.

Patients with diabetes are just as susceptible to skin cancer as the general population. However, sunburns not only increase the risk of carcinoma, but they can also cause the breakdown of fragile skin, leading to infection, hyperglycemia, and disruption of glucose control. The patient must be educated in sun protection guidelines to avoid these negative consequences.

REFERENCES

1. Reeves JRT: Skin changes associated with diabetes. In *Medical Management of Diabetes Mellitus*. Leahy JL, Clark NG, Cefalu WT, Eds. New York, Marcel Dekker, 2000, p. 539–558

2. Ferringer T, Miller OF: Cutaneous manifestations of diabetes mellitus. *Derm Clin North Am* 20:483–493, 2002

3. Paron NG, Lambert PW: Cutaneous manifestations of diabetes mellitus. *Prim Care* 27:371–383, 2000

4. Jelinek JE: Cutaneous markers of diabetes mellitus. In *The Skin in Diabetes*. Jelinek JE, Ed. Philadelphia, Lea and Febiger, 1986, p. 31–72

5. Sibbald RG, Landolt SJ, Toth D: Skin and diabetes. *Endocrinol Metab Clin North Am* 25:463–472, 1996

6. Habif TP, Campbell JL, Quitadamo MJ, Zug KA: Cutaneous manifestations of internal disease. In Skin Diseases: *Diagnosis and Treatment*. St. Louis, MO, Mosby, 2001, p. 458–471

7. Bello YM, Phillips TJ: Necrobiosis lipoidica. *Postgrad Med* 109:93–94, 2001

8. Reddy SG, Meffert JJ, Kraus EW, Becker LE: Dermatologic conditions in patients with diabetes. *Pract Diabetol* 27:6–10, 2008

9. Chakrabarty A, Norman RA, Phillips TJ: Cutaneous manifestations of diabetes. *Wounds* 14:267–274, 2002

10. Sibbald RG, Schachter RK: The skin and diabetes mellitus. *Int J Dermatol* 23:567–584, 1984

11. Wigington G, Binh N, Rendell M: Skin blood flow in diabetic dermopathy. *Arch Dermatol* 140:1248–1250,2004

Ms. Spollett is an Adult Nurse Practitioner at Yale Diabetes Center, New Haven, CT.

14. Peripheral and Autonomic Neuropathy

Wendy Kushion, RN, MSN, APRN-BC, CDE

Diabetic neuropathy is a chronic disorder that affects both the peripheral nervous system (sensory and motor) and the autonomic nervous system (ANS). It is the most common of all the long-term complications of diabetes and the least understood. Neuropathy usually has a slow progression. It may appear with obvious symptoms, sometimes as the presenting symptom of previously undiagnosed diabetes, or it may be hidden and discovered only by careful testing. Symptoms of peripheral neuropathy (PN) often start with numbness and paresthesia in the toes and feet and later appear in the fingers and hands. Autonomic neuropathy affects innervation to all of the organs of the body and can cause dysfunction in any body part (1,2).

The precise pathogenesis of neuropathy in diabetes is unknown. Chronic hyperglycemia, insulin deficiency, nerve ischemia, microvascular disease, and nonenzymatic glycation have been suggested as the major causative factors in the development of neuropathy (2–4). Chronic hyperglycemia has historically been blamed and is reported to cause oxidative stress, which may cause nerve injury (5). Neuropathy may be present at the time of diagnosis, or it may take years before symptoms arise. Most people with diabetes will develop symptoms of neuropathy over time, and these can cause minor to extreme physical symptoms.

PERIPHERAL NEUROPATHY

PN results from widely distributed lesions throughout the peripheral nerves. Distal symmetric polyneuropathy is the most widely recognized form of PN and the most easily recognized. The deficit is distributed over all sensorimotor nerves and starts in the most distal areas first, usually the toes and feet. PN usually begins with an early involvement of the long axons in the peripheral nerves, which is the

Signs and Symptoms of Peripheral Neuropathy

- Pain and numbness
- "Glove and stocking" sensory loss
- Diminished deep tendon reflexes
- Diminished sense of position and light-touch sensation
- Numbness, tingling, or feeling of cold feet
- Diminished or increased pain and temperature sensation
- Motor weakness
- Impaired balance
- Diminished proprioception and position sense
- Absent or reduced vibration sensation
- Ataxia
- Increased cutaneous hypersensitivity
- Extreme pain
- Distal muscle cramps
- Cranial nerve palsy
- Carpal tunnel or tarsal tunnel syndrome

characteristic lesion of neuropathy. Height plays a role because the longer the nerve fiber, the greater its vulnerability to injury (3,4).

Classes of PN are usually grouped into "diffuse" or "focal" types. Diffuse neuropathies include distal symmetric polyneuropathy and autonomic neuropathy. Focal neuropathies involve single or multiple peripheral nerves and are categorized as mononeuropathy, radiculopathy, or entrapment neuropathy.

DISTAL SYMMETRICAL POLYNEUROPATHY

This most common diffuse neuropathy begins in the toes and moves up the legs, causing a "stocking" pattern of sensory loss, with later upper-extremity "glove" sensory loss in the fingers and moving up the arms. Sensory deficits are more noticeable and common than motor deficits. Small-fiber sensory neurons are affected first, with loss of pain and temperature sensation. Large sensory fiber loss later occurs, with a loss of vibratory and light-touch sensation, proprioception, and then gait and balance deficits. A diminished Achilles tendon reflex is also an early symptom (2,4,6). Motor weakness can occur in PN and appears as wasting of the small muscles of the hands and feet.

Testing. Testing includes a clinical assessment of sensitivity to light touch, position, Achilles tendon reflex, vibratory sensation (tuning fork), and sensation using a 10-g monofilament (see also chapter 15). A thorough history of all symptoms and duration is essential to determine the extent of neuropathy. Nerve function tests may include quantitative sensory tests, nerve conduction studies, and electromyography. These tests evaluate the evidence of the specific sensory or motor nerve problem, its distribution and severity, and the underlying pathology (6).

Treatment. The initial and most effective treatment of PN is intensive glycemic control. The Diabetes Control and Complications Trial (DCCT) demonstrated that intensive insulin therapy decreases the development and progression of PN and may even reverse it (7). However in people who present with severe and chronic hyperglycemia, the symptoms of PN may become worse with rapid reduction in glucose levels. This is a transient effect but one of which patients and practitioners should be aware. Alcohol use and cigarette smoking can also affect painful neuropathy, and patients should be advised to discontinue both.

Pain management may include all forms of analgesics, including acetaminophen, nonsteroidal anti-inflammatory medications, and narcotics. Narcotics are typically avoided because of the risk of dependence. Tricyclic antidepressants may help with pain as well as insomnia, a frequent disturbance due to increased pain at night. Gabapentin has been demonstrated to be an effective treatment for painful PN, but should be monitored closely because high doses can cause dizziness, lethargy, and supine hypertension. The dosage of gabapentin can vary widely (200–800 mg t.i.d.). Pregabalin, which is FDA approved for treatment of PN, is dosed from 50 to 200 mg t.i.d. Duloxitine has also been approved for use in painful peripheral neuropathy.

The main treatment goal is the titration of medication to achieve efficacy with as few side effects as possible. Topical agents, such as capsaicin, a derivative of hot peppers, have been shown to be effective by releasing substance P from local nerve endings (8).

There is also evidence that α-lipoic acid and γ-linoleic acid can improve the sensory symptoms of diabetic polyneuropathy. α-Lipoic acid is a potent antioxidant and can be given both orally and intravenously. It has been used effectively in Germany for years and has been shown in international randomized controlled trials to effectively treat painful diabetic neuropathy (9,10). γ-Linoleic acid is a fatty acid found in evening primrose oil and has also been used to treat diabetic neuropathy. γ-Linoleic acid may improve problems with nerve membrane structure, impulse conduction, and nerve blood flow at doses of 360–480 mg/day (10). Although both of these acids have shown benefit in relieving the painful symptoms of diabetic neuropathy, further investigation is needed. For chronic unrelieved pain, referral to a pain management team may be appropriate.

ACUTE PAINFUL NEUROPATHY

The main symptoms of this diffuse small-fiber neuropathy are pain and paresthesia. These symptoms are worse at night and are found in the feet more often than in the hands. The pain can be intense and is described as a burning, stabbing, or deep aching sensation. Due to the chronic symptoms, anorexia, weight loss, and depression may also be present. This form of neuropathy is more common in men and often subsides spontaneously; it can also persist indefinitely and be debilitating, although the latter is rare (4).

NEUROPATHIC FOOT ULCER

Trauma and damage to the foot can occur in distal symmetrical polyneuropathy because of the loss of sensitivity to pain, decreased proprioception, loss of muscle, and vascular changes. Because of the loss of feeling in the foot and repetitive trauma, ulceration can occur. The metatarsal heads are the most common sites, but ulcers can form in other areas of pressure. In the absence of pain, calluses form over the metatarsal areas and become thickened. The overlying skin breaks down, ulceration occurs, and the foot may become infected. Treatment should be prophylactic and include foot care education and identifying abnormal foot shape and weight bearing. However, once ulcers occur, treatment includes mechanical measures to reduce (or eliminate) improper weight bearing and fitting of appropriate shoes. Debridement may be necessary to remove excess callus, and antibiotics will be needed if infection is present.

CHARCOT'S JOINTS

Neuropathic arthropathy, or Charcot's joints, also occurs with impaired pain recognition and proprioception but without motor loss. A picture is available on page 199 in chapter 15. The foot appears swollen and red, with a flattened arch, and is usually painless and warm. The gait becomes abnormal, and repeated trauma occurs as a result. On X-ray examination, there may be multiple fractures, osteopenia, bone lysis, and osteomyelitis. The pulses often are strong and bounding, but these pulses are due to the shunting of blood and may lead to more problems, such as excessive bone resorption and fractures. A podiatric or orthopedic referral is always necessary for the management of Charcot's joint and should be initiated as soon as possible to reduce foot disfiguration. Any symptoms of a red and hot foot in individuals with diabetes should be referred for X-ray and assessment of Charcot's joint.

Treatment. Treatment consists of reducing or eliminating weight bearing and preventing further structural damage. Antibiotics are needed if cellulitis or osteomyelitis is present. As in the treatment of neuropathic ulcers, proper shoes and mechanical devices will be necessary because the shape of the foot is usually grossly abnormal (3,4,6).

PROXIMAL MOTOR NEUROPATHY

Proximal motor neuropathy, or diabetic amyotrophy, affects a single or multiple peripheral nerves. It is characterized by severe muscle atrophy in the limb girdle, weight loss, weakness and wasting of lower-extremity muscles, and pain in the thigh muscles, lumbar regions, or perineal regions. This syndrome is uncommon and usually occurs in older adults, the onset is usually acute, and complete or partial recovery occurs.

CRANIAL NEUROPATHIES

Cranial neuropathies occur frequently, usually in older adults. The onset is abrupt, asymmetrical, and may be either painful or painless. The third cranial nerve is the most commonly affected. Symptoms often have a rapid onset and may include diplopia, sudden headache, ptosis, and eye pain. Femoral and thoracic nerve ischemias can cause hip, thigh, chest, and abdominal pain. Bell's palsy

PRACTICAL POINT	PRACTICAL POINT
Decreased pupil size may cause problems for individuals when entering a poorly lighted area or driving at night because pupils cannot dilate and adjust to darkness. Preventive education is necessary to avoid accidents or falls. Findings should be documented in the physical examination notes.	Take a detailed history and ask about the occurrence of unusual sweating, usually over the face and upper body during or after eating. Patients sometimes misinterpret these symptoms as hypoglycemic or hyperglycemic reactions and may treat them inappropriately.

(seventh nerve) can cause facial pain, drooping eyelid, and lacrimation. This occurs with more frequency and prognosis for recovery may be worse in patients with diabetes. Treatment is conservative and symptoms subside, although it can take at least 6–8 weeks (4,6).

RADICULOPATHY

Radiculopathy is a sensory neuropathy (intercostal or truncal) with a dermatomal pain and loss of cutaneous sensation. A single sensory nerve root is affected and is almost always unilateral and asymmetrical, with either hyperesthesia or paresthesia. This syndrome may be mistaken for acute abdominal crises, herniated disc, herpes zoster, or spinal cord compression. Spontaneous remission usually occurs within 3–6 months, and pain management will be necessary during that time (4,6).

ENTRAPMENT NEUROPATHIES

Entrapment neuropathies (mononeuropathy/multiplex) are isolated peripheral nerve palsies that can cause focal nerve damage at common entrapment sites such as the wrist and palm, upper arm and elbow, or thigh. The risk of developing carpal tunnel syndrome is twice as common in individuals with diabetes. Diagnosis is made by electrodiagnostic studies. Treatment may be conservative, such as immobilization with a splint, or surgical, which is often minor in nature. However, untreated entrapment injuries can often lead to muscle atrophy of the hand and permanent disability.

AUTONOMIC NEUROPATHY

Autonomic neuropathy is a serious form of neuropathy that often goes unrecognized because of its slow onset and confusing symptoms. In patients with PN, 50% have asymptomatic autonomic neuropathy (4). Autonomic control for each organ system is usually divided between opposing sympathetic and

---

PRACTICAL POINT

Identify voiding pattern, frequency of urinary tract infections, difficulty starting urinary stream, and presence/absence of bladder fullness. Obtain urinalysis if there is any suspicion of a urinary tract infection. Palpate and percuss the suprapubic area.

---

parasympathetic systems. Usually, the parasympathetic nerve fibers are affected first, and within 5 years, sympathetic nervous system dysfunction appears. The ANS is a complex entity that consists of a reflex arc made up of a sensor, afferent nerve, central nervous system (CNS) component efferent nerve, nerve ending, and effector organ. Because autonomic control of each organ is divided between opposing parasympathetic and sympathetic innervation, a symptom such as tachycardia could be attributed to either a decrease in sympathetic function or an increase in parasympathetic function (6).

The development of autonomic neuropathy is often considered ominous because the mortality rate over a 3- to 5-year period is as high as 50–60% (4,6). Although the involvement of the ANS is often diffuse, symptoms may often be confined to a single organ system (6). The organ systems most often affected by autonomic neuropathy are the cardiovascular system, gastrointestinal tract, genitourinary system, sweat glands, adrenal medulla, and ocular pupil (1).

ABNORMAL PUPILLARY FUNCTION

Decreased parasympathetic tone produces a smaller-than-normal pupil. This can be diagnosed during a routine eye examination and/or with the aid of a measuring device called a pupillometer. No specific treatment is needed (6).

GUSTATORY SWEATING

Abnormal profuse sweating that occurs when eating certain foods, particularly cheese or foods that are spicy, is thought to be of no risk, but it can be both bothersome and perplexing. It is frequently not recognized by health professionals as a diabetes related neuropathy. Anticholinergic drugs may alleviate symptoms, although this may require a high dose, which can produce unwanted side effects (6).

BLADDER DYSFUNCTION

A sensory abnormality of the detrusor muscle, the muscle that contracts to squeeze out urine while urinating, is the earliest autonomic symptom to occur and results in impaired bladder sensation. This decreased sensation of bladder fullness and decreased urinary frequency can lead to urinary tract infections. The parasympathetic involvement leads to decreased bladder contractions, causing individuals to have to strain to urinate. Urinary incontinence may also develop (6,7).

Asymptomatic urinary tract infections can occur. Periodic urinalysis is indicated to detect these. Also, symptoms of fever and rapid deterioration of blood glucose control may indicate urinary tract infections even in the absence of dysuria.

PRACTICAL POINT

Discuss or initiate discussion of ED to determine whether the condition exists. Often, reluctance on the part of the patient to discuss ED will result in this condition going untreated. It is important to consider psychological factors as a cause. Questions about ability to experience nighttime or early morning erections may also help differentiate between organic and psychogenic ED. Vardenafil and sildenafil may not be used if a patient is using a nitrate, e.g., nitroglycerin.

Tests of bladder function include postvoiding intravenous pyelogram, postvoiding catheterization, cystometry, sphincter electromyography, uroflometry, urethral pressure profile, and an electrophysiological test of bladder innervation (4,6). A postvoiding residual of >150 ml is diagnostic of abnormal bladder function. Suprapubic dullness to percussion over the bladder area can detect a full asymptomatic neurogenic bladder.

Treatment. Treatment should be aimed at reducing the number of urinary tract infections. Instructing individuals to urinate at least every 3–4 h, even though there may be no feeling of bladder fullness, will help to eliminate urinary tract infections. Medications such as bethanechol may help. If bladder emptying becomes difficult, self-catheterization may be necessary (6).

ERECTILE DYSFUNCTION

Erectile dysfunction (ED), or impotence, is a frequent and disturbing symptom and may affect at least 50% of all men with diabetes. It is defined as the consistent inability to achieve or maintain an erection that permits intercourse. ED is also characterized by the absence of erections during sleep and early morning. It can be the earliest symptom of autonomic neuropathy (3,6,11). There is no difference in the incidence of ED between patients with type 1 diabetes and those with type 2 diabetes when matched for age (12). The sympathetic nerves mediate both orgasm and ejaculation. The parasympathetic nerves control erectile function. Impotence caused by autonomic neuropathy progresses gradually but may be permanent within 2 years. Changes in the vasculature of the penis may also play a role in sexual dysfunction and will need to be evaluated as well (3).

PRACTICAL POINT

Careful history taking is important to begin appropriate therapy. It is important to consider psychological factors as a cause for the above symptoms, and psychological counseling may also be helpful.

Diagnosis. Diagnosis is made by a detailed sexual history including rapidity of onset of symptoms and time of day of occurrences. An assessment should also include history of sexual desire, orgasms, and erectile and ejaculatory function. Psychological sexual satisfaction is as important to assess as physical capabilities. It is important that possible adverse effects of drug therapy (e.g., some antihypertensives, antidepressants, tranquilizers), diseases (e.g., prostate, peripheral vascular), psychological problems, and other physical conditions (e.g., smoking, alcohol) be explored before diagnosing ED as caused by autonomic neuropathy.

Testing. Tests include nocturnal penile tumescence monitoring, which is used to differentiate between organic and psychogenic impotence. Other tests such as nerve conduction, vascular ultrasonography, pressure, and circumference measurements may also be used to obtain a diagnosis (6).

Treatment. Patients prefer to use oral medications for ED (see "Erectile Dysfunction Treatments," a patient handout in resources). Treatment may include the use of oral medications taken ~0.5–1 h before intercourse (vardenafil, sildenafil, or tadalafil). These medications work by inhibiting phosphodiesterase type 5 (PDE-5), which allows an increase in vasodilation and blood flow, resulting in penile rigidity. The cascade of chemical changes that lead to an erection is initiated during foreplay. Therefore, the PDE-5 inhibitors are only effective once sexual stimulation occurs. Most common side effects include flushing, headache, dyspepsia, and nasal congestion. High-fat-content meals eaten prior to the use of these drugs tend to slow the reaction time. Both vardenafil and sildenafil remain active in the system for ~4 h, and tadalafil at the 20-mg dose can remain active for up to 36 h. The FDA has now approved use of a 2.5-mg or 5-mg daily dose of tadalafil. Patients should not take the PDE-5 inhibitors more than once in a 24-h period unless using the daily dose of tadalafil. These drugs should not be prescribed for patients taking nitrate medications.

Papaverine and alprostadil are medicines that are injected into the corpus of the penis, resulting in increased blood flow. Alprostadil as an injected medication is considered the "gold standard" by urologists. If an erection cannot be achieved through the injection of alprostadil, then there is little chance of restoring erectile function by any other medications. Alprostadil in pellet form can be placed intraurethrally and has the same effect. The duration of the erection is from 0.5 to 2 h.

Mechanical vacuum devices and surgically implanted penile prostheses are also methods of treatment, but recently have been used less because oral medications are more easily used and are noninvasive (3,6). The vacuum device uses negative pressure to draw blood into the penis. A ring is then placed at the base of the penis to retain the engorgement of the cavernosa. Patients using this device can achieve satisfactory erections ~75% of the time (13). However, it is cumbersome and very mechanical, and many men find it psychologically unappealing.

Penile implants have improved markedly over the past few years, and the mechanical failures formerly associated with their use have been reduced. Infections resulting from the surgically implanted device are still of concern for men with diabetes.

PRACTICAL POINT

Assess heart rate for tachycardia, blood pressure orthostatic measurements (lying, sitting, and standing), and history of symptoms of lightheadedness, weakness, fatigue, visual blurring, and neck pain. A thorough list of all antihypertensive medications taken and changes in therapy should be noted, especially if new symptoms develop.

FEMALE SEXUAL DYSFUNCTION

The incidence of sexual dysfunction in women with diabetes is as high as 30%, and the symptoms are usually decreased vaginal lubrication, vaginal wall atrophy, and dyspareunia (painful intercourse). The sympathetic nervous system mediates orgasm, whereas the parasympathetic system affects vaginal lubrication (6).

It is more difficult to diagnose female sexual dysfunction because the symptoms can be due to hormonal changes of menopause as well as psychogenic. Diagnosis is made by careful history taking and report of painful intercourse and vaginal dryness. Treatment may include the use of vaginal lubricants and/or estrogen creams.

CARDIAC AUTONOMIC NEUROPATHY

The most frequent symptoms of cardiac autonomic neuropathy (CAN) are resting tachycardia and postural hypotension. Other notable symptoms are exercise intolerance, painless myocardial infarction (due to cardiac denervation), and heat intolerance. Increased heart rate is due to vagal cardiac neuropathy and may cause tachycardia to be at a fixed rate. Postural hypotension can be caused by a disturbance in the baroreceptors, which normally control blood pressure during a change in position. Symptoms may be lightheadedness and syncope on position change or extended standing. Sudden death may also occur. Cardiac arrest may occur in people with severe CAN, with the greatest risk occurring during surgery. Parasympathetic cardiac dysfunction is seen first, followed by sympathetic dysfunction (6,12). The increased frequency of sudden death in patients with CAN might be attributed to cardiac arrhythmias, silent cardiac ischemia, sleep apnea, and abnormal response to hypoxia (3).

Tests to detect CAN include

- Resting heart rate: >100 bpm, but over time may decrease to 80–100 bpm
- Beat-to-beat heart rate variation: measures variability of heart rate
- Valsalva maneuver: measures heart rate and peripheral vasoconstriction during strain
- Heart rate response to standing: measures heart rate (tachycardia at beat 15 is normal and bradycardia at beat 30 is normal)

- Systolic blood pressure response to standing: abnormal when blood pressure falls >30 mmHg within the first 2 min of standing
- Diastolic blood pressure rise with sustained exercise: using a hand-gripped meter, the diastolic blood pressure should rise
- QT interval on electrocardiogram: measured according to a normal standard (4,12)

Treatment includes careful management of hypertension medications and steps to improve glycemic control. In treating postural hypotension, wearing elastic support stockings, increasing salt intake, and elevating the head of the bed during sleep have been helpful. Drug therapy may include fludrocortisone, sympathomimetics (e.g., clonidine), and pressor agents.

GASTROPATHY

Neuropathy of the gastrointestinal (GI) tract may involve any portion of the system from the esophagus to the rectum. It is estimated that as many as 75% of people with type 1 or 2 diabetes have neuropathy of the GI tract (14). Delayed gastric emptying, or gastroparesis, can lead to abnormal absorption of glucose and oral medications. The undigested food may remain in the stomach for hours after a meal (6). The result is suboptimal glucose control, with hyperglycemia and/or hypoglycemia depending on the retention of food. Constipation is the most common lower-gastrointestinal symptom but can alternate with episodes of diarrhea.

Testing. Evaluation of gastric emptying should be done if symptoms are present. Barium studies or referral for endoscopy may be required. Endoscopy may be required to rule out other causes. Gastric emptying studies may be ordered, but it is important that testing occur with as near euglycemia as possible. The general consensus is that blood glucose should be under reasonable control on the day of the gastric emptying study. It is recommended that serum glucose be measured prior to the study and noted in the report. If the blood glucose is >275 mg/dl on the morning of the test, the glucose should be lowered with insulin to <275 mg/dl or the study should be rescheduled for another day (15). Some centers administer insulin to lower the blood glucose to less than 180 mg/dl prior to the study. Optimizing glucose control may improve gastric emptying and the resultant symptoms of gastroparesis.

PRACTICAL POINT

Individuals with hypoglycemia unawareness may have difficulty achieving glycemic control, and more frequent blood glucose monitoring is warranted. Situations that would put a person at high risk, such as driving, should not occur without a glucose check. Helping the patient recognize subtle symptoms that may indicate hypoglycemia, such as tingling around the mouth or a decreased ability to concentrate, and should prompt a glucose check is a critical component of patient education. Carrying glucose-monitoring equipment and portable hypoglycemia treatments, such as glucose gel, juice boxes, or glucose tablets, at all times is essential for safe management of this problem.

Treatment of this condition is aimed at controlling the potentially debilitating symptoms and improving glycemic control (14). Symptoms of gastropathy include heartburn or dysphagia, gastric esophageal reflux, early satiety, delayed gastric emptying and feelings of fullness, nausea and/or vomiting, constipation, diarrhea and/or incontinence of stool, and anorexia.

The treatment of diabetes gastropathy includes improving gastric emptying if necessary, as well as improving symptoms. Treatment may include exercise, smoking cessation, dietary management with small frequent meals, use of gastric prokinetic agents that assist with gastric emptying, excellent management of blood glucose, liquid feedings (which are emptied more easily from the stomach), and avoidance of fatty foods and fiber. A nutritional assessment and counseling with a dietitian to include a calorie count and dietary adjustments may be necessary to ensure adequate intake (16). The following drugs have been shown to be useful as antiemetics and increase action on the smooth muscle to increase the rate of gastric emptying of both solids and liquids: metoclopramide, erythromycin, and domperidone (not available in the U.S.) (14,16).

Gastric pacing has also been used in severe gastroparesis. Patients with gastroparesis often have depression. Antidepressants and psychotherapy are often successful and are important adjuncts to conventional therapy.

IMPAIRED HYPOGLYCEMIC AWARENESS AND HYPOGLYCEMIA UNAWARENESS

The response to hypoglycemia in people treated with insulin is mediated by the ANS. Impaired hypoglycemic awareness and hypoglycemia unawareness result in the inability of the person to recognize and treat hypoglycemia, with potential for injury or harm. The counterregulatory response consists of an increase in glucose production from the liver, a decrease in peripheral glucose uptake, and the secretion of glucagon and epinephrine. In individuals with type 1 diabetes, the glucagon response to low blood glucose deteriorates 1–5 years after diagnosis. Epinephrine responses may also decrease as the duration of the disease increases. The combined absence of glucagon and epinephrine responses decreases counterregulation. The usual signs and symptoms of hypoglycemia (sweating and tachycardia) may be absent but can include confusion, lethargy, amnesia, mental irritability, and seizures (3,6).

Impaired hypoglycemic awareness and hypoglycemic unawareness can occur as a result of very tight blood glucose control and/or frequent episodes of hypoglycemia. It may be necessary to adjust targets for glycemia in order to improve hypoglycemia unawareness. Research suggests that preventing all hypoglycemia for ~3 weeks will allow the individual to regain their hypoglycemia awareness (17). There are now "hypoglycemia awareness" training programs to aid people with this complication. (Blood glucose awareness training is described in chapter 17.)

SUMMARY

Neuropathy is the most common chronic disorder in diabetes and is both complex and difficult to understand. Diabetes care, education, and management require a thorough assessment of the person's history, symptoms, and limitations. An understanding of the complexity of the various neuropathies is important in caring for and educating the person with these conditions. It is often the nurse who performs the initial assessment, and by knowing the questions to ask and seeking further information, quality care can be achieved for the patient.

REFERENCES

1. Vinik AI: Diagnosing diabetic autonomic neuropathy [Internet], 2004. Available from http://www.medscape.com/viewarticle/473205. Accessed 4 January 2005

2. Bailes BK: Diabetes mellitus and its chronic complications. *AORN J* 76:266–276, 278–282 [quiz 283–286], 2002

3. Freeman R: The nervous system and diabetes. In *Joslin's Diabetes Mellitus*. 14th ed. Kahn CR, Weir GC, King GL, Jacobson AM, Moses AC, Smith RJ, Eds. Philadelphia, Lippincott Williams & Wilkins, 2005, p. 951–964

4. Boulton AJM, Vinik AI, Arezzo JC, Bril V, Feldman EL, et al.: Diabetic neuropathies: A statement by the American Diabetes Association. *Diabetes Care* 28:956–962, 2005

5. Ziegler D, Sohr C, Nourooz-Zadeh J: Oxidative stress and antioxidant defense in relation to the severity of diabetic polyneuropathy and cardiovascular autonomic neuropathy. *Diabetes Care* 26:2187–2183, 2004

6. Greene DA, Feldman EL, Stevens MJ, Sima AAF, Albers JW, Pfeifer MA: Diabetic neuropathy. In *Ellenberg & Rifkin's Diabetes Mellitus*. 5th ed. Porte D, Sherwin RS, Eds. Stamford, CT, 1997, p. 1009–1074

7. Nathan DM, E Cagliero: Fuel metabolism. In *Endocrinology & Metabolism*. 4th ed. Felig P, Frohman LA, Eds. New York, McGraw-Hill, 2001, p. 827–927

8. Ziegler D, Reljanovic M, Mehnert H, Gries FA: Alpha lipoic acid in the treatment of diabetic polyneuropathy in Germany: current evidence from clinical trials. *Exp Clin Endocrinol Diabetes* 107:421–430, 1999

9. SYDNEY Trial Authors: The sensory symptoms of diabetic polyneuropathy are improved with α-lipoic acid: the SYDNEY trial. *Diabetes Care* 26:770–776, 2003

10. Shane-McWhorter L: *Complimentary and Alternative Medicine (CAM) Supplement Use in People With Diabetes: A Clinician's Guide*. Alexandria, VA, American Diabetes Association, 2007

11. Munarriz R, Traish A, Goldstein I: Erectile dysfunction in diabetes. In *Joslin's Diabetes Mellitus*. 14th ed. Kahn CR, Weir GC, King GL, Jacobson AM, Moses AC, Smith RJ, Eds. Philadelphia, Lippincott Williams & Wilkins, 2005, 999–1013

12. Unger RH, Foster DW: Diabetes mellitus. In *Williams Textbook of Endocrinology*. 9th ed. Wilson JD, Foster DW, Kronenberg HM, Larsen PR, Eds. Philadelphia, W. B. Saunders Company, 1998, p. 973–1060

13. Snow KJ, Guay A: Erectile dysfunction in diabetes mellitus. In *Medical Management of Diabetes Mellitus*. Leahy JL, Clark NG, Cefalu WT, Eds. New York, Marcel Dekker, 2000, p. 427–442

14. Bernstein G: The diabetic stomach: management strategies for clinicians and patients. *Diabetes Spectrum* 13:11–15, 2000

15. Abell TL, Camilleri M, Donohoe K, Hasler W L, Lin H, et al.: Consensus recommendations for gastric emptying scintigraphy: joint report of the American Neurogastroenterology and Motility Society and the Society of Nuclear Medicine. *J Nucl Med Tech* 36:44–54, 2008

16. Mashimo H, Goyal RK: Effects of diabetes mellitus on the digestive system. In *Joslin's Diabetes Mellitus*. 14th ed. Kahn CR, Weir GC, King GL, Jacobson GC, Moses AC, Smith RJ, Eds. Philadelphia, Lippincott Williams & Wilkins, 2005, 1070–1086

17. Cryer PE, Childs B: Negotiating the barrier to hypoglycemia in diabetes. *Diabetes Spectrum* 15:20–27, 2002

Additional Resource:

Spollett GR: Diabetic neuropathies: diagnosis and treatment. *Nurs Clin N Am* 41:697–717, 2006

Ms. Kushion is the Manager and Clinical Nurse Specialist at Sparrow Regional Diabetes Center, Lansing, MI.

15. Evaluation and Management of the Diabetic Foot

George T. Liu, DPM, and John S. Steinberg, DPM

EPIDEMIOLOGY

The crude prevalence of diabetes in the U.S. increased 120% from 1980 to 2005 (1). Accordingly, the number of nontraumatic lower-extremity amputations increased comparably. Reports have estimated that ~15% of patients with diabetes will develop a diabetic foot ulcer in their lifetimes (2,3). In turn, 85% of nontraumatic lower-extremity amputations are preceded by the formation of a foot ulcer, making it the most common pivotal event (4,5). Foot complications account for 25% of diabetes-related admissions to hospitals (4–6), and an estimated 50% of those patients who undergo lower-extremity amputation will suffer a new amputation within 5 years (7,8).

Ulceration and amputation of the lower extremities pose a direct socioeconomic burden to both patients and society. Management of foot ulcers is estimated at $27,987 (U.S.) per occurrence for the 2 years following diagnosis (9), and the average hospital cost incurred for diabetes-related lower-extremity amputation ranges from $20,000 to $27,930 (10–13). Studies have demonstrated a relationship between the presence of ulceration/amputation and a negative impact on function, self-perception, emotional health, and quality of life (14–18).

The initial presence of a foot ulcer has been recognized as a marker of the diabetic disease state and not only as a local comorbid manifestation (19–21). In one study, 5-year mortality rates of diabetic patients with new-onset neuropathic, neuroischemic, and ischemic foot ulcers were 45%, 18%, and 55%, respectively (21). In a prospective study, diabetic patients with an ulcer were found to have a twofold increased risk of mortality compared with diabetic patients without a foot ulcer (19).

PATHOGENESIS OF DIABETIC FOOT PROBLEMS

Several pathological manifestations of diabetes contribute to ulceration and amputation of the diabetic foot. Sensory neuropathy is the most common reason for foot lesions encountered in the diabetic foot. This lack of protective sensation subjects the foot to increased risk of open injuries due to undetected trauma or repetitive low-grade stresses. Motor neuropathy causes muscle atrophy and subsequent imbalances of tendon-pull across the foot joints. The resultant foot deformities, such as hammertoes, claw toes, and prominent plantar metatarsal heads, may serve as areas of irritation and pressure within tight shoes (Fig. 15.1). Additionally, abnormal plantar pressures develop as a result of these foot deformities and altered mechanics. Increased plantar pressure combined with sensory neuropathy may predispose the foot to ulceration (Fig. 15.2). Autonomic neuropathy in the foot may manifest as decreased sweating of the feet, predisposing the dorsal and plantar skin to dryness and fissures. A more serious manifestation of autonomic neuropathy in the foot is Charcot neuroarthropathy, in which destruction of the foot joints can cause severe foot deformities (Fig. 15.3). Another pathologic manifestation of long-term diabetes is nonenzymatic glycosylation. This process of glycosylation in diabetes stiffens soft tissues such as ligaments and tendons, causing limited joint mobility, which also leads to increased plantar pressures. In addition, peripheral arterial disease in patients with diabetes is more advanced and prevalent compared with that in individuals without diabetes. Poor tissue oxygenation together with impaired blood flow may slow the healing of foot wounds, delay the delivery of antibiotics, and in severe cases, result in ischemic pain and gangrene.

FOOT ASSESSMENT AND EVALUATION

Assessment of high-risk conditions for ulceration and amputation in the diabetic foot is crucial in reducing the incidence of comorbid complications. A systems-based evaluation of the foot can identify early risk factors and identify appropriate interventions to prevent the progression toward ulceration and amputation.

VASCULAR ASSESSMENT: IS THERE ADEQUATE BLOOD FLOW TO THE FOOT?

Ischemia to the lower extremities impedes the immune response to infection, delivery of antibiotics, and healing of open wounds. Intermittent calf claudication, as identified by cramping of the calf muscles while walking, is an indication of relative ischemia, wherein the tissue demand for blood exceeds the available supply. Calf claudication is measured by city-block distances the patient is able to walk before intense cramping or tiredness of the leg ensues. Also measured is the amount of rest time required before walking can be comfortably initiated. Calf cramping during sleep (nocturnal leg cramping) is not intermittent calf claudication. Rest pain occurs in the advanced stages of ischemia and is characterized by intense pain and cramping primarily in the forefoot during sleep that is relieved

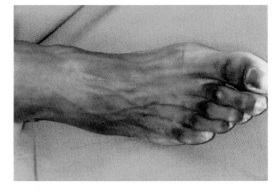

Figure 15.1
Retracted claw toes with prominent extensor tendons and depressed metatarsal head are a result of muscular imbalances from motor neuropathy.

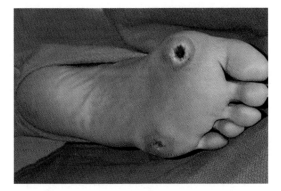

Figure 15.2
Depressed metatarsal heads create increased plantar pressures with walking. In the insensate foot, these focal pressures predispose skin to ulcerations.

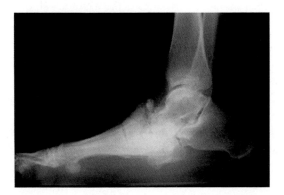

Figure 15.3
Clinically, Charcot foot presents with redness, swelling, heat, and severe deformity. Radiographic pictures demonstrate severe fracture dislocations accompanied with osteolysis and fragmentation in the foot joints.

Table 15.1 Examination of Vascular Status

Assessment	Potential Indication
Palpate femoral, popliteal, dorsalis pedis, and posterior tibial pulse.	Absent pedal pulse may be an indication of poor inflow to the foot. Palpating proximal arteries may help identify the level of lower-extremity arterial disease.
Feel for differences in skin temperature from proximal to distal; compare limbs.	Coolness may indicate diminished circulatory perfusion. Localized warmth may be an indication of infection or Charcot neuroarthropathy.
Inspect skin for atrophic, shiny, and taut appearance and digital hair growth.	Loss of turgor and digital hair growth may be signs of poor cutaneous perfusion.
Evaluate digital capillary filling time.	Normal refilling should be pink to color in 1–3 seconds. Refilling that is 3–5 seconds may indicate arterial insufficiency (28). Refilling that is immediate and bluish or purplish in color may indicate venous insufficiency.
Evaluate the following: ■ Elevational pallor by raising the leg above the level of the heart or 60° above horizontal for 1 min. ■ Dependent rubor by lowering and hanging the lower extremity.	In the elevated position, marked pallor to the sole and digits indicates arterial insufficiency. When lowering the extremity, if it takes >10 seconds for the pink color to return or vein filling takes >15 seconds, arterial insufficiency should be suspected.
Inspect for areas of gangrene.	Presence of gangrene is representative of end-stage vascular disease resulting in tissue death.

only by placing the limb in a dependent position. Gangrene, ischemic tissue death, signifies end-stage peripheral vascular disease or absolute ischemia, in which the blood supply is completely inadequate for tissue survival. If symptomatic peripheral vascular disease is present, lower-extremity noninvasive arterial examination consisting of arterial Doppler waveforms, ankle-brachial indices, segmental pressures, and digital plethysmography are indicated. Appropriate consultation with a vascular surgeon or interventional cardiologist with specific training in lower-extremity endovascular surgery is then made if the noninvasive arterial exam is abnormal. See Table 15.1.

NEUROLOGICAL ASSESSMENT: IS THERE ABSENCE OF PROTECTIVE SENSATION?

Indicators of clinical neuropathy may include the subjective presence of tingling, numbness, burning sensation, and/or formication (sensation of insects

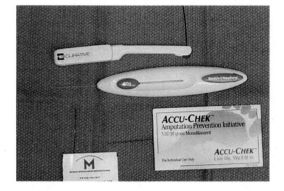

Figure 15.4
The 5.07 Semmes-Weinstein monofilament wire is used to detect loss of protective sensation.

crawling on skin) that typically begins at the toes and fingertips. In advanced cases of sensory neuropathy, the symptomatic sensations progress proximally to a "stocking-and-glove" distribution.

Evaluation for sensory neuropathy begins with assessment of protective sensation. The 5.07 Semmes-Weinstein monofilament wire (Fig. 15.4) has been the screening tool of choice for determining the loss of protective sensation with sensory neuropathy. This inexpensive and portable device can yield reproducible and predictive information regarding risk of ulcer formation (22). The 5.07 Semmes-Weinstein monofilament is calibrated to deliver 10 g of force to a designated testing site when sufficient force is applied, causing the wire to bend. The examination is performed with the subject's eyes closed. The patient is asked to respond "yes" if any pressure from the monofilament wire is detected. Demonstrating the monofilament on the patient's proximal leg or palm may assist in identifying the type of sensation he or she is to detect. Ten sites are tested: plantar first, third, and fifth digits; plantar first, third, and fifth metatarsal heads; plantar medial and lateral midfoot; plantar heel; and dorsal midfoot. A clinical finding of four insensate sites was found to be 97% sensitive and 83% specific for detecting a loss of protective sensation (23,24).

Another testing modality used to assess loss of protective sensation is the biothesiometer. This instrument delivers different levels of vibration through an application tip tactor, which is usually applied to the distal pulp of the hallux. Voltage is regulated by a dial that may be adjusted to deliver increasing vibration intensities. The tactor is applied to the toe while increasing the voltage, thereby increasing the intensity of the vibration, until the patient detects a vibratory sensation (Fig. 15.5). Patients who are only able to detect vibrations at 25 V are considered to have lost protective sensation. A decreased vibratory perception (>25 V) has a strong predictive value for ulcerations (25–27).

DERMATOLOGICAL ASSESSMENT: IS THERE SKIN PATHOLOGY?

Among the many vital functions of the integumentary system, the skin serves as a barrier to protect the body from foreign pathogens. As previously discussed, open lesions to the foot serve as pathways of infection to the body. In the diabetic

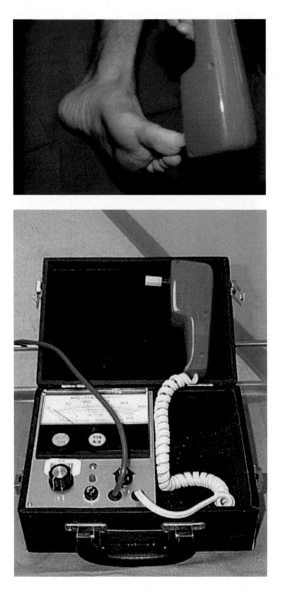

Figure 15.5
The tactor of biothesiometer is balanced on the toe pulp. Intensity of vibration is increased until detected by the patient.

foot, absent protective sensation and foot deformity leave the skin susceptible to mechanical injury, resulting in skin breakdown. The presence of an open wound is the pivotal event for development of infection. Examination of the skin should identify areas of open injury, such as laceration or ulceration, and areas of low-grade mechanical irritation, such as that seen with a callus or corn. See Table 15.2.

Table 15.2 Examination of Dermatologic Status

Assessment	Potential Indication
Observe the skin for cutaneous hydration with the skin texture and turgor.	■ Dry, rough, and scaling skin may be an indicator of poor cutaneous hydration. ■ In severe cases, this loss of moisture may lead to fissures, which can open and serve as a pathway for infection. ■ Chronic tinea pedis (athlete's foot) may cause scaling and thickening of the skin, which may also lead to fissures.
Inspect for corn and callus formation.	■ Formation of keratosis indicates areas subjected to repetitive pressure and shear stress. ■ Calluses are highly associated with areas of skin breakdown and potential ulcer formation.
Inspect nails.	■ Fungal infection of the nails (onychomycosis) presents with hypertrophy, dystrophy, discoloration, brittleness, and subungual debris (Fig. 15.6). ■ Thick nails may serve as a source of pressure within shoes, subjecting the nail bed to ulceration. ■ Inspect nail borders for ingrown toenails and for associated infection (paronychia).
Inspect for hemorrhage beneath calluses and toenails (Fig. 15.7).	■ Hemorrhage may indicate injury and presence of a preulcerative lesion. ■ Anecdotal evidence has indicated that painless bleeding beneath calluses and nails may be considered dermatological signs of clinically significant sensory neuropathy.
Inspect for open wounds.	■ Open wounds, such as ulcers, in the diabetic foot are pathways for infection. ■ Inspect the foot for abrasions, lacerations, blisters, ingrown nails, and ulcerations. ■ Inspect the web spaces between the digits for open lesions. Web space may become macerated, predisposing the skin to breakdown (Fig. 15.8). ■ Assess wounds for size; depth; location; exposure of tendon, joint capsule, or bone; presence of necrotic tissue; and signs of infection.
Inspect for areas of erythema.	■ Erythema may indicate inflammation associated with areas of irritation or pressure from poor-fitting shoes. ■ Erythema accompanied with pain, localized heat and swelling, and pus may indicate presence of infection.

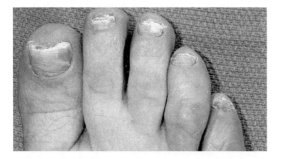

Figure 15.6
Fungally infected nails present with thickness, discoloration, and subungual debris. Thick nails may cause pressure to the nail bed within shoes, creating nail bed ulcerations.

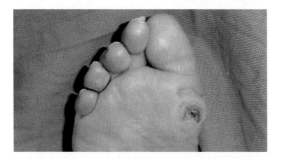

Figure 15.7
A hemorrhage beneath calluses may indicate the presence of a preulcerative lesion.

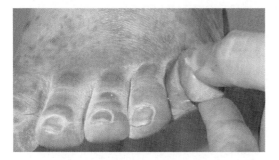

Figure 15.8
Web spaces of toes may retain moisture, which causes maceration. Chronic maceration may lead to skin breakdown.

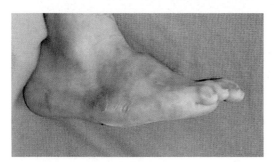

Figure 15.9
Collapse of the midfoot in Charcot foot will result in a "rocker bottom" deformity. The plantar bony prominence is subject to increased pressure and ulceration.

ORTHOPEDIC AND BIOMECHANICAL ASSESSMENT: IS THERE A FOOT DEFORMITY?

Structural and functional deformities of the foot, such as flat or high arched feet, bunions or hammertoes, may be sources of repetitive low-grade trauma within shoes during walking. In the insensate foot, this continual trauma may lead to ulceration of the skin. See Table 15.3.

SHOE ASSESSMENT: DOES THE PATIENT HAVE ADEQUATE PROTECTIVE FOOTWEAR AND COMPLY WITH ITS USE?

Ideally, the role of footwear is to protect the feet from injury. By accommodating deformity and off-loading pressure, a proper set of footwear can prevent ulcer occurrence and recurrence. Patients must understand the importance of prevention

Table 15.3 Orthopedic Examination of Musculoskeletal Status

Assessment	Potential Indication
Observe for digital deformities (e.g., hammertoes, claw toes, and mallet toes).	■ Determine whether the deformity is flexible or rigid. Rigid deformities are more prone to irritation and skin breakdown within shoes. ■ Inspect for associated callus or corn formation along the bony prominences, an indication of low-grade irritation within shoe gear.
Identify bunion or Tailor's bunion (fifth metatarsophalangeal joint) deformity.	■ Large bony protrusion of the metatarsal joint causing pressure in the area at risk of ulceration.
Inspect for prominent depressed metatarsal heads with an anteriorly displaced metatarsal fat pad.	■ Prominent plantar metatarsal areas with loss of fat pad protection are subject to increased pressures. Diffuse callus formation may be present.
Identify midfoot deformities: low arch and high arch.	■ Low arches may be seen with flatfoot deformities (pes planus). Inspect the plantar midfoot for any signs of callus formation or irritation. Collapse of the midfoot arch, with a "rocker bottom" deformity, may also be seen with Charcot neuroarthropathy (Fig. 15.9). This condition should be referred to a podiatrist or foot-and-ankle orthopedist for evaluation and treatment. ■ High arches may be seen with "intrinsic minus foot," in which atrophy of the intrinsic muscles of the foot and depression of the metatarsal heads gives a hollow appearance to the arch. This is accompanied with retracted digit and prominent extensor tendons. Observe the plantar metatarsal head area and heels for callus formation and irritation.

(continued)

Table 15.3 Orthopedic Examination of Musculoskeletal Status (*Continued*)

Assessment	Potential Indication
Identify rearfoot deformities: varus (inversion) or valgus (eversion).	■ Rigid varus or valgus rearfoot deformities at the heel may cause callus formation or irritation.
Identify prominences along joints or bones.	■ Bony prominence may be the result of arthritic joint changes or bony injury. ■ Severe deformity may be seen in Charcot neuroarthropathy.
Identify previous foot amputations.	■ Partial amputations of the foot alter the mechanics of gait and the normal distribution of plantar pressures, predisposing the foot to ulceration.
Assess the range of motion of joints for limited joint mobility.	■ First metatarsophalangeal joint: 65° in dorsiflexion in the sagittal plane. ■ Subtalar joint: 10° eversion and 20° inversion in the frontal plane. ■ Ankle joint: 10° of dorsiflexion in the sagittal plane. ■ Limited joint range of motion of the lower-extremity joints reduces shock absorption capacity and translates increased plantar pressures to the foot. Limited joint mobility has been associated with increased risk of ulcer formation.

and the role shoes and activity play. In the diabetic insensate foot, an ill-fitting shoe can be a source of repetitive injury. Examination of the shoe treads may reveal abnormal gait patterns and areas of increased pedal stress. Ideal footwear should be extra deep, with a wide toe box to accommodate digital deformities. Insoles should be custom molded and redistribute plantar pressures. Shoes should fit well, with little to no pistoning of the foot. See Table 15.4.

Compliance issues with therapeutic protective diabetic footwear are often related to shoe appearance (28,29). To address this problem with use, orthopedic shoe manufacturers have introduced various styles of diabetic compliant footwear to accommodate the social needs of the patient.

LABS AND TESTS

Few laboratory and advance testing modalities are used for routine assessment of the diabetic foot, and most ancillary tests are performed only when clinically indicated. Initial screening laboratory tests include glycated hemoglobin A1c (A1C) to assess long-term blood glucose control. Poor long-term glucose control has been

Table 15.4 Footwear Evaluation

Assessment	Potential Indication
Inspect interior of shoe for foreign objects and exterior of the shoe for impaled sharp objects (Fig. 15.10).	■ Sharp objects may injure the foot, predisposing to ulceration.
Inspect wear pattern of the shoe.	■ Wear patterns may be associated with abnormal gait and deformities of the foot.
Inspect shoe fit.	■ Shoes should be well-fitting. Tight shoes may create areas of pressure over the skin of bony prominences. Oversized or loose shoes will create pistoning within the shoe, which may produce areas of shear stress and irritation to the foot. ■ Toe box of the shoe should be deep and wide enough to avoid digital pressure and irritation. ■ Shoe fitting is best performed by certified pedorthist or health care professional with foot care training.
Inspect insoles for material fatigue and failure (bottoming out).	■ If inner soles cannot be visually inspected, place a hand into the shoe to assess worn spots or areas where padding is weak and worn.

shown to correlate with increased incidence of diabetes-related comorbidities, such as neuropathy, retinopathy, nephropathy, and peripheral vascular disease.

Oral temperatures, complete blood counts, and erthrocyte sedimentation rates are appropriate screening tests in cases of infection; however, these tests have been shown to correlate poorly with acute diabetic foot infections. One study demonstrated that in the presence of a clinically infected diabetic foot, oral temperature was elevated in only 18% of all cases and leukocytosis was seen in 46% of all infections. Only erthrocyte sedimentation rates, which were elevated in 96% of patients, were found to correlate well with diabetic foot infections (30).

Radiographic evaluation for underlying osteomyelitis of the foot should be performed in the presence of chronic foot ulcerations that probe deep soft tissue or bone. Severe and acute foot deformities should be radiographically evaluated for fracture/dislocation and Charcot neuroarthropathy. In cases of severe clinical infection, foot radiographs may detect soft tissue gas and bone involvement.

Additionally, nuclear and advanced diagnostic imaging, such as bone scan, computed tomography, and magnetic resonance imaging, may be used to evaluate the presence of osteomyelitis. Noninvasive vascular evaluation of the lower-extremity arteries (arterial Dopplers, digital plethysmography, pulse volume recordings, and ankle-brachial and toe-brachial indexes) may be used to evaluate the quality of physiological blood flow. This examination is commonly performed in patients with diabetes who present with clinical signs and symptoms of ischemia

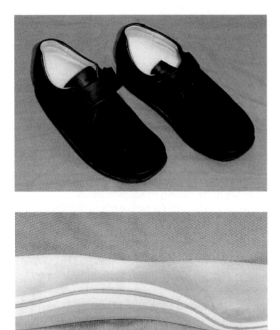

Figure 15.11
Extra-depth shoes with custom-molded inserts will accommodate minor foot deformities and attenuate focal plantar pressures.

EDUCATIONAL/BEHAVIORAL CONSIDERATIONS

Diabetes foot education has been shown to reduce foot complications associated with diabetes. Educating patients on daily monitoring and maintenance of the feet will aid in preventing complications and improve response time to potentially limb-threatening conditions.

Patients should be taught to perform a daily foot inspection as follows:

- Inspect feet, especially the soles, at least once per day for injury, callosities, and areas of redness. If the area of redness is associated with heat, swelling, pain, and pus accompanied by fever, chills, and night sweats, this condition should be reported immediately to a doctor or nurse. The use of a shatterproof mirror on the floor is recommended if the patient cannot bend his or her legs to visually inspect the feet.
- Inspect web spaces between toes for maceration and fissures.
- Inspect the interior and exterior of shoes for foreign objects before wearing and note areas of wear and tear. Worn-out shoes may not be supportive and therefore may be unable to evenly distribute foot pressure across the sole.

Patients should be taught the following daily maintenance:

- Do not walk barefoot (inside or outside the home). Always wear footwear recommended by a health care professional.

> ### PRACTICAL POINT
>
> A culmination of individual factors contributes to the cumulative risk of developing foot ulcers (31).
> - Approximately 85% of all diabetes-related lower extremity amputations are preceded by a preventable ulceration.
> - Patients with sensory neuropathy are 1.7 times more likely to develop an ulcer.
> - Patients with neuropathy and deformity are 12.1 times more likely to develop an ulcer.
> - Patients with neuropathy, deformity, and history of amputation are 36.4 times more likely to develop an ulcer.
> - Presence of a callus in the diabetic foot is strongly associated with the site of ulcer formation (32).

- Using lotions or creams recommended by a health care provider will help skin retain moisture and prevent cracking. Do not apply lotions to the web spaces between toes.
- Wash feet daily with mild soap and water. Test water temperature with an elbow before submerging the feet.
- After washing, dry feet well, especially the web spaces between toes, to prevent maceration. Apply lamb's wool to the web spaces as instructed to facilitate drying of macerated skin.
- Wear cotton socks to absorb perspiration from the skin. Wearing clean, light-colored socks will help identify the presence of pus or blood from an undetected injury. Do not wear tight socks that constrict the circulation to the feet.
- Trim toenails either straight across or along the contours of the toe pulp to maintain nail clearance from adjacent skin and to reduce potential ingrown toenail formation.
- Small calluses may be reduced with a pumice stone, ideally after bathing, when calluses are soft.
- Do not trim or cut nails or calluses if neuropathy is present; refer to a podiatrist or specialist with foot care training.
- Do not use over-the-counter "medicated" corn and callus pads because they contain salicylic acid, which can injure the insensate foot. Nonmedicated corn and callus pads are acceptable as directed by a health care professional.
- Do not self-treat ingrown nails and associated infections, and do not use sharp objects to reduce calluses. Seek the advice and help of a doctor or nurse.
- Open injuries of the foot should be cleansed with antiseptic solution and dressed. The condition should be reported immediately to the doctor or nurse for evaluation and treatment.
- Ulcer care should be performed as directed by a health care professional.

ADDRESSING BARRIERS TO TREATMENT AND LIFESTYLE CHANGES

Commonly reported reasons for poor patient adherence to treatment regimens are

- inability to understand physicians' instructions (33)
- difficulty remembering treatment regimen (34)
- lack of social support for healthy lifestyle changes (35)
- embarrassment when wearing protective therapeutic shoes because of appearance (36,37)

Detailed explanations of the disease process and the rationale for treatment have been shown to improve compliance rates (33). Therefore, educate both patients and family members regarding diabetes and foot maintenance. Understanding the rationale for the patient's lifestyle changes will encourage cooperative behavior and improve the support of family members. Enrollment in a diabetes self-management education course (that also provides instruction for foot maintenance) (38,39), provision of simple instructions in a handout, and recruitment of a family member's assistance during the patient visit may improve compliance and overall outcomes. Evaluate the patient's ability to perform the daily self-examination, which may be limited by the following conditions:

- inability to see his or her feet due to poor vision (40)
- inability to reach with hands to examine feet (in this situation, recruiting the assistance of family members or home health nursing services may help provide this necessary daily inspection and care) (41)

ROLE OF NURSING

With the increased attention drawn to the multidisciplinary model of health care delivery to patients with diabetes, nurses of all specialties have played an integral role as an extension of vital primary care services and have provided ancillary patient support mechanisms. This extension of nursing has been especially important as the patient health care delivery models have trended toward home health care, long-term assisted care, and skilled nursing services, where nurses are the primary screening professionals identifying high risk diabetic foot conditions.

ROUTINE FOOT SCREENINGS

Routine foot screenings for diabetic patients in primary care settings are a fundamental and inexpensive means of prevention that are often neglected (42–46). Reports have shown that in primary care practices, diabetic foot examinations are performed only 10–23% of the time during routine diabetes care visits (43,45,46). In a 78-chart review of six master's-level certified nurse practitioners in a primary ambulatory care center, a comprehensive foot examination based on American Diabetes Association foot care standards was documented for only

23.1% of diabetic patients (45). Additionally, a retrospective review of inpatient records revealed that a minimally acceptable evaluation of the acutely infected diabetic foot was performed for 14% of patients (47). Without routine screenings, high-risk conditions leading to diabetic foot complications cannot be identified. Altering practice patterns within the primary care setting, such as routinely removing the shoes and socks of patients during non-foot-related visits, has been shown to increase the likelihood of a foot examination more than threefold (48). Educational interventions have also been shown to be effective tools to increase probability of a foot exam. One retrospective study found that the percentage of proper diabetic foot examinations performed by physicians increased significantly, from 14 to 62% over a 6 month period, after an educational intervention consisting of two lectures and a quality assurance announcement (49). A routine foot screening program has been shown to statistically reduce lower-extremity major amputation rates in high-risk diabetic feet compared with a control group (50). Nurses play an important role in performing and facilitating foot screenings for high-risk conditions (51). Minimum requirements of the diabetic foot examination include evaluation of protective sensation, foot deformity and biomechanics, skin integrity, and vascular status (52).

DIABETIC FOOT EDUCATION

Studies have suggested that patient education improves foot care knowledge and behaviors that may reduce the incidence of complications in high-risk diabetic patients (38,39,53,54). In a randomized controlled study, patients attending a foot education session had a threefold decrease in ulceration and amputation rates after a 2-year follow-up period (38). Another randomized trial evaluating the outcome of diabetic patients who received group education compared with usual care by a general practitioner revealed a significant reduction in callus formation and minor skin injury at a 6-month follow-up (39). In addition, implementation of a support group that provides one-on-one or small-group interactive counseling and foot education to diabetic amputees and patients with chronic ulcerations has been shown to improve foot care behaviors, self-perceptions of health, and foot self-care practices (55,56).

THE TEAM APPROACH

A team approach to diabetic foot care is a coordinated method of addressing the multifaceted aspects of diabetic foot complications. Improved outcomes of diabetic foot care have been demonstrated with this organized approach. Patients who received intervention by a multidisciplinary diabetic foot team had 28% fewer reulcerations at a 2-year follow-up than did a group who received standard foot care (57). One study reported a 78% reduction in major amputations after implementation of a multidisciplinary program (58). Other studies have also demonstrated a lower incidence of major and minor amputations in patients who participated in a multidisciplinary intervention program for high-risk diabetic foot management (59). Team members have included primary care physicians, podiatrists, nurse educators, nutritionists, diabetes nurses, shoe specialists, and vascular and orthopedic surgeons (4,57–58,60–61).

Interest in the development of nursing-based models of diabetes care has grown (62–64). In a university health system, nurse-provided screening, education, and treatment has been shown to be a potential cost- and resource-effective method of decreasing the rate of diabetic foot complications (64). One reported measure of behavior improvement from this study was a reduction in improper footwear use from 73 to 43% at the first follow-up visit.

SUMMARY

Amputations of the lower extremities are among the most dreaded complications of diabetes. An estimated 85% of foot amputations are preceded by a preventable ulceration. The diabetic foot is best managed by a team approach. Screening for high-risk conditions of the diabetic foot is a basic and fundamental tool to prevent foot ulceration and amputation. Patient education in diabetic foot care may also encourage behaviors and lifestyle changes that would reduce the foot complications of diabetes. Referral to a podiatrist or foot-and-ankle orthopedist should be made for specialized treatment and management of diabetic foot complications. Despite best efforts, however, foot ulcerations and amputations may occur. Whether for prevention or treatment, nursing personnel can provide an extension of much-needed services in screening and management of the diabetic foot. Nurses have played increasingly vital roles in the multidisciplinary team through screening, patient education, and treatment. With the exhaustion of medical resources for diabetes care, the development of nursing-based models of comprehensive diabetic foot care needs to be evaluated and validated with further clinical investigations.

REFERENCES

1. Centers for Disease Control and Prevention: Crude and Age-Adjusted Prevalence of Diagnosed Diabetes per 100 Population, United States, 1980–2006 [Internet], 2007. Available from http://www.cdc.gov/diabetes/statistics/prev/national/figage.htm. Accessed on 13 February 2009

2. Palumbo P, Melton L: Peripheral vascular disease and diabetes. In *Diabetes in America*. 1st ed. Harris M, Hamman R, Eds. Washington, DC, U.S. Govt. Printing Office, 1985, p. 1–21

3. Reiber G, Boyko E, Smith D: Lower extremity foot ulcers and amputations in diabetes. In *Diabetes in America*. 2nd ed. Harris M, Cowie C, Stern M, Boyko E, Reiber G, Bennett P, Eds. Washington, DC, U.S. Govt. Printing Office, 1995, p. 409–428

4. Apelqvist J, Ragnarson-Tennvall G, Persson U, Larsson J: Diabetic foot ulcers in a multidisciplinary setting: an economic analysis of primary healing and healing with amputation. *J Intern Med* 235:463–471, 1994

5. Pecoraro RE, Reiber GE, Burgess EM: Pathways to diabetic limb amputation: basis for prevention. *Diabetes Care* 13:513–521, 1990

6. Reiber GE, Pecoraro RE, Koepsell TD: Risk factors for amputation in patients with diabetes mellitus: a case-control study. *Ann Intern Med* 117:97–105, 1992

7. Goldner M: The fate of the second leg in the diabetic amputee. *Diabetes* 9:100–103, 1960

8. Larsson J, Agardh CD, Apelqvist J, Stenstrom A: Long-term prognosis after healed amputation in patients with diabetes. *Clin Orthop* 350:149–158, 1998

9. Ramsey SD, Newton K, Blough D, McCulloch DK, Sandhu N, et al.: Incidence, outcomes, and cost of foot ulcers in patients with diabetes. *Diabetes Care* 22:382–387, 1999

10. Ashry HR, Lavery LA, Armstrong DG, Lavery DC, van Houtum WH: Cost of diabetes-related amputations in minorities. *J Foot Ankle Surg* 37:186–190, 1998

11. Bild DE, Selby JV, Sinnock P, Browner WS, Braveman P, Showstack JA: Lower-extremity amputation in people with diabetes: epidemiology and prevention. *Diabetes Care* 12:24–31, 1989

12. Fylling CP, Knighton DR: Amputation in the diabetic population: incidence, causes, cost, treatment, and prevention. *J Enterostomal Ther* 16:247–255, 1989

13. van Houtum WH, Lavery LA, Harkless LB: The costs of diabetes-related lower extremity amputations in the Netherlands. *Diabet Med* 12:777–781, 1995

14. Carrington AL, Mawdsley SK, Morley M, Kincey J, Boulton AJ: Psychological status of diabetic people with or without lower limb disability. *Diabetes Res Clin Pract* 32:19–25, 1996

15. Peters EJ, Childs MR, Wunderlich RP, Harkless LB, Armstrong DG, Lavery LA: Functional status of persons with diabetes-related lower-extremity amputations. *Diabetes Care* 24:1799–1804, 2001

16. Price P, Harding K: The impact of foot complications on health-related quality of life in patients with diabetes. *J Cutan Med Surg* 4:45–50, 2000

17. Ragnarson Tennvall G, Apelqvist J: Health-related quality of life in patients with diabetes mellitus and foot ulcers. *J Diabetes Complications* 14:235–241, 2000

18. Vileikyte L: Diabetic foot ulcers: a quality of life issue. *Diabetes Metab Res Rev* 17:246–249, 2001

19. Boyko EJ, Ahroni JH, Smith DG, Davignon D: Increased mortality associated with diabetic foot ulcer. *Diabet Med* 13:967–972, 1996

20. Chammas NK, Hill RL, Foster AV, Edmonds ME: Is neuropathic ulceration the key to understanding increased mortality due to ischaemic heart disease in diabetic foot ulcer patients? A population approach using a proportionate model. *J Int Med Res* 30:553–559, 2002

21. Moulik PK, Mtonga R, Gill GV: Amputation and mortality in new-onset diabetic foot ulcers stratified by etiology. *Diabetes Care* 26:491–494, 2003

22. Mayfield JA, Sugarman JR: The use of the Semmes-Weinstein monofilament and other threshold tests for preventing foot ulceration and amputation in persons with diabetes. *J Fam Pract* 49 (Suppl. 11):S17–S29, 2000

23. Armstrong DG, Lavery LA, Vela SA, Quebedeaux TL, Fleischli JG: Choosing a practical screening instrument to identify patients at risk for diabetic foot ulceration. *Arch Intern Med* 158:289–292, 1998

24. Mueller MJ: Identifying patients with diabetes mellitus who are at risk for lower-extremity complications: use of Semmes-Weinstein monofilaments. *Phys Ther* 76:68–71, 1996

25. Coppini DV, Bowtell PA, Weng C, Young PJ, Sonksen PH: Showing neuropathy is related to increased mortality in diabetic patients: a survival analysis using an accelerated failure time model. *J Clin Epidemiol* 53:519–523, 2000

26. Pham H, Armstrong DG, Harvey C, Harkless LB, Giurini JM, Veves A: Screening techniques to identify people at high risk for diabetic foot ulceration: a prospective multicenter trial. *Diabetes Care* 23:606–611, 2000

27. Young MJ, Breddy JL, Veves A, Boulton AJ: The prediction of diabetic neuropathic foot ulceration using vibration perception thresholds: a prospective study. *Diabetes Care* 17:557–560, 1994

28. Knowles EA, Boulton AJ: Do people with diabetes wear their prescribed footwear? *Diabet Med* 13:1064–1068, 1996

29. Macfarlane DJ, Jensen JL: Factors in diabetic footwear compliance. *J Am Podiatr Med Assoc* 93:485–491, 2003

30. Armstrong DG, Lavery LA, Sariaya M, Ashry H: Leukocytosis is a poor indicator of acute osteomyelitis of the foot in diabetes mellitus. *J Foot Ankle Surg* 35:280–283, 1996.

31. Lavery LA, Armstrong DG, Vela SA, Quebedeaux TL, Fleischli JG: Practical criteria for screening patients at high risk for diabetic foot ulceration. *Arch Intern Med* 158:157–162, 1998

32. Murray HJ, Young MJ, Hollis S, Boulton AJ: The association between callus formation, high pressures and neuropathy in diabetic foot ulceration. *Diabet Med* 13:979–982, 1996

33. Davis M: Variations in patients' compliance with doctors' orders. *J Med Educ* 41:1037–1048, 1966

34. Fitzgerald JT, Anderson RM, Funnell MM, Arnold MS, Davis WK, et al.: Differences in the impact of dietary restrictions on African Americans and Caucasians with NIDDM. *Diabetes Educ* 23:41–47, 1997

35. Tillotson LM, Smith MS: Locus of control, social support, and adherence to the diabetes regimen. *Diabetes Educ* 22:133–139, 1996

36. Breuer U: Diabetic patient's compliance with bespoke footwear after healing of neuropathic foot ulcers. *Diabete Metab* 20:415–419, 1994

37. Chantelau E, Kushner T, Spraul M: How effective is cushioned therapeutic footwear in protecting diabetic feet? A clinical study. *Diabet Med* 7:355–359, 1990

38. Malone JM, Snyder M, Anderson G, Bernhard VM, Holloway GA Jr, Bunt TJ: Prevention of amputation by diabetic education. *Am J Surg* 158:520–523, 1989

39. Pieber TR, Holler A, Siebenhofer A, Brunner GA, Semlitsch B, et al.: Evaluation of a structured teaching and treatment programme for type 2 diabetes in general practice in a rural area of Austria. *Diabet Med* 12:349–354, 1995

40. Crausaz FM, Clavel S, Liniger C, Albeanu A, Assal JP: Additional factors associated with plantar ulcers in diabetic neuropathy. *Diabet Med* 5:771–775, 1988

41. Thomson FJ, Masson EA: Can elderly diabetic patients co-operate with routine foot care? *Age Ageing* 21:333–337, 1992

42. Bailey TS, Yu HM, Rayfield EJ: Patterns of foot examination in a diabetes clinic. *Am J Med* 78:371–374, 1985

43. Chin MH, Cook S, Jin L, Drum ML, Harrison JF, et al.: Barriers to providing diabetes care in community health centers. *Diabetes Care* 24:268–274, 2001

44. Fain JA, Melkus GD: Nurse practitioner practice patterns based on standards of medical care for patients with diabetes. *Diabetes Care* 17:879–881, 1994

45. Wylie-Rosett J, Walker EA, Shamoon H, Engel S, Basch C, Zybert P: Assessment of documented foot examinations for patients with diabetes in inner-city primary care clinics. *Arch Fam Med* 4:46–50, 1995

46. Zoorob RJ, Mainous AG 3rd: Practice patterns of rural family physicians based on the American Diabetes Association standards of care. *J Community Health* 21:175–182, 1996

47. Edelson GW, Armstrong DG, Lavery LA, Caicco G: The acutely infected diabetic foot is not adequately evaluated in an inpatient setting. *Arch Intern Med* 156:2373–2378, 1996

48. Cohen SJ: Potential barriers to diabetes care. *Diabetes Care* 6:499–500, 1983

49. O'Brien KE, Chandramohan V, Nelson DA, Fischer JR Jr, Stevens G, Poremba JA: Effect of a physician-directed educational campaign on performance of proper diabetic foot exams in an outpatient setting. *J Gen Intern Med* 18:258–265, 2003

50. McCabe CJ, Stevenson RC, Dolan AM: Evaluation of a diabetic foot screening and protection programme. *Diabet Med* 15:80–84, 1998

51. Neil JA, Knuckey CJ, Tanenberg RJ: Prevention of foot ulcers in patients with diabetes and end stage renal disease. *Nephrol Nurs J* 30:39–43, 2003

52. American Diabetes Association: Preventive foot care in people with diabetes (Position Statement). *Diabetes Care* 27 (Suppl. 1):S63–S64, 2004

53. Litzelman DK, Slemenda CW, Langefeld CD, Hays LM, Welch MA, et al.: Reduction of lower extremity clinical abnormalities in patients with non-insulin-dependent diabetes mellitus: a randomized, controlled trial. *Ann Intern Med* 119:36–41, 1993

54. Ward A, Metz L, Oddone EZ, Edelman D: Foot education improves knowledge and satisfaction among patients at high risk for diabetic foot ulcer. *Diabetes Educ* 25:560–567, 1999

55. Neder S, Nadash P: Individualized education can improve foot care for patients with diabetes. *Home Healthc Nurse* 21:837–840, 2003

56. Ooi GS, Rodrigo C, Cheong WK, Mehta RL, Bowen G, Shearman CP: An evaluation of the value of group education in recently diagnosed diabetes mellitus. *Int J Low Extrem Wounds* 6:28–33, 2007

57. Dargis V, Pantelejeva O, Jonushaite A, Vileikyte L, Boulton AJ: Benefits of a multidisciplinary approach in the management of recurrent diabetic foot ulceration in Lithuania: a prospective study. *Diabetes Care* 22:1428–1431, 1999

58. Larsson J, Apelqvist J, Agardh CD, Stenstrom A: Decreasing incidence of major amputation in diabetic patients: a consequence of a multidisciplinary foot care team approach? *Diabet Med* 12:770–776, 1995

59. Rerkasem K, Kosachunhanun N, Tongprasert S, Khwanngern K, Matanasarawoot A, et al.: The development and application of diabetic foot protocol in Chiang Mai University Hospital with an aim to reduce lower extremity amputation in Thai population: a preliminary communication. *Int J Low Extrem Wounds* 6:18–21, 2007

60. Edmonds ME, Blundell MP, Morris ME, Thomas EM, Cotton LT, Watkins PJ: Improved survival of the diabetic foot: the role of a specialized foot clinic. *Q J Med* 60:763–771, 1986

61. Frykberg RG: The team approach in diabetic foot management. *Adv Wound Care* 11:71–77, 1998

62. Davidson MB: Effect of nurse-directed diabetes care in a minority population. *Diabetes Care* 26:2281–2287, 2003

63. Jones PM: Quality improvement initiative to integrate teaching diabetes standards into home care visits. *Diabetes Educ* 28:1009–1020, 2002

64. Pinzur MS, Kernan-Schroeder D, Emanuele NV, Emanuel M: Development of a nurse-provided health system strategy for diabetic foot care. *Foot Ankle Int* 22:744–746, 2001

ADDITIONAL READING

Apelqvist J, Bakker K, van Houtum WH, Nabuurs-Franssen MH, Schaper NC: International consensus and practical guidelines on the management and the prevention of the diabetic foot: International Working Group on the Diabetic Foot. *Diabetes Metab Res Rev* 16 (Suppl. 1):S84–S92, 2000

Boulton AJM, Armstrong DG, Albert SF, Frykberg R, Hellman R, et al.: Comprehensive foot examination and risk assessment: a report of the task force of the foot care interest group of the American Diabetes Association, with the endorsement of by the American Association of Clinical Endocrinologist. *Diabetes Care* 31:1679–1684, 2008

Frykberg RG, Armstrong DG, Giurini J, Edwards A, Kravette M, et al.: Diabetic foot disorders: a clinical practice guideline: American College of Foot and Ankle Surgeons. *J Foot Ankle Surg* 39 (Suppl. 5):S1–S60, 2000

Inlow S, Orsted H, Sibbald RG: Best practices for the prevention, diagnosis, and treatment of diabetic foot ulcers. *Ostomy Wound Manage* 46:55–68, 2000

Pinzur MS, Slovenkai MP, Trepman E, Shields NN: Guidelines for diabetic foot care: the Diabetes Committee of the American Orthopaedic Foot and Ankle Society. *Foot Ankle Int* 26:113–119, 2005

Schaper NC, Apelqvist J, Bakker K: The international consensus and practical guidelines on the management and prevention of the diabetic foot. *Curr Diabetes Rep* 3:475–479, 2003

Sykes MT, Godsey JB: Vascular evaluation of the problem diabetic foot. *Clin Podiatr Med Surg* 15:49–83, 1998

Dr. Liu is a Clinical Assistant Professor at the University of Texas Health Science Center at San Antonio, San Antonio, TX. Dr. Steinberg is an Assistant Professor at the University of Texas Health Science Center at San Antonio, San Antonio, TX, and Medical Director, Podiatry Clinic, at the Texas Diabetes Institute, San Antonio, TX.

DIABETES CARE
AND MANAGEMENT

16. Diabetes Education in the Management of Diabetes

Martha M. Funnell, MS, RN, CDE, and
Carolé R. Mensing, RN, MA, CDE

Diabetes self-management education (DSME), also referred to as diabetes self-management training (DSMT), has long been considered a cornerstone of diabetes care. Because ~99% of the care is provided by the person with diabetes and his or her family members, effective care requires a partnership between an actively involved patient and the health care team (1). Education is critical for the patient to become involved and to make informed self-management decisions on a daily basis.

Most nurses think of diabetes education as a comprehensive program offered in an outpatient setting or by an inpatient diabetes nurse educator. In fact, each encounter with a person who has diabetes is an opportunity for education, and every nurse shares the responsibility for that education. Even when time is limited, nurses can create "teachable moments" to provide and reinforce needed information. For example, giving insulin to a hospitalized patient is an excellent time to assess and review insulin injection technique, treatment of hypoglycemia, and the need to wear or carry diabetes identification and glucose tablets. Bathing a hospitalized or home care patient or doing a foot examination during an outpatient visit provides the opportunity to assess foot care self-management practices by asking, "What do you do to care for your feet at home?" and offering individualized foot care instruction based on the physical findings and the patient's response. In every setting, nurses not only teach information, but also help patients to develop strategies and overcome obstacles in order to effectively use that information to manage diabetes on a daily basis.

EVIDENCE FOR DSME

Multiple meta-analyses and reviews have documented the effectiveness of DSME in improving knowledge, psychosocial outcomes, and health outcomes (2–9). The greatest predictive factor of the effectiveness of DSME is the amount of time spent with the educator, typically a nurse (4,10). Table 16.1 summarizes the key findings from these studies (5).

It is important to note that although no single educational program is more effective than others, interventions that incorporate effective and behavioral aspects produce better outcomes (10–13). Tailoring the interventions to the age and culture of the participants (14–15) and including spouses and adult children may also increase DSME effectiveness, as has been shown for older African-American and Latino individuals with diabetes (14).

Table 16.1 Effectiveness of DSME

Characteristics of effective interventions
- Regular reinforcement is more effective than one-time or short-term education.
- Patient participation and collaboration appear to produce more favorable results than didactic interventions.
- Group education is more effective than one-on-one education for lifestyle interventions and appears to be equally effective for improving knowledge and accuracy of self-monitoring of blood glucose (SMBG).
- Studies with short-term follow up are more likely to demonstrate positive effects on glycemic control and behavioral outcomes than studies with long-term follow up.

Effectiveness in clinical settings
- In the short term (<6 months), DSME improves knowledge levels, SMBG skills, and dietary habits (per self-report).
- In the short term (<6 months), glycemic control improves.
- Improved glycemic control does not appear to correspond to measured changes in knowledge or SMBG skills.
- Weight loss can be achieved with repetitive interventions or with short-term follow up (<6 months).
- Physical activity levels are variably affected by interventions.
- Effects on lipids and blood pressure are variable but are more likely to be positive with interactive or individualized repetitive interventions.

Effectiveness in nonclinical settings
- Some evidence indicates that DSME is effective when given in community gathering places (e.g., churches and community centers) for adults with type 2 diabetes.
- The literature is insufficient to assess the effectiveness of DSME in the home for adults with diabetes (9).
- The literature is insufficient to assess the effectiveness of DSME in the workplace.

Reprinted with permission from Norris (5).

PRACTICAL POINT
The educational process includes assessment, provision of content using appropriate strategies, documentation, and outcome evaluation. Each of these steps is necessary whether DSME is part of a comprehensive program or focused education is provided during hospitalization, home care, or routine outpatient visits.

DSME is essential but not sufficient for the type of sustained behavior change required by a chronic illness such as diabetes (4,16). As a result, there is an increasing emphasis on the provision of ongoing diabetes self-management support (DSMS). Without this support, most outcomes return to pre-education levels in ~6 months (4). Strategies that can be used to provide ongoing self-management support include self-directed goal setting; nurse care management; use of lay or peer health workers; Internet, telephone, or e-mail systems; and support groups.

Diabetes education has evolved in recent years from a didactic format to more theoretically based empowerment models using approaches that recognize the principles of adult learning and acknowledge that the person with diabetes is the primary decision maker in his or her own care (3,17). Educational strategies have evolved as well to match this growing body of evidence and to meet quality standards to obtain reimbursement.

EDUCATIONAL PROCESS

The educational process parallels the nursing process. With assessment as the first step, the nurse and patient (or caregiver) identify the educational needs (nursing diagnosis), plan and implement the intervention, which in DSME involves the educational content and the educational strategies used, and then evaluates the process.

ASSESSMENT

Personalization, or developing a plan that incorporates and meets the needs of the individual, is a critical component of effective DSME. The first step in the process is assessment. (Examples of questions to ask during the assessment process are listed in Table 16.2.) The assessment is then used to develop the educational plan in collaboration with the participant and/or family members and caregivers. Areas of greatest concern and any questions identified by the patient need to be addressed at the beginning of the intervention. This helps tailor the educational program to that particular patient and increases both the efficiency and effectiveness of the DSME intervention. Beginning with "What questions do you have about . . ." or "What do you know about . . ." is an effective way to start even a brief educational encounter.

Table 16.2 Examples of Educational Assessment Questions

- In what language do you prefer to speak? To read?
- What is your favorite way to learn (e.g., reading, discussion, videos, computers, group class, individual teaching)?
- Where do you get most of your information about health and diabetes?
- Do you have difficulty with your hearing or vision, such as reading regular-size print?
- How far did you go in school?
- Do you have any cultural or religious practices or beliefs that affect how you care for your health and diabetes?
- Do you ever have difficulty paying for your diabetes supplies or medicines?
- Do you have trouble remembering things?
- Have you ever known other people with diabetes? How did it affect them?
- Do you have health problems that you manage other than diabetes? What helps you to manage them?
- Have you ever lost weight or increased your physical activity? What helped you to make those changes? What got in your way?
- What areas of diabetes are you most interested in learning more about?
- What are you currently doing to manage your diabetes at home?
- On a scale of 1 to 10, with 10 being the most important, how important is managing diabetes in your life?
- On a scale of 1 to 10, with 10 being the most sure, how confident are you that you can manage your diabetes?
- How much stress are you experiencing in your life?
- Have you felt sad and blue most of the time for the past 2 weeks? Two months?
- What kind of support do you want and need from your family and friends to care for your diabetes?
- What kind of support do you receive from your family and friends to care for your diabetes?
- Who helps you the most to care for your diabetes?
- What is your greatest concern about your diabetes?
- What is the hardest thing for you in caring for your diabetes?
- What were your thoughts/feelings when you first learned that you had diabetes? What are your thoughts/feelings now?
- How can I be most helpful to you?

A formal assessment needs to include developmental age, cultural influences, health beliefs and attitudes, diabetes knowledge, self-management skills and behaviors, readiness to learn, language, health literacy, cognitive ability, physical limitations, environment, family support, financial concerns (e.g., medication costs), and relevant medical history (18). It is equally important to find out what areas the patient wishes to learn or cause the greatest concerns or worries.

Assessment is appropriate whether the patient is newly diagnosed or has lived with diabetes for some time. Even newly diagnosed adults or parents of newly diagnosed children have some level of knowledge or experience with diabetes. A personal assessment not only is in keeping with adult learning principles, but also shows respect for the patient or the caregiver and allows a true partnership to begin. The assessment also provides the opportunity to clarify misconceptions, update old information, and involve patients in the creation of their personal educational objectives and plan. Including family members or caregivers in the planning process may also be desired by some patients.

CONTENT

Table 16.3 outlines topic-specific content areas to be addressed in a comprehensive educational program (18). These content areas are written in behavioral terms to allow maximum creativity and flexibility in the teaching process. Specific areas to address with each patient are identified during the assessment, and only the relevant areas need to be provided. Ideally, all patients with diabetes are referred to an in-depth, comprehensive educational program, either at diagnosis or at some point during their life with diabetes. Even patients who have had diabetes for a number of years can benefit from a refresher course or referral to a support group.

These content areas are applicable in all settings and can be provided at basic, intermediate, or advanced levels. Generally, the depth of the content needed determines the level rather than a particular topic. For example, basic or survival education for self-monitoring of blood glucose (SMBG) may include only the skills of checking glucose levels, recording the results, and setting standard goals. Intermediate SMBG education may include development of personal blood glucose goals and interpretation of the results, and advanced SMBG education may include pattern management. Standardized curricula and goals for diabetes education are available to help nurses create programs that address all of the recommended content areas and to ensure consistency among instructors (see RESOURCES and "Additional Reading" at the end of this chapter). Many nurses find adapting these curricula to be more efficient than developing their own. These can also be useful for nurses who provide education on an ongoing basis to be sure that they are consistently addressing all of the critical content areas.

The level of DSME is based on the assessment rather than the length of time since diagnosis. In addition, patients may be at a basic level in one area and at an advanced level in others based on their self-management experience and past education. When there is only the opportunity to provide limited education, such as with hospitalized patients, asking what they know and want to know about diabetes, current practices and concerns about managing it at home, fears about diabetes, and what is hardest for them helps the nurse provide relevant targeted information in a short period of time. Referral to a comprehensive DSME program is an important part of discharge planning and outpatient follow up for these patients.

Table 16.3 DSME Content Areas

- Describing the *diabetes disease process* and *treatment options*
- Incorporating *nutritional* management into lifestyle
- Incorporating *physical activity* into lifestyle
- Using *medication(s)* safely and for maximum therapeutic effectiveness
- *Monitoring blood glucose* and other parameters and interpreting and using the results for self-management decision making
- Preventing, detecting, and treating *acute complications*
- Preventing detecting, and treating *chronic complications*
- Developing personal strategies to address *psychosocial issues and concerns*
- Developing personal strategies to promote *health and behavior change*

Adapted from Funnell et al. (18).

EDUCATIONAL STRATEGIES

Multiple reviews and meta-analyses have been performed that are useful for understanding the underlying principles and critical elements of successful self-management education (4,5,8,10–12,16). Effective strategies include involving patients (or caregivers) in their own care; guiding them in actively learning about the disease by providing fewer lectures and more practice, interactive, or problem-based exercises; assessing and addressing feelings related to having diabetes; teaching the skills needed to adjust behavior (4,5,10,11,16,19); and tailoring the intervention to the age, culture, ethnicity, and health literacy of the participants (14,20–24). Framing information to meet patient-identified goals (e.g., have more energy, better quality of life) rather than focusing strictly on metabolic goals or risk reduction also helps to increase effectiveness.

Incorporating behavioral strategies into the education process by teaching patients how to use these skills to solve problems, respond to physical and self-management challenges throughout the course of their of their chronic illness, and make and sustain changes in their own behavior improves outcomes resulting from education (4,7,9,13,19,25,26). Training in self-directed goal-setting, problem solving, skill-building, action planning, healthy coping, stress-management, and self-monitoring and providing links to community resources have been effectively used in successful patient education programs (5,22,23,25,27). There is some evidence that using more than one of these strategies increases effectiveness (19,21–27).

Psychosocial issues affect behavior and can interfere with a person's ability to self-manage a chronic illness. For example, the Diabetes Attitudes, Wishes, and Needs (DAWN) study found that among 5,104 patients in 13 countries, diabetes-related distress was common among people with both type 1 and type 2 diabetes and that these issues interfered with their self-management efforts (28,29). A large majority of the patient participants (85.2%) reported a high level of distress at the time of diagnosis, including feelings of shock, guilt, anger, anxiety, depression, and helplessness. Many years after diagnosis (mean duration almost 15 years), problems of living with diabetes remained common, including fear of complications and immediate social and psychological burdens of caring for diabetes (28). Forty-one percent of patients reported poor well-being and indicated that they wanted greater acknowledgement and support for their distress (29). Teaching healthy coping and stress-management and exploring these feelings are strategies nurses can use to enhance self-efficacy and ultimately improve patients' ability to manage their chronic illnesses (19). Addressing these issues as part of group education, where other participants can help to normalize these feelings by sharing their own experiences and providing social support, is particularly useful (11,22–24).

Integrating the affective or emotional and behavioral components with clinical content increases effectiveness (4,10). For example, when teaching about SMBG, asking questions such as the following can help patients incorporate this behavior more easily:

- When will you check your blood glucose level?
- How will you check when you are away from home?

- How do others respond when you check your blood glucose in front of them?
- How would you like others to respond or show support?
- How do you feel/will you respond when a reading is higher or lower than you had hoped or anticipated?
- What can you do to help yourself check your blood glucose more faithfully?
- Would you like to set a goal for checking your blood glucose?

One strategy that has been used effectively is a question-based approach, with content presented in response to participant-identified issues (22–24,30). For example, a woman is concerned about how she will follow a specific meal plan while still providing her family the food they like. Teaching the woman to cook her family's favorite foods in a more healthy way is more likely to be helpful to her than giving her a preprinted meal plan. Content is monitored and recorded to be sure that all necessary areas are addressed. This approach helps ensure that participants remain engaged and actively involved in the discussion, take advantage of the experiences of other participants in the education program, and view it as "personal" (22).

DOCUMENTATION

Documentation of the educational assessment, plan, and actual education provided is necessary to meet quality and accreditation standards (18). The content areas presented in Table 16.3 are useful categories for documentation. In addition, documentation should include information about content presented, response of the patient, problems or barriers encountered, readiness to learn, and patient-selected goals. The documentation should provide enough information so that others can follow up and reinforce content as needed and assess goal attainment. Supplying this information to the referring provider helps promote a team approach and allows additional reinforcement during patient visits. Developing a specific form that includes content areas, level of education provided, problems identified, self-selected behavioral goals, and areas to reinforce helps promote consistent documentation and education by all health care providers. Once the education is completed, a written plan for ongoing diabetes self-management support is needed both to meet accreditation standards and to help ensure that it occurs (18).

OUTCOME EVALUATION

Outcomes to be evaluated include individual patient outcomes and programmatic outcomes. Attainment of self-selected behavioral goals is the most important individual outcome to assess (18). It is more effective if this follow-up occurs in <6 months (4). Programmatic outcomes can include pre- and postmetabolic measures, screening for complications, self-care behaviors, quality of life or other validated psychosocial measures, and patient satisfaction. Knowledge tests can be useful for helping patients identify areas that need more attention, but are generally not adequate for program evaluation.

It is important to choose programmatic outcomes that are likely to be affected by the content and format of the DSME intervention. For example, if foot care is an area that is of particular relevance to the population and emphasized throughout the program, pre- and post-assessment of foot care behaviors would be an appropriate outcome measure.

Continuous quality improvement provides ongoing monitoring and allows adjustments and improvements on an ongoing basis (18). A DSME program advisory group or committee made up of key staff members, stakeholders, and patients is often a useful mechanism to ensure that this process occurs and that the program is modified accordingly.

INDIVIDUAL VERSUS GROUP EDUCATION

The provision of DSME is constantly changing and is challenging for the nurse educator. Nurses are often most comfortable teaching patients individually at first, yet there are constraints with this approach. Time and money are two of the more compelling considerations in determining whether to provide a group or individual program. The time required for patients to attend such educational offerings and for nurse educators to set aside for the purpose of teaching is considerable, as are third-party reimbursement availability and self-payment abilities.

The group setting is being recognized more and more as an effective milieu for education (5,8,31–33). A recent meta-analysis (8) showed that group education was effective for improving metabolic and psychosocial outcomes among people with type 2 diabetes. Various community sites (e.g., places of worship, senior centers) can be used to increase accessibility (33,34). Little information on cost-effectiveness exists, yet this aspect is often used as justification for group education.

Group education is an important skill for nurses, and they are often encouraged by their patients, their own preferences, and their administrators to offer both individual and group teaching. Group programs provide the educator with a wider variety of experiences from which to learn and gain skills. Group sessions, like individual sessions, are based on the evidence, the nurse's personal style and teaching preferences, the patients who are in attendance, as well as the time available. Skills needed for effective group education include preparation (e.g., choice of teaching materials and resources), development of delivery options to enhance the content, assessment of the learners, and timely documentation (5,31). Nurses can provide counseling and problem solving in these settings without increasing the time spent (30–32).

Group education offers the nurse opportunities to learn a variety of new teaching and facilitation skills, learn new perspectives on how to deliver the "same old information," share team creativity, and expand the team as a coordinated working unit. Whether educating in groups or individually, the most important factor is not the setting, but the ability to provide interesting interventions, an efficient learning process, and empowerment for both the teacher and the patient.

OTHER DELIVERY METHODS

Print materials, videotapes, CDs, DVDs, and computer learning programs can be useful adjuncts to the educational process. Materials are more effective when they are based on the needs of the target audience and on a formative evaluation; tailored to the age, cultural background, and preferences of the target audience (33); written at a fifth- to sixth-grade reading level; and matched to a specific interest or need. Personalizing print materials by highlighting key areas or making handwritten notes helps increase their effectiveness. Print materials are available on the Internet from a variety of reputable sources, such as diabetes organizations (e.g., National Diabetes Education Program (NDEP) at http://ndep.nih.gov/). Downloading and providing these materials to patients has the advantage of offering more current information than keeping a number of booklets and brochures on hand.

Viewing a videotape or listening to a CD needs to be followed by asking patients if they have questions and evaluating their ability to apply the information to their own lives, situations, and treatment plans. Telephone follow-up for education, goal setting, and care management is also commonly used and effective (34–36).

Use of other technologies, such as the Internet and distance learning, shows promise in some studies but application of these programs has not been widespread (37). Ask patients who have questions based on Internet information to bring the material to their appointment or education session. This will help you better understand their questions and evaluate the validity of the information.

RECOGNITION OF DSME

Standards for DSME were first developed in 1983 by key diabetes organizations, including the American Diabetes Association (ADA) and the American Association of Diabetes Educators. These standards were most recently revised and published in 2007 (18). The standards were based on current evidence and best practices. There are 10 standards that address the structure, process, and outcomes of DSME. Nutrition education and counseling may be provided as part of the program, through a separate referral to a registered dietitian, or both.

The ADA created the Education Recognition Program (ERP) to recognize DSME programs that meet these national standards. Programs are required to apply and to document that they meet the established review criteria. Referring patients to recognized programs helps ensure that they receive comprehensive quality education that is likely to be reimbursed. Recognized programs can be found using a search page on ADA's web site (http://professional.diabetes.org/erp_zip_search.aspx). In addition to the national ADA ERP, the Indian Health Service offers certification for programs provided by that agency.

CERTIFICATION FOR DIABETES EDUCATORS

All nurses who interact with diabetic patients are diabetes educators in some form. Registered nurses and other health care professionals can become certified diabetes educators and use the designation CDE. Certification is available from the National Certification Board for Diabetes Educators (NCBDE) (www.ncbde.org). Nurses who wish to become certified must meet the educational and experiential requirements of the NCBDE and pass a multidisciplinary examination. Recertification is required every 5 years through continuing education credits or retaking the examination. Certification provides documentation that the educator is qualified to provide education but does not directly affect reimbursement for services.

Board Certified–Advanced Diabetes Management (BC-ADM) is the first advanced-practice certification offered to members of more than one discipline. Nurse practitioners, clinical nurse specialists, registered dietitians, and registered pharmacists may apply. It is conferred by the American Nurses Credentialing Center. While BC-ADM recognizes specialization and enhances professionalism and may indirectly influence financial reimbursement, this credential is not currently directly related to reimbursement. More information is available on the American Association for Diabetes Educators web site (http://www.diabeteseducator.org/ProfessionalResources/Certification/BC-ADM/).

REIMBURSEMENT FOR DSME

Insurance coverage for DSME is available and mandated by most states in the U.S. This reimbursement is the direct result of significant advocacy efforts by the major diabetes organizations and the growing body of evidence supporting the effectiveness of DSME. Although requirements vary according to the state and the individual's health plan, most require ADA recognition or state certification to ensure quality. Although coverage is not yet universal, it has become more available and accessible in recent years. Before referral, it is important for patients to check with their health insurance provider to determine the level of coverage available and the requirements for reimbursement. Most educational programs also have this information available.

Reimbursement for DSME was initiated by Medicare in 2001. Medicare requires a physician prescription and allows for 10 h of initial group training unless the patient has special needs, such as a hearing impairment, which create an additional allowance for individual education. One hour of this time is set aside for the assessment. Two hours of follow-up per year may be provided individually or in groups (38).

SUMMARY

DSME is a critical element of quality diabetes care (39). Patients and their caregivers must have information to actively manage in their own care and to form a partnership with the health care team. DSME is effective when provided by nurses using strategies and interventions that incorporate the current evidence for effective teaching. Providing ongoing self-management support using behavioral strategies, such as goal setting, helps patients maintain needed health behaviors. The national standards and recognition or certification help ensure quality and support reimbursement.

The future health and outcomes of people with diabetes depend on their ability to effectively manage diabetes on a daily basis. Nurses play a key role in ensuring that patients and those who care for and about them recognize the importance of their role in managing their diabetes, understand the need for education, and have the requisite skills to effectively control diabetes on a daily basis. Nurses need to take advantage of every encounter with patients to provide and reinforce education and the importance of self-management for their outcomes and future health. Providing information regarding third-party reimbursement and referring patients to programs that meet the national standards for DSME helps ensure that patients have access to this vital service.

REFERENCES

1. VonKorff M, Gruman J, Schaefer J, Curry SJ, Wagner EH: Collaborative management of chronic illness. *Ann Intern Med* 127:1097–1102, 1997

2. Brown S: Interventions to promote diabetes self-management: state of the science. *Diabetes Educ* 25 (Suppl.):52–61, 1999

3. Norris SL, Engelgau MM, Narayan KM: Effectiveness of self-management training in type 2 diabetes. *Diabetes Care* 24:561–587, 2001

4. Norris SL, Lau J, Smith SJ, Schmid CH, Engelgau MM: Self-management education for adults with type 2 diabetes: a meta-analysis of the effect on glycemic control. *Diabetes Care* 25:1159–1171, 2002

5. Norris SL: Self-management education in type 2 diabetes: what works? *Pract Diabetol* 22:7–13, 2003

6. Renders CM, Valk GD, Griffin SJ, Wagner EH, Eijk JThM van, Assendelft WJJ: Interventions to improve the management of diabetes mellitus in primary care, outpatient, and community settings (Cochrane Review). In *The Cochrane Library, Issue 4*. Chichester, UK, John Wiley & Sons, 2004

7. Gary TL, Genkinger JM, Guallar E, Peyrot M, Brancati FL: Meta-analysis of randomized educational and behavioral interventions in type 2 diabetes. *Diabetes Educ* 29:488–501, 2003

8. Deakin T, McShane CE, Cade JE, et al.: Review: group based education in self-management strategies improves outcomes in type 2 diabetes mellitus. *Cochrane Database Syst Rev* (2):CD003417, 2005

9. Ellis SE, Speroff T, Dittus RS, Brown A, Pichert JW, Elasy TA: Diabetes patient education: a meta-analysis and meta-regression. *Patient Educ Counsel* 52:97–105 2004

10. Polonsky WH, Earles J, Smith S, Pease DJ, Macmillan M, et al.: Integrating medical management with diabetes self-management training: a randomized control trial of the Diabetes Outpatient Intensive Treatment Program. *Diabetes Care* 26:3094–3053, 2003

11. Barlow J, Wright C, Sheasby J, Turner A, Hainsworth J: Self-management approaches for people with chronic conditions: a review. *Patient Educ Counsel* 48:177–187, 2002

12. Roter DL, Hall JA, Merisca R, Nordstrom B, Cretin D, Svarstad B: Effectiveness of interventions to improve patient compliance: a meta-analysis. *Med Care* 36:1138–1161, 1998

13. Skinner TC, Cradock S, Arundel F, Graham W: Lifestyle and behavior: four theories and a philosophy: self-management education for individuals newly diagnosed with type 2 diabetes. *Diabetes Spectrum* 16:75–80, 2003

14. Sarkisian CA, Brown AAF, Norris CK, Wintz R, Mangione CM: A systematic review of diabetes self-care interventions for older, African American or Latino adults. *Diabetes Educ* 28:467–479, 2003

15. Chodosh J, Morton SC, Mojica W, Maglione M, Suttorp MJ, et al.: Meta-analysis: chronic disease self-management programs for older adults. *Ann Intern Med* 143:427–438, 2005

16. Piette JD, Glasgow RE: Education and self-monitoring of blood glucose. In *Evidence-Based Diabetes Care*. Gerstein HC, Haynes RB, Eds. Ontario, Canada, Decker, 2001, p. 207–251

17. Funnell MM, Anderson RM, Nwankwo R, Gillard ML, Butler PM, et al.: A study of certified diabetes educators: influences and barriers. *Diabetes Educ* 32:359–372, 2006

18. Funnell MM, Brown TL, Childs BP, Haas LB, Hosey GM, et al.: National Standards for Diabetes Self-management Education. *Diabetes Care* 30:1630–1637, 2007

19. Kirchbaum K, Aarestad V, Buethe M. Exploring the connection between self-efficacy and effective diabetes self-management. *Diabetes Educ* 29:653–662, 2003

20. Glazier RH, Bajcar J, Kennie NR, Willson K: A systematic review of interventions to improve diabetes care in socially disadvantaged populations. *Diabetes Care* 26:1675–88, 2006

21. Schillinger D, Grumbach K, Piette J, Wang F, Osmond D, et al.: Association of health literacy with diabetes outcomes. *JAMA* 288:475–482, 2002

22. Anderson RM, Funnell MM, Nwankwo R, Gillard L, Oh M, Fitzgerald JT: Evaluating a problem based empowerment program for African Americans with diabetes: results of a randomized controlled trial. *Ethn Dis* 15:671–678, 2005

23. Tang TS, Gillard ML, Funnell MM, Nwankwo R, Parker E, et al.: Developing a new generation of ongoing diabetes self-management support interventions (DSMS): a preliminary report. *Diabetes Educ* 31:91–97, 2005

24. Deakin TA, Cade JE, Williams R, Greenwood DC: Structured patient education: the diabetes X-PERT Programme makes a difference. *Diabet Med* 23:944–954, 2006

25. Glasgow RE, Davis CL, Funnell MM, Beck A: Implementing practical interventions to support chronic illness self-management. *Jt Comm J Qual Patient Saf* 29:563–574, 2003

26. Peyrot M, Rubin RR: Behavioral and psychosocial interventions in diabetes: a conceptual review. *Diabetes Care* 30:2433–2440, 2007

27. Bodenheimer T, MacGregor K, Sharifi C: *Helping Patients Manage Their Chronic Conditions*. Oakland, CA, California Healthcare Foundation, 2005

28. Skovlund SE, Peyrot M, on behalf of the DAWN International Advisory Panel: The Diabetes Attitudes, Wishes, and Needs (DAWN) program: a new approach to improving outcomes of diabetes care. *Diabetes Spectrum* 18:136–142, 2005

29. Peyrot M, Rubin RR, Lauritzen T, Snoek FJ, Matthews DR, Skovlund SE: Psychosocial problems and barriers to improved diabetes management: results of the cross-national Diabetes Attitudes, Wishes, and Needs study. *Diabet Med* 22:1379–1385, 2005

30. Funnell MM, Nwankwo R, Gillard ML, Anderson RM, Tang TS: From DSME to DSMS: developing empowerment-based diabetes self-management support. *Diabetes Spectrum* 20:221–226, 2007

31. Mensing CR, Norris SL: Group education in diabetes: effectiveness and implementation. *Diabetes Spectrum* 16:96–103, 2003

32. King EB, Schlundt DG, Pichert JW, Kinzer CK, Backer BA: Improving the skills of health professionals in engaging patients in diabetes-related problem solving. *J Contin Educ Health Prof* 22:94–102, 2002

33. Caballero AE: Cultural competence in diabetes mellitus care: an urgent need. *Insulin* 2:80–91, 2007

34. Norris SL, Nichols PJ, Caspersen CJ, Glasgow RE, Engelgau MM, et al.: Increasing diabetes self-management education in community settings: a systematic review. *Am J Prev Med* 22 (Suppl. 4):39–66, 2002

35. Brownson CA, O'Toole ML, Sherry G, Anwuri VV, Fisher EB: Clinic-community partnerships: a foundation for providing community supports for diabetes care and self-management. *Diabetes Spectrum* 20:209–213, 2007

36. Norris SL, Nichols PJ, Caspersen CJ, Glasgow RE, Engelgau MM, et al.: The effectiveness of disease and case management for people with diabetes: a systematic review. *Am J Prev Med* 22 (Suppl. 4):15–38, 2002

37. Piette JD: Interactive behavior change technology to support diabetes self-management. *Diabetes Care* 30:2425–2432, 2007

38. Bourgeois P: Insurance: what our patients need to know. *Diabetes Spectrum* 18:62–64, 2005

39. American Diabetes Association: Standards of medical care in diabetes—2009 (Position Statement). *Diabetes Care* 32 (Suppl. 1):S13–S61, 2009

ADDITIONAL READING

Franz MJ, Reader D, Monk A: *Implementing Group and Individual Medical Nutrition Therapy for Diabetes.* Alexandria, VA, American Diabetes Association, 2003

Funnell MM, Lasichak AJ, Burkhart NT, Gillard ML, Nwankwo R: *101 Tips for Diabetes Self-Management Education.* Alexandria, VA, American Diabetes Association, 2002

Funnell MM, Lasichak AJ, Arnold MS, Barr PB: *Life with Diabetes: A Series of Teaching Outlines.* 3rd ed. Alexandria, VA, American Diabetes Association, 2004

Kanzer-Lewis G: *Patient Education: You Can Do It!* Alexandria, VA, American Diabetes Association, 2003

Marrero DG, Anderson R, Funnell MM, Maryniuk MD: *1000 Years of Diabetes Wisdom.* Alexandria, VA, American Diabetes Association, 2008

Siminerio L, McLaughlin S, Polonsky W: *Diabetes Education Goals.* 3rd ed. Alexandria, VA, American Diabetes Association, 2003

Ms. Funnell is a Clinical Nurse Specialist at the Michigan Diabetes Research and Training Center, University of Michigan, Ann Arbor, MI. Ms. Mensing is a Manager, Clinical and Education Programs, Strategic Initiatives, at the Joslin Diabetes Center, Boston, Massachusetts.

Work on this chapter was supported in part by grant numbers NIH5P60 DK20572 and 5 R18 DK070020 from the National Institute of Diabetes and Digestive and Kidney Diseases of the National Institutes of Health.

17. Behavioral Strategies for Improving Self-Management

KATIE WEINGER, EDD, RN, AND SHEILA J. McMURRICH GREENLAW, BA

M any health care professionals now recognize that health education involves more than just providing information. Diabetes education is a perfect example. The goal of diabetes education is to help individuals with diabetes live well. This goal is met by assisting those with diabetes as they integrate diabetes care into their lifestyles and, when necessary, adapt their lifestyles to healthy living guidelines and treatment requirements.

Accordingly, diabetes care and education are all about behavior, i.e., helping reinforce some behaviors and change others. Because change can be slow and frustrating, nurses caring for individuals with diabetes face the important challenge of effectively supporting patients in their efforts to manage their diabetes. This chapter discusses several aspects of behavioral approaches in the treatment of diabetes: general principles that apply to most interventions and strategies, useful tools and strategies for diabetes and education, four phases of psychological responses to diabetes, and examples of validated behavioral programs.

GENERAL PRINCIPLES IMPORTANT TO BEHAVIORAL STRATEGIES FOR DIABETES

UNDERSTAND THAT DIABETES IS A CHRONIC ILLNESS

Diabetes treatment and education do not fit neatly into the acute care model (1). Although acute episodes may arise and need immediate attention, diabetes is primarily a chronic illness that requires lifestyle adjustments and long-term prevention strategies to ensure maintenance of health. Much of the education and training for nurses occurs in hospital environments and is

236

centered on an acute care model. However, several general principles, outlined below, may help these health care professionals make the transition to a chronic care model.

USE EMPOWERMENT IN DIABETES

Empowerment in diabetes differs from the more community-oriented public health model of empowerment. Empowerment in this case is a more philosophical approach to clinical practice that emphasizes "helping people discover and use their innate abilities to gain mastery over their diabetes" (2). Empowerment means that individuals with diabetes have the tools, such as knowledge, control, resources, and experience, to implement and evaluate their self-management practices (2). Most therapeutic communication skills and principles of adult learning described here are consistent with this philosophy of empowerment.

PEOPLE WITH DIABETES ARE IN CHARGE OF THEIR OWN CARE

One of the most important underlying principles of diabetes treatment is that individuals with diabetes, not their health care teams, provide all the self-care and make the everyday decisions for their diabetes. Once this fact is accepted, behavioral approaches become logical methods to support patients in their diabetes self-management. Some health care professionals, particularly those schooled in an acute care approach, may struggle with this concept. Nurses need to conceptualize their role as being one who helps the patient learn to solve problems rather than one who solves problems for the patient.

HEALTH EDUCATION, LIKE ADULT EDUCATION, MUST BE DIRECTLY RELEVANT TO THE LEARNER

Nurses must remember that patients are learning about diabetes because they have it. Patients are more likely to remember information that they see as relevant to them and that affects how they live, work, play, and relate to others. The key is their perception; information must be presented in such a way that individuals with diabetes can immediately understand how information and recommended self-care tasks apply to them.

HEALTH LITERACY

Literacy is often viewed as the ability to read and comprehend and is obviously very important in self-management. However, health literacy also includes numeracy, which refers to quantitative skills or the ability to understand and calculate numbers. Even someone who is literate and educated may lack these skills. Successful diabetes self-management includes the ability to understand target ranges of glucose and to make frequent calculations of carbohydrates and insulin doses. Yet low numeracy skills have been seen to be common among people with diabetes (3), which could affect self-management and glycemic control.

STRATEGIES AND TOOLS

ORIENTING PATIENTS TO THE HEALTH CARE SYSTEM

Although health care professionals spend years training for their profession, patients receive no formal instruction in how to be a patient. Yet being a patient is a distinct and important role that will affect their lives. Over time, patients will develop ideas of their roles based on information from their own prior experience, the media, and intended and unintended cues from their health care providers and support staff. For example, if someone with diabetes has had a negative experience when dealing with a physician or nurse, she may "learn" that the health care team should only be contacted for dire emergencies. Without any guidelines as to when it is appropriate to contact the health care team, she may become reluctant to contact the health care team for help or advice. Therefore, orienting patients to diabetes treatment and providing guidelines on how best to use the health care team are important.

BUILDING A RESPECTFUL COLLABORATIVE RELATIONSHIP

The philosophy of empowerment and many of the tools described below contribute to the establishment of a mutually respectful relationship with patients (2). The health care provider and the patient should jointly agree on the agenda for an education appointment. As an educator, you may want to cover specific topics, but the patient will not be able to devote full attention to the issues you want to cover if he or she is concerned about other issues. Listening to a patient's concerns and validating your understanding through reflection and summarization are extremely important tools to use in developing a collaborative relationship. Table 17.1 lists several useful communication techniques.

Remember that the patient's task is to learn self-management, not simply to receive advice. People with diabetes must learn how to manage diabetes and to problem solve. They will not benefit from having problems solved for them. Although advice is often important, before giving advice, consider whether first clarifying the problem through discussion and then allowing the patient to practice problem solving would better serve the patient. Giving advice too quickly may stifle the relationship by emphasizing the nurse as the knowledgeable one whose job is to solve problems and the patient as the passive recipient of knowledge. In this case, the health care professional, not the person with diabetes, is in control; passive knowledge rarely translates to behavior change.

ASSESSMENT

The goal of behavioral assessment is to understand patients' points of view and their specific questions and perceptions about diabetes, its treatment, and their health status. The behavioral assessment begins with open-ended questions that elicit knowledge of treatment recommendations and self-care tasks as well as attitudes, barriers, and support for diabetes self-management (Table 17.2). Reflection as a follow-up to open-ended questions often helps the patient verbalize issues and identify barriers to successful self-care (4).

Table 17.1 Useful Communication Techniques

Setting a mutually acceptable agenda	Begin an appointment by finding out what the patient wants to talk about. An agenda should include items important to the patient as well as items that you think are important. Be sure the number and depth of the agenda items fit within the time frame of the meeting. Although there may be multiple items to discuss, it may be necessary to prioritize and arrange additional appointments.
Open-ended questions	Allow the patient to verbalize feelings and provide information in their own words by asking open-ended questions. Some examples are ■ "Tell me about. . . ." ■ "How are you doing with taking your medications?" ■ "What about your meal plan is working?" ■ "What problems are you having taking care of your diabetes?"
Active listening	Actively listen while consciously focusing on what the person means. This is not as easy as it sounds. Many people tend to think about what they will say next instead of focusing on what the patient is actually saying. Two useful tools for listening are reflection and summarizing. Reflection (4) Repeat or paraphrase the statement back to the person but in the tone of a question. ■ "You are having trouble with your exercise plan?" ■ "You are frustrated with your treatment recommendations?" Summarizing (4) Summarizing the general idea of the patient's conversation shows that you have been listening and that you understand. It also provides an opportunity to correct any misunderstandings. If the patient has outlined a plan or made other positive steps, summarizing can help reinforce their progress.

GOAL SETTING

When asked what their goals for diabetes care are, most people think in broad, sweeping terms. Commonly stated goals are to "lose weight," "improve glycemic control," or "check glucose more often." However, sweeping goals often do not affect behavior because they are long term and difficult to put into operation. Such broad goals should be acknowledged and used to set more specific, short-term goals that are realistic, achievable, and measurable (5,6). Identifying the steps to be taken to achieve the broader goal is important. Effective evaluation recognizes the amount or percentage of the goal achieved rather than simply

Table 17.2 Important Behavioral Assessment Areas

Area	Comments
Knowledge of self-care recommendations	The rationale for and frequency of doing self-care behaviors is central, rather than knowledge of pathophysiology.
Attitudes toward diabetes and self-care tasks	Does the patient perceive self-care tasks as important? On a scale of 1 to 10, how important is it for the patient to take care of his or her diabetes? Is the person feeling overwhelmed? The Problem Areas in Diabetes survey (15,16) can be used to start conversation.
Depression	Depression is common in diabetes but is underrecognized and undertreated (see chapter 22). If a person is tearful, sad, or extremely angry, a referral to a mental health professional may be necessary.
Cognitive status	Over time, diabetes may affect memory, and aging certainly affects memory. Be aware of signs of lack of understanding. Have the person summarize important points before leaving, providing key points in writing.
Readiness, ability, and intention to make necessary changes	Does the patient feel that changing behavior is necessary or important? Until a person is ready, behavior is difficult to change, and maintenance of a behavior change is even more difficult.
Family and other support	Does the person feel alone with their diabetes or overwhelmed by family nagging ("diabetes police")? Does the person with diabetes receive the amount of emotional support and the amount of help that he or she wants (14)?
Health literacy	Assess whether and in what language(s) the person can read. Remember that most people read at least one to two grade levels below their highest grade achieved. Reading ability is not necessarily equated with level of intelligence. Numeracy, the ability to understand, calculate and manipulate numbers must also be assessed.

determining whether the goal was met. For example, a patient who walked for 30 min 3 days a week instead of the desired 5 days achieved 60% of his or her goal. Evaluation, more than just a check to see whether goals are met, should also be an opportunity for patients to assess their plan. Did they meet their goals because of their plan or in spite of it? If the latter is true, then they need to think about revising their plan. Once goals are met, patients need to develop a maintenance plan or set new goals.

SELF-EFFICACY

Self-efficacy has been associated with improvement in self-care behaviors in a number of chronic illnesses (7,8,9), including diabetes (10). It refers to the ability to feel confident enough in oneself to act and make behavior changes. This requires knowledge and motivation. While the belief in importance of changing a behavior may be high, if confidence is low, it can present a barrier to change. Meeting goals and being successful in changing one's behavior can boost self-efficacy. It is therefore helpful to assess self-efficacy when developing goals and to support confidence in self-management behavior.

USE OF STRUCTURED ACTIVITIES

Several tools, such as glucose monitors and pedometers, help engage people in their diabetes self-care. If used correctly, these tools can improve self-management because they help people learn about the body's response to diabetes and its treatment. In order to maximize the benefits of this type of equipment, two important rules apply. First, all information is valuable and should not be judged as good or bad. Thus, when a glucose reading is high, patients must learn to acknowledge the importance of knowing that information so they can take action. Similarly, knowing that a treatment is not working is important. If a patient's eating habits are not healthy, then that is also important to know. Only with knowledge can changes be made. Inadvertent negative verbal and nonverbal messages about high glucose readings may foster avoidance of glucose monitoring. The second rule is that patients must understand what to do with the information; if they do not, they will not use it. Pedometers are very popular among people with diabetes as well as the general population, mainly because they are easy to use and provide information that is relatively easy to understand. On the other hand, glucose monitoring is not as intuitive, particularly for individuals with type 2 diabetes. However, if they use a glucose meter to learn how medications, food, or exercise affects their blood glucose, monitoring can be more relevant and less frustrating.

FOUR PHASES OF PSYCHOLOGICAL RESPONSE TO DIABETES

The emotional or psychological response of a person with diabetes can influence the success of behavioral approaches. Psychological responses follow a general progression of four phases from the time of diagnosis until complications are so dominant that they may overshadow diabetes care (11,12). Knowing about these phases can help nurses tailor their educational approach to the mindset of the patient.

DIAGNOSIS

A person with newly diagnosed diabetes struggles to learn about this chronic illness, to figure out how life will change, and to incorporate the diagnosis into his or her persona. Meanwhile, the individual also strives to maintain life as it is already known.

A person recently diagnosed with type 1 diabetes can be so overwhelmed trying to process the fact of the diagnosis that he or she may not be able to internalize any additional information provided. Repetition of all information is important. A contact telephone number and a clearly written handout that repeats all key points are extremely useful for the person to have at home. Schedule follow-up sessions within 1 month to assess how the person is doing and to reinforce important self-care behaviors.

For individuals with newly diagnosed type 1 diabetes, survival skills are important. Patients must learn how to handle equipment and give themselves injections with either a syringe or a pen. Repetitive practice is very helpful. Although one demonstration by the educator may be adequate, many practice sessions under the watchful guidance of an educator are typically more useful. Patients should feel comfortable handling the equipment and drawing up the correct dose before leaving the office.

The ability to learn new information and skills may also be compromised in individuals newly diagnosed with type 2 diabetes if the diagnosis is accompanied by other severe comorbidities. Depending on the patient's age, support systems, and cognitive status, several educational sessions may be necessary to help the patient understand the care and implications of diabetes. Individuals with type 2 diabetes without comorbidities may consider the diagnosis of diabetes to be a normal part of aging, simply "taking another pill." Such individuals may lack the motivation to make important lifestyle changes.

PREVENTION PERIOD

During this phase, the person with diabetes is expected to implement lifestyle changes to stay healthy and prevent complications. However, the patient experiences no immediate distressful symptoms. This lack of symptoms may diminish motivation for lifestyle adjustments, particularly for individuals whose coping styles include procrastination and denial. Several validated behavioral interventions may be useful during this phase. Training in coping skills helps healthy adolescents who are receiving intensive treatment improve their diabetes self-management skills. Motivational interviewing may be used to help patients recognize the importance of self-management tasks and thus move toward improving their self-care behaviors (13) (Table 17.3).

WORRY ABOUT COMPLICATIONS/EARLY COMPLICATIONS

Individuals who have not maintained glycemic control within targets may begin to worry about complications, particularly if they have signs of early complications. This phase often triggers patients to take action to regain control of their diabetes; this response, if unfulfilled or unstructured, may result in burnout (14). Being able to recognize the signs of burnout is key to effective care of the patient with diabetes. These signs include feelings of being overwhelmed by diabetes self-care, of being controlled by diabetes, of constantly worrying about taking care of diabetes, and lack of motivation or willingness to continue with diabetes self-care practices. Cognitive behavioral techniques and motivational interviewing are useful interventions to help address negative attitudes and perceptions that interfere with self-care (Table 17.3).

Table 17.3 Examples of Successful Behavioral Intervention Programs

Program Name	Description
Blood Glucose Awareness Training (17)	Eight-week group education with homework assignments designed to help participants with type 1 diabetes prevent glucose fluctuations by early recognition or anticipation and treatment of hypoglycemia and hyperglycemia. Blood glucose awareness training is helpful for individuals with hypoglycemia unawareness.
Coping Skills Training (18)	Small-group program designed to help adolescents develop more positive coping strategies to help them manage the stresses of diabetes and its treatment. Coping skills training uses role-playing and scenarios to engage teens in learning how to cope with typical life situations.
Motivational Interviewing (4,13,19,20,21)	Developed in the treatment of addictions, motivational interviewing is effective in the treatment of diabetes. This approach uses interviewing techniques and therapeutic approaches to help patients become more ready to change their self-management behaviors. Motivational interviewing is mainly used in one-on-one interactions and requires special training.
Cognitive Behavioral Therapy (22,23)	In the treatment of diabetes, this type of therapy is used in group education sessions to help people with diabetes change their negative attitudes and thought habits to more positive approaches to diabetes self-management.

COMPLICATIONS DOMINATE

When individuals with diabetes develop one or more serious complications, they may seek treatment from subspecialists who treat the complication but not the underlying diabetes. Thus, the patient is faced with several different illnesses with which to cope instead of focusing on one integrated diabetes treatment program.

SUMMARY

Reinforcing some behaviors and changing others is a key component of diabetes care and education. Endorsing the philosophy that the patient is in charge of his or her diabetes and providing the person with the tools and knowledge necessary to manage his or her own care provide the foundation for the nurse's role in the treatment of diabetes. Supporting others in the management of their diabetes requires that nurses develop skillful communication techniques and use other behavioral interventions.

PRACTICAL POINT

People with diabetes may exhibit a variety of symptoms and may flow in and out of these phases of psychological response at different times. Simply labeling an individual as "noncompliant" when he or she is having difficulty coping with the disease and self-management regimen does a disservice to patients and does little to assist in improving their health. An assessment of behavior and emotions can help identify problem areas for intervention or referral.

REFERENCES

1. Anderson RM, Funnell MM: Using the empowerment approach to help patients change behavior. In *Practical Psychology for Diabetes Clinicians*. 2nd ed. Anderson BJ, Rubin RR, Eds. Alexandria, VA, American Diabetes Association, 2002, p. 3–12

2. Anderson B, Funnell M: *The Art of Empowerment: Stories and Strategies for Diabetes Educators*. 2nd ed. Alexandria, VA, American Diabetes Association, 2005

3. Cavanaugh K, Huizinger MM, Wallston KA, Gebretsadik T, Shintani A, et al.: Association of numeracy and diabetes control. *Ann Intern Med* 148:737–746, 2008

4. Rollnick S, Mason P, Butler C: *Health Behavior Change: A Guide for Practitioners*. Edinburgh, UK, Churchill Livingstone, 1999

5. Davis M, Eshelman ER, McKay M: *The Relaxation and Stress Reduction Workbook*. Oakland, CA, New Harbinger Publications, 1988

6. Strecher VJ, Seijts GH, Kok GJ, Latham GP, Glasgow R, et al.: Goal setting as a strategy for health behavior change. *Health Educ Q* 22:190–201, 1995

7. Osborne RH, Wilson T, Lorig KR, McColl GJ: Does self-management lead to sustainable health benefits in people with arthritis? *J Rheumatol* 34:906–907, 2007

8. Sol BGM, van der Graaf Y, van der Bijl JJ, Goessens N, Visseren FL: Self-efficacy in patients with clinical manifestations of vascular diseases. *Patient Educ Couns* 61:443–448, 2006

9. Marks R, Allegrante JP, Lorig K: A review and synthesis of research evidence for self-efficacy–enhancing interventions for reducing chronic disability: implications for health education practice. *Health Promot Pract* 6:37–43, 2005

10. Sarkar V, Fisher L, Schillinger D: Is self-efficacy associated with diabetes self-management across race/ethnicity and health literacy? *Diabetes Care* 29:823–829, 2006

11. Hamburg BA, Inoff GE: Coping with predictable crises of diabetes. *Diabetes Care* 6:409–416, 1983

12. Jacobson AM, Weinger K: Psychosocial complications in diabetes. In *Medical Management of Diabetes Mellitus*. Leahy JL, Clark NG, Cefalu WT, Eds. New York, Marcel Dekker, 2000, p. 559–572

13. Miller WR, Rollnick S: *Motivational Interviewing: Preparing People for Change*. 2nd ed. Miller WR, Rollnick S, Eds. New York, Guilford Press, 2002, p. 3–198

14. Polonsky WH: *Diabetes Burnout: What To Do When You Can't Take It Anymore*. Alexandria, VA, American Diabetes Association, 1999

15. Polonsky WH, Anderson BJ, Lohrer PA, Welch G, Jacobson AM, et al.: Assessment of diabetes-related distress. *Diabetes Care* 18:754–760, 1995

16. Welch GW, Jacobson AM, Polonsky WH: The Problem Areas in Diabetes (PAID) scale: an examination of its clinical utility. *Diabetes Care* 20:760–766, 1997

17. Cox D, Gonder-Frederick L, Polonsky W, Schlundt D, Julian D, Clarke W: A multicenter evaluation of blood glucose awareness training II. *Diabetes Care* 18:523–528, 1995

18. Grey M, Boland EA, Davidson M, Li J, Tamborlane WV: Coping skills training for youth with diabetes mellitus has long-lasting effects on metabolic control and quality of life. *J Pediatr* 137:107–113, 2000

19. Zweben A, Zuckoff A: Motivational interviewing and treatment adherence. In *Motivational Interviewing: Preparing People for Change*. 2nd ed. Miller WR, Rollnick S, Eds. New York, Guilford Press, 2002, p. 299–319

20. Channon SJ, Huws-Thomas MV, Rollnick S, Hood K, Cannings-John RL, et al.: A multicenter randomized controlled trial of motivational interviewing in teenagers with diabetes. *Diabetes Care* 30:1391–1395, 2007

21. West DW, DiLillo V, Bursac Z, Gore SA, Greene PG: Motivational interviewing improves weight loss in women with type 2 diabetes. *Diabetes Care* 30:1081–1087, 2007

22. Van der Ven N, Weinger K, Snoek F: Cognitive behavior therapy in diabetes: an opportunity to help people with diabetes improve their self-management. *Diabetes Voice* 47:1013, 2002

23. Snoek FJ, van der Ven NC, Lubach CH, Chatrou M, Ader HJ, et al.: Effects of cognitive behavioral group training (CBGT) in adult patients with poorly controlled insulin-dependent (type 1) diabetes: a pilot study. *Patient Educ Couns* 45:143–148, 2001

Dr. Weinger is Assistant Professor, Department of Psychiatry, at Harvard Medical School, Boston, MA, and an Investigator at the Section on Behavioral and Mental Health Research, Joslin Diabetes Center, Boston, MA. She also directs the Center for Innovation in Diabetes Education and the Office of Research Fellow Affairs at Joslin Diabetes Center, Boston, MA. Sheila McMurrich Greenlaw is a medical student at University of Massachusetts Medical School, Worcester, MA.

18. Cultural Context of Diabetes Education and Care

Gail D'Eramo Melkus, EDD, C-ANP, CDE, FAAN, and
Kelley Newlin, DNSc, C-ANP, CDE

Diabetes affects individuals across the lifespan from infancy to old age, independent of sex, socioeconomic status, and ethnicity. This diversity is represented in the increasing number of individuals living with diabetes in the U.S. and worldwide. Although diabetes does not discriminate in terms of whom it affects, type 2 diabetes and its related complications are disproportionately present among American ethnic minorities (1). In fact, recent studies on health disparities provide evidence that ethnic minority and vulnerable populations often do not receive adequate care, including diabetes care (2). Disparate care may result from a mismatch in illness experiences between patients and providers that are based on a range of cultural factors, such as religion, ethnic background, and personal history. The Institute of Medicine report on health disparities identified factors associated with health care delivery specific to cultural or linguistic barriers that may contribute to the current state of health disparities in the U.S. (3). Also, the context of the patient health care provider interaction may be compromised by health care provider bias.

Diabetes self-management and related metabolic outcomes are associated with the development of diabetes-related complications (4,5). Thus, optimal glycemic control is the goal of diabetes care and patient education interventions. The complexity of disease management necessitates the active involvement of the patient (and often the family as well) in daily decisions regarding dietary intake, physical activity, and medications in an effort to achieve optimal glycemic control and prevent complications. Individual and family response to these daily demands of living with diabetes is central to self-management and its related outcomes. Participation that results in successful adherence to the therapeutic regimen depends on a number of important factors, such as patient satisfaction with the provider and setting and perceived benefit of adherence on health status (6). An individual's personal response and participation in self-management are often based on a complex set of health beliefs, perceptions, and practices that are culturally embedded (7). Because of increasing cultural diversity among Americans, rising incidence and prevalence of diabetes, and complexity of self-management, cultural considerations must be addressed in the context of delivering quality diabetes care and education.

The American Diabetes Association (ADA), the American Association of Diabetes Educators (AADE), and the Centers for Disease Control and Prevention (CDC) strongly recommend that diabetes education and care address cultural factors. The ADA and CDC clinical care guidelines and the AADE standards for diabetes education underscore the significant influence that cultural factors may have in adherence to prescribed regimens of self-care and, in turn, physiological outcomes (8,9).

CONCEPTUAL PERSPECTIVES

Culture is a concept that is derived from anthropological and sociological concepts. Leininger, a nursing anthropologist, defines culture as the "learned and shared beliefs, values, and lifeways of a designated or particular group that are generally transmitted intergenerationally and influence one's thinking and action modes" (10). Mechanic, a medical sociologist, proposes that great variation exists in behaviors among people within a particular cultural group; therefore, observed cultural patterns may be considered only rough approximations of how people act in specific contexts (11). Thus, among any ethnic or cultural group, there is a great degree of within-group variation in terms of socioeconomic status, traditions, concepts of health and illness, and personal identity. Based on both anthropological and sociological concepts, the Office of Minority Health, U.S. Department of Health and Human Services, defines culture as "integrated patterns of human behavior that include language, thoughts, communications, actions, customs, beliefs, values, and institutions of racial, ethnic, religious, or social groups" (12). It is important to note, however, that membership within a given cultural group may or may not delineate a person's ethnic affiliation.

Often, the term cultural competence is used interchangeably with *cultural sensitivity*, *cultural awareness*, *cultural congruence*, *cultural relevance*, and other related terms, suggesting that these terms are synonymous. They are in fact conceptually distinct.

ETHNICITY

Ethnicity more specifically defines a person's race, religion, national or geographic origin, or symbolic identification. It is important to note that although there is no scientific or biological basis of race, the terms race and racism have meaning as social constructs and therefore have social connotations that differ from ethnicity (13). Although cultural competency is necessary for providing diabetes care and education to any given group, cultural assessment of each patient is necessary to prevent cultural stereotyping.

Cultural sensitivity or awareness refers to the examination of a person's own assumptions regarding other cultural groups and becoming aware of how these notions might affect perceptions and prejudices of culturally different groups (14). Cultural congruence refers to a match between the delivery of care and the cultural values, beliefs, and patterned behavior of the care recipients (15). Cultural relevance involves the perception of the care recipient in terms of the cultural appropriateness of the delivery of health services. Cultural competence, as suggested by the Office of Minority Health (12), involves the actual integration of consistent behaviors, attitudes, and policies in the delivery of health care in cross-cultural situations. This involves blending congruent behaviors, attitudes, and policies in systems, in agencies, among professionals, and in therapeutic interventions to effectively work within cross-cultural contexts involving the beliefs, behaviors, communication patterns, and needs of health care consumers and their communities (16). In a review of the literature on culturally competent health care interventions, results showed a compelling number of studies that demonstrated significantly improved outcomes for patients with diabetes and other health problems after receiving culturally competent or relevant interventions compared with others who did not receive such care (17). Recently, a new term, *cultural leverage*, has been defined. Cultural leverage is a strategy that engages and facilitates target communities of interest by including key aspects of their cultural heritage, practices, philosophies and the environment and uses the processes of cultural competence (18). Using the concept of cultural leverage and related strategies, a recent review of thirty-eight interventions aimed at decreasing health disparities found similar results with the majority of the outcomes being significantly improved (18).

CULTURAL HEALTH BELIEFS AND PRACTICES

Beliefs of health and illness are derived from heritage and cultural phenomena that vary among cultural, religious, and ethnic groups. As already stated, there is great within- and between-group diversity among any given group, lending to a multicultural identity for many individuals. Thus, the domains of culture may vary based on the extent to which an individual has become acculturated to the dominant culture and the degree to which individuals have maintained their traditional heritage (19). Studies have shown that the more acculturated an individual is, the more likely he or she is to exhibit autonomy in the patient role and with patient-provider interactions (20,21), consistent with the American model of health care delivery. However, even when patient autonomy is present, individuals from different ethnic groups often rely on family involvement in the context of illness, regardless of their personal cultural identity. This is particularly true of Native Americans, whose family-centeredness is constant regardless of acculturation level, tribal affiliation, and family lifestyle (traditional or bicultural) (22).

SPIRITUAL AND RELIGIOUS BELIEFS AND PRACTICES

Spirituality and religion are prominent cultural factors across American ethnic groups, demonstrating constancy independent of other culturally related factors. In fact, most Americans (97%) consider themselves spiritual, religious, or both (23). Furthermore, many Americans indicate spirituality and/or religion are important components of health, reporting the use of prayer in a medical context (67%) and the desire that physicians be "spiritually attuned to them" (70%) (24).

Spirituality and religion, although often used interchangeably, are conceptually different but related terms. Spirituality, as a broader term, is often defined by such attributes as transcendence, hope, strength, identification of meaning and purpose in life, and interconnectedness with others, God, or a higher power (25–28). Spirituality is further referred to as a source of peace, coping, and guidance (27). Religion may be conceived of as an organized system of beliefs and practices that provides intellectual, behavioral, and social forms to spiritual expression and thereby nurtures a relationship with God or a higher power (25,26,28).

Religion and/or spirituality may contribute to diabetes self-management in terms of both psychosocial and physiological outcomes. Accumulating research indicates religion and spirituality are related to psychological well-being, coping styles or strategies, and glycemic control levels (29–35). The theoretical literature suggests psychosocial factors may mediate the significant associations observed between religion/spirituality and glycemic control, although beginning quantitative research in this area is inconclusive (35,36). According to the qualitative literature, religious/spiritual beliefs may limit or enhance confidence in the effectiveness of daily diabetes self-management (37–41). For some, religious/spiritual beliefs may foster deferring coping styles with relinquishment of diabetes self-management to God. For others, religious/spiritual beliefs may promote responsibility for diabetes self-management with increased psychological well-being and active or constructive coping styles and strategies (33,37–39,41–43).

Hence, in clinical practice, increased awareness of specific spiritual and religious health beliefs and practices (Table 18.1) is warranted because they may inform an individual's approach to, preferences for, and behaviors in daily self-management of diabetes. Yet across and within ethnicities, religious/spiritual health beliefs and practices may be interfused with ethnically based values and traditions to varying degrees, further influencing a person's orientation to health and illness.

Native Americans, although belonging to >300 individual tribal traditions, tend to view health/wellness as harmony with natural, social, and supernatural environments (44). Illness is thus viewed as disharmony or disruption in the delicate balance among these environments. Health maintenance or restoration may be achieved with traditional religious or spiritual practices, including cleansing sweats, prayer, and intervention of a medicine man or woman (44–47). However, certain illnesses, such as diabetes, may be considered "non-Indian" diseases. In such cases, traditional Western medicine may be preferred and integrated with religious healing practices (46). Some Native Americans with diabetes, however, may rely on spiritual practices, such as those performed by a medicine man, especially when Western approaches have failed (48).

Ethnically diverse black American populations with diabetes often share common Protestant beliefs and practices, while distinctly integrating them into their orientation toward diabetes self-management. For many Protestants, God or Jesus is believed to be the supreme healer or divine physician (49,50). His healing powers may be realized through faith and related religious and/or spiritual practices, such as prayer, scripture reading, and laying on of hands (50,51). Although often sharing common religious beliefs and practices, Protestant black Americans,

Table 18.1 Religious Health Beliefs, Practices/Restrictions, and Dietary Habits Relevant to Diabetes Care

Religious Groups	Religious Health Beliefs	Religious Health Care Practices/Restrictions Relevant to Diabetes Care	Religious Dietary Habits Relevant to Diabetes Care
Adventist, Seventh Day	■ Body is the temple of God ■ Healthy living is essential (77) ■ Healing may be achieved through both divine and medical interventions (44,78)	■ Prayer ■ Anointing of the Sick, involving prayer and anointing with oil by the clergy ■ Holy Communion (50) ■ No restrictions on medications ■ Some sects may prohibit narcotics and/or stimulants (44) ■ No restrictions on surgical procedures, including amputations ■ Emphasis on physical medicine, rehabilitation, and therapeutic diets (44,78)	■ Vegetarian diet is common ■ Nonvegetarian members may refrain from pork, shellfish, and some birds (44,78) ■ Alcohol, coffee, and tea are proscribed (44) ■ Fasting may be practiced by individual churches to varying degrees ■ Fasting is not recommended if it is likely to have an adverse effect on health (78)
American Indian religions	■ Wellness reflects harmony (47) ■ Illness reflects disharmony with nature, social, and supernatural environments (44) ■ Creator reveals guidance to achieve restoration of harmony ■ Individual responsible for following Creator's guidance and thereby personal health (44,47)	■ Varies according to tribe ■ Some tribes participate in sweat ceremonies, involving singing, sharing, prayer, and contemplation. Participation in sweat ceremonies promotes spiritual and physical cleansing, physical transcendence, and receptivity to ancestral wisdom ■ Peyote used as a sacrament within the Native American Church. Peyote promotes spiritual guidance and may stimulate inner cleansing/release (44) ■ Prayers for harmony with nature and for health (47)	■ Blessed food is believed to be free of harmful substances (46) ■ Following spiritual rituals, berries, corn, and dried meats may be consumed (44)

Table 18.1 Religious Health Beliefs, Practices/Restrictions, and Dietary Habits Relevant to Diabetes Care (*Continued*)

Religious Groups	Religious Health Beliefs	Religious Health Care Practices/Restrictions Relevant to Diabetes Care	Religious Dietary Habits Relevant to Diabetes Care
		■ Use of a Medicine Man or Woman to heal through prayers, ceremonies, and/or spiritual powers of ancestors, often complementing traditional western medicine (44,79)	
Buddhism	■ Illness due to karma or the result of actions in this or a previous life (44) ■ Healing not achieved through faith ■ Healing and recovery promoted by peace and liberation from anxiety experienced through awakening to Buddha's wisdom (44,78)	■ Specific practices and restrictions not dictated ■ Practices determined on an individual basis (44,78) ■ Practices that contribute to Enlightenment are encouraged ■ Medical procedures that may prolong life and attainment of Enlightenment are encouraged (78)	■ Moderate diet is encouraged (78)
Catholicism	■ Body is the temple of the Holy Spirit ■ Health is a gift from God ■ Illness may result from sin (44) ■ Christ has the power to forgive sins and heal illness ■ Christ's healing presence is active through the sacraments and prayer	■ Sacrament of the Sick (anointing, communion, and blessing by a priest) (78) ■ Sacrament of Holy Communion (receiving the Eucharist—a consecrated wafer—for health and healing) ■ Prayer and/or laying on of hands (77,78)	■ Foods and beverages to be used in moderation and in a manner not detrimental to health ■ Healthy adults are encouraged to abstain from meat and meat products on Ash Wednesday, Good Friday, and all Fridays during Lent (77)

(continued)

Table 18.1 Religious Health Beliefs, Practices/Restrictions, and Dietary Habits Relevant to Diabetes Care (*Continued*)

Religious Groups	Religious Health Beliefs	Religious Health Care Practices/Restrictions Relevant to Diabetes Care	Religious Dietary Habits Relevant to Diabetes Care
	■ Care for personal health and the health of others is encouraged	■ Medications encouraged if benefits exceed risks (78) ■ Amputations are acceptable if they are for the good of the whole person (78)	
Islam	■ Life is a gift from God, or Allah ■ Illness reflects God's will ■ Illness may serve as a means for expiating sin and strengthening character ■ God shows mercy and compassion by providing cures (44,80)	■ Daily prayer and reading or listening to the Qur'an in combination with medical treatment (80) ■ Faith healing is acceptable in the context of deteriorating physiological and mental health as a supplement to medical treatment (44,78) ■ Prescribed medications are not restricted, including pork derivatives ■ Amputations are not restricted (78) ■ Feminine modesty and feminine preference for female clinicians (77) ■ During the month of Ramadan, a patient may not take medication between dawn and sunset (81)	■ Pork, alcohol, and some shellfish are proscribed (44,77) ■ Permissible meat must be blessed and properly slaughtered (77) ■ Dietary moderation is expected (44) ■ Fasting from dawn to sunset during the entire *month* of Ramadan. Children, elderly, infirm, and pregnant or nursing women are exempt (77)
Judaism	■ Illness may result from sin ■ God's given wisdom responsible for medical discoveries that modify/eliminate disease or suffering ■ Jewish law requires Jews to seek medical services to	■ Praying independently or in community to God ■ Commandment of visiting the sick (44,82) ■ No medication restrictions (44) ■ On the weekly Sabbath (sunset Friday to sunset Saturday), ultra-Orthodox Jews may	■ Wine is appropriate and acceptable in moderation (82) ■ Orthodox and some Conservative and Reform Jews follow kosher laws, including no consumption of predatory fowl, pork products, shellfish,

Table 18.1 Religious Health Beliefs, Practices/Restrictions, and Dietary Habits Relevant to Diabetes Care (*Continued*)

Religious Groups	Religious Health Beliefs	Religious Health Care Practices/Restrictions Relevant to Diabetes Care	Religious Dietary Habits Relevant to Diabetes Care
	promote health and healing (44,82)	refrain from taking medications if viewed as not life threatening (82) ■ Consultation with a Rabbi in health care decisions is encouraged (44) ■ Beliefs related to amputations vary widely (78)	fish without fins or scales, and animal products not ritually slaughtered (77) ■ Rosh Hashanah may be initiated by eating apples and honey (82) ■ On Yom Kippur, Jews fast for 24 h unless prevented by medical reasons ■ During Passover, leavened products are not eaten (77)
Protestantism	■ Varied beliefs about health and illness ■ Individuals are encouraged to formulate beliefs according to conscious and not formal religious authority (44)	■ Scripture reading and personal prayer common among many Protestants ■ Holy Communion ■ Anointing of the Sick (e.g., Church of Brethren and Lutheran traditions) ■ Prayer and/or laying on of hands for divine healing often in conjunction with medical treatment (e.g., Assemblies of God and Church of Nazarene traditions) (77,78)	■ Abstinence from alcohol is encouraged by some Protestant faiths (e.g., Baptist, Church of Nazarene, and Mennonite traditions) ■ Fasting is not required among the Protestant faiths ■ Episcopalians may abstain from meat on Fridays (77)

including those with African and/or Hispanic ethnic roots, may approach diabetes self-management differently based on conceptualization of God's healing powers. Studies suggest black Americans often assume responsibility for diabetes self-management, believing God's healing powers are made manifest through application of medical knowledge with divine guidance and support in managing the daily complexities of diabetes to foster amelioration of its trajectory. However, reports also suggest some black Americans may prefer to surrender responsibility for diabetes self-management to God with demonstration of faith in His healing powers to cure disease (37–40,43,48).

Within any given ethnic group, spiritual and/or religious health beliefs and practices are similarly diverse. America's Hispanic population, for example, consists of individuals of Mexican, Cuban, Puerto Rican, Central American, and South American descent, among others. Within this broadly defined ethnic population, spiritual and/or religious health beliefs and practices may be heterogeneous, despite the predominance of Catholicism. Mexican Americans, for example, may mix elements of Catholicism with Native American traditions, practicing *Curanderismo*. Curanderismo is a folk medicine aimed at restoring balance among the spiritual, psychological, and physical through prayers, rituals, herbal remedies, and/or states of consciousness. Traditionally, *curanderos* are lay community members with expertise in treating folk and non-folk illnesses, but increasingly professional nurse-curanderos are emerging (52,53). Some Cuban Americans blend Catholicism with West African (Yoruba) tribal beliefs and practices into a religion called *Santeria* (also known as *Regla de Ocha*). Believers of this religion may view illness as caused by natural or spiritual intrusions into the body. Spiritual rebirth, protection, and cleansing may be sought with assistance from a *santero*, or spiritual healer, which may involve ritualistic spells, magic, and animal sacrifice (53–55). Likewise, some Cuban and Puerto Rican Americans may integrate elements of Catholicism with both African and Indian beliefs, practicing *Espiritismo*. According to this religious tradition, spirits may influence the health of individuals. Spiritual healers, or *espiritistas*, communicate with spirits to restore physical and emotional well-being (53). Related rituals may involve topical herbs, aromatic ointments or liquids, and prayers (56,57). Although some Hispanics may integrate elements of Curanderismo, Santeria, or Espiritismo into their health practices, more traditional Christian beliefs and practices are reported as a source of guidance, support, and strength in self-managing diabetes (39,41,42,53).

Although religious/spiritual beliefs and practices are well-documented salient aspects of diabetes self-management across varying ethnicities, research suggests religion and spirituality may not be addressed adequately in the provision of diabetes care (38,42,48). The diversity of cultural health beliefs and practices, including those related to religion and spirituality, necessitates that a comprehensive cultural assessment be conducted as part of the diabetes education and care process.

CULTURAL ASSESSMENT

A cultural assessment addresses patient beliefs and practices in the context of the larger reference group, the family, and the individual. Culturally competent education and care requires skills of individualized cross-cultural communication, assessment, interpretation, and intervention (58). These skills are based on the cultural and linguistically competent care recommended by the Office of Minority Health in newly published guidelines aimed at decreasing health disparities (59) (Table 18.2).

Table 18.2 Standards for Culturally and Linguistically Appropriate Services Summarized by Themes

Standards 1–3: Culturally Competent Care
- Ensure diverse staff
- Ongoing training of staff

Standards 4–7: Language Access Services
- Bilingual staff
- Interpreter services
- Printed patient materials

Standards 8–14: Operational Support for Cultural Competence
- Community collaborations
- Demographic database
- Organizational assessment

From U.S. Office of Minority Health, Department of Health and Human Services (59).

SELF-ASSESSMENT

The first step in cross-cultural communication and counseling is self-assessment. Health care providers will have to identify cultural assumptions by reviewing their own social, religious, and personal beliefs and practices, particularly those related to health and illness. Diabetes education and care are focused on self-management of dietary intake, physical activity, medications, and screening and care practices for prevention of complications, e.g., eye examinations, foot care, dental care. Therefore, nurses and other health care providers who are involved in diabetes education and care must evaluate their own attitudes, beliefs, values, and norms that are related to having a chronic illness such as diabetes.

RELIGION AND SPIRITUALITY

As a component of the cultural assessment, the patient's individual religious/spiritual health beliefs and practices may be assessed. Several religious/spiritual clinical assessment frameworks have been advanced across health-related disciplines (60–65). When considered collectively, key components of a religious/spiritual assessment relevant to diabetes self-management emerge: *1*) religious and/or spiritual identity and community; *2*) religious and/or spiritual health beliefs and practices/rituals; and *3*) integration of religion and/or spirituality into diabetes care (see Table 18.3). In new health care relationships, some patients may perceive a religious/spiritual assessment as intrusive, while others may not. Those in an established health care relationship may welcome and appreciate clinical acknowledgement of their religion/spirituality, engaging in discussion of associated health beliefs and practices. Certain patients may find it challenging to articulate their religious/spiritual health beliefs and practices as they pertain to diabetes. Pursuing verbal and nonverbal indicators may prove helpful in such instances (60). In any case, the religious/spiritual assessment process should be

Table 18.3 Religious/Spiritual Assessment Relevant to Diabetes Self-Management: Key Components and Related Questions (61–65)

Religious and/or Spiritual Identity and Community	Religious and/or Spiritual Health Beliefs and Practices/Rituals	Integration of Religion and/or Spirituality into Diabetes Care
■ Do you identify yourself as religious or spiritual? ■ Is your religion or spirituality important to you in your daily life? ■ Is your religious or spiritual life a source of hope, meaning, strength, or comfort? ■ Do you belong to or participate in a religious or spiritual community? ■ Does your religious or spiritual community serve as a source of support?	■ Do your religious or spiritual beliefs influence how you perceive health and illness? ■ Do your religious or spiritual beliefs influence how you perceive or cope with diabetes, including managing your diabetes (diet, exercise, taking medications, and monitoring your blood sugar)? ■ Do you have religious or spiritual practices/rituals that assist or help you with managing your diabetes (diet, exercise, taking medications, and monitoring your blood sugar)? ■ Do you have religious or spiritual practices/rituals or restrictions that might affect how you manage your diabetes (diet, exercise, taking medications, and monitoring your blood sugar)?	■ With consideration of your religious or spiritual beliefs and practices/rituals, how may a health care provider personalize your diabetes care and education? ■ With consideration of your religious or spiritual beliefs and practices/rituals, how may a health care provider help you to manage your diabetes?

conducted in a nonthreatening, nonjudgemental manner to convey respect for and encourage open responses from the patient (66). The religious/spiritual assessment process may yield information suggestive of religious struggle or conflict. Clinicians without expertise in religious counseling may refer patients to professional religious or secular counselors as indicated (67).

Performing a religious/spiritual assessment may promote development or refinement of diabetes self-management plans congruent with the cultural orientation and preferences of care recipients. Research suggests addressing religion/

spirituality in the context of diabetes care and education may foster greater motivation and responsibility for daily disease management while fostering greater confidence and trust in the health care provider (37,48).

DIETARY PRACTICES

Diet and nutrition therapy is a core component of education and care for people with diabetes, and for the majority of individuals with type 2 diabetes, such care is focused on dietary modification for the purpose of weight loss and maintenance. Attitudes and beliefs about eating, body shape, and weight will influence the process and outcomes of nutrition therapy as well as physical activity recommendations. In conducting an assessment of personal attitudes toward patterns of food use, shape, and weight, health care providers should acknowledge their own cultural assumptions and preferences, which may differ from those of other ethnic groups. In terms of weight and shape, white women often experience the greatest social pressure for thinness, whereas black women may not perceive weight as a problem when compared with a reference group of other black women (68,69). In some cultures, eating and overweight are equated with good health and thinness with illness. Based on such assumptions, suggestions to change dietary patterns and food preferences may be met with resistance.

Attitudes and practices related to types of food also differ among groups, and taking time to learn about a patient's culture is another important aspect of cross-cultural counseling. For example, in certain European countries, corn is animal feed unfit for human consumption, whereas corn is a core food with spiritual connotations for some Native-American groups (lending to the belief by Americans

---

PRACTICAL POINT

Four steps to cross-cultural counseling
1. Self-evaluation of own culture
   - Review past and present social, religious, and personal beliefs and attitudes about health, illness, food, and food use
2. Learn patient culture
   - Research written materials
   - Talk with friends or colleagues of the same ethnic group as the patient
   - Eat in a restaurant or visit a food store of the patient's ethnic background
3. Interview patient
   - Offer opportunities for family and/or significant other(s) to participate as appropriate
4. Analyze information and plan intervention
   - Identify cultural beliefs, practices, traditions, food preferences, meals, and patterns of eating
   - Incorporate findings into management strategy
   - Involve the patient in setting goals

in general that corn is used as both livestock feed and human food). Core foods and conventional methods of preparation are important factors for consideration in planning cross-cultural dietary interventions. Japanese, Chinese, Korean, and other Asian groups, like many Hispanic groups, use rice as a core food, whereas Italians use pasta and Native Americans use cornmeal. Many African Americans, including those of Caribbean descent, enjoy fried foods, whereas West Africans use stews. It is important to note, however, that many African Americans, like various other groups living in or from the southern U.S. region, may be accustomed to fried foods because they are conventional for southern-style cooking. The cultural context of regional cooking needs to be considered in addition to ethnic and religious practices to avoid making generalized assumptions of food practices.

In many ethnic cultural groups, dietary practices and religious and/or spiritual beliefs are related. Chinese people with chronic illness, for example, use dietary manipulation based on the concepts of Yin-Yang to restore balance and health (70). Yin conditions (negative, dark, and cold) of Yin organs, such as the heart, lung, liver, spleen, and kidney, are treated with Yang, or hot, foods, such as ginger or beef. Yang conditions (positive, light, and warm) of the Yang organs, such as the stomach, gallbladder, intestines, and bladder, are treated with Yin, or cold, foods, such as coconut or pork. This association of hot and cold foods with health and illness is also found among Mexican and Filipino people. For instance, chest pain is considered a cold disease brought on by cold air or cold foods, such as tropical fruits, fresh vegetables, or dairy products, and is treated with hot foods, such as herbal teas, soups, and temperate-zone fruit. Some African Americans rely on folk medicine remedies, such as blueberry tea, peach tree leaves tea, lemon juice, vinegar, and aloe vera, to lower blood glucose or prevent diabetes-related complications (71,72).

COMMUNICATION AND INTERACTION

Interactions between patients and health care providers are heavily influenced by the personal beliefs and communication strategies of both parties. This communication consists of both verbal and nonverbal expression. Cultural differences in eye contact, touching behaviors, and personal space vary among cultures. For example, some Native Americans believe that avoidance of eye contact is a sign of respect and that a handshake is a sign of courtesy (22). The goals of communication between the patient and health care provider are to 1) create a good interpersonal relationship; 2) exchange information, which consists of both giving and receiving information; and 3) make treatment decisions. These goals of communication are difficult to achieve when language and cultural barriers exist, underscoring the need for cultural literacy and linguistic competency (73). A recent study to identify barriers in the provision of diabetes care in 42 Midwestern community health centers found that providers frequently identified language or cultural barriers as elements that hinder the quality of patient education (74). Health care providers can evaluate their cultural and linguistic competencies by using the Inventory for Assessing the Process of Cultural Competence Among Health Care Professionals (75) (see also the "Additional Reading" provided at the end of this chapter).

SUMMARY

The goal of diabetes patient education and care is to assist the patient and family with self-management that results in optimal glycemic control and improved quality of life. In recognizing the increasing diversity of individuals affected by diabetes, culturally competent care must be incorporated into clinical practice and education programs. It has been written that "although the knowledge of differences between cultures may be useful, the knowledge of the what of health and illness in different cultures does not reveal the how of being in the care experience as it is actually lived" (76). Cross-cultural counseling is an opening step in the long process of understanding and facilitating cultural diversity and specificity in the context of culturally competent diabetes education and care. Such may be facilitated through cultural leverage that involves individuals with the "lived experience" and employs strategies and processes of cultural competence. The goal of equitable health care for all people can only be met through a combination of approaches that minimizes the barriers for individuals from different cultural, ethnic, racial, and socioeconomic backgrounds and results in the delivery of culturally competent care.

REFERENCES

1. National Center for Health Statistics, Division of Health, Promotion Statistics: Data 2010: The Healthy People 2010 Database [Internet]. Available from http://wonder.cdc.gov/data2010. Accessed 25 February 2009

2. Flaskerud JH, Lesser J, Dixon E, Anderson N, Conde F, et al.: Health disparities among vulnerable populations: evolution of knowledge over five decades in Nursing Research publications. *Nurs Res* 5192:74–84, 2002

3. Institute of Medicine: *Unequal Treatment: Understanding Racial and Ethnic Disparities in Health Care.* National Academies Press, Washington, DC, 2002

4. Diabetes Control and Complications Trial Research Group: The effect of intensive diabetes treatment on the development and progression of long-term complications in insulin-dependent diabetes mellitus. *N Engl J Med* 329:977–986, 1993

5. UK Prospective Diabetes Study Group: Tight blood pressure control and risk of macrovascular and microvascular complications in type 2 diabetes (UKPDS 38). *BMJ* 317:703–723, 1998

6. Haynes RB, McKibbon KA, Kanani R: Systematic review of randomized trials of interventions to assist patients to follow prescriptions for medications. *Lancet* 348:383–386, 1996

7. Steffenson MS, Colker L: Intercultural misunderstandings about health care: recall of descriptions of illness and treatment. *Soc Sci Med* 16:1949–1954, 1982

8. American Diabetes Association: Standards of medical care in diabetes—2009 (Position Statement). *Diabetes Care* 32 (Suppl. 1):S13–S61, 2009

9. Centers for Disease Control and Prevention: The prevention and treatment of complications of diabetes mellitus: a guide for primary care practitioners [Internet], 1991. Available from http://wonder.cdc.gov/wonder/prevguid/p0000063/p0000063.asp. Accessed 25 February 2009

10. Leininger M: What is transcultural nursing and culturally competent care? *J Transcult Nurs* 10:9, 1999

11. Mechanic D: *Medical Sociology: A Selective View*. New York, The Free Press, 1968

12. Goode T: Promoting cultural diversity and cultural competency. *Closing the Gap: Newsletter of the Office of Minority Health* 6–7 January 2000

13. Tripp-Reimer T: Cultural interventions for ethnic groups of color. In *Handbook of Clinical Nursing Research*. Hinshaw AS, Feetham SL, Shaver JL, Eds. Thousand Oaks, CA, Sage, 1999

14. Brach C, Fraser I: Can cultural competency reduce racial and ethnic health disparities? A review and conceptual model. *Med Care Res Rev* 57 (Suppl. 1):181–217, 2000

15. Cross TL, Bazron BJ, Dennis KW, Isaacs MR: *Towards a Culturally Competent System of Care: A Monograph on Effective Services for Minority Children Who Are Emotionally Disturbed*. Washington, DC, Child and Assistance Center, Georgetown University Child Development Center, 1989

16. Meleis A: Culturally competent care (Letter). *J Transcult Nurs* 10:12, 1999

17. Kehoe KA, Melkus GD, Newlin K: Culture within the context of care: an integrative review. *Ethn Dis* 13:344–353, 2003

18. Fisher TL, Burnet DL, Huang ES, Chin MH, Cagney KA: Cultural leverage. Interventions using culture to narrow racial disparities in health care. *Med Care* 64 (Suppl. 5):243S–282S, 2007

19. Spector RE: *Cultural Diversity in Health and Illness*. 4th ed. Stamford, CT, Appleton and Lange, 1996

20. Blacknall L, Murphy S, Frank G, Michel V, Azen S: Ethnicity and attitudes toward patient autonomy. *JAMA* 274:820–825, 1995

21. Degazon C: Ethnic identification, social support and coping strategies among three groups of ethnic African elders. *J Cult Divers* 1:79–86, 1994

22. Seideman R, Jacobson S, Primeaux M, Burns P, Weatherby F: Assessing American Indian families. *MCN Am J Matern Child Nurs* 21:274–279, 1996

23. Gallup News Service: Religion and Values: New Index Tracks Spiritual State of the Union. 28 January 2003

24. Gallup News Service: Religion and Values: Religion May Do a Body Good. 28 May 2002

25. Burkhardt M: Spirituality: an analysis of the concept. *Holist Nurs Pract* 3:69–77, 1989

26. Meraviglia M: Critical analysis of spirituality and its empirical indicators. *J Holist Nurs* 17:18–33, 1999

27. Newlin K, Knafl K, Melkus GD: African-American spirituality: a concept analysis. *Adv Nurs Sci* 25:57–70, 2002

28. Emblen J: Religion and spirituality defined according to current use in nursing literature. *J Prof Nurs* 18:41–47, 1992

29. Newlin K, Melkus GD, Knafl G, Laing N, Jefferson V: The relationship of quality of life to spiritual, emotional, and physiologic factors in black American women with type 2 diabetes. *Diabetes Metab* 59 (Suppl. 29):2809, 2003

30. Fitchett G, Davis JA, Quinn L: Examining the role of spiritual and religious dimensions in living with diabetes. *Ann Behav Med* 25:S173, 2003

31. Fitchett G, Murphy PE, Kim J, Gibbons JL, Cameron JR, Davis JA: Religious struggle: prevalence, correlates and mental health risks in diabetic, congestive heart failure, and oncology patients. *Int J Psych Med* 34:179–196, 2004

33. Newlin K, Melkus G, Chyun D: The relationships of coping strategies to religious, spiritual, and psychosocial factors in black American women with type 2 diabetes. (Manuscript in preparation.)

34. Landis BJ: Uncertainty, spiritual well-being, and psychosocial adjustment to chronic illness. *Issues Ment Health Nurs* 17:217–31, 1996

35. Newlin K, Melkus GD, Tappen R, Chyun D, Koenig H: Relationships of religion and spirituality to glycemic control in black women with type 2 diabetes. *Nurs Res* 57:331–339, 2008

36. Koenig HG, McCullough ME, Larson DB: *Handbook of Religion and Health*. New York, Oxford University Press, 2001

37. Polzer RL, Miles SM: Spirituality in African Americans with diabetes: self-management through a relationship with God. *Qual Health Res* 17:176–188, 2007

38. Polzer RL: African Americans and diabetes: Spiritual role of the health care provider in self-management. *Res Nurs Health* 30:164–174, 2007

39. Newlin K, Mclean Y, Melkus GD: Developing a church-based diabetes program for black Nicaraguans: exploration of faith values and health beliefs related to diabetes self-care (Abstract). In press

40. Egede LE, Bonadonna RJ: Diabetes self-management in African Americans: an exploration of the role of fatalism. *Diabetes Educ* 29:105–115, 2003

41. Rivera C: Lessons learned from urban Latinas with type 2 diabetes mellitus. *J Transcult Nurs* 14:255–265, 2003

42. Carbone ET, Rosal MC, Torres MI, Goins KV, Bermudez OI: Diabetes self-management: perspectives of Latino patients and their health care providers. *Patient Educ Counsel* 66:202–210, 2007

43. Samuel-Hodge C, Headen S, Skelly A, Ingram A, Keyserling T, Jackson E, Ammerman A, Elasy T: Influences on day-to-day self-management of T2DM

among African-American women: spirituality, the multi-caregiver role, and other social context factors. *Diabetes Care* 23:928–933, 2000

44. Minarik PA: Diversity among spiritual and religious beliefs. In *Culture & Nursing Care: A Pocket Guide*. Lipson JG, Dibble SL, Minarik PA, Eds. San Francisco, CA, UCSF Nursing Press, 1996, p. B1–B21

45. Broome B, Broome R: Native Americans: Traditional healing. *Urologic Nurs* 27:161–163, 2007

46. Kramer J: American Indians. In *Culture & Nursing Care: A Pocket Guide*. Lipson JG, Dibble SL, Minarik PA, Eds. San Francisco, CA, UCSF Nursing Press, 1996, p. 11–22

47. Still O, Hodgins D: Navajo Indians. In *Transcultural Health Care*. 2nd ed. Purnell LD, Paulanka BJ, Eds. Philadelphia, FA Davis, 2003, p. 284–306

48. Devlin H, Roberts M, Okaya A, Xiong YM: Our lives were healthier before: focus groups with African American, American Indian, Hispanic/Latino, and Hmong people with diabetes. *Health Promot Pract* 7:47–55, 2006

49. Glanville CL: People of African American heritage. In *Transcultural Health Care*. 2nd ed. Purnell LD, Paulanka BJ, Eds. Philadelphia, FA Davis, 2003, p. 40–53

50. Gerardi R: Western spirituality and health care. In *Spiritual Dimensions of Nursing Practice*. Carson V, Ed. Philadelphia, W.B. Saunders, 1989, p. 76–112

51. Morgan MG: African Americans and culture care. In *Transcultural Nursing: Concepts, Theories, Research and Practice*. 3rd ed. Leininger M, McFarland MR, Eds. New York, McGraw-Hill, 2002, p. 313–324

52. Luna E: Las que curan at the heart of Hispanic culture. *J Holist Nurs* 21:326–342, 2003

53. Murguía A, Peterson RA, Zea MC: Use and implications of ethnomedical health care approaches among Central American immigrants. *Health Soc Work* 28:43–51, 2003

54. Varela L: Cubans. In *Culture & Nursing Care: A Pocket Guide*. Lipson JG, Dibble SL, Minarik PA, Eds. San Francisco, CA, UCSF Nursing Press, 1996, p. 91–100

55. Purnell LD: People of Cuban heritage. In *Transcultural Health Care*. 2nd ed. Purnell LD, Paulanka BJ, Eds. Philadelphia, FA Davis, 2003, p. 122–137

56. Juarbe T: Puerto Ricans. In *Culture & Nursing Care: A Pocket Guide*. Lipson JG, Dibble SL, Minarik PA, Eds. San Francisco, CA, UCSF Nursing Press, 1996, p. 222–228

57. Juarbe TC: People of Puerto Rican heritage. In *Transcultural Health Care*. 2nd ed. Purnell LD, Paulanka BJ, Eds. Philadelphia, FA Davis, 2003, p. 307–326

58. Lipson JG: Culturally competent nursing care. In *Culture & Nursing Care: A Pocket Guide*. Lipson JG, Dibble SL, Minarik PA, Eds. San Francisco, CA, UCSF Nursing Press, 1996, p. 1–6

59. Department of Health and Human Services, U.S. Office of Minority Health: Standards for culturally and linguistically appropriate services (CLAS). *Closing The Gap: Newsletter of the Office of Minority Health*. February/March 2001, p. 3

60. Quinn MT, Cook S, Nash K, Chin MH: Addressing religion and spirituality in African Americans with diabetes. *Diabetes Educ* 27:643–644, 647–648, 655, 2001

61. Polzer R, Miles MS: Spirituality and self-management of diabetes in African Americans. *J Holistic Nurs* 23:230–250, 2005

62. Puchalski C, Romer AL: Taking a spiritual history allows clinicians to understand patients more fully. *J Palliat Med* 3:129–137, 2000

63. Stoll R: Guidelines for spiritual assessment. *Am J Nurs* 1574–1577, 1979

64. Anandarajah G, Hight E: Spirituality and the medical practice: using HOPE questions as a practical tool for spiritual assessment. *Am Fam Phys* 63:81–89, 2001

65. Hodge DR: Spiritual assessment: a review of major qualitative methods and a new framework for assessing spirituality. *Soc Work* 46:203–214, 2001

66. McSherry W, Ross L: Dilemmas of spiritual assessment: considerations for nursing practice. *J Adv Nurs* 38:479–488, 2002

67. Astrow AB, Puchalski CM, Sulmasy DP: Religion, spirituality, and health care: Social, ethical, and practical considerations. *Am J Med* 110:283–287, 2001

68. Cassell J: Social anthropology and nutrition: a different look at obesity in America. *J Am Diet Assoc* 95:424–427, 1995

69. Kumanyika SK, Wilson JF, Guilford-Davenport M: Weight-related attitudes and behaviors of black women. *J Am Diet Assoc* 93:416–422, 1993

70. Hwu Y, Coates V, Boore J: The health behaviours of Chinese people with chronic illness. *Int J Nurs Stud* 28:629–641, 2000

71. Anderson-Loftin W, Moneyham L: Long-term disease management needs of Southern African Americans with diabetes. *Diabetes Educ* 26:821–832, 2000

72. Anderson-Loftin W, Barnett S, Sullivan P, Summers Bunn P, Tavakoll A: Culturally competent dietary education for southern rural African Americans with diabetes. *Diabetes Educ* 28:245–257, 2002

73. Vandervort EB, Melkus GD: Linguistic services in ambulatory clinics. *J Transcult Nurs* 14:358–366, 2003

74. Chin M, Auerbach SB, Cook S, Harrison J, Koppert J, et al.: Quality of diabetes care in community health centers. *Am J Public Health* 90:431–434, 2000

75. Campinha-Bacote J: *Inventory for Assessing the Process of Cultural Competence Among Health Care Professionals*. Cincinnati, OH, Transcultural C.A.R.E. Association, 1998

76. Smith C: The lived experience of care within the context of cultural diversity. *J Holist Nurs* 12:282–290, 1994

77. Gerardi R: Western spirituality and health care. In *Spiritual Dimensions of Nursing Practice*. Carson V, Ed. Philadelphia, W.B. Saunders, 1989, p. 76–112

78. Andrews MM, Hanson PA: Religion, culture, and nursing. In *Transcultural Concepts in Nursing Care*. 4th ed. Andrews MM, Boyle JS, Eds. Philadelphia, Lippincott Williams & Wilkins, 2003, p. 432–502

79. Tom-Orme L: Transcultural nursing and health care among Native American peoples. In *Transcultural Nursing: Concepts, Theories, Research and Practice*. 3rd ed. Leininger M, McFarland MR, Eds. New York, McGraw-Hill, 2002, p. 429–440

80. Kulwicki AD: People of Arab heritage. In *Transcultural Health Care*. 2nd ed. Purnell LD, Paulanka BJ, Eds. Philadelphia, FA Davis, 2003, p. 90–105

81. Henley A, Schott J: *Culture, Religion, and Patient Care in a Multi-Ethnic Society*. London, Age Concern England, 1999

82. Selekman J: People of Jewish heritage. In *Transcultural Health Care*. 2nd ed. Purnell LD, Paulanka BJ, Eds. Philadelphia, FA Davis, 2003, p. 234–248

ADDITIONAL READING

Mason JL: *Cultural Competence Self-Assessment Questionnaire: A Manual for Users*. Portland, OR, Portland State University, 1995

Dr. D'Eramo Melkus is the Independence Foundation Professor of Nursing at Yale University School of Nursing, New Haven, CT. Dr. Newlin is a Post-Doctoral Fellow at Florida Atlantic University, FL.

19. Economic Costs of Diabetes

Geralyn Spollett, MSN, C-ANP, CDE

D iabetes is a costly disease. The expenditure of health care dollars, the reduction in productivity with an increase in disability, as well as other indirect expenses are estimated to be five times greater among people with diabetes than health-related expenses among the general population. According to a 2008 American Diabetes Association (ADA) statement (1), direct and indirect expenditures attributable to diabetes were estimated at $174 billion in 2007. While this is a conservative estimate that does not reflect many of the associated costs of diabetes care, it does represent a significant increase of nearly 33% over the $132 billion cost in 2002 (2). Furthermore, the $174 billion signifies that one-tenth of the nation's $2 trillion health budget goes to diabetes care. Data regarding the cost of diabetes care can also be found on the ADA web site (www.diabetes.org).

Diabetes is the sixth leading cause of death by disease in the U.S. At present, it is estimated that there are more than 17.5 million people diagnosed with this disease, an increase of more than 5 million from the 2002 report of 12.1 million individuals diagnosed with diabetes. These incidence figures do not include individuals who do not know they have the disease or who did not report their diagnosis to the U.S. Census Bureau. It also does not include women with gestational diabetes. A study conducted in 2006 projects that during the years 2005–2050 the prevalence of diagnosed diabetes will more than double, growing from 5.6 to 12% of the population (3). The cost of care for this increased population will place a significant burden on the health care budget.

Lost productivity, based on lost workdays, restricted activity days, prevalence of permanent disability, and mortality attributable to diabetes cost the U.S. economy an estimated $40 billion in 2002. By 2007, the cost grew to $58 billion (1). However, these figures may be underestimated. Men and women with diabetes are less likely to be in the labor force than those without diabetes because a higher proportion of individuals with diabetes have disabilities, such as vision loss, kidney failure, and amputations, that prohibit full-time or part-time employment. For example, a 2005 Centers for Disease Control and Prevention (CDC) fact sheet reports that ~82,000 lower-limb amputations are performed each year in people with diabetes (4).

Currently, the age-group with the largest incidence of diabetes comprises individuals >55 years old. The prevalence of diabetes continues to increase with age. The number of individuals age 65 and older with diabetes is currently estimated to be about 8.5 million (1). Of this age-group, roughly 50% have Medicare as their primary health insurance. They also have the highest premature mortality rates and have higher incidences of diabetes-associated complications (1).

Certain ethnic and racial minority groups are also disproportionately affected by diabetes, and the growth rates of disease within these groups continue to rise. This includes their children, who have an increasing incidence of type 2 diabetes. The number of people with diabetes continues to grow in epidemic proportions as the rate of obesity, a factor in the development of type 2 diabetes, rises. Worldwide there are ~1 billion people who are overweight or obese, compared with the 850 million who are chronically underweight (5). The U.S. leads the world in rates of overweight and obesity, followed closely by Mexico, the U.K., and Australia.

Both the ADA and the CDC project the rate of growth in the net number of those diagnosed with diabetes to ~1 million cases per year (1). The economic burden of diabetes will become greater over time. By 2020, the size of the population with diabetes was projected to increase by 44%. Given the current rate of growth, this may be a gross underestimation. The rates of racial and ethnic minorities affected by diabetes will most likely double, and the incidence of diabetes among individuals aged 45–64 years is projected to increase by 46%. Since this age-group is considered a mainstay for the workforce, the increasing number of individuals with diabetes will affect the nation's productivity and further increase the indirect costs attributable to diabetes.

In breaking down the total cost of $174 billion reported in 2008, $116 billion were direct costs that went to excess medical expenditures for diabetes, and the remaining $58 billion was attributed to the lost of productivity. Of the $116 billion, $27 billion went to direct care, $58 billion to the treatment of complications, and $31 billion to the excess medical costs associated with diabetes care (1).

USE OF HEALTH CARE RESOURCES

Use of health care resources is higher among individuals with diabetes than in the general population. People with diabetes are at greater risk for a host of medical complications that are directly or indirectly related to diabetes. Various neurological, cardiovascular, peripheral, vascular, renal, endocrine, and ophthalmic diseases can be associated with diabetes, and underlying diabetes may worsen their presentation and/or progression. The number of inpatient stays, nursing home occupancies, and home health care visits are all higher in the diabetic population. It is also estimated that inpatient days and outpatient visits for treatment of diabetes and its comorbidities tend to be more expensive than those for other disease states. The complexities of caring for individuals with multiple illnesses, complications, and medications that require frequent and periodic monitoring, observation, and follow-up make caring for diabetes a very costly disease. These comorbidities not only increase care costs, but they limit the earning potential of the person with diabetes, resulting in higher health care bills and reduced income with which to pay them.

The Social Security Disability Insurance (SSDI) program assists disabled workers by providing benefits to them, their spouses, and/or their children. In 2002, the calculated number of individuals aged 18–64 years who received SSDI attributed to diabetes-related disability topped 230,000; of those, 122,000 listed diabetes as the primary basis of disability. The U.S. government estimates that each case of permanent disability results in an average of $42,462 in lost earnings per year.

In a study of economic costs in diabetes conducted by the ADA (2), three trends were identified:

- Most of the health care use attributable to diabetes is for the treatment of general medical conditions in which the primary diagnosis is neither diabetes nor a related chronic complication.
- Of the chronic complications associated with diabetes, cardiovascular disease accounts for the largest proportion of health care use attributable to diabetes.
- Diabetes accounts for a sizable increase in the use of health care services.

In 2002, $23.2 billion was spent for health care events with a primary diagnosis of uncomplicated diabetes. This figure also included dollars spent for diabetes-related supplies. By 2008, that figure had increased significantly (Table 19.1). One in every five health dollars was spent caring for the person with diabetes. In looking at the cost of health care attributable to diabetes and its complications, one in ten health dollars was spent. Unlike the figures in the 2002 report, the 2007 figures include services such as podiatry, dentistry, optometry, and nutrition counseling, which are necessary components of diabetes care.

In 2007, more than 50% of the $27 billion in direct care costs for diabetes was spent on inpatient care. Diabetes-specific medications and supplies made up 12% of the cost, and medications for complications associated with diabetes another 11%. Office visits to medical providers constituted 9% of the direct care cost (1).

The 2007 mortality rates for various health problems associated with diabetes are similar to those reported in 2002. Of those who died, 58% had cardiovascular disease listed as the primary cause. Renal disease accounted for ~2,000 deaths. Other causes listed were cerebrovascular disease or diabetes (Table 19.2). Dialysis, coronary bypass surgeries, stroke, and cardiac rehabilitation are expensive tertiary care interventions aimed at extending life. As evidenced by the rate of mortality in these areas, people with diabetes, many of whom have cardiovascular, renal, or cerebrovascular complications, use a high proportion of health care dollars and resources. These costs do not factor in pain and suffering, family sacrifice and support, care by non-paid caregivers, or excess medical costs associated with undiagnosed diabetes. The costs of clinical training programs, health care administration, and research and development of new infrastructures do not figure into the total expenditure.

Table 19.1 Average Cost of Medical Events Related to Diabetes in 2007

Medical event	Unit cost ($)
Prescription (excluding insulin and oral agents)[*]	72
Oral agents (per user per year)[*]	697
Insulin (per insulin user per year)[*]	751
Diabetic supplies (per person with diabetes per year)[*, a]	102
Home health visits (cost per person per day of use)[*, a]	204
Hospice care day[†]	147
Nursing facility day[‡] (excluding food and rent) [b]	131 (120)
Other medical supplies (excess cost per person with diabetes per year)[*, a]	
Glasses/contacts	5.57
Ambulance services	5.92
Orthopedic items	5.52
Hearing devices	9.02
Prosthesis	4.09
Bathroom aids	1.52
Medical equipment	7.09
Disposable supplies	10.85
Alterations/modifications	7.10
Other	0.14

Sources for figures: [*]2003–2005 MEPS. [†]Hospice Association of America 2006. [‡]Average of cost for semi-private room and private room per the Genworth Financial 2007 Cost of Care Survey (http://longtermcare.genworth.com/comweb/consumer/pdfs/long_term_care/Cost_Of_Care_Survey. pdf). Note: [a] Cost estimate varies by age and sex. [b] An estimated 38% of the cost per day in a nursing home is for food and rent. For long-term residents, excluded from the cost estimates are expenses for room and board that would still have been incurred if the person were living at home. Estimates are adjusted to 2007 dollars. From ADA (1).

COST TO THE INDIVIDUAL

The person with diabetes can expect to spend approximately $11,744 per year on diabetes treatment and other related costs. In comparison with the person without diabetes, medical costs are two to three times greater for person with diabetes. Similarly, European studies have found that medical expenditures of people with diabetes are roughly twice those of a matched population without diabetes (6).

Financial costs of treating and controlling diabetes influence the ability of patients to self-manage the disease. Insurance premiums, whether employer supported or privately funded, are costly. Those who are uninsured or do not have a prescription clause in their insurance find the cost of medications and testing supplies prohibitive. Even those with medication support find the co-pay for drugs in the second and third tier a financial burden. In the over 65 group, the management of type 2 diabetes can place an undue burden on the finances of individuals living on fixed incomes.

Table 19.2 Mortality Costs Attributed to Diabetes in 2007

Primary cause of death	Total U.S. deaths (thousands)	Deaths attributed to diabetes		
		Deaths (thousands)	% of total U.S. deaths	Value of lost productivity (millions of dollars)
Diabetes	77	77	100.0	9,520
Renal disease	43	25	57.4	2,116
Cerebrovascular disease	155	59	37.6	3,849
Cardiovascular disease	739	123	16.5	11,417
Grand total	NA*	284	NA*	26,902

*Grand total comprises mortality for reasons other than diabetes, renal disease, cerebrovascular disease, and cardiovascular disease. From ADA (1).

The Translating Research Into Action for Diabetes (TRIAD) study, which is an ongoing multi-site longitudinal study, has examined factors related to the underuse of medications among insured adults with diabetes. In a survey, 14% of 5,000 respondents answered that in the past 12 months they had used less medication than they wanted to or were prescribed because of the cost. Level of income and out-of-pocket costs were stronger predictors of underuse than race/ethnicity (7).

The patient with type 2 diabetes on average is prescribed seven or eight medications for disease-related treatment: two or three oral hypoglycemic agents, two or three antihypertensive drugs, a cholesterol-lowering medication, and aspirin (Table 19.3). If the patient has another chronic illness, such as asthma, or must be treated for chronic complications associated with diabetes, such as peripheral or autonomic neuropathy or renal disease, the total number of daily medications can easily reach 10 to 12. In addition, the patient may need to purchase testing supplies, glucose tablets, or other products for health problems associated with diabetes complications, such as special footwear.

ADDRESSING THE PROBLEM

Prevention and early detection of diabetes is the first step to lowering health care costs. The skyrocketing overweight and obesity statistics indicate that there is an ever increasing population at significant risk for diabetes. If the goal is to lower economic costs related to diabetes, then nations around the world, and the U.S. in particular, must take a more aggressive stance in addressing the problems underlying the rise in obesity.

Improving diabetes care outcomes, thereby decreasing the incidence of chronic complications, can reduce the devastatingly high socioeconomic burden of diabetes. Research such as that from the Diabetes Control and Complications

Table 19.3 Example of Monthly Medication Costs* for Treating Type 2 Diabetes

Oral Agents	1-Month Supply	Retail Cost
Glipizide ER (generic) 10 mg b.i.d.	60	$10.99
Metformin (generic) 1,000 mg b.i.d.	60	$31.97
Actos 45 mg q.d.	30	$189.99
Antihypertensives		
Lisinopril 5 mg q.d.	30	$9.99
Norvasc 5 mg q.d.	30	$43.99
Hydrochlorothiazide 25 mg q.d.	30	$9.99
Lipid-lowering		
Atorvastatin 20mg q.d.	30	$145.99
Enteric coated aspirin 81 mg q.d.	100 (over-the counter)	$5.29
Example of Costs Associated with Insulin Use		
Insulin Analogs Glargine, Glulisine, Levemir, Lispro, Aspart	1 vial	$72–89
Insulin syringes	Box of 100	$30
Glucose tabs	Bottle of 50	$6.50
Glucose test strips	Bottle of 50	~$50
Lancets	Box of 100	$9–14
Meter kit (lancing device included)	1 kit	$25–80

*Costs listed reflect an averaging of retail prices from two major pharmacy chains. In some cases the cost was identical and that is then the listed price.

Trial and the U.K. Prospective Diabetes Study has demonstrated the importance of glycemic control in reducing the rates of many chronic complications, such as renal and eye disease. Each 10% increase in glycated hemoglobin A1c (A1C) is associated with a 20% increase in the rate of microalbuminuria and a 56% increase in the rate of retinopathy (8).

Because cardiovascular disease accounts for ~50% of deaths attributable to diabetes, control of cardiovascular risk factors will reduce health care costs and increase productivity among individuals with diabetes. Improved blood pressure control has a significant impact on preventing vascular and renal disease and may be equal to glycemic control in preventing chronic complications. Lipid screening and treatment of dyslipidemias can prevent myocardial and cerebrovascular mortality. Smoking cessation is critical to preserving cardiovascular health. More time and energy need to be dedicated to informing people with diabetes of the high health risks associated with smoking.

Countries that have adopted diabetes care programs that include prevention strategies taught by health care teams at the national, provincial, or county levels were able to improve the quality of care and optimize human and economic resources (9). For the U.S. to adequately meet the economic challenge of preventing and treating diabetes in the next decade, the current health care delivery system will need to shift care practices toward more fully encompassing the lifestyle issues and cardiovascular risk factors that contribute so heavily to the incidence of diabetes (see also "Keeping Medicine Costs Under Control," a patient handout in RESOURCES).

REFERENCES

1. American Diabetes Association: Economic costs of diabetes in the U.S. in 2007 (Position Statement). *Diabetes Care* 31:596–615, 2008

2. American Diabetes Association: Economic costs of diabetes in the U.S. in 2002 (Position Statement). *Diabetes Care* 26:917–932, 2003

3. Narayan KMV, Boyle JP, Geiss LS, Saaddine JB, Thompson TJ: Impact of recent increases in incidence on future diabetes burden. *Diabetes Care* 29:2114–2116, 2006

4. Centers for Disease Control and Prevention: National diabetes fact sheet: General information and national estimates on diabetes in the United States [Internet], 2005. Available from http://www.cdc.gov/diabetes/pubs/factsheet.htm. Accessed 16 February 2009

5. Runge CF: Economic consequences of the obese. *Diabetes* 56:2668–2672, 2007

6. Bottomley JM on behalf of the T2ARDIS Steering Committee: Managing care of type 2 diabetes: learning from T2ARDIS. *Br J Diabetes Vasc Dis* 1:68–72, 2001

7. Tseng CW, Tierney EF, Gerzoff RB: Race/ethnicity and economic differences in cost-related medication underuse among insured adults with diabetes: the Translating Research Into Action for Diabetes Study. *Diabetes Care* 31:261–266, 2008

8. Vijan S, Hofer TP, Hayward RA: Estimated benefits of glycemic control in microvascular complications in type 2 diabetes. *Ann Intern Med* 127:788–795, 1997

9. Gagliardino JJ, Williams R, Clark CM: Using hospitalization rates to track the economic costs and benefits of improved diabetes care in the Americas: a proposal for health policy makers. *Diabetes Care* 23:1844–1846, 2000

Ms. Spollett is an Adult Nurse Practitioner at Yale Diabetes Center, New Haven, CT.

20. Alternative and Complementary Medicine

Diana W. Guthrie, PHD, FAAN, ARNP, BC-ADM, CDE

Complementary and alternative medicine (CAM) has existed throughout time. The use of CAM therapies in diabetes dates back centuries. An early Greek treatise, which described diabetes as a "melting down" into the urine, stated that diabetes was treated with fasting, specific food choices, water restriction, or herbs. Any treatment that reduced the flow of urine was included in the early treatments.

People have tried numerous remedies or treatments for various ailments, some with success and some to the detriment of the recipient. CAM therapy, as it is commonly known, has increased in popularity because of recognition that it can be useful and perhaps even cost-effective. Senator Thomas Harkin of Iowa became a supporter of CAM after he had health problems related to allergies (1). After a series of treatments in the 1980s provided no relief, he was goaded into trying a CAM therapist. According to Senator Harkin, the results were positive and his "allergies [were] cured." He cosponsored a bill in Congress that created the Office of Alternative Medicine (OAM). The first call for grants by OAM resulted in the submission of 455 proposals, 30 of which were subsequently funded. Gradually, CAM centers took their place not only as centers for research training, but also as grantees for specific research proposals. At the end of the 1990s, OAM was renamed the National Center for Complementary and Alternative Medicine (NCCAM).

Two significant papers showed that the public had an interest in using alternative therapies. The benchmark article by Eisenberg et al. (2) in 1993 titled "Unconventional Medicine in the United States" was followed 5 years later by another publication from the same group that focused on changes in the use and opinions of CAM over time (3). CAM use was working its way into the minds, if not the hearts, of more health care professionals (4).

Complementary therapies are those used along with standard practices. Therapies (modalities) such as any of the energy therapies, massage, acupuncture, and the use of various herbs, vitamins, and/or minerals alongside standard practice are considered complementary therapy. These might include the more familiar medical nutrition therapies, exercise, and relaxation techniques. Using these modalities in place of standard practice, particularly medication, is considered alternative therapy. Meal planning and exercise can be considered an alternative form of medicine, one that was found to be more effective than medication in the prevention of type 2 diabetes in the Diabetes Prevention Program (5). In that study, appropriate food choices and exercise were successfully used in place of medication in the earliest forms of type 2 diabetes.

The trend towards more widespread use of CAM therapies has resulted in schools of medicine and nursing beginning to teach CAM therapies as either required or elective courses, some blend CAM with traditional care and some provide credentials for practitioners (6).

CATEGORIES OF CAM

The NCCAM has divided CAM therapies into five categories (Table 20.1). These therapies cover the use of nutrition (e.g., herbs, vitamins, minerals) and various modalities (e.g., from Chinese medicine to magnetic therapy). Each of these therapeutic areas may directly or indirectly have an effect on diabetes or its complications. Some may counteract a medication or foster higher blood glucose levels rather than having the desired lowering effect. Factors such as renal and hepatic clearance need to be considered when prescribing these therapies for a person with diabetes. Certain herbal therapies may not be excreted properly from the body and over time build up to toxic levels. It is unknown how some of these herbs might affect the diabetes medications currently being used. This requires further study.

Table 20.2 describes some common types of energy- and body-based CAM modalities and will help the health care professional decide which therapeutic modality will be most effective in the plan of care. No single CAM modality will be appropriate for every patient. Choosing one or two specific modalities depends on the need(s) as determined by the assessment of the person. If the person is in

Table 20.1 NCCAM Therapy Categories

1. Alternative medical systems: Chinese medicine, Ayurveda
2. Mind-body interventions: prayer, meditation, music, support groups
3. Biologically based therapies: dietary supplements, herbal products
4. Manipulative and body-based methods: chiropractic, massage
5. Energy therapies: yoga, healing touch
   a. Biofield therapies: qigong, Reiki, therapeutic touch
   b. Bioelectromagnetic-based therapies: electromagnetic fields, alternating or direct current fields

Table 20.2 Common Types of CAM

CAM Type	Description
Acupuncture	Insertion of very fine needles into or along various pathways called meridians to enhance the flow of energy.
Aromatherapy	The use of various oils to aid in, depending on the oil, antibacterial action, antiviral action, mood harmonization, relaxation, joint and muscle improvement, and diuretic action, among others.
Biofeedback	Any type of information that enhances the learning process and supports healing, e.g., body temperature, an indicator of relaxation and improved blood circulation.
Healing touch	A variety of techniques that increase the body's energy output or modulate this energy into more useful patterns.
Hypnotherapy	A technique for self-learning to assist in peace of mind and of body through the use of suggestion.
Magnetic therapy	Altering the body's responses through the use of magnetic energy.
Massage	Manipulation of the muscles, joints, and, indirectly, the nerves to promote healing, e.g., various forms of massage using body meridians (shiatsu), a particular pattern of massage (Swedish), or a greater focus on the joints and muscles attached to such joints (Thai).
Reflexology	Massage and manipulation of the reflexes of the feet (or hands) to correspond to the needs in various parts of the body for the purpose of rebalancing the body.
Reiki	Supporting the flow of energy throughout the body for the purpose of healing.
Therapeutic touch	A set use of physical and nonphysical contacts for the purpose of relieving pain, reducing inflammation, and enhancing relaxation, i.e., centering, assessing, modulating, and smoothing.
Yoga	Another energy therapy with the purpose of uniting the flow of physical, mental, and spiritual energy for improving health and well-being.

pain, one of the energy or massage therapies might be in order and could be accompanied by an herb for use in aromatherapy. Less pain and lowered blood glucose levels may be the outcome.

CAM EFFECTS ON BLOOD GLUCOSE

Today, there are over 400 herbs known to lower blood glucose levels and some that actually raise blood glucose levels (Table 20.3) (7). Much of the concern regarding the use of CAM therapies is centered on the self-administration of herbs without adequate knowledge of their efficacy and safety. In addition, the

Table 20.3 Effects of Plants and Herbs on Blood Glucose

Plants That May Lower Blood Glucose	Plants That May Raise Blood Glucose
Aloe: dried exudates	Cocoa: seeds
Banana: flowers and roots	Coffee: seeds
Barley: sprouts	Cola: seeds
Bilberry: leaves	Mahuang: plant
Bitter melon: fruit	Rosemary: leaves
Carob: bean gum	Tea: leaves
Cashew: leaves	Cucumber: fruit
Cumin: seed	
Dandelion: plant	
Eucalyptus: leaves	
Fenugreek: seeds	
Garlic: cloves	
Ginseng: roots	
Guar gum: seeds and pods	
Juniper: berries	
Kidney beans: immature pods	
Mulberry: leaves	
Onion: bulbs	
Prickly pear: cactus plant	
Reijshi mushroom: body	
Spinach: leaves	
Wheat: leaves	

purity and concentration of packaged herbs is not regulated and may be inconsistent.

Herbs and plants that lower blood glucose levels do so through a variety of physiological responses. Some, such as guar gum, were thought to decrease the absorption of food and increase the feeling of fullness (7). Others, such as ginseng, increase metabolism but may also add weight from increased muscle growth (8). Cinnamon was thought to decrease blood glucose levels, but in five highly controlled and randomized trials, cinnamon did not improve glycated hemoglobin A1c (A1C), fasting blood glucose levels, or lipid parameters whether the person had type 1 or type 2 diabetes (9). Increasing fiber in the meal plan using fenugreek seeds might aid in lowering blood glucose levels and has been demonstrated to be especially beneficial for someone who has type 2 diabetes, whereas agar or a pectin meal did not affect the postprandial glucose profile even though they were both found to delay gastric emptying (10).

Pain is known to raise blood glucose levels, and fever may further raise blood glucose levels. Anything that reduces pain, such as standard medication, massage, or acupuncture, could also lower blood glucose levels. In one study in which the parents of children with type 1 diabetes were asked about CAM use in their children, 18.4% ($n = 42$) indicated they had used CAM, most commonly homeopathy, vitamins and minerals, and modified diets. The parents did not question the need for insulin, but instead had hopes of improved well-being and diabetes control (11). Anxiety and its corresponding stressors are known to have effects on various body functions (12). Usually, blood glucose levels become elevated during periods of stress; however, they have also been known to decrease in the face of increased agitation. Relaxation therapies or energy therapies might aid in lowering glucose levels. Massage- or biofeedback-enhanced relaxation training may result in less labile blood glucose levels or overall lowered blood glucose levels in both type 1 and type 2 diabetes. The use of biofeedback to speed up the learning process when teaching relaxation techniques has also been found to lower blood glucose levels and to aid in increased circulation (13).

CAM EFFECT ON COMPLICATIONS

CAM therapy may be of some use when the associated complications of diabetes are present. For example, if polyneuropathy is present, then a trial of α-lipoic acid might be helpful, especially if normalization of blood glucose levels has not fully relieved the burning or tingling sensation in the extremities. Milk thistle, which is known to have hepatoprotective effects, might be very useful if the person has developed some mild liver enzyme changes with the use of statin medication.

SAFETY ISSUES

The patient should discuss all herb use with the health care team. Some patients may be reluctant to admit to their use of herbs for fear of being looked upon negatively by their health care provider. In fact, in one study of people in the U.S. using CAM therapies, fewer than half of the thousands of survey respondents told their health clinicians that they used CAM therapy for fear of reprimand or ridicule (3). The nurse should try to elicit information about use of herbs in such a way that the patient does not feel judged.

It is important that patients understand safety issues in the use of some herbs. Overuse or increased amounts of certain herbs can cause unfavorable reactions. Examples are impaction from the use of guar gum, diarrhea from the use of dandelion, or various other toxic responses.

The following tables are helpful in at least determining what is safe and unsafe in our present state of knowledge: Table 20.4 lists unsafe herbs (14), Table 20.5 lists moderately unsafe herbs (8), and Table 20.6 lists modalities that have been shown to be useful for people with diabetes (15).

Caution should be exercised when recommending use of herbs or dietary supplements because some are not standardized for purity or for strength. Safe dosages should be considered when advising the use of these products. (One useful web site is www.prescribersletter.com, which has a natural medicine database on the usage of herbs and supplements and safety issues.) Additionally, these supplements may be regulated by state practice acts; check your local guidelines before prescribing.

Some CAM modalities have not been adequately studied or not studied in relation to diabetes. The American Diabetes Association (ADA) has established guidelines regarding the use of unproven therapies (16). Therapies are classified

Table 20.4 Unsafe Herbs

Chaparral: liver damage
Chitosan: potentiates an anticoagulant effect
Ephedra (Mahuang): raises blood glucose, raises blood pressure, toxic
Hydrangea: leaves contain cyanide
Poke root: vomiting
Sassafras: carcinogenic, liver damage
Yohimbine: raises blood pressure, increases anxiety

Table 20.5 Moderately Unsafe Herbs

Bearberry: not to be used in pregnancy or for prostate disorders
Black/blue cohosh: not to be used during pregnancy or chronic illnesses (might affect blood glucose levels)
Boneset: toxicity possible in large doses
Comfrey: liver damage
Juniper: kidney disease, not for use in pregnancy
Licorice: not for use in pregnancy, diabetes, heart disease, or hypertension
Lobelia: not to be used in pregnancy
Wormwood: not to be used in pregnancy

Table 20.6 Potentially Useful Modalities for People with Diabetes

Nutrients: ω-3 and -6 fatty acids (γ-linolenic acid), bulk laxatives (such as bran, psyllium, and methylcellulose)
Vitamins: B, C, D, E (dosage not >400 IU)
Minerals: chromium, magnesium, vanadium, zinc
Herbs (topical or oral): basil, bilberry, bitter melon, capsaicin, fenugreek, ginko biloba, panax ginseng, gymnema sylvestre, milk thistle, nopal
Body-based methods: massage, chiropractic, reflexology
Energy therapies: acupressure (acupuncture), healing touch, Reiki, therapeutic touch

PRACTICAL POINT

Factors to consider when evaluating a CAM therapy for someone with diabetes:
■ Is the kidney and hepatic function normal?
■ Will there be an effect on blood pressure?
■ How will the therapy affect blood glucose levels?

as clearly effective, somewhat effective, unknown or unproven but possibly promising, or clearly ineffective. Operationally, the ADA considers the therapeutic modality to be safe and effective if it has been approved by the U.S. Food and Drug Administration, supported by at least two independent well-controlled studies that have been published in a peer-reviewed scientific publication, endorsed or recommended by the ADA Professional Practice Committee, or endorsed by a relevant or appropriate medical specialty organization.

EDUCATIONAL AND BEHAVIORAL CONSIDERATIONS

The Internet has become a source of information and education, but not necessarily in a way that is safe for someone with a chronic condition. Most CAM information on the Internet is at an eleventh-grade reading level (17). Greater misunderstanding can occur when the language is not thoroughly understood by the patient. Reviewing these materials with the patient is necessary to ensure adequate understanding.

Patient education should accompany any chosen modality and include an explanation of what it is, its intended therapeutic effect, and the time needed to achieve the expected outcome (see "A Step-by-Step Approach to Complementary Therapies" and "Guidelines for Using Vitamin, Mineral, and Herbal Supplements," patient handouts in RESOURCES). Side effects and possible adverse reactions must also be discussed, and the person should be alerted to signs or symptoms that require immediate action. In people with diabetes, the effect of the CAM modality on both acute and chronic complications will need to be reviewed.

The physical, mental, and emotional state of the person should be weighed against the chosen therapy. Treatment should include a team effort among the health care professional, the person with diabetes, and, if needed, a certified professional in the field of CAM therapy (such professionals can be found through

Assessing a Person for CAM

When assessing a person for CAM use, the nurse should do the following:
- Take a thorough history of daily intake of food and fluids.
- Include current or past use of herbs, supplements, or other types of CAM.
- Determine whether there are problems with various body systems.
- List stressors that might be found at home, school, or work.
- Identify and explore religious and social beliefs.
- Aid the person in identifying coping mechanisms that are already in use.
- Determine what might be of use or acceptable for the individual, e.g., daily meditation to lower blood pressure, lower pulse rate, and lead to the more effective use of oxygen (13).

Once this assessment is complete, the health care professional can determine which modalities are best suited for the patient.

Future Nursing Research

Sociological research on the use of CAM therapies has emerged (26). This development leads to the need for relevant research to clearly determine the use, problems, and promises of this field. Resources such as useful books and Internet sites as well as monographs and literature databases may be found (27). Not only is rigorous research needed from the standpoint of the effective use of these therapies, but it is especially salient for the field of diabetes, wherein potential problems might occur due to the diabetes disease state (28). NCCAM is supportive of such research and welcomes proposals, especially those that document the specific needs found in diabetes care.

the American Holistic Nurses Association [www.ahna.org] and the Healing Touch International [www.healingtouch.net]). Education should be updated as new treatments become available or as new information regarding current CAM is discovered. The therapeutic plan may need to be adjusted when any new CAM modality is introduced.

OTHER CONSIDERATIONS

Determining the effectiveness of a CAM therapy requires a trial period. For instance, if a person begins taking α-lipoic acid for polyneuropathy, a trial period of 2–3 months is needed using therapeutic levels. If no response is seen in that time, there is no value in continuing the therapy, and another therapy may be tried. No single CAM modality is appropriate or effective for all people. In a 2001 survey of health care professionals who recommend CAM therapy, the providers indicated that they prescribed the same therapy for a specific condition 34% of the time. This survey would indicate that health care professionals are individualizing CAM prescriptions (18).

Reimbursement has become an area of concern. Even though third-party payment is increasing for such modalities as chiropractic, acupuncture, and therapeutic massage (19), there are still many more modalities that are not supported by insurance carriers. According to a 2002 article (20), Medicaid reimbursement for the use of CAM therapies is increasing. This increase allows individuals who are unable to pay out of pocket to also experience appropriate complementary or alternate treatments for their diabetes management.

Ethical considerations must also be taken into account when using CAM. The patient has the right to be informed of the various therapeutic modalities available for the treatment of his or her disease. The health care professional must be open to discussion of CAM modalities and allow the patient to pursue alternative methods, if appropriate. The health care professional also has the responsibility to inform the patient of unintended consequences or deleterious effects caused by the initiation of CAM or the discontinuation of proven medical therapies (21). As public interest increases, more patients and health care professionals will turn to the use of CAM, and these ethical considerations must be met (22).

SUMMARY

CAM has had a significant impact on today's medicine and nursing care (23). Patients seek information regarding CAM and its use in their health care regimen. They expect that their health care professional will be able to respond appropriately. Although only 20% of individuals with diabetes reported that they were using CAM therapy to treat their diabetes (24), physicians and nurses will need to foster communication with their patients about CAM therapy and provide sufficient information for adequate and safe decision making (25). For safe use of such modalities, health care professionals should have a working knowledge of the prescribed CAM or be able to consult or refer to a certified professional in that field.

REFERENCES

1. NCCAM web site. Available from http://nccam.nih.gov. Accessed 20 March 2008

2. Eisenberg DM, Kessler RC, Foster C, Norlock RE, Calkins DR, DelBance TL: Unconventional medicine in the United States: prevalence, cost and patterns of use. *N Engl J Med* 328:246–252, 1993

3. Eisenberg DM, Davis RB, Ettner SL, Appel S, Wilkey S, Van-Rompay MI, Kessler RC: Trends in alternative medicine use in the United States. *JAMA* 280:1569–1575, 1998

4. Eisenberg DM, Kessler RC, Van-Rompay MI, Kaptchuk TJ, Wilkey SA, et al.: Perceptions about complementary therapies relative to conventional therapies among adults who use both: results from a national survey. *Ann Intern Med* 135:344–351, 2001

5. Pastors JG, Warshaw H, Daly A, Franz M, Kulkarni K: The evidence for the effectiveness of medical nutrition therapy in diabetes management. *Diabetes Care* 25:608–613, 2002

6. Peck S: Integrating CAM therapies into NP practice. *Am J NP* 12:10–18, 2008

7. Shane-McWhorter L: Biological complementary therapies: a focus on botanical products in diabetes. *Diabetes Spectrum* 14:199–208, 2001

8. Vuksan V, Sievenpiper JL, Koo VY, Francis T, Beljan-Zdravkovic U, et al.: American ginseng (*Panax quinquefolius* L) reduces postprandial glycemia in nondiabetic subjects and subjects with type 2 diabetes mellitus. *Arch Intern Med* 160:1009–1013, 2000

9. Baker WL, Gutierrez-William G, White CM, Kluger J, Coleman CL: Effect of cinnamon on glucose control and lipid parameters. *Diabetes Care* 31:41–45, 2008

10. Sanaka M, Yamamoto T, Anjiki H, Nagasawa K, Kuyama Y: Effects of agar and pectin on gastric emptying and post-prandial glycaemic profiles in healthy human volunteers. *Clin Exp Pharmacol Physiol* 34:1151–1155, 2007

11. Dannemann K, Hecker W, Haberland H, Herbst A, Galler A, et al.: Use of complementary and alternative medicine in children with type 1 diabetes mellitus-prevalence, patterns of use, and costs. *Pediatric Diabetes* 9:228–235, 2008

12. Benson H, Steward EM: *The Wellness Book: The Comprehensive Guide to Maintaining Health and Treating Stress Related Illness.* New York, Simon & Shuster, 1993

13. Rice BI, Schindler JV: Effect of thermal biofeedback assisted relaxation training for blood circulation in lower extremities of a population with diabetes. *Diabetes Care* 15:853–858, 1992

14. Tyler VE: *The Honest Herbal.* New York, Pharmaceutical Products, 1993

15. Guthrie D, Huebscher R, Shuler P, Rauckhorst L, Miller H: Endocrine concerns. In *Natural, Alternative, and Complementary Health Care Practices.* Huebscher R, Shuler P, Eds. St. Louis, MO, Mosby, 2004, p. 658–713

16. American Diabetes Association: Unproven therapies (Position Statement). *Diabetes Care* 27 (Suppl. 1):S135, 2004

17. Sagaram S, Walji M, Bernstam E: Evaluating the prevalence, content and readability of complementary and alternative medicine (CAM) web pages on the Internet. *Proc AMIA Symp* 672–676, 2002

18. Long L, Huntley A, Ernst E: Which complementary and alternative therapies benefit which conditions? A survey of the opinions of 223 professional organizations. *Complement Ther Med* 9:178–185, 2001

19. Cleary-Guida MB, Okvat HA, Oz MC, Ting W: A regional survey of health insurance coverage for complementary and alternative medicine: current status and future ramifications. *J Altern Complement Med* 7:269–173, 2001

20. Steyer TE, Freed GL, Lantz PM: Medicaid reimbursement for alternative therapies. *Altern Ther Health Med* 8:84–88, 2002

21. Kaler MM, Ravella PC: Staying on the ethical high ground with complementary and alternative medicine. *Nurse Pract* 27:38–42, 2002

22. Jonas WB: Advising patients on the use of complementary and alternative medicine. *Appl Psychophysiol Biofeedback* 26:205–214, 2001

23. Egan CD: Addressing use of herbal medicine in the primary care setting. *J Am Acad Nurse Pract* 14:166–171, 2002

24. Yeh GY, Eisenberg DM, Davis RB, Phillips RS: Use of complementary and alternative medicine among persons with diabetes mellitus: results of a national survey. *Am J Public Health* 92:1648–1652, 2002

25. Corbin-Winslow L, Shapiro H: Physicians want education about complementary and alternative medicine to enhance communication with their patients. *Arch Intern Med* 162:1176–1181, 2002

26. Tovey P, Adams J: Nostalgic and nostophobic referencing and the authentication of nurses' use of complementary therapies. *Soc Sci Med* 56:1469–1480, 2003

27. Kiefer D, Shah S, Gardiner P, Wechkin H: Finding information on herbal therapy: a guide to useful sources for clinicians. *Altern Ther Health Med* 7:74–78, 2001

28. Kinsel JF, Straus SE: Complementary and alternative therapeutics: rigorous research is needed to support claims. *Ann Rev Pharmacol Toxicol* 43:463–484, 2003

ADDITIONAL READING

Dossey BM, Keegan L, Guzzetta CE: *Holistic Nursing: A Handbook for Practice*. 3rd ed. Gaithersburg, MD, Aspen, 2000

Guthrie DW: *Alternative and Complementary Diabetes Care*. New York, Wiley, 2002

Guthrie DW: *Diabetes Self-Management's Hidden Secrets of Natural Healing*. New York, Rappaport, 2007

Geil P, Shane-McWhorter L: Dietary supplements in the management of diabetes: potential risks and benefits. *J Am Diet Assoc* 108: s59–s65, 2008

Huebscher R, Shuler P: *Natural, Alternative, and Complementary Health Care Practices*. St. Louis, MO, Mosby, 2004

Kuhn MA: *Complementary Therapies for Health Care Providers*. Baltimore, MD, Lippincott Williams & Wilkins, 1999

Physicians' Desk Reference for Herbal Medicines. 3rd ed. Montvale, NJ, Thompson PDR, 2004

Snyder M, Lindquist R (Eds.): *Complementary/Alternative Therapies in Nursing*. 4th ed. New York, Springer, 2002

Shane-McWhorter L: *Complementary and Alternative Medicine (CAM) Supplement Use in People With Diabetes: A Clinician's Guide*. Alexandria, VA, American Diabetes Association, 2007

Yeh GY, Eisenberg DM, Kaptchuk TJ, Phillips RS: Systematic review of herbs and dietary supplements for glycemic control in diabetes. *Diabetes Care* 26:1277–1294, 2003

Dr. Guthrie is a Diabetes Nurse Specialist/Practitioner at Mid-America Diabetes Associates, Wichita, KS, and Professor Emeritus, the University of Kansas School Medicine. Along with being a CDE and BC-ADM, she is certified in Healing Touch and Advanced Certified in Holistic Nursing. As Adjunct Professor at the Wichita State University, School of Nursing, she teaches an enhanced computer course on CAM therapies.

21. Living with Diabetes

Diana Rhiley, LCMFT, CDE

Living with diabetes is a daily challenge. The nature of the regimen—frequent blood glucose monitoring, meal planning, exercising, and scheduling medication—creates the need for constant vigilance on the part of the person with diabetes. There are tremendous payoffs for these efforts, including fewer and less frequent complications of diabetes, but such efforts are not without cost. Patients often express a sense of loss of freedom, spontaneity, or food choices and the feeling that diabetes management is taking over their lives. Diabetes may affect relationships, limit social interactions, and present the fear that even with hard work, bad things can happen.

The health care professional becomes part of the individual's health care team and support system. This may be a short-term relationship for nurses in a short-stay hospital or a long-term relationship for the nurse in the clinic or home health care setting. The role of the nurse may be pivotal in assisting the patient in self-care management skills and in the psychosocial adaptation to a life-changing illness. Many courageous people successfully live with diabetes because of the skills, relationships, and strategies they have developed to cope with the day-to-day challenges of diabetes.

The individual with diabetes sometimes feels more comfortable confiding in a nurse or nonphysician health care professional. Therefore, the role of the nurse is important in assessing an individual's ability to adjust, cope, and manage his or her diabetes effectively. Assessment involves careful observation, probing questions, and attention to the types of responses.

Diabetes does not take a day off. Diabetes is a disease of many details. It is not surprising that it is difficult to maintain vigilance to the regimen day in and day out. The nurse plays an important role as coach and advocate.

Table 21.1 Specific Assessment Questions for the Newly Diagnosed Patient

Assessment Areas	Questions and Observations
Education	Who will provide the patient's education? Does the patient have access to certified diabetes educators (CDEs)? If hospitalized, will there be more intensive education after discharge? If a CDE is providing inpatient education, ask the patient about what he or she is learning. Is the patient retaining the information? Are family members involved in the education?
Patient structure	Does the patient appear to have a way of organizing him/herself? Does the patient have a schedule and routine in his/her daily life? Or does a schedule feel confining and something that the patient will come to resent? Is this a chaotic time in the patient's life when structure is changing, e.g., new job, moving, breakup of a relationship?
Ability to change	Where is the client in the change cycle? Is the patient beginning to process change? Is he/she talking about what will be different and how such changes will be implemented?
Support system	Who makes up the patient's support system? Can the patient easily access them? What is their geographical proximity to the patient? Are they willing to be involved? Will they be present for education?
Ability to ask for help	Is the patient good at asking for help when needed? Or does something prevent him/her from asking for support or information from others? If the patient is unclear about something, will he/she ask for clarification? If the patient is having a hypoglycemic event, does he/she recognize the symptoms and will he/she seek assistance?

ASSESSING THE NEWLY DIAGNOSED

The patient who is newly diagnosed has special needs and considerations. Table 21.1 provides suggested questions and observations to assist in supporting the patient who has recently been diagnosed with diabetes. This is a critical time for supporting and empowering the patient in preparation for self-care management. The messages that the patient with newly diagnosed diabetes receives at this moment will be remembered for a lifetime. It is important to provide accurate, positive information to the patient and family.

EVALUATING LEVEL OF ADAPTATION

Table 21.2 identifies several key questions that the nurse can use to assess the individual's level of knowledge about diabetes, perceived stress level, family dynamics, attitudes about life, and potential for depression, diabetes burnout, or denial.

> ### PRACTICAL POINT
>
> Burnout may create feelings of being alone or overwhelmed and of failure. Poor self-care and poor follow-up with the health care professional are other common symptoms. The patient may feel that diabetes controls his or her life.

Table 21.2 Key Questions and Observations Regarding Adaptation

Assessment Areas	Specific Questions and Observations
Knowledge and attitude toward diabetes	What can the patient tell you about his/her regimen? Is he/she able to describe the diabetes regimen accurately? What is the patient's attitude when talking about diabetes and the diabetes regimen? What is this discussion's effect on the patient? Does he/she get tearful or angry? Is he/she proud of the ability to self-manage? Are there past personal or family experiences that are meaningful to the patient and influence attitudes toward diabetes and self-care issues?
Current stress level	What are the current stressors in the patient's life in addition to diabetes? Work? Finances? Relationships?
Family dynamics and support systems	What are the family dynamics? Are interactions pleasant and loving or are they cold and distant? Do other family members show knowledge of the regimen and take part in it? Are family members overly protective and indulgent? Do family members tend to nag, creating a situation in which the patient may resist doing the things that are in his/her best interest? If the patient lives alone, where does the support come from? Is there a close extended family, helpful neighbors, supportive friends, and a supportive health care team or health care professionals?
Attitude about life	What is the patient's overall attitude toward life? Does he/she make reference to his/her faith or spiritual life? How has the person coped with personal challenges in the past?
Depression	Do you see any signs of depression or anxiety? Is the patient sleeping through the night? Has the patient's eating pattern changed beyond just what the diabetes recommendations include? Has the patient lost interest in the things he/she would have been excited about previously? Has the patient restricted social activities or withdrawn from friends, significant others, etc.? Does the patient talk of worrying about things?
Denial or burnout	Does the patient show any signs of denial or burnout or express feelings of being overwhelmed? Is the patient unable to incorporate changes in his or her treatment program? Does he/she tend to minimize diabetes? Or does the patient justify or rationalize away the poor choices he/she has made?

Table 21.3 Strategies to Assist in Reducing Diabetes Burnout

Skills	Suggested Strategies
Establish a strong collaborative relationship	It may be very helpful to the patient for the health care professional to acknowledge the patient's struggles, applaud successes, and strive for frequent visits to help the patient through the time of burnout.
Increase commitment	Encourage patient to do a cost analysis. A table format can help the patient review the benefits and costs of choosing or not choosing to follow a prescribed diabetes regimen.
Negotiate goals	The health care professional can help the patient reestablish goals that are measurable and achievable. Start with what the patient is already doing and add to it in small steps. Make sure to help the individual develop simple goals that are realistic.
Pay attention to strong negative feelings	Listen intently and acknowledge or validate. Acknowledging the patient's feelings is a very powerful tool. This means that the health care professional must listen intently to identify and label those feelings and then normalize those feelings when possible. If this continues to be a roadblock after repeated attempts by the health care professional, consider a referral to a mental health professional.
Optimize social support	Loving, supportive relationships with others who take an interest in diabetes management can be a great antidote to diabetes burnout. Other parts of this chapter also address the role of the support system.
Engage the patient in active problem solving	1. Implement only one change at a time. 2. Focus on a behavior that can become a habit. 3. When possible, use the environment as a reminder to do a behavior, e.g., putting vitamins next to the coffeemaker (2).

REDUCING DIABETES BURNOUT

The term diabetes burnout is accepted as the description for a feeling of failure and chronic frustration developed by an individual with diabetes. One study reported that ~60% of patients sampled reported at least one serious diabetes-related concern (1,2). Burnout may lead to poor-self care. Strategies identified to alleviate diabetes burnout are included in Table 21.3.

ADAPTING TO COMPLICATIONS

The patient with complications from diabetes has special considerations. It will be important to assess the level of pain and his or her ability to cope with the complications. Table 21.4 lists assessment areas and questions and observations for individuals with complications.

Table 21.4 Specific Questions and Observations for a Patient with Diabetes Complications

Assessment Areas	Questions and Observations
Severity	What is the complication? How severe is the complication? Does it interfere with the patient's lifestyle? If so, how has the patient adapted?
Pain level	Is the patient experiencing physical discomfort in relation to the complication? If so, how much? It may be necessary to use a pain severity scale.
Support system and coping skills	It is crucial to assess the patient's coping skills and support system. These will be key indicators as to how the client will handle the complication and assimilate it into his/her future.

Individuals who develop diabetes-related complications face many challenges, particularly in accommodating to limitations and loss, such as alterations in vision or mobility. The process of adjusting to a complication may be similar to the individual's adjustment to the diagnosis of diabetes. Many of the assessment items used at the time of diagnosis may be useful when assessing a patient with a new complication, such as the onset of renal failure or the significant visual changes associated with retinopathy.

The psychological implications of a diabetes-related complication might be devastating and result in self-blame and feelings of failure or depression. Complications increase the risk factors for depression (3). Individuals with complications of diabetes may have greater need for psychological support to assist with adaptation (4). The RESOURCES section of this book has a list of organizations that can provide materials and support for the patient dealing with visual changes or amputations.

DEPRESSION

At some point during the process of dealing with diabetes, many patients will experience depression (see chapter 22). It may not be recognized, particularly because some of the symptoms of depression, e.g., fatigue, feelings of hopelessness, and lack of appetite, resemble poorly controlled diabetes or hyperglycemia. There is a tendency to underdiagnose or undertreat depression in patients with chronic illness. Because depression has been shown to contribute independently to the complications of diabetes, in addition to contributing to hyperglycemia, health care professionals must be aware of its presence (5). Using a simple and quick screening tool for depression, such as the Beck Depression Scale or Zung Depression Scale, gives the provider an opportunity to recognize, refer, or provide treatment (see RESOURCES for an online screening tool).

The health care provider must be supportive and help the patient recognize that depression is a medical problem and must be treated as such. For some patients, being diagnosed with depression carries a stigma, and they may resist counseling and medication therapy. In these cases, it is critical that the health care provider help the patient understand that the stress of living with a chronic illness can result in depression and that this is neither unusual nor a reflection of his or her character (see RESOURCES for information on these tools and the patient handout, "How Can We Help You?").

SUPPORT SYSTEMS

It is difficult to face a chronic disease and make and maintain numerous lifestyle changes without a support system. Affirmation and validation by others can assist the individual with diabetes in continuing effective health care behaviors.

At the same time, diabetes can cause a strain on relationships. A support person may begin to resent an individual who does not follow all of the recommendations and is not the "perfect patient." Some individuals may feel that it is their responsibility to make sure the person with diabetes takes better care of himself or herself. They may begin to nag and constantly watch the person with diabetes. Keeping in mind the degree of dependency present, the support person and the person with diabetes need to talk about their mutual expectations in the management of diabetes. Without open, honest communication, the relationship can evolve into a game and a tool with which to hurt each other. The support person needs to be aware of his or her feelings about diabetes, such as fear, resentment, anger, etc. It is often these kinds of feelings that drive one toward overprotective or smothering behavior. If a codependent or other unhealthy relationship is suspected, referral to a mental health professional is recommended.

COPING SKILLS

Coping skills are a necessary tool for a person to acknowledge and accept the difficulties of managing diabetes. Table 21.5 outlines specific skills that may be beneficial to the individual with diabetes and his or her family.

Table 21.5 Behaviors to Enhance Coping Skills

Skill	Specific Behaviors
Self-talk as a foundation for attitude	Listen to the patient's exact language; it is a direct link to his or her attitude: ■ Encourage motivating and successful speech: Does the patient use words that include hope and are encouraging? A patient's self-efficacy is crucial to his/her success, so it is important to know if the patient feels able to do the things asked of him/her and to do them over the long term.

Table 21.5 Behaviors to Enhance Coping Skills (*Continued*)

Skill	Specific Behaviors
	■ Words lead to attitude: The patient's words are a good clue as to how he/she sees this process playing out. Encourage patients to change their words to match a successful attitude.
Assertiveness	Assertiveness is an extremely important skill for people with diabetes. Assertiveness includes the following behaviors: ■ Expressing feelings rather than holding them in, and taking ownership of these feelings: Encourage discussion about feelings of frustrations or resentment. ■ Saying "no" when he/she really means it: Patients need to set and maintain protective limits around their time and energy in order to preserve good health. ■ Asking questions: The patient needs to be able to ask for clarification. Not asking may be a sign of being overwhelmed or depressed. ■ Asking for assistance when needed: The ability to ask for assistance demonstrates that the patient has balanced the dependence/independence behavior dichotomy and knows how and when to seek help.
Problem solving	Problem solving is a skill that helps the patient maintain a sense of empowerment. Problem solving includes the following steps, which are done together with the patient: ■ Develop a clear definition of the problem: What is the issue? What does the patient want to happen? ■ Brainstorm possible solutions: Identify realistic goals, and guide the patient toward selecting his/her own resolution. ■ Use reasonable solutions: Identify what is possible within the patient's power and implement that plan. Engage in active problem solving: Include the three steps used for active problem solving in Table 21.3.
Goal setting and time management	Diabetes requires a significant amount of time for self-care activities; therefore, the priority given it by a patient is tantamount to the success of the treatment regimen: ■ Assess the priority of diabetes self-care: Where on the patient's priority list is diabetes care? Is it high enough to make a commitment to it? It will be difficult for the patient to make a time commitment to these tasks unless these goals are given significant priority. ■ Determine an approach for reluctant individuals: The use of motivational interviewing and skills, such as agenda setting, rapport building, negotiating, building readiness to change, and assessment of importance and confidence, may be helpful when working with a reluctant patient (6,7).

(*continued*)

Table 21.5 Behaviors to Enhance Coping Skills (*Continued*)

Skill	Specific Behaviors
Support system	Help the patient identify the person or people who can play the following roles in his/her life: ■ Someone who can help with the day-to-day "mechanics" of diabetes, e.g., cooking and meal planning, keeping prescriptions filled, being an exercise partner? ■ Someone with whom the patient can share frustrations and achievements? ■ Someone who can run interference in situations that wear the patient down or that the patient continually finds frustrating?
Manage stress	Help individuals identify different methods for coping or managing stress (see also "Stress Management Tools," a patient handout in RESOURCES). For example, ask them what they like to do to relax or what they do when they feel very stressed. Some people like to listen to music, read a book, or talk with a friend. Other types of stress management skills are: ■ Exercise: Exercise creates many benefits for everyone. Not only is it a large part of a successful diabetes-management regimen, but it also pays huge rewards as part of a stress-management program. The more consistent the exercise, the greater the benefit. ■ Relaxation: Begin with progressive relaxation. This is the alternate tensing and relaxing of muscle groups to know the difference between tense and relaxed muscles. Work with large motor muscles and progress to fine motor muscles. Autogenic relaxation focuses on producing physical sensations that are associated with relaxation. Imagining body parts as feeling heavy and warm can reduce the tension in the body. Imagery is the creation of a relaxing scene in the mind in which the person feels free and relaxed and totally removed from pressure and worry. Using relaxation successfully requires practice sessions of ~20 min twice daily for 6 weeks. Before that, it may be difficult to implement the benefits of relaxation in the middle of a stressful moment. ■ Biofeedback: Biofeedback is the monitoring of a bodily function such as heart rate, brain waves, or hand temperature. In the learning process, it is coupled with relaxation so that a patient can learn to create the conditions that help calm the body.

SUMMARY

A nurse can play a key role in assisting the individual to live successfully with diabetes. To help individuals with diabetes, it is essential that nurses provide current and accurate diabetes information or be able to refer the patient to someone with appropriate expertise. The American Diabetes Association, the American Association of Diabetes Educators, and a local certified diabetes educator are good resources.

Interactions with the patient may only be for a limited time. Unless the patient has requested that information be kept confidential, the health care team should be apprised of any changes or concerns regarding individual patients. It is important that the patient receive the same messages from each of his or her health care professionals. Any information obtained from the assessments that causes concern should be directed to the patient's primary health care provider and certified diabetes educators. Interactions with the patient may broaden the primary health care provider's understanding of the patient and help him or her better meet the patient's needs. It may be appropriate to encourage a social services or mental health consultation.

Frequent interactions with patients, however brief, may also be vital in encouraging the patient to maintain a continued commitment to diabetes care. Because of the investment of time and interest on the part of the health care provider, the patient may find that living with diabetes can be easier.

REFERENCES

1. Anderson B, Rubin R (Eds.): *Practical Psychology for Diabetes Clinicians*. 2nd ed. Alexandria, VA, American Diabetes Association, 2002

2. Polonsky WH: Understanding and treating patients with diabetes burnout. In *Practical Psychology for Diabetes Clinicians*. 2nd ed. Anderson B, Rubin R, Eds. Alexandria, VA, American Diabetes Association, 2002, p. 219–228

3. Vileikyte L, Leventhal H., Gonzalez JS, Peyrot M, Rubin RR, et al.: Diabetic peripheral neuropathy and depressive symptoms: the association revisited. *Diabetes Care* 28:2378–2383, 2005

4. Egede LE, Nietert PJ, Zheng D: Depression and all-cause and coronary heart disease mortality among adults with and without diabetes. *Diabetes Care* 28:1339–1345, 2005

5. Lustman PJ, Singh PK, Clouse RE: Recognizing and managing depression in patients with diabetes. In *Practical Psychology for Diabetes Clinicians*. 2nd ed. Anderson B, Rubin R, Eds. Alexandria, VA, American Diabetes Association, 2002, p. 229–238

6. Rollnick S, Mason P, Butler C: *Health Behavior Change: A Guide for Practitioners*. London, Churchill Livingstone, 1999

7. Miller WR, Rollnick S (Eds.): *Motivational Interviewing: Preparing People for Change*. 2nd ed. New York, Guilford Press, 2002

ADDITIONAL READING

American Diabetes Association: *Caring for the Diabetic Soul*. Alexandria, VA, American Diabetes Association, 1997

Anderson B, Funnell M: *The Art of Empowerment: Stories and Strategies for Diabetes Educators*. 2nd ed. Alexandria, VA, American Diabetes Association, 2005

Polonsky W: *Diabetes Burnout: What to Do When You Can't Take It Anymore* (book and audiotape). Alexandria, VA, American Diabetes Association, 1999

Ms. Rhiley is a Certified Diabetes Educator, an Adjunct Supervisor in the Marriage and Family Therapy Program at Friends University, Wichita, KS, and is in private practice as a marriage and family therapist specializing in medical family therapy.

22. Depression, Anxiety, and Eating Disorders

Ann Goebel-Fabbri, PHD, and John Zrebiec, MSW, CDE

> ## PRACTICAL POINT
>
> Depression is two to three times more prevalent in patients with diabetes. It is very important to screen patients at each visit and to look for cues that suggest the presence of depression. Examples of such cues are *1*) lack of interest in self-care behaviors, *2*) increased forgetfulness in taking medications or self-monitoring glucose, and *3*) change in dress or appearance.

The Diabetes Control and Complications Trial (DCCT) and the U.K. Prospective Diabetes Study demonstrated that intensive management of type 1 and type 2 diabetes improves long-term health outcomes (1,2). However, the goal of achieving near-normal blood glucose values requires a complex set of daily behaviors and problem solving involving dietary control, exercise, blood glucose monitoring, and oral anti-hyperglycemic medications or multiple daily insulin injections. Over the long term, it is not uncommon for patients to have difficulty sustaining the burden of these daily self-care demands and numerous lifestyle changes. It is therefore not surprising that the stress of coping with diabetes is a major risk factor for psychiatric illnesses and problems related to adhering to complex treatment recommendations.

DEPRESSION AND DIABETES

The prevalence of depression in diabetes patients is two to four times higher than that found in the general population (3,4). Several studies suggest that patients with depressive disorders develop worse glycemic control problems and have a

Symptoms of Depression

At least five of the following symptoms have been present during the same 2-week period (including at least one of the first two):
- Depressed mood
- Loss of interest or pleasure
- Significant weight (appetite) loss or weight gain
- Insomnia or hypersomnia
- Psychomotor agitation or retardation
- Fatigue, loss of energy
- Feelings of worthlessness or guilt
- Difficulty concentrating or indecisiveness
- Thoughts of death or suicide

heightened risk of diabetes complications, such as retinopathy, nephropathy, hypertension, cardiac disease, and sexual dysfunction (5). Although depression is related to complications and disease duration, it has been found to occur relatively early in the course of diabetes, before the onset of complications (6). Therefore, the increased rate of depression and diabetes cannot be explained solely by emotional reactions to the onset of complications. Indeed, the relationship may be bidirectional because symptoms of depression, such as decreased motivation, poor energy, and hopelessness, likely interfere with adherence to diabetes treatment, leading to worse glycemic control.

In a meta-analysis of 24 studies of depression, hyperglycemia, and diabetes, Lustman et al. (7) reported a consistent, strong association between elevated glycated hemoglobin A1c (A1C) values (indicating chronic hyperglycemia) and depression. However, they were unable to determine the direction of the association, so it remains unclear if hyperglycemia causes depressed mood or if hyperglycemia is a consequence of depression. Furthermore, Lustman et al. (7) noted that the relationship might be a reciprocal one in which hyperglycemia is provoked by depression, independently contributing to the exacerbation of depression, like a feedback loop.

Studies of type 2 diabetes clearly indicate that depression and diabetes are associated, but the direction of the association is still unclear. Depression may occur as a consequence of having diabetes (8). However, in some instances, the increased rates of depression seen in patients with type 2 diabetes appear to precede the onset of illness, thereby raising an entirely different hypothesis about the etiological relationship, i.e., depressive disorders themselves may place patients at risk of developing type 2 diabetes. Depressed patients often decrease physical activity, increase cardiovascular risk factors by smoking, and eat high-calorie and fatty foods, placing them at higher risk of developing type 2 diabetes (9,10).

Furthermore, Jacobson and colleagues (11) hypothesized that the metabolic problems of diabetes (increased rates of hypoglycemia and/or hyperglycemia) could themselves play a causal role in the development of depression. In a recent study, they found a similar prevalence of white-matter lesions in both diabetic patients and nondiabetic control subjects. However, preliminary evidence using more sensitive techniques suggests that diabetes may lead to changes in white matter in the brain and that these white-matter abnormalities (if present in regions of the brain involved in affect regulation, e.g., the limbic system) may play a causal role in the development of depression. Their research team also demonstrated that diabetic patients show lower gray-matter density than nondiabetic patients in several regions of the brain (12). Differences in gray-matter density were also observed in the brains of type 1 diabetes patients with histories of depression compared with those of patients without depression. These early studies suggest an association between brain structural changes (in both white and gray matter) and depression in patients with diabetes that may be related to the underlying metabolic fluctuations of diabetes. Finally, in a functional MRI study conducted to evaluate brain function responses to acute hypoglycemia in both diabetic and non-diabetic individuals, they found a network of common activated brain regions in both groups, as well as several regions that responded in one group only, suggesting that the two groups may respond differently to hypoglycemia (13).

Evidence indicates that treatment for depression can lead to improvements in diabetes regimen adherence and improved glycemic control. The combination of high rates of depression in patients with diabetes and the known effectiveness of treatments for depression reinforces how critical it is to identify and treat depression early in its onset. The possibility of comorbid depression should also be considered when treating patients with worsening glycemic control and trouble adapting to diabetes. A small number of studies have demonstrated that treatment of depression, including cognitive behavior therapy and antidepressants (particularly selective serotonin reuptake inhibitors [SSRIs]), has equivalent efficacy in depressed patients with diabetes and patients with depression alone. The mutual identification, support, and problem solving offered by other people with diabetes makes group therapy an increasingly popular option for treatment of depression. Thus, whatever the causal links between depression and diabetes, psychiatric treatment can improve glycemic control and reduce depressive symptoms (7–14).

> **PRACTICAL POINT**
>
> Treatment of depression will help people with diabetes have longer, more enjoyable, healthier lives.

ANXIETY DISORDERS AND DIABETES

All patients are anxious about their diabetes at one time or another. Whether anxiety is normal or abnormal depends on its intensity and on the duration, consequences, and circumstances that caused it. A recent prospective study found that anxiety was a significant risk factor for the onset of type 2 diabetes independent of lifestyle factors and indicators of the metabolic syndrome (15). Of course, anxiety can have negative effects on regimen adherence and glycemic control. Panic episodes, in particular, have been associated with higher A1C values, more diabetic complications, and higher levels of disability and dysfunction (16).

Diagnostically, anxiety disorders encompass generalized anxiety disorder, panic disorder, obsessive-compulsive disorder, post-traumatic stress disorder,

Symptoms of Anxiety

Excessive worry associated with at least three of the following symptoms, with some symptoms present for more days than not in the past 6 months:
- Restless, keyed-up, on edge
- Easily fatigued
- Difficulty concentrating
- Irritability
- Muscle tension
- Sleep disturbance

and various phobias. In addition to depression, they are some of the most disabling psychiatric illnesses and often coexist with depression. These illnesses are notorious for their chronicity, negative impact on quality of life, and interference with receiving medical care. In a review of 18 studies, Grigsby et al. (17) reported that generalized anxiety disorder was present in 14% of patients with diabetes compared with 4% for the general population. Elevated anxiety levels were present in 40% of subjects, with no difference in prevalence between individuals with type 1 diabetes and those with type 2 diabetes. Women with diabetes were more likely to have higher levels of anxiety than men with diabetes.

Anxiety commonly focuses on fears of hyperglycemia and complications or fears of hypoglycemia and feeling out of control. Less frequently, there may be phobic avoidance of needles and fingersticks or compulsive monitoring of blood glucose levels. Ordinarily, chronic anxiety (commonly called stress) is created simply by the effects of diabetes on day-to-day life. The demands of self-care are complex, never-ending, and often frustrating. Patients can feel overwhelmed, guilty, angry, fearful, or unmotivated, particularly when blood glucose levels are high or unpredictable despite their best efforts.

PRACTICAL POINT

Anxiety about diabetes tends to peak at distinct periods of stress, which can include the initial crisis of diagnosis, the onset of major complications, and failure to achieve the desired therapeutic response. These crises give the nurse a unique opportunity to have an enormous impact on patients and their families, who are likely to be more receptive to outside support at these times.

The psychophysiological effects of stress on blood glucose levels have also been studied. Although most people with diabetes report that stress affects their blood glucose levels, the results of research have been inconsistent, with some studies reporting blood glucose responses (usually hyperglycemic) to stress and others have finding no response (18). Thus, while there is no conclusive evidence reporting the effects of stress on blood glucose, its potential as a factor influencing the achievement of self-care goals in diabetes should be considered in the treatment of diabetes patients.

Diabetes is a disease that affects the family, and the behavior of the family can have an effect on the person with diabetes. Family members may add stress by being overprotective, accusatory, unrealistic, or uninvolved with diabetes care. The person with diabetes may complicate these family dynamics by rejecting family support or becoming overly dependent, leaving family members feeling frustrated and worried. Once again, the nurse plays a crucial role in helping families find effective ways to communicate about diabetes management.

TREATMENT RECOMMENDATIONS

Psychopharmacological treatments for anxiety, including the SSRIs, appear to be effective for patients with diabetes, although they have not been closely studied with either type of diabetes. Likewise, while there has been limited formal research done on other forms of psychotherapeutic intervention and diabetes per se, it is reasonable to assume that other accepted forms of psychotherapy would be equally effective in diabetes (19). A recent systematic review by Fisher et al. (20) found that a wide range of interventions improved quality of life and healthy coping skills, including cognitive-behavioral, cognitive-analytic, family systems, and multisystemic therapies, as well as support groups and problem-solving interventions. Stress-management training holds promise as a cost-effective treatment for improving glycemic control (21). Cognitive behavioral treatments are being used successfully with a range of anxiety disorders. In general, this approach identifies maladaptive thought patterns and troublesome behaviors and instructs patients in developing more adaptive substitute thoughts and behaviors. Relaxation training and hypnotic suggestion have potential for individuals suffering from needle phobias. (See chapter 21 for more on helping the patient deal with his or her diabetes.)

EATING DISORDERS AND DIABETES

Despite the promise of risk reduction for the long-term complications of type 1 diabetes, one negative side effect of intensive diabetes management is weight gain. For example, during the first 6 years of follow-up in the DCCT, the patients in the intensively treated group gained an average of 10.45 lb more than patients in the standard treatment cohort (22). The most recent follow-up of these patients, 9 years after the completion of the DCCT, indicated that once patients on intensive treatment gained weight, this weight was difficult to lose (23). A survey of patients' responses to the recommendations of the DCCT documented that women with type 1 diabetes were especially concerned about tight glucose control causing weight gain (24,25). Researchers and

> **PRACTICAL POINT**
>
> Researchers estimate that 10–20% of girls in their midteen years and 30–40% of late teenaged girls and young adult women skip or alter their insulin doses to control their weight (see "Diabetes and Eating Disorders" in RESOURCES).

Symptoms of Anorexia

- Refusal to maintain normal body weight
- Intense fear of becoming fat, even though underweight
- Disturbance in the way weight or shape is experienced
- Absence of at least three consecutive menstrual cycles

clinicians have argued that the attention to food portions, blood glucose levels, and risk of weight gain associated with intensive diabetes management parallels the rigid thinking about food and body image characteristic of women with eating disorders and may place women with diabetes at heightened risk of developing eating disorders. Women with type 1 diabetes may use insulin manipulation (i.e., administering reduced insulin doses or omitting necessary doses altogether) as a means of caloric purging. Intentionally induced glycosuria is a powerful weight loss behavior and a symptom of eating disorders unique to people with type 1 diabetes. This behavior is more common in women but can also occur in men, especially during adolescence (see also "Diabetes and Eating Disorders," a patient handout in RESOURCES).

The most recent controlled studies suggest an increased risk of eating disorders among female patients with type 1 diabetes. Jones et al. (26) report that young women with type 1 diabetes have 2.4 times the risk of developing an eating disorder and 1.9 times the risk for subclinical eating disorders (i.e., when symptoms of disordered eating do not meet the level of severity to warrant a formal diagnosis) of age-matched women without diabetes (26). Intermittent insulin omission and reduction for weight loss purposes has been found to be a common practice among women with type 1 diabetes. For example, in women and girls with type 1 diabetes between the ages of 13 and 60 years, Polonsky et al. (27) found that 31% reported intentional insulin omission. Rates of omission peaked in late adolescence and early adulthood, with 40% of women and girls between the ages of 15 and 30 years reporting intentional omission. A recent report by Peveler et al. (28) indicates that eating problems continue to increase past age 30. Additionally, studies show that this behavior, even at a subclinical level of severity, places women at heightened risk for the medical complications of diabetes. Women reporting intentional insulin misuse had higher A1C levels, higher rates of hospital and emergency room visits, and higher rates of neuropathy and retinopathy than women who did not

Symptoms of Bulimia

- Recurrent episodes of binge eating
- Recurrent inappropriate compensatory behavior to prevent weight gain
- Binge eating or compensatory behaviors occur at least twice per week for 3 months
- Self-evaluation is unduly influenced by body shape and weight

report insulin omission (27). In a longitudinal study, Rydall et al. (29) reported that after 4 years of eating disordered behavior, 86% of patients classified as highly eating disordered had retinopathy, compared with 43% and 24% of women with moderate or no reported eating disturbance, respectively. Women with diabetes and eating disorders are in poorer glycemic control, with A1C levels approximately two or more percentage points higher than those of similarly aged women without eating disorders (29). The chronic hyperglycemia found in women with diabetes who intentionally omit or reduce their insulin doses places these women at much greater risk for frequent episodes of diabetic ketoacidosis and the long-term onset of macro- and microvascular complications of diabetes (30).

Disordered eating behaviors are often well hidden, and because these patients may not use other means of purging (such as self-induced vomiting or laxative abuse), their eating disorders may go undiagnosed. Once established as a long-standing behavior pattern, the problem of frequent insulin omission may be particularly difficult to treat. For this reason, early detection and intervention appears to be crucial. Questions such as "Do you take less insulin than you should?" (30) or "Do you ever change your insulin dose or skip insulin doses to influence your weight?" or "Tell me about your weight issues and how you feel insulin affects them" can be helpful in screening for insulin omission, especially when patients present with persistently elevated A1C levels or unexplained diabetic ketoacidosis.

Because obesity is a significant risk factor in type 2 diabetes, recurrent binge eating may increase the chances of developing this form of diabetes. Research indicates that among obese adults, there is a distinct subgroup (20–46%) who report engaging in recurrent binge eating, defined as consumption of a large amount of food while feeling out of control of the behavior (31).

The literature on binge eating in type 2 diabetes is still in its infancy, with initial studies relying on small, nonrepresentative samples. Kenardy et al. (32) found that 14% of the patients with newly diagnosed type 2 diabetes experienced problems with binge eating, compared with 4% of the age-, sex-, and weight-matched control subjects. A newer study examined prevalence rates of binge eating disorder (BED) and night eating syndrome (NES) among a subset of the large group of Look AHEAD participants (33). This study reports lower rates of both BED (1.4%) and NES (3.8%) than previously reported, which the authors attribute to the older age range of their study cohort. Participants with BED were younger than participants without eating disorders and reported that their weight problems began earlier in life. Based on this report, it may be that recurrent binge eating is a risk factor for developing type 2 diabetes earlier in life.

TREATMENT RECOMMENDATIONS

A multidisciplinary team approach is considered the optimal treatment for both eating disorders and diabetes. When designed to treat a patient with both diabetes and an eating disorder, such a team should include an endocrinologist/diabetologist, nurse educator, nutritionist with eating disorder and/or diabetes training, and psychologist or social worker to provide weekly individual therapy. Depending on the level of comorbid depression and anxiety and the frequency of binge eating, a psychiatrist may also be needed for psychopharmacological

Helpful questions to ask:
- Do you feel sad or blue?
- What part of diabetes management is the hardest for you?
- What aspects of diabetes do you worry about most?
- Do you ever change your insulin dose or skip insulin doses to influence your weight?

For more on eating disorders, review the Spring 2002 (volume 15) issue of *Diabetes Spectrum* (available from http://spectrum.diabetesjournals.org).

evaluation and treatment. At this time, little research has examined treatment efficacy for eating disorders in the context of diabetes; however, a large volume of research on treatment outcomes in bulimia nervosa supports the use of cognitive behavioral therapy in combination with antidepressant medications as the most effective treatment (34). These approaches would need to be adapted slightly in order to directly address the role of insulin omission as the means of caloric purging.

Weekly psychotherapy is strongly recommended. Early in the treatment, monthly appointments with the endocrinologist, nurse educator, and nutritionist may be necessary to maintain medical stability. Laboratory tests (especially A1C and electrolytes) and weigh-ins should occur at each of the medical appointments. Some patients may require a medical or psychiatric inpatient hospitalization until they are medically stable and emotionally ready to engage in treatment as outpatients.

With regard to diabetes management, the treatment team must be willing to set incremental goals that the patient feels ready to achieve. Early in treatment, intensive glycemic management of diabetes is not an appropriate target for a person with diabetes and an eating disorder. The first goal must be to establish medical safety for the patient. Gradually, the team can build toward increased doses of insulin, increases in food intake, greater flexibility in meal plans, regularity of eating routines, and more frequent blood glucose monitoring.

Additionally, newer insulin analogs show some evidence of improved weight profiles. Research is needed to develop additional insulin analogs that do not promote weight gain. As newer agents come to market and as more research is done to understand their impact, we will learn more about how to use these tools to optimize treatment. Matching patients with appropriate tools will remain challenging as many of these newer agents have the same potential for misuse as older insulin analogs (35).

SUMMARY

Nursing takes a holistic approach to chronic care, seeing the physical, emotional, and spiritual issues that contribute to the health problems of an individual. Many times, a patient will see the nurse as the safest person to talk with to share feelings of anger, depression, or anxiety. The role of the nurse can be pivotal in helping patients to seek treatment (medication and/or counseling) to address these mental health problems.

When psychiatric problems are suspected by the nurse, it can be helpful to remind the patient, the family, and the treatment team that diabetes management is burdensome and requires support. This support can come from family members, friends, coworkers, and a multidisciplinary diabetes treatment team. Both the patient and treatment team must be encouraged to work collaboratively to set small, attainable diabetes treatment goals that can increase in complexity over time. Because of the interplay of psychological factors and diabetes control, it is crucial to include mental health treatment in the multidisciplinary treatment approach, especially when adherence problems arise.

REFERENCES

1. Diabetes Control and Complications Trial Research Group: The effect of intensive treatment of diabetes on the development and progression of long-term complications in insulin-dependent diabetes mellitus. *N Engl J Med* 329:977–986, 1993

2. Krentz AJ: UKPDS and beyond: into the next millennium: United Kingdom Prospective Diabetes Study. *Diabetes Obes Metab* 1:13–22, 1999

3. Barnard KD, Skinner TC, Peveler R: The prevalence of co-morbid depression in adults with type 1 diabetes: systematic literature review. *Diabet Med* 23:445–448, 2006

4. Ali S, Stone MA, Peters JL, Davies MJ, Khunti K: The prevalence of co-morbid depression in adults with type 2 diabetes: a systematic review and meta-analysis. *Diabet Med* 23:1165–1173, 2006

5. de Groot M, Anderson R, Freedland KE, Clouse RE, Lustman PJ: Association of depression and diabetes complications: a meta-analysis. *Psychosom Med* 63:619–630, 2001

6. Jacobson AM, Samson JA, Weinger K, Ryan CM: Diabetes, the brain, and behavior: is there a biological mechanism underlying the association between diabetes and depression? *Int Rev Neurobiol* 51:455–479, 2002

7. Lustman PJ, Anderson RJ, Freedland KE, de Groot M, Carney RM, Clouse RE: Depression and poor glycemic control: a meta-analytic review of the literature. *Diabetes Care* 23:934–942, 2000

8. Knol MJ, Twisk JW, Beekman AT, Heine RJ, Snoek FJ, Pouwer F: Depression as a risk factor for the onset of type 2 diabetes mellitus: meta-analysis. *Diabetologia* 49:837–845, 2006

9. Pirraglia PA, Gupta S: The interaction of depression and diabetes: a review. *Curr Diabetes Rev* 3:249–251, 2007

10. Egede LE: Effect of depression on self-management behaviors and health outcomes in adults with type 2 diabetes. *Curr Diabetes Rev* 1:235–243, 2005

11. Weinger K, Jacobson AM, Musen G, Lyoo IK, Ryan CM, et al.: The effects of type 1 diabetes on cerebral white matter. *Diabetologia* 51:1554–1555, 2008

12. Musen G, Lyoo IK, Sparks CR, Weinger K, Hwang J, et al.: Effects of type 1 diabetes on gray matter density as measured by voxel-based morphometry. *Diabetes* 55:326–333, 2006

13. Musen G, Simonson DC, Bolo NR, Driscoll A, Weinger K, et al.: Regional brain activation during hypoglycemia in type 1 diabetes. *J Clin Endocrinol Metab* 93:1450–1457, 2008

14. Lustman PJ, Griffith LS, Freedland KE, Kissel SS, Clouse RE: Cognitive behavior therapy for depression in type 2 diabetes mellitus: a randomized, controlled trial. *Ann Intern Med* 129:613–621, 1998

15. Engum A: The role of depression and anxiety in the onset of diabetes in a large population-based study. *J Psychosom Res* 62:31–38, 2007

16. Ludman E, Katon W, Russo J, Simon G, Von Korff M, et al.: Panic episodes among patients with diabetes. *Gen Hosp Psychiatry* 28:475–481, 2006

17. Grigsby AB, Anderson RJ, Freedland KE, Clouse RE, Lustman PJ: Prevalence of anxiety in adults with diabetes: a systematic review. *J Psychosom Res* 53:1053–1060, 2002

18. Rubin RR, Peyrot M: Psychological issues and treatments for people with diabetes. *J Clin Psychol* 57:457–478, 2001

19. Anderson BJ, Rubin RR (Eds.): *Practical Psychology for Diabetes Clinicians.* 2nd ed. Alexandria, VA, American Diabetes Association, 2002

20. Fisher EB, Thorpe CT, Devellis BM, Devellis RF: Healthy coping, negative emotions, and diabetes management: a systematic review and appraisal. *Diabetes Educ* 33:1104–1106, 2007

21. Surwit RS, Bauman A: *The Mind-Body Diabetes Revolution: A Proven New Program for Better Blood Sugar Control.* New York, Free Press, 2004

22. Diabetes Control and Complications Trial Research Group: Weight gain associated with intensive therapy in the Diabetes Control and Complications Trial. *Diabetes Care* 11:567–573, 1988

23. Diabetes Control and Complications Trial Research Group: Influence of intensive diabetes treatment on body weight and composition of adults with type 1 diabetes in the Diabetes Control and Complications Trial. *Diabetes Care* 24:1711–1721, 2001

24. Thompson CJ, Cummings JF, Chalmers J, Gould C, Newton RW: How have patients reacted to the implications of the DCCT? *Diabetes Care* 19:876–879, 1996

25. Jones J, Colton P: Prevalence of eating disorders in girls with type 1 diabetes. *Diabetes Spectrum* 15:86–89, 2002

26. Jones JM, Lawson ML, Daneman D, Olmsted MP, Rodin G: Eating disorders in adolescent females with and without type 1 diabetes: cross sectional study. *BMJ* 320:1563–1566, 2000

27. Polonsky WH, Anderson BJ, Lohrer PA, Aponte JE, Jacobson AM, Cole CF: Insulin omission in women with IDDM. *Diabetes Care* 17:1178–1185, 1994

28. Peveler RC, Bryden KS, Neil HAW, Fairburn CG, Mayou RA, et al.: The relationship of disordered eating habits and attitudes to clinical outcomes in young adult females with type 1 diabetes. *Diabetes Care* 28:84–88, 2005

29. Rydall AC, Rodin GM, Olmsted MP, Devenyi RG, Daneman D: Disordered eating behavior and microvascular complications in young women with insulin-dependent diabetes mellitus. *N Engl J Med* 336:1849–1854, 1997

30. Goebel-Fabbri AE, Fikkan J, Franko DL, Pearson K, Anderson BJ, Weinger K: Insulin restriction and associated morbidity and mortality in women with type 1 diabetes. *Diabetes Care* 31:415–419, 2008

31. de Zwaan M, Mitchell JE, Seim HC, Specker SM, Pyle RL, et al.: Eating related and general psychopathology in obese females with binge eating disorder. *Int J Eat Disord* 15:43–52, 1994

32. Kenardy J, Mensch M, Bowen K, Pearson SA: A comparison of eating behaviors in newly diagnosed NIDDM patients and case-matched control subjects. *Diabetes Care* 17:1197–1199, 1994

33. Allison KC, Crow SJ, Reeves RR, Smith West D, Foreyt JP, et al.: Binge eating disorder and night eating syndrome in adults with type 2 diabetes. *Obesity* 15:1287–1293, 2007

34. Peterson CB, Mitchell JE: Psychosocial and pharmacological treatment of eating disorders: a review of research findings. *J Clin Psychol* 55:685–697, 1999

35. Goebel-Fabbri AE: Diabetes and eating disorders. *J Diabetes Sci Tech* 2:530–532, 2008

Dr. Goebel-Fabbri is a Psychologist at Joslin Diabetes Center, Boston, MA, and an Instructor in Psychiatry at Harvard Medical School, Boston, MA. Mr. Zrebiec is Associate Director, Behavioral and Mental Health Unit, at Joslin Diabetes Center, Boston, MA, and a Lecturer in Psychiatry at Harvard Medical School, Boston, MA.

23. Polypharmacy

Barbara Kocurek, PharmD, BCPS, CDE

Many patients with diabetes will be on multiple medications and have "polypharmacy." This is because medications are considered the standard of care for diabetes and its related complications (Table 23.1) (1–3). A recently published editorial suggested that it may even be time for a polypill of aspirin and a statin because of their benefits in both the primary and secondary prevention of coronary artery disease in patients with diabetes (4). Since the use of multiple medications is usually required in patients with diabetes, the goal is for patients to use the most appropriate medication regimen to improve their health and quality of life with minimal adverse events. Inappropriate medication regimens can and often do result in adverse events, such as drug reactions, drug-drug interactions, decreased adherence to medications, and increased medical costs (5).

POTENTIAL ADVERSE EFFECTS OF POLYPHARMACY

In 2000, the cost of drug-related morbidity and mortality was estimated to exceed $177.4 billion, with hospital admissions accounting for nearly 70% ($121.5 billion) of total costs, followed by long-term-care admissions, which accounted for 18% ($32.8 billion) (6). Drug-related problems can include side effects, adverse drug reactions, and drug interactions. The risk of an adverse drug event has been estimated to be 13% for two drugs, 58% for five drugs, and 82% for seven or more (1). Evaluating a patient's medication regimen for drug interactions (this includes prescription medications, over-the-counter medications and alternative

Table 23.1 Drug Therapy for the Prevention and Management of Diabetes and Its Complications

- Hyperglycemia (oral and injectable antihyperglycemic medications or combination of both)
- Cardiovascular disease
  - Hypertension (blood pressure medications, often two or more are needed)
  - Dyslipidemia (statins and other lipid-lowering agents)
  - Coronary heart disease (antiplatelet, ACE inhibitor, and statin therapy recommended)
- Nephropathy (ACE inhibitors or ARBs)
- Neuropathy (tricyclic drugs, anticonvulsants, and other agents often needed)
- Smoking cessation (smoking cessation products)

From the American Diabetes Association (3).

therapies) requires time and knowledge of medications. Resources for medication information include:

- Pharmacists (many large hospitals and schools of pharmacy have drug information centers)
- Package inserts (which can usually be located on the manufacturer's website)
- Drugs@FDA (http://www.accessdata.fda.gov/scripts/cder/drugsatfda/index.cfm; a site providing therapeutic equivalents, approval history, labeling information, and consumer information)
- Drug Interaction Checker (available at www.drugs.com)

EFFECTS OF MEDICATIONS ON DIABETES CONTROL

Some medications can affect glucose levels themselves. Glucocorticoids, for example, commonly cause an increase in blood glucose levels (see chapter 28 for a discussion of the impact of glucocorticoid use on glucose levels and management issues). Other medications that are known to raise blood glucose levels are thiazide diuretics, phenytoin (Dilantin), estrogen compounds, and atypical antipsychotics (e.g., clozapine, olanzapine, risperidone) (7). Individuals should be counseled to monitor their blood glucose levels when initiating these medications. If the patient is taking atypical antipsychotics, he or she should routinely be monitored for the development of hyperglycemia (8). Some medications may decrease blood glucose levels, including some antibiotics (e.g., Levaquin, Biaxin) and large doses of salicylates. It is prudent to counsel patients to frequently monitor blood glucose levels when treating any infection with an antibiotic (7).

> **PRACTICAL POINT**
>
> The use of multiple medications (polypharmacy) is often required and beneficial in helping patients with diabetes achieve optimal blood glucose, blood pressure, and lipid control and manage other diabetes-related complications and comorbidities.

Some commonly used prescription and over-the-counter medications can raise blood pressure and/or interfere with the effectiveness of blood pressure medications (9). These include:

- glucocorticoids
- nonsteroidal anti-inflammatory drugs (NSAIDs), such as ibuprofen
- nasal decongestants and other cold remedies
- diet pills
- cyclosporine
- erythropoietin
- tricyclic antidepressants
- monoamine oxidase inhibitors
- oral contraceptives

If these medications are used, the patient's blood pressure should be monitored more frequently. If the medication causes an increase in blood pressure, this should be communicated to the physician.

EFFECTS OF POLYPHARMACY ON ADHERENCE

For a medication to work, it needs to be taken. Unfortunately, accurate measurement of medication adherence is difficult, and currently there is no generally accepted "Gold Standard" for measuring adherence (10). Self-reporting of medication adherence is often used; however, it tends to be overestimated, making it difficult for the patient and health care professional to effectively and safely manage diabetes and its comorbidities. A recent systematic review on medication taking and diabetes reported adherence rates to diabetes medications varied from 31 to 87% in retrospective studies and from 53 to 98% in prospective studies (11). Despite the known issues with adherence, there is little data on specific interventions to improve adherence rates to medications (11).

> **PRACTICAL POINT**
>
> Patients should be asked about medication-related side effects or adverse effects at every encounter. If a patient is experiencing an adverse reaction that necessitates a change in medication, this should be discussed with the patient's physician. Serious adverse drug reactions should be reported to MedWatch, the FDA Safety Information and Adverse Events Reporting Program (www.fda.gov/medwatch).

As with other health care behaviors, there are barriers to taking medications. Common reasons patients give for not taking medications as directed include unacceptable side effects, lack of perceived effectiveness, and cost of the medications. In addition, cultural groups may have differing beliefs regarding the use of medications or certain herbs or have incorrect perceptions about what different medications can do. Patients may not understand the chronic nature of diabetes and may see the medication as a temporary measure. Or patients may discontinue medications once they have achieved blood pressure or cholesterol level goals. Patients may also add cultural or folk

Common Factors Affecting Medication Adherence (11,13)
- Regimen complexity
- Dosing frequency greater than twice a day
- Remembering doses and refills
- Depression
- Adverse effects or fear of them
- Lack of belief that the medication will help

remedies that may interact or cause side effects when combined with prescription medications. Patients may seek care from nontraditional sources that prohibit the use of allopathic medications and may resist adding medications to the treatment. Financial barriers may be more important for some groups than for others (12).

STEPS TO ENSURE APPROPRIATE MEDICATION USE IN PATIENTS WITH DIABETES

Nurses are in a position to help ensure appropriate medication use and can do the following to decrease the risks associated with drug use:

1. Review the patient's medication regimen to identify potential problems, if appropriate. Consider the following [adapted from Good (2)]:
   - Can nonpharmacological measures be used to treat the medical condition?
   - Is the medication list complete? Does it include all prescription medications, over-the-counter drugs, herbal products, and vitamin and mineral supplements?
   - Are the medications prescribed by different providers? Filled at different pharmacies? If so, is there clear communication among providers and pharmacies?
   - Are there any duplicate medications (brand/generic or drugs from the same drug class)?
   - Is their an indication for each medication?
   - Is the medication having a positive therapeutic response?
   - Is there a way to simplify the regimen (e.g., use a combination pill)?
   - Is a medication being used to treat symptoms that are related to an adverse drug reaction?
2. If possible, discuss the medication regimen with the patient at every visit. Assess adherence and any barriers the patient may be experiencing. Discuss ways the patient can address barriers. This will be easier if open-ended questions are used, such as:
   - How do you manage to take your medications on a consistent basis?
   - What gets in the way of taking your medications?
   - What do you do when you miss a dose?
3. Suggest pillboxes, calendars, watch alarms, or some other system that will help patients remember when to take their medications if needed.
4. Encourage patients to keep an up-to-date list of all their medications, including vitamins, over the counter medications, and herbal products. Patients can often obtain a list of their prescription medications from their pharmacy and develop a complete list from there.

Resources for Safe Medication Use

- Check Your Medicines: Tips for Taking Medicines Safely
  (http://www.ahrq.gov/consumer/checkmeds.htm)
- Be An Active Member of Your Health Care Team
  (www.fda.gov/cder/consumerinfo/)
- Medication Use Safety Training for Seniors
  (www.mustforseniors.org)

5. Include the purpose for each medication on the directions for use if you are a prescriber. For example, "Take one tablet two times a day with breakfast and dinner for diabetes."
6. Encourage patients to use just one pharmacy to get their prescriptions, vitamins, and over-the-counter medications filled. This can help decrease the potential for drug-drug interactions, and the pharmacist is one of the best sources of information for over-the-counter medications.
7. Encourage patients to discuss their medications with their health care providers. There are several medication-related handouts and websites that can be given to patients to encourage them to be active members of their health care teams.
8. Communicate any potentially drug-related problems to the patient's health care provider.

SUMMARY

The use of multiple medications has become the standard of care for diabetes. Nurses are in a key position to promote improved medication adherence by assessing for potential barriers and assisting the patient in implementing strategies to overcome these barriers. Nurses need to be knowledgeable about medications, both prescription and over-the-counter, as well as nutritional supplements, herbal products, and other complementary therapies to assist the patient in understanding the purpose, benefits, and potential risks of the medications. Because of the increasing number of medications available, it is imperative that the nurse have a good resource for drug information.

REFERENCES

1. Fulton MM, Allen ER: Polypharmacy in the elderly: a literature review. *J Am Acad Nurse Pract* 17:123–131, 2005

2. Good CB: Polypharmacy in elderly patients with diabetes. *Diabetes Spectrum* 15:240–248, 2002

3. American Diabetes Association: Standards of medical care in diabetes—2009 (Position Statement). *Diabetes Care* 32:S13–S61, 2009

4. Wienbergen H, Senges JS, Gitt AK: Should we prescribe statin and aspirin for every diabetic patient? *Diabetes Care* 31 (Suppl. 2):S222–S225, 2008

5. Austin RP: Polypharmacy as a risk factor in the treatment of type 2 diabetes. *Diabetes Spectrum* 19:13–16, 2006

6. Ernst FR, Grizzle JA: Drug-related morbidity and mortality: updating the cost-of-illness model. *J Am Pharm Assoc* 41:192–199, 2001

7. Harmel AP, Mathur R: *Davidson's Diabetes Mellitus: Diagnosis and Treatment.* 5th ed. Philadelphia, W. B. Saunders, 2004

8. American Diabetes Association, American Psychiatric Association, American Association of Clinical Endocrinologists, North American Association for the Study of Obesity: Consensus development conference on antipsychotic drugs and obesity and diabetes. *Diabetes Care* 27:596–601, 2004

9. American Heart Association: Your High Blood Pressure Questions Answered— Over-the-Counter Drugs [Internet], 2008. Available from www.americanheart. org. Accessed 17 February 2009

10. Vik, SA, CJ Maxwell, DB Hogan: Measurement, correlates, and health outcomes of medication adherence among seniors. *Ann Pharmacother* 38:303–312, 2004

11. Odegard PS, Capoccia K: Medication taking and diabetes: a systematic review of the literature. *Diabetes Educ* 33:1014–1029, 2007

12. Tseng CW, Tierney EF, Gerzoff RB, Dudley RA, Waitzfelder B, et al.: Race/ ethnicity and economic differences in cost-related medication underuse among insured adults with diabetes: the Translating Research Into Action for Diabetes Study. *Diabetes Care* 31:261–266, 2008

13. Grant RW, Devita NG, Singer DE, Meigs JB: Polypharmacy and medication adherence in patients with type 2 diabetes. *Diabetes Care* 26:1408–1412, 2003

Dr. Kocurek is the Diabetes Education Coordinator at Baylor Health Care Diabetes Services, Irving, TX.

24. Continuous Subcutaneous Insulin Infusion (Insulin Pump Therapy)

Donna Tomky, MSN, RN, C-ANP, CDE

In search of optimal insulin delivery, technological advances have led to the development of small portable devices that mimic physiological insulin replacement. An insulin pump is an alternative to multiple daily insulin injections that allows for intensive insulin therapy when used in conjunction with blood glucose monitoring and carbohydrate counting or a similar approach of matching food and insulin. These portable devices continuously infuse insulin under the subcutaneous tissue through a pumping mechanism. Continuous subcutaneous insulin infusion (CSII) via an insulin pump has allowed people with diabetes to attain improved blood glucose control. Attaining and maintaining blood glucose control on a sustained basis requires habitual and frequent monitoring of blood glucose levels by the pump wearer because these devices do not continuously monitor blood glucose. CSII therapy gives people with diabetes the ability to make sensible alterations to their insulin regimen to attain targeted blood glucose levels. Successful CSII therapy requires appropriate candidate selection, intense diabetes education, skill building, and training by a knowledgeable diabetes care team that results in consistent attention to details and competent self-care behaviors. This chapter discusses essential elements that all nurses need to consider in delivering safe and effective care to patients who use or are considering using an insulin pump.

THE TECHNOLOGY

An insulin pump is a small battery-operated mechanical device containing a reservoir or syringe of fast- or rapid-acting insulin. The reservoir is attached to plastic tubing called an infusion set. At the end of the infusion set is a detachable

25- or 27-gauge needle or soft plastic catheter. The catheter (with needle) is inserted into the subcutaneous tissue and stays in place with adhesive tape or a Bioclusive dressing. The pump wearer changes the infusion site every 24–72 h using an aseptic technique. When insulin pumps became available for clinical use in the early 1980s, they weighed slightly less than 1 lb, with simple delivery of basal and bolus insulin. Current models weigh as little as 3 oz and can be worn discreetly under clothing or on a belt like a pager or cell phone. The newer models contain miniature computers that provide an array of basal and bolus functions.

Some pumps link to a PDA (personal digit assistant) for calculating insulin doses, while others link to a continuous glucose monitoring (CGM) sensor or a glucose meter. Sensors are inserted into subcutaneous tissue and read glucose levels in the interstitial fluid. The electron activity is converted to a number that corresponds to a glucose value. This is transmitted to a "receiver." The MiniMed 722 pump (Medtronic) can act as the receiver so the continuous glucose level appears on the screen of the insulin pump. There are other sensor models (DexCom and Navigator) that are not associated with an insulin pump at this time but have the same sensor-and-receiver concept.

Advanced features in the pump can calculate insulin-correction factors, deduct active insulin on board, and recommend fractionated, specific insulin doses to be delivered. This level of sophistication in glucose analysis and insulin delivery make the "closed-loop" system seem very close to reality. The insulin pump has safety features that require manual initiation of the bolus of insulin if the individual agrees with the data calculations from the pump program.

At this time, CGM is primarily prescribed for patients with type 1 diabetes who are having issues with hypoglycemia. Insurance reimbursement is limited. Many individuals are choosing to purchase CGM systems out of pocket and may use the sensor technology intermittently, e.g., wearing it one week out of a month.

Every year the American Diabetes Association's magazine, *Diabetes Forecast*, publishes a resource guide in which all the current technologies are listed. This would be an excellent resource for anyone interested in reviewing the features of all the technologies. The *Diabetes Forecast Resource Guide* is available online at http://www.diabetes.org/diabetes-forecast/resource-guide.jsp.

Pump therapy and the use of a CGM sensor require a professional staff knowledgeable about the unique and special requirements of diabetes patients who wear pumps and sensors. Ideally, CSII therapy should be prescribed, implemented, and followed by a skilled professional team familiar with CSII therapy and capable of supporting the patient (1). Pump therapy is considered a subspecialty in the milieu of diabetes care. Typically, the pump therapy team consists of at least an endocrinologist (or physician with diabetes expertise), a nurse, and a dietitian familiar with CSII therapy. Before initiating pump therapy, potential pump candidates must have basic and advanced knowledge and skills regarding intensive insulin therapy. They must also demonstrate safe and consistent behavior in the regular tasks of diabetes self-management, including frequent blood glucose monitoring, injection of insulin, carbohydrate counting, problem solving for high and low blood glucose levels, and sick-day management.

PRINCIPLES OF PUMP THERAPY

CSII therapy is the modality that most closely duplicates the fully functioning pancreas. The Diabetes Control and Complications Trial conclusively demonstrated the beneficial effects and impact of optimal glycemic control (2). Insulin is needed for using food to fuel the body and for storing energy for future needs. During the fasting state, insulin is released at a slow and steady rate (basal), with larger amounts (bolus) released during the fed state (Fig. 24.1). Only rapid- or fast-acting insulin (insulins aspart, glulisine, or lispro or regular insulin) is used in the pump. Intermediate- and long-acting insulins are never used. Insulin is delivered by either the basal rate or a bolus.

The benefits of CSII therapy are derived from the pharmacological advantage of using rapid-acting insulin that is delivered as a continuous infusion with incremental bolus administration at meals. Rapid-acting insulin is associated with the least amount of variation in day-to-day absorption. Bolus insulin activated by the wearer is given in anticipation of food or to correct an elevated blood glucose level. Meals can be skipped, delayed, or altered without loss of glycemic control. Bolus insulin activated by the pump user is given just before eating food or as needed to correct high blood glucose levels (Fig. 24.2). The bolus can be given all at once to cover carbohydrate intake or over time to mimic the insulin release for a more slowly digested meal. Most pumps are equipped with internal calculators to recommend a corrective or carbohydrate (food) coverage dose of insulin based on predetermined insulin sensitivity and insulin-to-carbohydrate ratios of the pump wearer.

Basal insulin, or metabolic/background insulin, supplies the body's continuous fasting or basic insulin needs. The basal delivery mode is preprogrammed with a continuous infusion of insulin for 24 h/day. Usually, the basal rate approximates

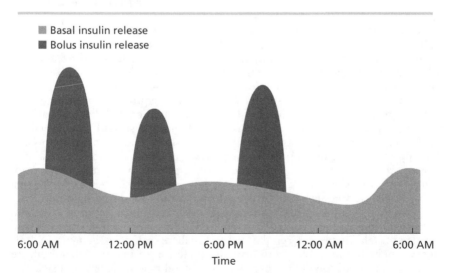

■ Basal insulin release
■ Bolus insulin release

6:00 AM   12:00 PM   6:00 PM   12:00 AM   6:00 AM

Time

Figure 24.1 Normal insulin secretion in nondiabetic individuals.

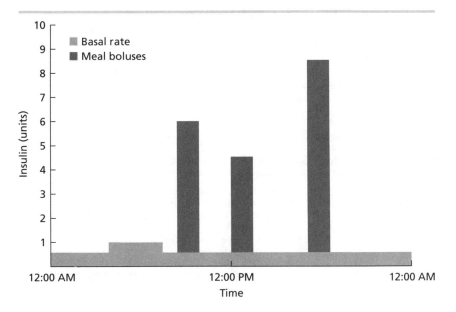

Figure 24.2 Pump insulin delivery.

50% of the total daily insulin needs. If basal rates are set appropriately, the pump wearer can fast and does not need to eat to maintain fairly level blood glucose values. The basal rate is prescribed by the pump therapy team and can be set or changed by the pump wearer. Basal infusion can be programmed to coincide with the diurnal variation of insulin sensitivity and the requirements at different times of day. Programmed basal rates can vary throughout the day and are usually determined after wearing the pump for a few days. Temporary basal rate adjustments can be made during exercise, after exercise, during stress, or during illness, when lower or higher insulin requirements may exist. Often pumps are equipped to allow multiple basal rate patterns to accommodate change in the pump wearer's routine, e.g., a profile for usual work days versus weekend activities.

WHO IS A PUMP CANDIDATE?

Successful CSII therapy depends in part on appropriate candidate selection and preparation for initiating pump therapy. It is generally accepted that highly motivated patients who use insulin and have well-established diabetes self-care behaviors, including problem-solving skills and frequent self-monitoring of blood glucose, are most successful at insulin pump therapy. Some pump therapy teams believe a structured screening protocol (with a trial pump that infuses saline) increases safety when initiating therapy in an outpatient setting and lowers discontinuation rates (3). A saline pump trial before initiating insulin pump therapy allows the candidate to understand the challenges of being continuously tethered to the pump before going forward with CSII. Many pump therapy teams would agree on the candidate selection criteria identified in Table 24.1 (3–5). (See also "Is an Insulin Pump Right for Your Child and Family?" a patient handout in RESOURCES.)

Most individuals using CSII have type 1 diabetes. Although less common, it can be used in individuals with insulin-treated type 2 diabetes. Criteria for coverage of CSII set forth by most health insurance plans require that the individual have type 1 diabetes or insulin-requiring type 2 diabetes. Medicare requires

Table 24.1 Candidate Selection Criteria for CSII

Medical/metabolic indications	■ Suboptimal glycemic control ■ Wide blood glucose excursions ■ Dawn phenomenon with elevated fasting blood glucose levels ■ Frequent severe hypoglycemia ■ Nocturnal hypoglycemia ■ Pregnant or planning conception ■ Inconsistent daily schedule not well managed with injections ■ Insulin sensitivity and requirement of low doses of insulin
Cognitive/psychomotor criteria	■ Has sound rationale for pursuing and realistic expectations of CSII therapy ■ Capacity to learn the technical and cognitive components of the pump ■ Has appropriate problem-solving skills for troubleshooting hyper- and hypoglycemic events and sick days ■ Able to match insulin with food using carbohydrate-counting skills ■ Adaptability of behavior or aspects of the regimen in response to outcome evaluation
Motivational ability	■ Perform frequent blood glucose monitoring as a lifetime behavior ■ Comply with recommendations for safe insulin pump use ■ Pay attention to details regarding the insulin regimen and the needed adjustments ■ Anticipate insulin needs as situations change
Technical/physical ability	■ Perform blood glucose monitoring accurately and frequently, up to 6–10 times daily ■ Perform the technical components of insulin pump use or have necessary support if visually impaired ■ Absence of serious disease that could impair technical performance
Financial resources	■ Can obtain adequate financial resources to cover the initial and ongoing costs of CSII therapy (approximately $6,400 for setup and $1,500–3,000 for yearly supplies)

Data are from Refs. 3–5, 13, and 14.

documentation of the pump candidate's type 1 status by requesting verification of low C-peptide levels or presence of glutamic acid decarboxylase (GAD_{65}) or insulin antibodies (6).

CSII therapy has not been fully evaluated in patients with type 2 diabetes. A limited number of clinical studies show that CSII therapy can safely improve glycemic control and β-cell function in a relatively short period. Pump therapy may be particularly useful in treating patients with type 2 diabetes who do not satisfactorily respond to intensive insulin treatment strategies (7). Usually, higher insulin doses are required for individuals with type 2 diabetes because both insulin deficiency and insulin resistance are common.

Characteristics of Pump Therapy in Type 2 Diabetes Compared with Type 1 Diabetes (7)

- Patients with type 2 diabetes usually need a higher basal rate.
- Meal-related boluses are larger in type 2 diabetes.
- The time between reservoir refills is shorter in type 2 diabetes.
- Battery life may be shorter in type 2 diabetes.
- Pump therapy may improve endogenous insulin secretion and resistance in type 2 diabetes.
- Patient acceptance and satisfaction are similar in type 2 diabetes.

Benefits of Pump Therapy

Research has shown that using pump therapy to maintain normal or near-normal blood glucose levels can improve health and reduce the long-term complications of diabetes (1).

- Improvement in blood glucose levels is possible with pumps.
  - Pumps do not use long-acting insulin, but instead use rapid- or short-acting insulin, which is more predictable and can be delivered more physiologically.
  - Pump wearers often experience fewer and less severe hypoglycemic events.
  - Insulin dosing can be precise, to within one-hundredth of a unit.
  - There is more predictable insulin absorption from a continuous insulin depot.
  - Dawn phenomenon effects are easier to manage with the basal rate and can be set to accommodate the rise in insulin requirements overnight.
  - Basal rates can be quickly changed to accommodate growth spurts in children or increased insulin needs during pregnancy.
- Improvement in the safety profile is possible.
  - Reducing the basal rate during periods of low physiological requirements can minimize nocturnal or daytime hypoglycemia.
  - Using a temporary basal rate that meets short-term physiological needs can accommodate the patient when sick.

Benefits of Pump Therapy *(Continued)*

- Improvement in lifestyle flexibility and patient satisfaction is possible.
  - Meals and food can be customized to fit the individual's schedule and preference in timing, size of meal, and type of food.
  - Carbohydrate counting using an insulin-to-carbohydrate ratio is one method of matching appropriate amounts of (bolus) insulin to the food consumed.
  - Weight loss may be more easily achieved in motivated patients, although initial improved glycemia may promote weight gain.
  - Pumps can deliver insulin to coincide with travel or work schedules.

PROBLEM SOLVING AND SAFETY CONCERNS IN CSII

HYPERGLYCEMIA

Because the insulin pump uses only short- or rapid-acting insulin, even a partial interruption of insulin flow can result in hyperglycemia in patients with severe or total endogenous insulin deficiency. Complete interruption can result in ketosis or ketoacidosis within a few short hours. High blood glucose can occur for various reasons, including infection, illness, stress, menstrual cycle, battery failure, infusion set or catheter occlusion, leaking connection, inadequate or missed meal

Limitations of Pump Therapy

- The risks or drawbacks of pump therapy must be fully understood by the wearer and the health care team.
  - Pumps are not for everyone, and patients must maintain a high degree of motivation before and throughout pump therapy.
  - Patients must be willing to maintain habitual and frequent self-monitoring of blood glucose.
  - The learning curve is steep, and some patients struggle with the concepts and problem-solving skills required for CSII.
  - Being connected to a pump is a visual reminder of having diabetes.
  - Technical or mechanical failure is possible with a pump and, if not corrected in a timely manner, can quickly lead to diabetic ketoacidosis in individuals with type 1 diabetes.
  - Skin irritations and infections are possible.
  - Weight gain is possible with improved glycemic control.
  - Some patient populations, such as children or the visually impaired, may require assistance from a caregiver.
- Many physicians and health care providers are unfamiliar with pump therapy and may not provide the necessary training and support.
- The cost of insulin pumps is usually over $5,000, and supplies (not including blood glucose monitoring items) cost $1,500–3,000 per year. Insurance companies typically cover only 80% of pump expenses, and coverage varies from state to state and plan to plan. Reimbursement for diabetes education to support the patient also varies (13).

Contraindications to Pump Therapy

- Some individuals have unrealistic expectations that pump therapy will cure their diabetes and automatically control it.
- Severe depression or other serious mental health disorders may distract patients from paying attention to details that are critical to successful pump therapy.
- A history of poor self-care behaviors and health care practices, such as failure to perform self-monitoring of blood glucose, keep appointments, weigh and estimate portions of food to appropriately match food with insulin, and apply problem-solving skills, will signal failure.
- Financial resources are needed for initiating and maintaining optimal pump therapy practices.

bolus, or poor absorption of insulin from the site. Immediate replacement of subcutaneous or intravenous insulin is required. Usually this is accomplished by injecting rapid-acting insulin to correct high blood glucose and restarting CSII therapy or long-acting basal insulin (glargine, detemir, or NPH).

HYPOGLYCEMIA

Hypoglycemia is the main side effect of insulin, regardless of delivery method. Insulin pump therapy does not seem to have a higher rate of hypoglycemia than

PRACTICAL POINT

Troubleshooting Hyperglycemia in Insulin Pump Therapy

- Red, tender, and swollen catheter site (The insulin is not being absorbed correctly and leads to high blood glucose levels, which indicates that the site needs to be changed.)
- Leakage, breakage, or kinking of tubing
- Battery failure
- Empty reservoir or cartridge
- Improper positioning of reservoir or piston rod
- Improper basal rate programming
- Air in tubing
- Illness
- Menstrual cycle fluctuations
- Omitted bolus or improper amount given
- Ineffective insulin (expired date, exposure to heat or cold)
- Crimped catheter or needle not penetrating skin
- Change in usual routine
- Suspect site not absorbing, if no other apparent reason for high blood glucose

CAUTION: Any of these can occur even if the infusion site/set was recently changed.

PRACTICAL POINT

When assessing a patient on pump therapy:
- Correct known problems immediately.
- Advise the patient to change infusion sites with each new reservoir or cartridge, infusion set, and catheter.
- Check blood glucose.
- Check urine for ketones.
- If ketotic, check serum for bicarbonate to determine the severity of diabetic ketoacidosis.
- If hyperglycemic, patient may need to take supplemental insulin with a conventional insulin syringe.
- Provide nursing support for symptoms of nausea, dehydration, or infection.

---

multiple daily injections. In fact, pump therapy has been shown to reduce severe hypoglycemia, particularly in children, because it pumps small amounts of insulin (8).

There is a danger of losing consciousness with severe hypoglycemia. Not everyone gets warning signs of low blood glucose (e.g., in hypoglycemia unawareness); therefore, reinforcing to pump wearers the importance of frequent blood glucose monitoring, especially before driving or when operating equipment, is essential. Testing blood glucose is the only dependable way to verify blood glucose levels at any time. Family members, friends, and coworkers, among others, need education and training on how to administer intramuscular glucagon in the event that the pump wearer experiences a severe hypoglycemic event.

CGM systems offer alarms warning individuals of low and high blood glucose levels with thresholds that are preprogrammed in the pump. Real-time sensing of interstitial fluid has a lag time of 5–15 min (9–11). The individual's ability to recognize symptoms and interstitial fluid lag time must be considered when setting pump alarms based on CGM data.

OTHER CONSIDERATIONS

Insulin dosages vary from person to person and can be significantly altered by changes in diet, physical activity, stress levels, and many other variables. Performing frequent blood glucose testing is necessary to safely use a pump. Blood glucose levels can be maintained near the normal range after individualized basal rates and bolus requirements have been determined based on blood glucose results. A basic rule is to always check blood glucose before dosing with an insulin bolus.

REIMBURSEMENT ISSUES

Most insurance plans provide reimbursement for insulin pump therapy because physicians prescribe pumps in response to specific clinical issues, e.g., the inability to safely achieve adequate blood glucose control, low glucose levels during sleep, work/shift schedules that require flexible insulin delivery.

Most health insurance plans follow the Centers for Medicare and Medicaid Services (CMS) guidelines for coverage of insulin pumps. These policies were updated in 2005. Medicare covers the costs of an external insulin infusion pump and related items for treating diabetes. Under this provision, patients must be *1)* insulinopenic as verified by fasting C-peptide testing or *2)* positive for β-cell autoantibodies. The requirement to meet these criteria is a fasting serum C-peptide level ≤110% of the lower limit of normal of the laboratory's measurement method. For patients with renal insufficiency and a creatinine clearance ≤50 ml/min, this level is ≤200% of the same limit. Additionally, fasting C-peptide measurements are valid only if a simultaneously obtained fasting blood glucose measurement is ≥225 mg/dl (6). Thus, if the normal range for C-peptide in a laboratory is 0.9–4.0 ng/ml, a C-peptide level of ≤0.99 ng/ml (i.e., 0.9 × 1.10) would qualify for coverage. If the patient has renal insufficiency and a qualifying creatinine clearance, the level would be ≤1.80 ng/ml (i.e., 0.9 × 2.00). For more information on the criteria, go to the CMS website at http://search.cms.hhs.gov and search on "insulin pump."

MANAGING CSII DURING TESTS, PROCEDURES, AND HOSPITALIZATIONS

The insulin pump may be continued in the hospital if the staff is competent in insulin pump therapy or the patient and family are able to safely operate the insulin pump. Local endocrinologists or diabetes educators are excellent resources to contact if questions or concerns arise about insulin pump therapy during the patient's hospitalization. The insulin pump should be discontinued during X-rays, MRIs, and other procedures that might affect a pump's reliability for insulin delivery. If a person is going to be off of the insulin pump for >1 h, compensatory insulin should be administered. For short surgical procedures, the pump can be left on, infusing at the basal rate. However, it is important during surgical procedures to place the pump catheter in subcutaneous tissues away from the surgical site.

Each hospital should establish a policy for use of the insulin pump depending on the expertise of the staff within the facility. Potential contraindications for continuing CSII during hospitalization include altered mental status, inability to operate the insulin pump safely, impaired decision making, risk of suicide, failure to follow medical advice, and subcutaneous insulin absorption issues, e.g., hypotensive, edematous (12). If the hospital staff is not familiar with insulin pump therapy and a family member is not available to assist with the safe operation of the insulin pump, alternative insulin replacement should be maintained, i.e., intravenous infusion or basal-bolus injection therapy.

When patient using an insulin pump is hospitalized for diabetic ketoacidosis (DKA), pump malfunction or poor absorption of insulin is usually the culprit. Immediate replacement of insulin is required. CSII therapy may be restarted once DKA is corrected and the cause is determined. If equipment malfunction or unsuitable patient self-care behaviors are the cause, initiating multiple daily injection therapy is always a safe option for establishing metabolic control.

SUMMARY

In general practice, nurses, unless they are diabetes pump specialists, will likely not be trained in operating CSII pumps. However, they should be able to access resources for the patient in any health care setting to assist with pump management. Nurses should recognize that most patients on CSII are very knowledgeable and that the patient's expertise should be acknowledged. When feasible, the pump therapy should be maintained. It is paramount that each institution or setting have a policy on insulin pump therapy. Interrupted CSII therapy can disrupt the glucose control of the patient and lead to rapid deterioration in metabolic status. Continuing pump therapy during hospitalization helps to maintain target glucose levels and reduce risk factors for infection and increased length of stay.

REFERENCES

1. American Diabetes Association: Continuous subcutaneous insulin infusion (Position Statement). *Diabetes Care* 27 (Suppl. 1):S110, 2004

2. Diabetes Control and Complications Trial Research Group: The effect of intensive treatment of diabetes on the development and progression of long-term complications in insulin dependent diabetes mellitus. *N Engl J Med* 329:977–985, 1993

3. Sanfield JA, Hegstad M, Hanna RS: Protocol for outpatient screening and initiation of continuous subcutaneous insulin infusion therapy: impact on cost and quality. *Diabetes Educ* 28:599–607, 2002

4. Klingensmith GJ (Ed.): *Intensive Diabetes Management.* 3rd ed. Alexandria, VA, American Diabetes Association, 2003

5. Brooks AM, Kulkarni K: Insulin pump therapy and carbohydrate counting for pump therapy: carbohydrate-to-insulin ratios. In *A Core Curriculum for Diabetes Education: Diabetes Management Therapies.* Franz MJ, McCloskey BA, Nath CR, Polonsky W, Eds. Chicago, IL, American Association of Diabetes Educators, 2001, p. 249–278

6. Department of Health and Human Services, Centers for Medicare & Medicaid Services: Infusion pumps: C-peptide levels as a criterion for use [Internet], 2005. Available from http://www.cms.hhs.gov/MLNMattersArticles/downloads/MM3705.pdf. Accessed 17 February 2009

7. Mudaliar S: Insulin therapy in type 2 diabetes. *Endocrinol Metab Clin North Am* 30:935–982, 2001

8. Litton J: Insulin pump therapy in toddlers and preschool children with type 1 diabetes mellitus. *J Pediatr* 141:490–495, 2002

9. Wentholt M, Vollebregt M, Hart A, Hoekstra J, and Hans DeVries J: Comparison of a needle-type and a microdialysis continuous glucose monitor in type 1 diabetic patients. *Diabetes Care* 28:2871–2876, 2005

10. Steil G, Rebrin K, Mastrototaro J, Bernaba B, Saad M: Determination of plasma glucose during rapid glucose excursions with a subcutaneous glucose sensor. *Diabet Technol Ther* 5:27–31, 2003

11. Wilhelm B, Forst S, Weber M, Larbig M, Pfützner A, Forst T: Evaluation of CGMS® during rapid blood glucose changes in patients with type 1 diabetes. *Diabet Technol Ther* 8:146–155, 2006

12. Cook CB, Boyle ME, Cisar NS, Miller-Cage V, Bourgeois P, et al.: Use of continuous insulin infusion (insulin pump) therapy in the hospital setting: proposed guidelines and outcome measures. *Diabetes Educ* 31:849–857, 2005

13. Kanakis SJ, Watts C, Leichter SB: The business of insulin pumps in diabetes care: clinical and economic considerations. *Clinical Diabetes* 20:214–216, 2002

14. Lenhard MJ, Reeves GD: Continuous subcutaneous insulin infusion: a comprehensive review of insulin pump therapy. *Arch Intern Med* 161:2293–3000, 2001

ADDITIONAL READING

American Diabetes Association, American Dietetic Association: *Basic Carbohydrate Counting*. Alexandria, VA, American Diabetes Association, 2003

Bode BW, Tamborlane WV, Davidson PC: Insulin pump therapy in the 21st century: strategies for successful use in adults, adolescents, and children with diabetes. *Postgrad Med* 111:69–77, 2002

Bolderman KM: *Putting Your Patients on the Pump*. Alexandria, VA, American Diabetes Association, 2002

Fredrickson L, Rubin RR, Rubin S: *Optimal Pumping: A Guide to Good Health with Diabetes*. Northridge, CA, Medtronic MiniMed, 2001

McCarren M: *Counting Carbs Made Easy for People with Diabetes* (Fast Fact Series). Alexandria, VA, American Diabetes Association, 2002

Walsh J, Roberts R: *Pumping Insulin: Everything You Need for Success With an Insulin Pump*. 3rd ed. San Diego, CA, Torrey Pines Press, 2000

Warshaw HS, Bolderman KM: *Practical Carbohydrate Counting: A How-to-Teach Guide for Health Professionals*. Alexandria, VA, American Diabetes Association, 2001

Ms. Tomky is a Certified Adult Nurse Practitioner and Diabetes Educator at Lovelace Sandia Health Systems, Albuquerque, NM.

SPECIAL POPULATIONS

25. Women and Diabetes

CAROL J. HOMKO, RN, PHD, CDE

D iabetes is a serious chronic illness that affects ~20 million people in the U.S. Although men and women are equally affected by type 1 diabetes, the prevalence of type 2 diabetes is higher in women than in men. More women die each year from diabetes and its complications than from breast cancer, making diabetes a significant "women's health issue" (1). Women with diabetes face special health challenges throughout their lives (see "Making Time for Diabetes Care in a Woman's Busy Life," a patient handout in RESOURCES). This chapter examines the available data concerning the impact of diabetes on women, beginning with the implications for childbearing and ending with its effects in later life on the risks of cardiovascular disease (CVD) and osteoporosis.

PREGNANCY IN DIABETES

PRECONCEPTION COUNSELING

Diabetes is generally classified into the following categories: type 1 diabetes, type 2 diabetes, and gestational diabetes mellitus (GDM). It is estimated that 150,000 pregnancies are complicated by diabetes each year in the U.S. GDM accounts for 135,000 of these pregnancies, type 2 diabetes for 12,000, and type 1 diabetes for 7,000 (2). Additional data from the 2002 edition of *Diabetes in America* estimate that maternal diabetes complicates 2–3% of all pregnancies (3). White's classification remains the most commonly accepted system for categorizing diabetes during pregnancy (Table 25.1). This system relates the onset of disease, disease duration, and presence of vascular complications to pregnancy outcome. Women in the highest categories and their offspring are at the greatest risk of

Table 25.1 White's Classification of Diabetes in Pregnancy

Class A	GDM
Class B	Onset at ≥20 years of age and <10 years' duration
Class C	Onset between 10 and 19 years of age or 10–19 years' duration
Class D	Onset <10 years of age or >20 years' duration
Class F	Diabetic nephropathy
Class R	Proliferative retinopathy
Class FR	Nephropathy and proliferative retinopathy
Class H	Coronary artery disease
Class T	Renal transplantation

diabetes-related adverse pregnancy outcomes (Table 25.2) (i.e., a class A pregnancy is at least risk, whereas a class T pregnancy is at highest risk).

FUEL METABOLISM

Pregnancy is recognized as having a profound effect on maternal carbohydrate metabolism. These pregnancy-related alterations are necessary to meet the demands of the developing fetus. Early pregnancy is characterized by greater-than-normal insulin sensitivity, which produces a milieu that favors maternal fat accumulation in preparation for the increasing energy requirements of late gestation and lactation. Late pregnancy is characterized by accelerated growth of the feto-placental unit, increasing plasma concentrations of several diabetogenic hormones, including human placental lactogen and estrogens, and increasing insulin resistance. Studies have demonstrated that insulin sensitivity is reduced by 33–50% by the third trimester of pregnancy (4,5). The cause or causes of this decline in insulin sensitivity are not entirely clear. However, the parallel development of insulin resistance and increases in blood levels of human placental lactogen and other diabetogenic hormones, including cortisol, progesterone, and estrogens,

Table 25.2 Pregnancy Complications

Maternal	Fetal/Neonatal
Preterm labor	Stillbirth
Infectious morbidities	Congenital malformations
Polyhydramnios	Altered fetal growth
Pregnancy-induced hypertension	Metabolic abnormalities
Worsening of diabetic retinopathy, nephropathy	Cardiomyopathy
Hypoglycemia, ketoacidosis	Respiratory distress syndrome

suggest that these hormones are responsible for much of the observed insulin resistance. In healthy pregnant women, insulin secretion must be increased by 200–300% in late gestation to overcome the resistance and maintain euglycemia. Women who are unable to increase their insulin secretion to compensate for the physiological changes of advancing gestation go on to develop impaired glucose tolerance (IGT) and GDM.

DIABETES-RELATED CONGENITAL MALFORMATIONS

Congenital malformations continue to complicate between 6 and 10% of all diabetic pregnancies and account for ~40% of the perinatal mortality among these infants (6). The malformations associated with diabetes can involve multiple organ systems, but the cardiovascular and nervous systems are most frequently involved. The defects most often associated with diabetes occur before the seventh week of gestation. Both animal and human studies have demonstrated that diabetes-associated malformations are related to hyperglycemia during the period of organogenesis (6–9). In addition, numerous clinical trials in humans have demonstrated that strict glycemic control before and during early pregnancy can, in most cases, reduce the rate of structural defects to the background level (10,11). Despite this evidence, ~60% of women with diabetes still only seek medical care after they learn that they are pregnant (12).

PRECONCEPTION CARE

Care of women with type 1 or type 2 diabetes ideally begins 3–6 months before conception to allow sufficient time to evaluate the mother's heath status and to maximize glycemic control. The prepregnancy assessment includes a careful history and thorough physical examination to assess the patient's vascular status. Baseline creatinine clearance and protein excretion levels are evaluated, and an electrocardiogram is performed. Ideally, these women are referred for an ophthalmologic consultation. Care should include counseling about the risks associated with hyperglycemia. Achieving low-risk glycemia requires a plan for reaching glycated hemoglobin A1c (A1C) levels <1% above the normal range of 4–6%, and lower if possible (13). This level of blood glucose control needs to be achieved before the woman is advised to become pregnant, and women need to receive appropriate contraceptive therapy while they are preparing for pregnancy. For patients who have not met treatment goals, an extensive period of education and the initiation of self-blood glucose monitoring are also necessary (14). Women

Preconception Assessment

- Maximize glucose control
- History and physical examination for vascular status
- Electrocardiogram
- Baseline creatinine clearance
- Baseline urine total protein
- Fundoscopic examination

with type 2 diabetes controlled with oral antihyperglycemic agents that are classified as teratogenic need to begin insulin therapy.

GESTATIONAL DIABETES

GDM is a common problem. It complicates ~5–7% (2) of all pregnancies in the U.S., and data demonstrate that the prevalence is increasing (15). The likelihood of developing GDM is significantly increased among certain subgroups, including individuals with a family history of type 2 diabetes, advancing maternal age, obesity, and nonwhite ethnicity. Excess risks for both GDM and IGT have been demonstrated in African-American, Hispanic, and Native American women, as well as women from the Indian subcontinent and the Middle East (16).

Glucose testing is recommended for women in all high-risk groups and should be done as early as feasible. However, there are certain populations of low-risk women in whom it may not be cost-effective to routinely screen for GDM. This low-risk group includes women who are not members of the previously highlighted ethnic groups and have all of the following characteristics: age <25 years, normal body weight, and no family history of diabetes (15). Screening should be performed between the 24th and 28th week of gestation for those of average risk and in women at high risk whose initial screening did not lead to diagnosis of GDM (see chapter 1).

The presence of fasting hyperglycemia (>105 mg/dl [>5.8 mmol/l]) may be associated with an increase in the risk of intrauterine fetal death during the last 4–8 weeks of gestation. GDM is also associated with an increased incidence of maternal hypertensive disorders (17).

MANAGEMENT OF PREGNANCY COMPLICATED BY DIABETES

The main goal of management for pregnancies complicated by diabetes is to achieve and/or maintain euglycemia throughout gestation. The treatment approach requires a combination of medical nutrition therapy, exercise, insulin therapy, and daily multiple blood glucose determinations. The goals of nutrition therapy are to provide adequate maternal and fetal nutrition, to achieve appropriate gestational weight gain, and to minimize glucose excursions. For both women with preexisting diabetes and those with GDM, guidelines suggest that the composition of the meal plan be based on an individualized nutritional assessment. In GDM, it is generally accepted that the amount and type of carbohydrate be adjusted to achieve postprandial glucose targets (18).

Evidence regarding the risk and/or benefits of either periodic or regular exercise in pregnant women with preexisting diabetes is limited. However, mild exercise in the form of walking is possible for most women and has been reported to improve lipid profiles and blood glucose control (19). In GDM, exercise has been recommended as an adjunct to nutritional therapy. Regular aerobic exercise has been shown to lower fasting and postprandial glucose concentrations. Several randomized controlled trials have demonstrated that upper-extremity exercise for 20 min three times a week can significantly lower blood glucose levels in women with GDM (20,21). In addition, these trials found no significant increase in either maternal or neonatal complications.

In the U.S., until very recently, insulin was the only therapy recommended to treat diabetes during pregnancy. There is now evidence from one randomized controlled trial (22) and several observational studies demonstrating that glyburide is a useful and clinically effective alternative to insulin for women with GDM (15). The goal of pharmacotherapy is to achieve blood glucose levels that are nearly identical to those observed in healthy pregnant women.

Human insulin is the least immunogenic of all insulins and is exclusively advised for use in pregnancy. There are several approaches to insulin administration that can be used during pregnancy, and the superiority of one regimen over another has never been fully demonstrated. The rapid-acting insulin analogs with peak hypoglycemic action 1–2 h after injection offer the potential for improved postprandial glucose control. Studies support their safety during pregnancy and their ability to improve glycemic control (23,24). Continuous subcutaneous insulin infusion pumps are another treatment option that has been successfully used during pregnancy (25).

Diabetes control is monitored through blood glucose levels, ketone measurements, and A1C concentrations. Although it is widely accepted that the level of metabolic control achieved in the pregnancy complicated by diabetes significantly affects perinatal outcome, what constitutes optimal control has not been established. Emerging evidence suggests that a continuum of risk exists between carbohydrate intolerance and both perinatal and neonatal morbidity. The logical approach is to achieve as near-normal glucose levels as possible without undue severe hypoglycemia. The most recent recommended plasma blood glucose goals in pregnancy are 60–90 mg/dl before breakfast, lunch, supper, and bedtime snack; <120 mg/dl after meals (1 h); and 60–90 mg/dl overnight (2:00 a.m. to 6:00 a.m.) (26).

ANTEPARTUM AND INTRAPARTUM MANAGEMENT

Guidelines for the antepartum management of pregnant women with diabetes can be found in Table 25.3. Early enrollment in prenatal care is encouraged for all women with preexisting diabetes. The frequency of prenatal visits will depend on the level of glycemic control. Maternal blood pressure should be evaluated at each visit, and all pregnancies complicated by diabetes require additional fetal evaluation and assessment. Fetal ultrasonography in the first trimester or early in the second trimester allows confirmation of gestational age and helps to verify the absence of any malformations. A fetal echocardiogram in midpregnancy is used to screen for congenital heart defects. Serial ultrasounds thereafter are used to assess fetal growth, measure amniotic fluid volume, and evaluate the placenta (27).

During labor and delivery, optimal blood glucose control should be maintained to prevent neonatal hypoglycemia. Maternal blood glucose levels should be maintained at a level <100 mg/dl by using an insulin/glucose infusion. After delivery, maternal insulin requirements tend to dramatically fall as a result of the significant decrease in the level of placental hormones.

POSTPARTUM MANAGEMENT

The primary goal of the postpartum period for women with preexisting diabetes is continued maintenance of euglycemia. An immediate decrease in insulin

Table 25.3 Monitoring a Pregnancy Complicated by Diabetes

Class A	■ Daily self-monitoring of blood glucose (fasting and 1–2 h after meals) ■ Serial ultrasound examinations in third trimester ■ Nonstress test at 34–36 weeks, then weekly ■ A1C every 4–6 weeks ■ No 24-h urine, ophthalmologic evaluation, or fetal electrocardiogram necessary ■ Daily fetal movement counts
Classes B and C	■ Daily self-monitoring of blood glucose (5–7 times/day) ■ Level II ultrasound and fetal electrocardiogram at ~20 weeks, then follow-up every 4–6 weeks ■ A1C every 4–6 weeks ■ Nonstress test at 32 weeks, then weekly ■ Ophthalmologic evaluation, follow-up according to findings ■ 24-h urine, initially and in each trimester ■ Daily fetal movement counts (beginning at 28 weeks' gestation)
Classes D to FR	■ Above, plus electrocardiogram initially ■ Uric acid, liver function test, fibrinogen, fibrin split products (may repeat in each trimester)

> **PRACTICAL POINT**
>
> Because of the high risk of developing type 2 diabetes after GDM, women should have their glycemic status retested at least 6 weeks after delivery according to standard diagnostic criteria and every 1–3 years thereafter (17).

requirements will be noted in women with type 1 and type 2 diabetes and GDM. Typically, the woman with GDM who required insulin during pregnancy will no longer need insulin after delivery. The woman with type 1 diabetes may need very little insulin for up to 48 h after the delivery. Lack of a reduction in insulin requirement may signal an underlying infection.

In some instances, it is difficult to determine whether the woman had underlying type 2 diabetes that was diagnosed during pregnancy or whether the change in glucose metabolism experienced during pregnancy was related to GDM. If type 2 diabetes is present, hyperglycemia will persist after the delivery of the infant and the mother will continue to need medication/insulin to maintain euglycemic levels.

Women who breastfeed are more likely to need less insulin than mothers who do not breastfeed. Mothers should be encouraged to monitor blood glucose regularly. Breastfeeding mothers expend more energy and require more calories than non-breastfeeding mothers. Education on the prevention of hypoglycemia should be provided. Additional blood glucose testing and snacks may be required before, during, or after breastfeeding (28).

For women with GDM, the goal is to prevent subsequent diabetes. An individualized reproductive health plan will need to be developed that addresses contraception, importance of planning future pregnancies, and lifestyle changes aimed at preventing diabetes or its long-term complications. The risk of GDM occurring in subsequent pregnancies has been reported to be 60–90%, depending on the woman's weight in the first trimester (29).

The use of contraception in all women with diabetes or a prior history of GDM cannot be emphasized strongly enough. Contraception is the only way to ensure that preconception care can be provided. A variety of family planning methods are currently available. Natural family planning is a contraceptive method that requires that women abstain from intercourse during the fertile phase of the menstrual cycle. Barrier methods of contraception create mechanical and/or chemical barriers to fertilization and include diaphragms, male and female condoms, spermicidal foam, jelly or foam, and cervical caps. Although both of these methods pose no health risks to women with diabetes, they are user-dependent and therefore have a high failure rate, particularly in the first year.

Oral contraceptives remain the most popular form of birth control despite controversy over potential side effects. The main reasons for their popularity are their failure rate of generally <1% and ease of use. Low-dose formulations are preferred and are recommended only for patients without vascular complications or additional risk factors, such as smoking or a strong family history of myocardial disease. Their effects on carbohydrate and lipid metabolism are minimal. Progestin only ("minipill") oral contraceptives are an option for women with contraindications to the estrogen component, such as hypertension or thrombosis (30,31).

An IUD (intrauterine device) is the most effective nonhormonal contraceptive device. It should only be offered to women with diabetes who have a low risk of sexually transmitted diseases because any infection might place the patient with diabetes at risk for sepsis and ketoacidosis. Patient education should include the early signs of sexually transmitted diseases, such as increased and abnormal vaginal discharge; dyspareunia; heavy, painful menses; lower abdominal pain; and fever (30,31).

Depo-Provera is a long-acting progestin that provides highly effective pregnancy prevention. It is administered intramuscularly every 3 months and works by inhibiting ovulation. The high efficiency and long period of action of Depo-Provera make it an attractive option for women with a history of poor medication compliance (30,31). Unfortunately, this long-acting progestin has not been studied in women with diabetes.

Permanent sterilization, including tubal ligation or vasectomy, may be considered by the patient or her partner when they desire no more children.

INFANTS OF WOMEN WITH DIABETES

The offspring of women with diabetes have an increased risk for perinatal mortality and morbidity. The two major causes of perinatal mortality are unexplained fetal death and congenital malformations (32). The causes of unexpected death are not well understood. In animal models, sustained hyperglycemia has been associated with increased insulin secretion, elevated fetal oxygen consumption, acidosis, and death. It has been postulated that fetal polycythemia and increased platelet aggregation could explain the increased incidence of intravascular thrombosis in infants of diabetic mothers and that thrombotic episodes could be the underlying cause of late unexplained intrauterine deaths (32–35).

Macrosomia is a hallmark of the pregnancy complicated by diabetes and is reported to occur in 20–25% of pregnancies complicated by diabetes. Macrosomia is defined as excessive birth weight (>90%) for gestational age or birth weight >4,000 g. Increased adiposity is the primary cause of the increased birth weight seen in offspring of women with diabetes. Numerous studies have established a relationship between macrosomia and the level of maternal glucose control achieved during pregnancy. Other factors associated with an increased risk for fetal macrosomia include increased maternal weight, increased parity, previous delivery of a macrosomic infant, and insulin requirements >80 units/day (32,33). Perinatal mortality is associated with macrosomia. These infants also have an increased demand for oxygen, and asphyxia can occur, which may account for the increased death rate for macrosomic infants.

Hypoglycemia occurs in infants when plasma glucose levels fall below 40–45 mg/dl (34). Infants of mothers with diabetes can develop hypoglycemia during the first few hours of life, particularly in cases of poor glycemic control. Macrosomic infants and infants with elevated cord-blood C-peptide or immunoreactive insulin levels are also at increased risk. The incidence of hypoglycemia is reported to range from 25 to 40% in infants of mothers with diabetes. Both poor glycemic control during pregnancy and elevated maternal plasma glucose levels at the time of delivery increase the risk of its occurrence.

The incidence of hypocalcemia is also significantly increased in infants of women with diabetes. Hypocalcemia generally occurs in association with hyperphosphatemia and occasionally with hypomagnesemia. Neonatal hypocalcemia is defined as a calcium level <7 mg/dl. Serum calcium levels are usually lowest on the second or third day of life.

Polycythemia is defined as a venous hematocrit that exceeds 65% and is reported to occur in one-third of neonates born to women with diabetes. Polycythemia is believed to occur as a result of chronic intrauterine hypoxia, which leads to an increase in erythropoietin and consequently results in an increase in red blood cell production. Neonates born to women with diabetes also have a higher incidence of hyperbilirubinemia compared with nondiabetic control subjects (32–35).

Offspring born to women with diabetes are also at increased risk of developing various hypertrophic types of cardiomyopathies and congestive heart failure. The exact incidence is not known, but one study reported that 10% of infants born to women with diabetes might have evidence of myocardial and septal hypertrophy. Thickening of the interventricular septum as well as the left or right ventricular wall

> **PRACTICAL POINT**
>
> Women who are anovulatory may ovulate when metformin and/or glitazone are prescribed. Premenopausal women without appropriate contraception may be at risk for pregnancy. All premenopausal women should be counseled regarding the risk for pregnancy and provided guidance regarding appropriate contraception.

can occur and is thought to be a result of the fetal hyperinsulinemic state. In most cases, these infants are asymptomatic and the myocardial abnormalities regress by 6 months of age.

Respiratory distress syndrome (RDS) is another common complication associated with diabetes. In the past, offspring born to women with diabetes had a four- to sixfold greater incidence of RDS, but this incidence has dramatically decreased with the initiation of strict metabolic control. More recent studies, in fact, seem to indicate that stringent metabolic control may reduce the incidence of RDS in neonates of women with diabetes to near the background level in the population (32–35). Last, there may be long-term consequences of diabetic pregnancies, including childhood obesity, neuropsychological deficits, and increased tendency to develop overt diabetes.

OTHER WOMEN'S HEALTH ISSUES

EFFECTS OF THE MENSTRUAL CYCLE ON GLUCOSE CONTROL

Menstrual cycle-related alterations in blood glucose control have been reported in some women with type 1 diabetes. Most of these women describe deterioration in glycemic control around the time of menstruation, although some women have reported improvements (36). As a result, both diabetic ketoacidosis and mild and severe hypoglycemia have been noted to occur more frequently at this time. The exact mechanism of these changes in glucose homeostasis in women with diabetes is unknown, but it is presumed to be related to changes in levels of estrogen, progesterone, and other reproductive hormones.

Studies examining this phenomenon have yielded controversial results. Some studies have demonstrated decreased insulin sensitivity during the luteal phase compared with the follicular phase, but other studies have not found these differences (36–38). Data from Widom, Diamond, and Simonson (39) suggest that there is a subgroup of women with type 1 diabetes who exhibit worsening premenstrual (luteal phase) hyperglycemia and a decline in insulin sensitivity. In these studies, this deterioration in glucose utilization was associated with greater increments in estradiol levels from the follicular to the luteal phase. From a clinical perspective, women with diabetes need to be counseled regarding the possibility of altered glucose control at various points in the menstrual cycle. They will need to monitor blood glucose levels more frequently and adjust insulin dosages accordingly. In some women, increases in cravings for high-carbohydrate food during the premenstrual phase may further accentuate the loss of glucose control; therefore, attention to dietary changes is also important.

POLYCYSTIC OVARY SYNDROME

Polycystic ovary syndrome (PCOS) is an endocrine disorder that affects 4–6% of all women and is the leading cause of infertility in the U.S. There is no firm consensus as to the definition of PCOS. However, the diagnosis is based on findings of hyperandrogenism and ovulatory dysfunction after all other known causes of androgen excess or ovulatory dysfunction are excluded. The presence of polycystic ovaries on sonography is suggestive of PCOS but not diagnostic because these can be present in women without PCOS. The vast majority of women with PCOS will demonstrate frank elevations in circulating androgens, particularly free testosterone, and ~60% of these women are obese (40). Although not part of the diagnostic criteria, many women with PCOS are also insulin resistant and exhibit secondary hyperinsulinemia.

PCOS should be suspected in women who present with infertility, amenorrhea or irregular menses, hirsutism, acne, and obesity. Acanthosis nigricans may be present, as well as dyslipidemia (41). PCOS tends to develop shortly after menarche and persists throughout most of the woman's reproductive life. The menstrual irregularities and hyperandrogenism appear to normalize as women approach perimenopause. However, the associated metabolic abnormalities, especially glucose intolerance, actually worsen with age. The inherent insulin resistance present in PCOS that is aggravated by the high prevalence of obesity places these women at increased risk of IGT. Approximately 40% of individuals with PCOS develop either type 2 diabetes or IGT (42).

The most common reason that women with PCOS present to the gynecologist is infertility, secondary to chronic anovulation. Treatment with thiazolidinediones has been shown to decrease both androgen and insulin levels. Resumption of ovulation has been reported to occur in ~60% of women (42). Other approaches to improve insulin sensitivity and restore ovulation have included weight reduction and metformin therapy. Women with PCOS are at increased risk for the development of GDM during pregnancy. Treatment of PCOS with metformin throughout pregnancy in one study was associated with a 10-fold reduction in the incidence of GDM (43); however, metformin in pregnancy is not currently recommended. Counseling for women with PCOS should emphasize the importance of lifestyle interventions to prevent diabetes.

DIABETES IN OLDER WOMEN

CARDIOVASCULAR DISEASE

CVD is the leading cause of death in women with diabetes, surpassing both breast and ovarian cancers (1). Women without diabetes are generally protected from heart disease before menopause. However, for women with diabetes, this protective effect is absent. Studies have found that individuals with diabetes are at greater risk for CVD than individuals without diabetes and that the risk for women with diabetes actually exceeds that of men with diabetes. In a population-based study of ~2,500 men and women, Lundberg et al. (44) found that the relative risk for CVD was 2.9 in men with diabetes but 5.0 in women with diabetes. In addition, the mortality rate from myocardial infarction was four times higher in men with diabetes and seven times higher in women with diabetes compared with healthy individuals. Both the Strong Heart Study (45) and the Rancho Bernardo Study (46) reported similar increases in mortality.

Not only are women with diabetes at increased risk for CVD compared with their nondiabetic female counterparts, but they also appear to fare worse in terms of morbidity and mortality compared with men with diabetes (47–49). Other sex-based differences have been found in the management of modifiable CVD risk factors (50) and in the presentation and treatment of coronary heart disease in women. Studies have found that women are more likely to have their initial manifestation as angina pectoris, are more likely to be referred for diagnostic tests at a more advanced stage of disease, and are less likely than men to have corrective invasive procedures (47). Early and ongoing assessment of cardiovascular risk factors coupled with intense intervention and education is needed for all women with diabetes.

OSTEOPOROSIS

Osteoporosis is the most prevalent metabolic bone disease in the U.S. Although more common in white women, it does affect both sexes and all ethnic groups. Whether there is an increased risk of osteoporosis in individuals with type 1 or type 2 diabetes remains controversial. Most studies in women with type 1 diabetes have reported lower bone mineral density (BMD) levels than in either nondiabetic control subjects or women with type 2 diabetes (51). Why these differences occur is not well understood. Moreover, it is not clear whether the low BMD in type 1 diabetes is the result of reduced peak bone mass or of increased bone loss. All women with diabetes should be evaluated for the risk of osteoporosis and related fractures. Consensus is lacking on when to begin BMD testing, but screening is recommended for all postmenopausal women >65 years of age or those who are considered at high risk (52). In addition, they should be counseled regarding appropriate preventive measures, which include adequate dietary calcium and vitamin D intake, regular exercise, and avoidance of smoking and other potential risk factors (see also "Are You at Risk for Osteoporosis?" a patient handout in resources).

HORMONE REPLACEMENT THERAPY

Conventional wisdom based on cross-sectional data is to prescribe hormone replacement therapy (HRT) for postmenopausal women with the goal of reducing CVD, preventing osteoporosis, preserving memory, promoting sexual well-being, and maintaining overall health and vitality. Data specific to HRT in women with diabetes are scarce but of potential interest because these women are at high risk of developing CVD. The Third National Health and Nutrition Examination Survey (53) found that postmenopausal women with diabetes had increased dyslipidemia compared with nondiabetic counterparts. Among women with diabetes in that trial, individuals using HRT had significantly better lipoprotein profiles and glycemic control than women with diabetes who had never used or previously used HRT. However, recent trials in women without diabetes have not supported the safety or benefits of HRT. The Heart and Estrogen/Progestin Replacement Study (HERS), published in 1998 (54), demonstrated that HRT had an early adverse effect in women with preexisting coronary disease. Most recently, the Woman's Health Initiative (55), which investigated the health risks and benefits of combined estrogen and progestin replacement therapy in healthy postmenopausal women, was concluded early because increased risk of breast cancer as well as increased risk of coronary heart disease, stroke, and pulmonary embolism outweighed the evidence for benefits in the rates of fracture and possibly colon cancer. Unequivocally, the conclusion from the Women's Health Initiative is that HRT should not be recommended for primary prevention of CVD or fractures in women with or without diabetes. HRT may still be appropriate for short-term therapy for menopausal symptoms, including vasomotor instability with hot flushes, sleep disturbance, night sweats, and mood lability.

SUMMARY

Nursing plays a key role in the education and care of women throughout the life cycle. In women with diabetes, health concerns begin at puberty and continue through preconception and pregnancy, culminating in menopause-related issues. Anticipatory guidance and education in each phase of development can help avoid health care problems and achieve desired outcomes.

Frequently, women who see specialists for health care management do not have primary care providers. As a consequence, they may not receive routine screenings, such as Pap smears and mammograms. As practitioners of preventive care, nurses need to remind women of the need for these screening tests.

Future nursing research is needed in the treatment of women with diabetes:

- Identification of the modifiable barriers to preconception care and strategies to increase the proportion of women with diabetes who plan their pregnancies is needed.
- The development and testing of innovative programs and strategies to prevent CVD and reduce excessive risk for poor outcomes among women with diabetes should be explored.
- The effects of various treatment modalities on the psychosocial impact of high-risk pregnancy require investigation.
- The impact of the patient-provider relationship on compliance and self-care behaviors in women with diabetes is important to determine the success of any treatment regimen.

Key Points

- Diabetes is a significant health problem that affects women throughout their life cycles.
- Strict blood glucose control before conception and throughout gestation can reduce and/or eliminate the excess risk for both mother and baby.
- All women with diabetes of childbearing age should be counseled regarding the importance of preconception glycemic control and of planning their pregnancies.
- All pregnant women except for those deemed at low risk should be screened for GDM between 24 and 28 weeks' gestation.
- Women with PCOS are at increased risk for developing IGT and diabetes.
- Not only are women with diabetes at increased risk for CVD compared with their nondiabetic female counterparts, but they also appear to fare worse in terms of morbidity and mortality compared with men with diabetes.

REFERENCES

1. Giardina EG: Call to action: cardiovascular disease in women. _J Womens Health_ 7:37–43, 1998

2. Engelgau NM, Herman WH, Smith PJ, German RR, Aubert RE: The epidemiology of diabetes and pregnancy in the U.S., 1988. _Diabetes Care_ 18:1029–1033, 1995

3. Buchanan TA: Pregnancy in preexisting diabetes. In _Diabetes in America_. 2nd ed. Harris MI, Cowie CC, Stern MP, Boyko EJ, Reiber GE, Bennett PH, Eds. Available from http://diabetes.niddk.nih.gov/dm/pubs/america/pdf/chapter36.pdf. Accessed 19 February 2009

4. Homko CJ, Sivan E, Reece EA, Boden G: Fuel metabolism during pregnancy. _Semin Reprod Endocrinol_ 17:119–125, 1999

5. Catalano PM, Tyzbir ED, Roman NM, Amini SB, Sims EAH: Longitudinal changes in insulin release and insulin resistance in nonobese pregnant women. _Am J Obstet Gynecol_ 165:1667–1672, 1991

6. Reece EA, Homko CJ, Wu YK: Multifactorial basis of the syndrome of diabetic embryopathy. _Teratology_ 54:171–182, 1997

7. Eriksson UJ: Congenital malformations in diabetic animal models: a review. _Diabetes Res_ 1:57–61, 1984

8. Rose BI, Graff S, Spencer R, Hensleigh P, Fainstat T: Major congenital anomalies in infants and glycosylated hemoglobin levels in insulin-requiring diabetic mothers. _J Perinatol_ 8:309–311, 1998

9. Ylinen K, Aula P, Stenman UH, Kesaniemi-Kuokkanen T, Teramo K: Risk of minor and major fetal malformations in diabetics with high hemoglobin A1c values in early pregnancy. _Br Med J_ 289:345–346, 1984

10. Fuhrmann K, Reiher H, Semmler K, Fischer F, Fischer M, Glockner E: Prevention of congenital malformations in infants of insulin-dependent diabetic mothers. _Diabetes Care_ 6:219–223, 1983

11. Kitzmiller JL, Gavin LA, Gin GD, Jovanovic-Peterson L, Main EK, Zigrang WD: Preconception care of diabetes: glycemic control prevents congenital anomalies. _JAMA_ 265:731–736, 1991

12. Janz NK, Herman WH, Becker MP, Charron-Prochownik D, Shayna VL, et al.: Diabetes and pregnancy: factors associated with seeking pre-conception care. _Diabetes Care_ 18:157–165, 1995

13. American Diabetes Association: Preconception care of women with diabetes (Position Statement). _Diabetes Care_ 27 (Suppl. 1):S76–S78, 2004

14. Kitzmiller JL, Buchanan TA, Kjos S, Combs CA, Ratner RE: Pre-conception care of diabetes, congenital malformations, and spontaneous abortions. _Diabetes Care_ 19:514–541, 1996

15. Metzger BE, Buchanan TA, Coustan DR, de Leiva A, Dunger DB: Summary and recommendations of the Fifth International Workshop-Conference on Gestational Diabetes. *Diabetes Care* 30 (Suppl. 2):S251–S260, 2007

16. Marshall JA, Hamman RF, Baxter J, Mayer EJ, Fulton DL, et al.: Ethnic differences in risk factors associated with prevalence of non-insulin dependent diabetes mellitus: the San Luis Valley Diabetes Study. *Am J Epidemiol* 137:706–718, 1993

17. American Diabetes Association: Gestational diabetes mellitus (Position Statement). *Diabetes Care* 27 (Suppl. 1):S88–S90, 2004

18. Reader DM: Medical nutrition therapy and lifestyle interventions. *Diabetes Care* 30 (Suppl. 2): S188–S193, 2007

19. Hollingsworth DR, Moore TR: Postprandial walking exercise in pregnant insulin dependent (type I) diabetic women: reduction of plasma lipid levels but absence of a significant effect on glycemic control. *Am J Obstet Gynecol* 157:1359–1363, 1987

20. Jovanovic-Peterson L, Peterson CM: Exercise and the nutritional management of diabetes during pregnancy. *Obstet Gynecol Clin North Am* 23:75–86, 1996

21. Bung P, Artal R, Khodiguian N, Kjos S: Exercise in gestational diabetes: an optional therapeutic approach? *Diabetes* 40 (Suppl. 2):182–185, 1991

22. Langer O, Conway DL, Berkus M, Elly M, Xenakis J, Gonzales O: A comparison of glyburide and insulin in women with GDM. *N Engl J Med* 343:1134–1138, 2000

23. Bhattacharyya A, Brown S, Hughes S, Vice PA: Insulin lispro and regular insulin in pregnancy. *QJM* 94:255–260, 2001

24. Jovanovic L, Ilic S, Pettitt DJ, Hugo K, Gutierrez M, et al.: Metabolic and immunologic effects of insulin lispro in gestational diabetes. *Diabetes Care* 22:1422–1427, 1999

25. Jornsay DL: Pregnancy and continuous insulin infusion therapy. *Diabetes Spectrum* 11:26–32, 1998

26. American Diabetes Association: Pregnancy. In *Medical Management of Type 1 Diabetes*. 4th ed. Bode BW, Ed. Alexandria, VA, American Diabetes Association, 2004, p. 146–157

27. Conway DL: Obstetric management in gestational diabetes. *Diabetes Care* 30: S175–S179, 2007

28. Riordan J: Women's health and breastfeeding. In *Breastfeeding and Human Lactation*. Sudbury, MA, Jones and Bartlett, 2005, p. 459–461

29. Jovanovic L, Pettitt D: Gestational diabetes mellitus. *JAMA* 286:2516–2518, 2001

30. Kjos SL: Contraception in women with diabetes mellitus. *Diabetes Spectrum* 6:80–86, 1993

31. Kjos SL: Postpartum care of women with diabetes. *Clin Obstet Gynecol* 43:46–55, 2000

32. Weintrob N, Karp M, Hod M: Short- and long-range complications in offspring of diabetic mothers. *J Diabetes Complications* 10:294–301, 1996

33. Schwarz R, Teramo KA: Effects of diabetic pregnancy on the fetus and newborn. *Semin Perinatol* 24:120–135, 2000

34. Kalhan S, Peter-Wohl S: Hypoglycemia: what is it for the neonate? *Am J Perinatol* 17:11–18, 2000

35. Reece EA, Homko CJ: Infant of the diabetic mother. *Semin Perinatol* 18:459–469, 1994

36. Case A, Reid RL: Effects of the menstrual cycle on medical disorders. *Arch Intern Med* 158:1405–1412, 1998

37. Jarrett RJ, Graver HJ: Changes in oral glucose tolerance during the menstrual cycle. *BMJ* 2:528–529, 1968

38. Moberg E, Kollind M, Lins PE, Adamson U: Day-to-day variation of insulin sensitivity in patients with type 1 diabetes: role of gender and menstrual cycle. *Diabet Med* 12:224–228, 1995

39. Widom B, Diamond MP, Simonson DC: Alterations in glucose metabolism during menstrual cycle in women with IDDM. *Diabetes Care* 15:213–220, 1992

40. Legro RS, Azziz R: Androgen excess disorders. In *Danforth's Obstetrics and Gynecology*. 9th ed. Scott JR, Gibbs RS, Kaplan BY, Haney AF, Eds. Philadelphia, Lippincott Williams and Wilkins, 2003, p. 669–672

41. Hill KM: Update: the pathogenesis and treatment of PCOS. *Nurse Pract* 28:8–23, 2003

42. Bloomgarden ZT: Diabetes issues in women and children. *Diabetes Care* 26:2457–2463, 2003

43. Glueck CJ, Wang P, Kobayashi S, Phillips H, Sieve-Smith L: Metformin therapy throughout pregnancy reduces the development of gestational diabetes in women with polycystic ovary syndrome. *Fertil Steril* 77:520–525, 2002

44. Lundberg V, Stegmayr B, Asplund K, Eliasson M, Huhtasaari F: Diabetes as a risk factor for myocardial infarction: population and gender perspectives. *J Intern Med* 241:485–492, 1997

45. Howard BV, Cowan LD, Go O, Welty TK, Robbins DC, Lee ET: Adverse effects of diabetes on multiple cardiovascular disease risk factors in women: the Strong Heart Study. *Diabetes Care* 18:1258–1265, 1998

46. Barrett-Connor E, Ferrara A: Isolated postchallenge hyperglycemia and the risk of fatal cardiovascular disease in older women and men. *Diabetes Care* 21:1236–1239, 1998

47. Kaseta JR, Skafar DF, Ram JL, Jacober SJ, Sowers JR: Cardiovascular disease in the diabetic woman. *J Clin Endocrinol Metab* 84:1835–1838, 1999

48. Berra K: Women, coronary heart disease and dyslipidemia: does gender alter detection, evaluation or therapy? *J Cardiovasc Nurs* 14:59–78, 2000

49. Gregg EW, Gu Q, Cheng YJ, Narayan V, Cowie CC. Mortality trends in men and women with diabetes, 1971 to 2000. *Ann Intern Med* 147:149–155, 2007

50. Ferrara A, Mangione CM, Kim C, Marrero DG, Curb D, et al.: Sex Disparities in control and treatment of modifiable cardiovascular disease risk factors among patients with diabetes. *Diabetes Care* 31:69–74, 2008

51. Tuominen JT, Impivaara L, Puukka P, Ronnemaa T: Bone mineral density in patients with type 1 and type 2 diabetes. *Diabetes Care* 22:1196–1200, 1999

52. Chau DL, Goldstein-Fuchs J, Edleman S: Clinical decision making: osteoporosis among patients with diabetes: an overlooked disease. *Diabetes Spectrum* 16:176–182, 2003

53. Crespo CJ, Smit E, Snelling A, Sempos CT, Anderson RE: Hormone replacement therapy and its relationship to lipid and glucose metabolism in diabetic and nondiabetic postmenopausal women: results from the Third National Health and Nutrition Examination Survey (NHANES III). *Diabetes Care* 25:1675–1168, 2002

54. Hulley S, Grady D, Bush T, Furberg C, Herrington D, et al.: Randomized trial of estrogen plus progestin for secondary prevention of coronary heart disease in postmenopausal women: Heart and Estrogen/Progestin Replacement Study (HERS) research group. *JAMA* 280:605–613, 1998

55. Women's Health Initiative Investigators Writers' Group: Risks and benefits of estrogen plus progestin in healthy postmenopausal women: principal results from the Women's Health Initiative randomized controlled trial. *JAMA* 288:321–333, 2002

Dr. Homko is an Associate Research Professor in the Department of Medicine, Temple University School of Medicine, Philadelphia, PA.

26. Children with Diabetes

Barbara Schreiner, RN, MN, CDE, BC-ADM

Having diabetes during childhood and adolescence poses distinct challenges and requires unique solutions. Although the child with diabetes will typically have type 1 diabetes, increasing numbers of children and teens are developing type 2 diabetes.

Children with type 1 diabetes typically present with the classic symptoms of diabetes: polyuria, polydipsia, ketonuria, and weight loss. In the very young child, early symptoms of diabetes, such as lethargy, irritability, and dehydration, are often mistaken for flu or gastroenteritis. The child with type 2 diabetes will classically have a BMI >85th percentile and have a strong family history of diabetes, display features of insulin resistance, and/or belong to a high-risk population, e.g., Latino, African American, Native American, or Pacific Islander (1). Overweight children should be screened for type 2 diabetes with fasting plasma glucose every 2 years if they meet these criteria (2). In addition to type 1 and type 2 diabetes, there are other metabolic disturbances of glucose metabolism in children. Cystic fibrosis–related diabetes (see chapter 29) and maturity-onset diabetes of the young (MODY) are two types seen in children. Cystic fibrosis–related diabetes is neither an autoimmune disease nor a disease of insulin resistance. Rather, it results from β-cell dysfunction caused by pancreatic fibrosis and fatty infiltration. MODY is also a distinct type of metabolic disorder. Occurring mostly in children, it is a type of familial diabetes characterized by autosomal-dominant inheritance. MODY results in an insulin-secretion defect that leads to hyperglycemia. The child has neither insulin resistance nor insulin antibodies. Children with MODY have mild hyperglycemia with no ketones and generally are lean. The term MODY has often been incorrectly used to label type 2 diabetes in children. A comparison of type 1 and type 2 diabetes is presented in Table 26.1.

Table 26.1 Comparison of Type 1 and Type 2 Diabetes in Children

	Type 1 Diabetes	Type 2 Diabetes
Mean age at onset (years)	10	13.5
Ethnicity	Caucasian	African American Latino Native American Pacific Islander
Fasting plasma glucose	≥126 mg/dl (≥7.0 mmol/l)	≥126 mg/dl (≥7.0 mmol/l)
Random plasma glucose	≥200 mg/dl (≥11.1 mmol/l)	≥200 mg/dl (≥11.1 mmol/l)
Body shape	Lean	Obese, often central
Acanthosis nigricans	None	Possible
Genetics	Possible	Probable
Primary treatment	Insulin	Diet and exercise
Additional treatment	Diet and exercise	Metformin and insulin
Underlying pathophysiology	Autoimmune destruction of β-cells	Insulin resistance, β-cell exhaustion, and excess hepatic glucose production
Progression of disease	From honeymoon period (remission) in the first year, for some, to β-cell destruction	From β-cell hypertrophy to β-cell exhaustion
Comorbidity	Other autoimmune diseases	Other insulin-resistance diseases

Adapted from Rosenbloom and Silverstein (2).

INITIATING TREATMENT

When managing diabetes in children, a health care professional must consider a number of issues unique to the pediatric population.

GOALS OF CARE

Managing diabetes for the child and family includes goals for achieving normal physical growth and psychosocial development, including family and peer relationships and school interactions. These goals are in addition to the typical objectives for gaining glycemic control, delaying and preventing chronic complications, and minimizing acute complications.

THE HONEYMOON PERIOD AND TYPE 1 DIABETES

As many as 62% of children with type 1 diabetes experience a partial remission of their disease (3). Known as the "honeymoon period," this is a time of decreased demand for injected insulin because the child's pancreas produces some insulin. Insulin doses decrease, and the patient's diabetes may be a bit easier to manage (4). The honeymoon period may last 6 weeks to 2 years (5). Some children never seem to have a remission. Once the honeymoon period is finished, the β-cells stop producing insulin, and the child's need for injected insulin increases. Families must be prepared for the beginning and end of the honeymoon because many believe their child's diabetes has been cured.

LINEAR GROWTH

Monitoring height and weight and pubertal development is a necessary component to pediatric care. Although now rare, Mauriac syndrome, a diabetes-related growth disorder, may affect children who have long-term suboptimal control (6). Features of this condition include delayed linear growth and sexual maturity, joint contractures, and hepatomegaly.

Children should be weighed and measured quarterly. Their growth should be plotted not only on age-appropriate standardized height and weight charts, but also on BMI charts, which are available from the Centers for Disease Control and Prevention at http://apps.nccd.cdc.gov/dnpabmi/Calculator.aspx. BMI is used differently in assessing children versus adults. Body fat differs in girls and boys as they mature. BMI charts are thus based on sex and age. Percentile cutoffs are used to identify overweight children (Table 26.2).

The growing child who has diabetes requires an ongoing source of nutrients. Parents of the child with type 1 diabetes will sometimes try to limit carbohydrate intake to control blood glucose or limit insulin doses. But appropriate calories are necessary for linear growth. The more reasonable approach is to adjust (increase) insulin doses as the child grows. The growing child may require an insulin dose adjustment every 3–4 days during growth spurts.

GROWTH OF SPECIFIC ORGANS

In addition to linear growth, the young child experiences rapid development of organs, such as the central nervous system (CNS) and the gastrointestinal

Table 26.2 Classification of Children Based on BMI

Classification	BMI for Age
Underweight	<5th percentile
Healthy weight	5th percentile to <85th percentile
At risk of overweight	85th to <95th percentile
Overweight	≥95th percentile

From http://www.cdc.gov/nccdphp/dnpa/bmi/childrens_BMI/about_childrens_BMI.htm.

system. The CNS requires a constant supply of glucose, with the brain requiring about 6 g glucose per hour. Because glycogen stores are limited in the young child, this glucose requirement must be met by consumed calories. Having limited glycogen stores also means that young children using insulin are at increased risk of hypoglycemia. Such physiological changes have implications for the child's meal plan. Meals and snacks must be spaced throughout the day, especially for the infant, toddler, and preschooler.

COGNITIVE DEVELOPMENT

The growing child is also in the process of developing cognitive skills. This process will affect the child's health beliefs and problem-solving skills. For the very young child, illness is often viewed as punishment and temporary. A young child hospitalized at onset might believe that his or her diabetes will go away once he or she returns home. Preschoolers might believe that they will lose all of their blood through a fingerstick. The infant responds to the parent's anxiety and sadness during injection time. Abstract concepts such as causes of hyperglycemia are not understood until later childhood, and the math skills required for dose adjustments and carbohydrate counting are not honed until young adolescence.

PSYCHOSOCIAL DEVELOPMENT

Another difference for the child with diabetes involves developing psychological and social skills. As the child matures, his or her psychosocial focus changes. The infant, for example, depends on his or her parents, whereas the school-aged child begins to form relationships with peers and other adults, such as teachers and school nurses. Adolescents focus on individuation while maintaining a peer-group relationship. Diabetes will affect each developmental stage (7,8). Table 26.3 summarizes the issues pertinent to each age and stage of development.

MEDICAL NUTRITION THERAPY

Medical nutrition therapy for the infant with type 1 diabetes focuses on providing adequate calories for rapid growth. The infant will need to feed every 3–4 h. Parents eventually learn how to coordinate meals with insulin and naps. The toddler with type 1 diabetes poses particular meal-planning challenges. Typical behaviors include food jags (eating only one or a few foods rather than a variety) and negativity. A young child may prefer to eat only one food for the whole week and refuse to eat anything else. The preschooler's appetite will often increase immediately before a growth spurt. Toddlers and preschoolers will need morning, afternoon, and bedtime snacks to build and maintain an available source of glycogen. However, they are easily distracted by other activities and often do not complete a meal or snack. Parents may find it nearly impossible to predict what the child will eat, making it difficult to plan a safe insulin dose. Fortunately, the rapid-acting insulin analogs make it possible to give the insulin dose after a meal. Parents can then more safely decide a dose based on what is truly consumed.

Table 26.3 Impact of Diabetes at Different Ages

Characteristics	Impact of Diabetes	Approaches
Infants		
Developing trust	Parents must perform invasive procedures; leads to parental anxiety, tension, guilt	Coaching and counseling parents: diabetes is not their fault; anticipatory guidance for parents; parents should cuddle and comfort child after each procedure; parents must interact with child outside of times for diabetes care
Interactions with caregivers around food	Mealtime may become a battleground; parents fear giving insulin and baby not eating; difficult to quantify carbohydrate intake in breast-fed infants	Loosen overall blood glucose control goals (100–200 mg/dl [5.5–11.1 mmol/l] is more safe); injections after meals
Immunizations	May have high blood glucose with or without ketones	More frequent monitoring for 24 h after immunizations
Physical development	Activity and exercise are inconsistent and unpredictable; hypoglycemia is dangerous to the developing CNS; small stomach; small liver glycogen stores (must be replenished frequently); limited tissue for subcutaneous injections	Loosen blood glucose target; frequent feedings; use legs, arms, and hips for injection sites; watch sites carefully; use short, fine (31-gauge) insulin syringes; do not reuse needles, use a fresh, sharp needle each time
Parenting issues	Symptoms of diabetes may have been ignored or misdiagnosed (diabetes is rare in infants); parents feel guilty about delay in treatment; parents are overwhelmed and lonely, with added responsibility and tasks	Counseling for parents: focus on parents' success in controlling diabetes; simplify the treatment plan as much as possible; parent support groups
Developing motor, speech, and social skills	Difficulty differentiating hypoglycemia from normal distress	Use blood glucose testing to learn infant's symptoms; feed before naps

Toddlers

Developing autonomy	Balkiness or stubborn around shots, testing, and food; regressive behaviors (speech, toilet training); temper tantrums may be symptom of hypoglycemia	Be matter-of-fact with tasks; use blood glucose tests to distinguish hypoglycemia from behavior; use usual behavior management approaches
Exploring environment	Caregivers may be overprotective of toddler; excitement may result in hypoglycemia (rather than hyperglycemia)	Counseling/coaching parents; watch for signs of low blood glucose at parties, holidays, etc.
Food jags and rituals are common	Picky eaters may result in parents becoming "short-order" cooks, doing anything to get the child to eat; parental anxiety about hypoglycemia; illness may result in poor appetite and hypoglycemia (rather than hyperglycemia)	Three meals/three snacks; use nutrient-dense foods (raisins instead of an apple); injections after the meal; creative insulin programs, minidose glucagon; do not focus on "cheating," instead say, "Did you want that extra cookie because you were hungry?"
Rapid physical growth	Frequent, routine insulin and food adjustments are needed; limited liver glycogen stores; activity and exercise are inconsistent and unpredictable	Parents should be taught to adjust insulin doses; snacks are important; record in a log book particularly active or inactive days—such notes may help in interpreting blood glucose patterns

Preschoolers

Concerned about body integrity and strength, fear of body mutilation	Invasive aspects of care become a problem; child may use procrastination to avoid injections and fingersticks	Use injection devices and lots of Band-Aids; needle/medical play; behavioral charts
Moody	May mimic hypoglycemia	Blood glucose tests to help distinguish
Imitation and symbolic play	May want to participate in aspects of self-care	Gradually add portions of the tasks, e.g., pick and wipe the injection site, turn on meter
Limited attention span; gets easily distracted	May not finish meals and snacks	Behavioral approaches to limit mealtime; use carbohydrate-dense foods
Needs to feel in control	Diabetes increases dependence	Create a log book for the child to keep, with stickers to identify blood glucose within target; encourage child in aspects of self-care; offer reasonable choices with diet

(continued)

Table 26.3 Impact of Diabetes at Different Ages (*Continued*)

Characteristics	Impact of Diabetes	Approaches
Preschoolers (continued)		
Egocentrism and absolutism	Reasoning with the child about the need for testing and shots will not work; in the child's mind, injections either hurt or don't hurt (nothing in between)	Perform skills quickly with assistance from child if possible; recognize that shots hurt; try comments such as, "It's time for your insulin—insulin will keep you healthy."
Magical thinking	May believe that diabetes goes away when you leave the hospital or clinic; views illness as the result of misdeeds or as being transferred magically	Use care with phrases such as "taking your blood glucose" or "taking a test"; children interpret these phrases literally
Parenting issues	Parents view child as vulnerable or endangered because of diabetes; daycare/preschool/babysitting challenges	Counseling and guidance from diabetes care team; support groups; mentoring from other parents; educate parents about the rights of children in daycare and schools
School-Aged Children		
Development of motor, intellectual, and social skills	Involved in athletics, PE, sports—requires planning/adjustment of food and/or insulin; may become sedentary after school, with TV, computers, increased snacking; lack of activity has impact on blood glucose control; has appropriate psychomotor skills to perform self-care skills, but needs supervision	Keep records of impact of activity on blood glucose patterns; child should learn injections and blood glucose testing skills; parents cannot abdicate their diabetes care roles yet; encourage family to engage in exercise
Attachment shifts from family to peers	Food choices may be difficult at parties; diabetes care may interfere with sleepovers; child may have trouble telling friends, teachers, coaches, etc., about diabetes; parents may become overprotective	Snack lists are helpful; encourage self-care skills; explore options for increasing the child's independence; science fair projects are a good way to share knowledge about diabetes

Sensitive to feeling adequate	Child may feel different, especially if care is required at school; hypoglycemia may happen in front of friends; childhood depression; may be more aware of genetic factors of diabetes	Simplify the care program; role-play managing hypoglycemia; educate about the causes of diabetes
Physical growth	Needs frequent food and insulin adjustments	Parents should know how to use blood glucose data to make dose and food adjustments
Development of concrete thought; understands cause and effect	Can recognize and treat hypoglycemia; typically receptive to diabetes education, but will be bored with didactic approaches	Diabetes education; role-play anticipated problems and solutions; use interactive approaches to diabetes education
School demands	Lunch and snack schedule may be variable (timing and amount of carbohydrate); testing at lunch may be a hassle; need for knowledgeable school personnel; PE schedule and diabetes knowledge of coach	Diabetes education; encourage problem solving; educate school personnel; educate parents about the rights of children with diabetes in schools; decrease care required at school

11- to 14-Year-Old Adolescents

Worries about appearance, self-consciousness	Doesn't want fingersticks to show; won't wear medical ID tag; self-conscious about injection sites; worries that hypoglycemia will happen with friends or during sports; may skip injections to manage weight	Alternatives to traditional ID tags; use self-consciousness as a motivator to rotate sites; use hypoglycemia worry to motivate blood glucose testing; understand that such concern may motivate the teen to keep blood glucose high
Hormonal changes	Blood glucose fluctuations; insulin resistance of puberty; mood changes may mimic hypoglycemia	Creative medical management; modify sick-day rules
Asserts independence from family	Experiments with diabetes management; may skip insulin; ignores diet/meal plan; choices and decisions may not always be best; may not be ready for diabetes care independence; deals with overprotective parents	"Personal scientist" approach—use personal experimentation in a safe way; see diabetes team alone at office visits; modify diabetes plan; work with parents on their changing roles; if teen was diagnosed as infant or child, complete reeducation about diabetes care is important
Rebellious, defiant	Refuses diabetes self-care; hates reminders	Counseling; communication skills; how to deal with anger

(continued)

Table 26.3 Impact of Diabetes at Different Ages (*Continued*)

Characteristics	Impact of Diabetes	Approaches
11- to 14-Year-Old Adolescents (continued)		
Peers are more important	Peers have priority over diabetes care; may want to hide diabetes or use it to establish role within a group	Talk about priority setting and how priorities change over time; talk about when diabetes care will take precedence
Strong sense of justice; hard to compromise	"Why me?" questioning; adolescent depression	Support groups; peer support; assess for depression and intervene
Oriented to the present	Little thought to long-term complications	Scare tactics have little value; focus on immediate concerns
Emerging sexuality	Wonders if more at risk for sexually transmitted diseases and AIDS because of diabetes	Education
15- to 16-Year-Old Adolescents		
Increased ability to compromise	Can make more choices about diabetes care	Include the teen more fully in management decisions; use negotiation; use behavioral contracting
Increased independence and decision making	Can begin to adjust all aspects of management: exercise, diet, insulin; understands the relationship of exercise, diet, and insulin; increased stress from social, school, and family responsibilities	Diabetes education can be more sophisticated; stress management; assertive communication training
Experiments to determine self-image	Begins to define self as an individual with diabetes, not as a "diabetic"	Support positive self-image and ways to integrate self-care into active lifestyle
Tests boundaries, takes risks; sense of invulnerability	May try drugs, alcohol, smoking, unprotected sex, etc.; skips doses; may not take risks because of diabetes (too scared to try)	Educate about teen issues; discuss logical consequences

Builds set of values, personal sense of morality	Determines how diabetes fits into life	Values clarification
Starts to make more lasting friendships	Determines who and when to tell about diabetes	Role-playing; communication skills
Accepts own sexuality	May become sexually active; worries how diabetes may affect sexual performance	Sexuality education; decision making
Wider interests; abstract thinking	Can participate in intensive management protocols	Diabetes education; interact directly with teen
Increased mobility	Obtaining driver's license: telling motor vehicle department about diabetes; driving safely with diabetes	Diabetes education: focus on driving responsibly
17- to 18-Year-Old Adolescents		
Idealistic	May be interested in political side of health care; may wish to participate in diabetes research; "If I do everything right, it won't happen to me"	Involve in support groups, camps, American Diabetes Association activities
Increased involvement with work and relationships; preparing to set off on own	Diabetes may cause career goals to change; what to tell employers; preparing for college life: dorm living/roommate, cafeteria food, erratic schedules, "all-nighters," etc.	Vocational counseling; role-play college issues; values clarification; diabetes education with focus on transitioning to adult care
Set course for financial or emotional independence	Health insurance; obtaining supplies	Diabetes education
Increased self-reliance	Finding an adult doctor; doctor visits on own	Diabetes education: standards of care

For the school-aged child, medical nutrition therapy challenges include school lunches, snacks, parties, and eating out. Parents begin to have less control over their child's food choices and less knowledge about what the child is eating. School-aged children must begin to develop their own meal-planning skills, including carbohydrate counting, food choices, and portion control. Planning and schedules become increasingly important as these children participate in more activities away from home. As the school-aged child begins to participate in activities outside of the home, parents will need to plan more carefully and consider

- whether the child eats a school lunch or packs a lunch from home
- changes in the child's overall schedule with each new school year
- types of food that are provided to the child at school
- planned exercise, such as physical education or after-school activities
- possible overnights, sleepovers, or school trips

Planning the school-aged child's day means considering the schedule for lunchtime, physical education and exercise time, after-school snacks, and after-school athletics. Timing of meals and snacks may vary considerably from weekday to weekend. Schedules become particularly important when the child's insulin program uses a split-mixed regimen (for example, two injections per day of NPH with Humalog). Snacks should be planned if meals are >4 h apart.

The adolescent with diabetes also finds meal planning demanding. Teens desperately want to be part of the crowd, and their nutrition habits may include frequent fast food meals, attempts at a vegetarian diet, or disordered eating behaviors. Regular soft drinks and sports drinks are favorites in this age-group and must be limited to maintain glycemic control. Teens typically do not get enough calcium or other important nutrients in their diet. At this age, boys are interested in building muscle and bulk, whereas girls are concerned about weight gain. The focus, therefore, for the teen with diabetes is controlling portion sizes, consuming fewer calorie-dense foods, and increasing fruits, vegetables, and calcium in the meal plan. Eating disorders are more common in adolescents with diabetes than in other teens (9,10). Warning signs of such problems include binge eating, skipped insulin doses, family stress, frequent hypoglycemia or diabetic ketoacidosis (DKA), and concerns about being weighed.

Medical nutrition therapy for the child with type 2 diabetes focuses on calorie reduction in the context of a healthy diet. Simple ways to decrease calories are to eliminate sugar-filled drinks, such as soda and sports drinks, and limit fruit juice portions. The entire family should limit weekly or daily visits to fast food restaurants and avoid super-sizing servings. The food-guide pyramid and the plate method are helpful teaching tools (11).

EXERCISE

As the young child with diabetes becomes more active and mobile, insulin and nutrition plans must be adjusted. For the toddler, play and erratic activity patterns are the norm. While encouraging the child's physical activity, it is important to monitor blood glucose carefully to avoid hypoglycemia. School-aged children have more predictable activity patterns, including school physical education and sports. For the child with type 1 diabetes, a snack will be necessary before exercise if his or her blood glucose level is <100 mg/dl (<5.6 mmol/l). For the child with type 2 diabetes, pre-exercise snacks are usually not necessary. For the athletic child using insulin, adjusting meals, snacks, and insulin doses is required to accommodate practice days versus game days.

Despite the importance of sports and after-school exercise, more children are leading inactive, sedentary lives. Computer games and television have replaced softball games and bike riding. The prevalence of childhood obesity is highest in children who watch about 4 hours of television per day (12), and obesity risk increases 6% for each additional hour of television viewing per day (13). Diabetes self-management education includes recommendations to limit such sedentary activities. The family should model and encourage physical activity; counseling for the obese child must include the entire family.

Case Study

Jerry is a 12-year-old who takes two injections a day, with NPH and Humalog at breakfast and supper. He has swim practice 4 days a week immediately after school. On Fridays, he has a swim meet from 6:00 to 8:00 p.m. His afternoon snack is at 3:00 p.m., and his supper is at 6:00 p.m. On Fridays, he does not want to eat a meal before swimming. After discussing his concerns with his diabetes team, he and his parents made the following adjustments for swim meet days:

- 6:00 p.m.: Have a snack (equivalent of bedtime amount of carbohydrate).
- Go to swim meet: Take blood glucose meter, insulin, and glucose gel.
- After swim meet: Dinner with the team, taking usual supper insulin dose before eating.
- Before bed: Check blood glucose. If <100 mg/dl (<5.6 mmol/l), eat a 30-g carbohydrate snack.

MEDICATIONS

There are distinct issues concerning insulin injections for the infant with diabetes. First, the infant has less surface area and thus fewer potential injection sites. Site rotation is important, with the arms, legs, and buttocks as preferred sites. Commonly available syringes and insulin pens have half-unit markings, allowing for much more precise dosing for the young child. Parents need to receive instruction in the use of half-unit syringes because the unit and half-unit markings are opposite each other on the syringe barrel on some models. Some infants require very small amounts of insulin, necessitating dilution of the insulin. Most insulin manufacturers have diluting fluid specific to the brand and type of insulin; a pharmacist is a great resource for help with diluting insulin to U10 or U25. For example, to dilute U100 insulin to U10 insulin, 0.9 cc of diluting fluid would be added to 0.1 cc of U100 insulin in a sterile mixing bottle. To administer 1 unit of insulin, 10 units (0.1 cc) is drawn into the syringe, i.e., 10 units/cc insulin.

The young child's insulin requirement will vary considerably as he or she grows. At onset, most children with type 1 diabetes require between 0.5 and 0.8 units/kg body wt/day. During the honeymoon phase, insulin requirements may drop to near zero. As the child enters puberty, insulin needs may soar to 1.0–1.5 units/kg body wt/day. Parents need to be aware that their child may require two or three dose changes per week during growth spurts. Most children will need ~50–60% of their daily dose as basal insulin. Because of the need for flexibility in dosing, commercially premixed insulins are not recommended for the child with type 1 diabetes.

Young children may be exquisitely sensitive to fast-acting insulins. Some insulin programs use only intermediate-acting insulin given several times during the day, thus providing basal requirements only. Insulin glargine may also be used as the basal insulin. For young children, rapid-acting insulin is often given after meals. This allows the parent to determine a correct dose based on what the child actually ate.

Knowing when to transfer self-care is another issue for parents and is unique to pediatric diabetes. Most children can begin to help with injections at an early age (as young as 4 years old) (14). They can select the injection site, wipe the skin with an alcohol swab, and push in the plunger after the parent has injected the needle. Many 8- to 10-year-old children have the skills to completely give an injection. Some can even accurately draw a mixed dose of insulin. How quickly a child gains these skills is highly individual. Parents can facilitate self-care by encouraging the child to participate in some small way. By the age of 10–12 years, children with diabetes are able to draw the insulin, mix doses, and inject without assistance (15). However, parental supervision is still required throughout childhood. Parents may need help with knowing when it is safe to transfer to self-care. Chronological age should not be the sole factor.

For the older child and adolescent, multiple daily injections and insulin pumps are increasingly more common forms of insulin delivery (see chapter 24 and "Is an Insulin Pump Right for Your Child and Family?" a patient handout in RESOURCES). Both systems require more involvement, skill, and knowledge from the child. Math skills become important, for instance. Even though the children may demonstrate these skills, they commonly forget meal boluses or guess at a dose. Newer pumps have reminder alarms and are able to communicate directly with blood glucose meters to calculate recommended doses for the child based on a preprogrammed algorithm.

Insulin pumps have also been successfully implemented in toddlers and preschoolers. In these children, pump therapy provides a more consistent delivery of insulin and has been associated with less hypoglycemia. Parents who are conscientious and have a strong health care team knowledgeable in pump therapy are those whose children are most successful (16).

For the child with type 2 diabetes, there are limited medication choices. Currently, only metformin is approved for children 10 years of age and older (17). Most pediatric diabetes centers are using this drug as initial therapy and adding insulin as required later.

MONITORING

Blood glucose monitoring for the young child requires some adaptation. Very-fine-gauge lancets and adjustable tips on the lancing devices are important tools. The young child's body has less surface area for fingersticks. Parents should use shallow-depth settings on the lancet devices, rotate fingerstick sites, inspect the sites for soreness, and consider alternate site testing. Alternate site testing is a good option for children but has some limitations. Blood glucose from a site other than the fingertip can vary as much as 10–15% if proper technique is not used. Testing from the forearm or other site should not be used if blood glucose is rapidly changing, if the child is having hypoglycemia, or during illness (18,19).

Blood glucose monitoring is generally recommended before each meal and at bedtime for the child with type 1 diabetes. This means that the child will be checking blood glucose at school or at daycare. Parents, school or daycare personnel, and the diabetes team will need to develop a plan that addresses *1)* location of testing, *2)* frequency of testing, *3)* management of glucose level, and *4)* safe disposal of sharps (20,21).

Additional glucose checks are needed overnight at times when the child has been unusually active in the evening, has not eaten a bedtime snack, has required extra insulin at bedtime, has been ill, or has had hypoglycemia at bedtime. Overnight testing is also helpful when evening insulin doses are being adjusted. Parents may also check a young child's blood glucose to determine the cause of behaviors such as sleepiness, crankiness, or crying. Parents want to discipline unacceptable behaviors but need to distinguish these behaviors from hypoglycemia. Postprandial blood glucose level may need to be tested to determine the adequacy of the insulin-to-carbohydrate ratio.

Goals for blood glucose levels are not standardized for children. Most diabetes teams will loosen blood glucose control in the infant or very young child. This avoids undetected hypoglycemia in the child and protects the developing CNS. On the other hand, an adolescent using an insulin pump will often have fairly tight blood glucose targets. Because blood glucose goals may be more liberal for the child with diabetes, so will the glycated hemoglobin A1c (A1C) goals. An example of modifying blood glucose and A1C targets based on age is given in Table 26.4. These goals are adjusted if the child begins to have frequent or severe hypoglycemia.

There are distinct psychosocial issues related to monitoring in children. The preschooler, for example, relies on magical thinking to explain his or her world and may, for example, believe that all of his or her blood will be lost with a fingerstick. Children this age will often insist on a Band-Aid for every fingerstick and insulin injection. School-aged children may find that peers confuse blood glucose monitoring with HIV or AIDS. Teens may avoid monitoring altogether or falsify their record books. Table 26.5 lists suggestions for assessing the child whose blood glucose logs do not match his or her A1C values.

Some parents are so anxious about their child's blood glucose that they check levels seven or eight times a day. This behavior especially occurs after a child has had severe hypoglycemia (22). These parents need time to build self-confidence

Table 26.4 Plasma Blood Glucose and A1C Goals for Type 1 Diabetes by Age-Group

Age-group (years)	Plasma blood glucose goal range		Target A1C (%)	Rationale
	Before meals (mg/dl)	Bedtime/ overnight (mg/dl)		
Toddlers and preschoolers (0–6)	100–180	110–120	≤8.5 (but ≥7.5)	High risk and vulnerability to hypoglycemia
School age (6–12)	90–180	100–180	<8	Risks of hypoglycemia and relatively low risk of complications prior to puberty
Adolescents and young adults (13–19)	90–130	90–150	<7.5	Risk of severe hypoglycemia; developmental and psychological issues; lower goal (7.0%) is reasonable if it can be achieved without excessive hypoglycemia

Key concepts in setting glycemic goals:

■ Goals should be individualized and lower goals may be reasonable based on benefit-risk assessment.

■ Blood glucose goals should be higher than those listed above in children with frequent hypoglycemia or hypoglycemia unawareness.

■ Postprandial blood glucose values should be measured when there is a disparity between preprandial blood glucose values and A1C levels.

From American Diabetes Association: Standards of medical care in diabetes—2009 (Position Statement). *Diabetes Care* 32 (Suppl. 1):S13–S61, 2009.

and to feel less scared. Strategies for helping these families include ongoing reassurance, frequent contact with the diabetes team, and adjustment of glucose targets to avoid further severe hypoglycemia (23,24).

MANAGING ROUTINE PROBLEMS

HYPOGLYCEMIA

The mechanisms for hypoglycemia in children with diabetes are similar to those in adults. However, in the very young child, limited glycogen stores or unrecognized hypoglycemia can lead to more severe or frequent episodes. For the

---

Table 26.5 Troubleshooting When the Blood Glucose Log and A1C Value Do Not Correlate

Meter factors	■ Meter coded improperly ■ Strips outdated ■ Battery low ■ Control solution outdated
User factors	■ Errors recording in log book ■ Not testing when blood glucose may be high ■ Technique errors in meter use ■ Avoiding negative responses from parents and health care professionals for having high blood glucose readings ■ Fabricating log book entries
Physiological factor	■ High postprandial or nocturnal blood glucose levels occur when testing is not done

---

toddler, excitement may lead to hypoglycemia. Illness may also be a cause of hypoglycemia in the child who is not eating well when sick. The longer a child has diabetes, the more risk for severe hypoglycemia, possibly because of defects in glucagon secretion (25).

Parents and children fear hypoglycemia, particularly overnight. They worry that the hypoglycemia will be undetected and result in seizures or death. The incidence of mild-to-moderate nocturnal hypoglycemia in children has been reported to be 14–35% (26), whereas 6.6–22% of pediatric patients will experience a hypoglycemic seizure (27). The mortality associated with hypoglycemia in children with diabetes is not well documented but may be as low as one-tenth of the mortality associated with DKA (28). Predictors of nighttime hypoglycemia include younger age and lower A1C levels. More recent studies using continuous glucose monitoring (see chapter 6) in children have found that nocturnal hypoglycemia is a common occurrence, can be prolonged, tends to happen in the early part of the night, and is associated with bedtime glucose values of <150 mg/dl (<8.3 mmol/l) (29).

There is controversy about the impact of hypoglycemia on the child's later cognitive functioning. The DCCT study group (27) in general found no association between severe hypoglycemia and decrease in memory skills. Wysocki et al. (30) also found no adverse effects on cognitive function after severe hypoglycemia.

For the adolescent who is driving, assessing and treating hypoglycemia is particularly important. Adults with type 1 diabetes have reported driving even when their blood glucose level was <40 mg/dl (31). Adolescents may make similar errors in judgment. Thus, patient education should include a discussion about responsible self-care when driving: checking blood glucose before driving, having testing supplies in the vehicle, wearing a medical identification tag, and having snacks available.

PRACTICAL POINT
Hypoglycemia in the child is treated with 10–15 g carbohydrate, with the dose repeated every 15 min as needed; this is known as the rule of 15. This treatment often needs to be followed with a snack if the next meal or snack is >1 h away. Insulin regimen, however, primarily determines the need for a snack, e.g., a child using insulin glargine likely will not need follow-up calories.

For the ill child who refuses to eat or drink and is having hypoglycemia, small doses of glucagon may be given (32). This minidose glucagon treatment is outlined in Table 26.6. Glucagon is mixed according to the package insert. The parent then uses a standard insulin syringe to withdraw an amount of glucagon appropriate for the child's age. The dose may be repeated if blood glucose does not improve.

Parents and caregivers must also know how to administer glucagon for severe hypoglycemia. The dose of glucagon for adults and children >20 kg is 1.0 mg. For children <20 kg, the glucagon dose is 0.5 mg or the equivalent of 20–30 µg/kg (33).

HYPERGLYCEMIA AND SICK DAYS

Management for the child with type 1 diabetes during illness involves fluid replacement and glucose control. When ill, infants and young children are at increased risk of dehydration, so fluid replacement is crucial to preventing DKA. Illness, colds, and infections are the main causes of hyperglycemia. But in the infant, hyperglycemia may follow routine immunizations or even teething. For the adolescent, hyperglycemia and ketosis may result from missed insulin doses (34), emotional stress, or the impact of insulin resistance due to pubertal hormones (35).

Although urine glucose testing is no longer used, urine ketone testing is still the most common tool for monitoring sick days. When blood glucose is >300 mg/dl (>16.7 mmol/l), urine ketones should be checked. Oral fluids are important at this point. The child should be encouraged to drink 0.5–1.0 cup sugar-free liquid every hour. If ketones are moderate or large, the child will also need additional fast-acting insulin. The child will need as much as 10% of the total daily dose or 0.1 units/kg of additional fast-acting insulin. This dose is repeated every 2–4 h until the blood glucose level is <300 mg/dl (16.7 mmol/l) and/or ketones fall below moderate levels. If the child is not eating, sugar-containing liquids may be needed with the frequent fast-acting insulin injections.

Parents need to know when to call for help during a sick-day episode. DKA is a medical emergency that may be avoided with early and aggressive management (36). Signs that the child will need medical attention include prolonged vomiting or diarrhea, refusing to drink, lethargy, rapid and deep (Kussmaul) breathing, signs of moderate to severe dehydration, or persistent hyperglycemia and ketosis.

Repeated episodes of DKA, often seen during adolescence, merit further assessment. These children may be depressed and often live in chaotic or stress-filled families. Family counseling and close follow-up by the diabetes team are important interventions for these children (37).

Table 26.6 Using Minidose Glucagon

Step 1: Assess Dose Amount

Age	Initial Minidose of Glucagon
0–3 years	3 "units" (amount drawn on syringe) of glucagon (i.e., 30 µg glucagon/year of age)
>3 years	1 "unit" (amount drawn in syringe) per year of age, i.e., 10 µg glucagon/year of age. The initial dose is not to exceed 15 "units."

Step 2: Observe

Check blood glucose and record values immediately before the injection and at 30 and 60 min postinjection.	The glucagon dose may be repeated every 30–60 min as long as the child is at risk of hypoglycemia and blood glucose is <60 mg/dl (3.3 mmol/l).

Step 3: Respond

Blood Glucose at 30 or 60 min After Initial Injection	Immediate Action	Follow-Up
Blood glucose >60 mg/dl (>3.3 mmol/l) and taking carbohydrate	Observe	Repeat dose if blood glucose decreases again
Blood glucose <60 mg/dl (<3.3 mmol/l), but has increased >15 mg/dl (>0.8 mmol/l)	Repeat initial dose	Measure blood glucose every 30–60 min and treat as needed
Blood glucose <60 mg/dl (<3.3 mmol/l), has increased <15 mg/dl (<0.8 mmol/l), and no severe symptoms	Double the previous dose	Measure blood glucose every 30–60 min and treat as needed
Blood glucose <60 mg/dl (<3.3 mmol/l) and severe symptoms, e.g., coma or seizure	Give 500–1,000 µg subcutaneously or intramuscularly	Call diabetes center for further instructions or call Emergency Medical Services for transport to local emergency room

PRACTICAL POINT

An easy way to collect enough urine from an infant or toddler is to place several cotton balls in the child's diaper. This will prevent the sample from being wicked into the diaper. Serum ketones provide a measurement of the more abundant β-hydroxybutyrate and may be useful in managing ketosis in the child.

CHRONIC COMPLICATIONS

When do chronic complications happen in the child with type 1 diabetes? Some believe that the clock begins to tick at puberty. One longitudinal study found that children diagnosed with type 1 diabetes before puberty, especially those diagnosed before age 5 years, have a longer time free from complications, such as retinopathy and albuminuria (38). Elevated A1C values during adolescence seem to accelerate the onset of complications.

For children with type 2 diabetes, however, cardiovascular risk factors and comorbidities may be present at diagnosis (39). The child with type 2 diabetes should therefore be assessed for hypertension and dyslipidemia.

Diabetes education for both children with type 1 diabetes and those with type 2 diabetes must include information about complications, especially detection and prevention. The nurse should provide information in a nonthreatening way and avoid scare tactics. A good approach is to focus on the positive impact of maintaining near-target blood glucose and A1C values. Having near-normal blood glucose levels may avoid future complications, but will also give the child energy to play and participate in sports. Having near-normal A1C levels will allow the child to reach maximal height potential. Maintaining euglycemia may allow parents to feel more confident and thus allow the child more independence.

SPECIAL ISSUES FOR THE CHILD WITH DIABETES

PARENTS AND OTHER FAMILY MEMBERS AND CAREGIVERS

Parents of a newly diagnosed child will grapple with confusion and guilt. They will wonder if they were responsible for their child's diabetes and how they could have prevented it (40). They will be confused and concerned. A hundred questions will arise: How did this happen? Where did it come from? What did I do or not do? Is it my fault? What about my other children? What is going to happen? They will deal with family members who have the same questions. They will find themselves explaining to and, eventually, educating anyone who comes into contact with their child. They will fear hypoglycemia and other complications. They will fear making mistakes. They will have to learn to trust other caregivers. Their parenting skills will be tested.

Threatening Versus Nonthreatening Approaches

Threatening

"Do you want to end up on dialysis or have your leg amputated? Because that's going to happen if you don't do what the doctor tells you."

Nonthreatening

"Lowering your overall blood glucose levels will help prevent the complications from diabetes. What is the hardest thing to do when taking care of your diabetes?" Give them time to answer. "Maybe together we can find a way to make that a little easier."

The diabetes team can best help parents by providing consistent, accurate information and encouraging hope and optimism. Parents need to have their efforts and successes recognized. They need role models and support from other families. They need accurate information about the risk of diabetes for their other children (41). Families that are most successful in raising a child with diabetes are highly cohesive and organized. The parents share open communication and provide consistent guidance and problem solving. Successful parents are typically warm and nurturing (42–44).

The sibling's response to diabetes may range from feeling guilty and responsible to being fearful of also developing the disease. Some nondiabetic children hope they do get diabetes so they will get as much attention as their sibling with diabetes. Older siblings often feel extraordinarily responsible for the care of their brother or sister. They worry about hypoglycemia and monitor the child's food choices. Siblings are often forgotten in the care plans and teaching sessions. It is important to prepare families for the typical reactions of siblings to the child's diabetes.

Diabetes is also a concern for others outside of the child's immediate family. As the child grows, he or she will be in the care of many other adults: teachers, school nurses, daycare workers, babysitters, and so forth. Any care plan or teaching plan must include these other individuals. Babysitters in particular must be educated about basic diabetes care. Instructions should include how and when to prepare meals and snacks, how to detect and treat hypoglycemia, and how to check blood glucose and urine ketones. Other instructions may include who to call and when to call for help.

SCHOOL

Returning to school after diagnosis or starting a new school year can mark new challenges for the family and child with diabetes. While parents want a knowledgeable and trained adult to be available for their child, school administrators may struggle with competing demands on personnel and resources. In this case, parents will need to be leaders and advocates for the child (45). Federal laws and some state laws protect children with diabetes from discrimination in daycare settings and schools. However, parents will have to educate each new school or caregiver about the particular needs of their child.

First, parents should meet with the appropriate school personnel and be prepared to identify resources that will help educate them about diabetes in children and to provide child-specific training and information on how to best meet the needs of their child. Many schools do not have a full-time nurse on staff, and many times a school nurse is not available, so a small group of school staff members should be trained to provide routine and emergency care. While many teachers, coaches, and principals are familiar with diabetes in adults, they often lack an accurate appreciation for the differences in safely managing diabetes in children.

At the meeting, parents should collaborate with the school nurse and school administrator to implement a Diabetes Medical Management Plan (DMMP). This plan should address blood glucose targets and checking, insulin and pump management, identifying and treating hypoglycemia and hyperglycemia, supplies to be kept at school, and ability of the student to provide self-care. The DMMP should be prepared and signed by the child's health care provider.

In addition to the DMMP, the parents should ask that a 504 Plan or Individual Education Program (IEP) be implemented for their child. The 504 Plan (a plan for services under Section 504 of the Rehabilitation Act of 1973) and the IEP (a plan for services under the Individuals with Disabilities Education Act) complement the DMMP by assuring that the child's rights and needs are being appropriately and formally addressed. Samples of both a DMMP and a 504 plan are available from the American Diabetes Association (ADA) at www.diabetes.org.

At times, parents may run into resistance and need to advocate at a more aggressive level. It may be necessary to contact school officials with more authority. In such cases, parents should be knowledgeable about the law and legal rights and stay calm and confident as they advocate for their child. Parents may also seek other support from elected officials, their health care team, or the ADA.

A valuable resource for the school nurse and other school personnel, titled "Helping the Student with Diabetes Succeed: A Guide for School Personnel," has been developed by the National Diabetes Education Program (NDEP), in partnership with over 200 other organizations. This guide is available online at http://www.diabetes.org/for-parents-and-kids/diabetes-and-the-law/ndep.jsp and provides valuable information for the school nurse in guiding others in understanding diabetes and in providing a safe environment for all children with diabetes. In addition to the NDEP school guide, ADA's two-disk training set *Diabetes Care Tasks at School: What Key Personnel Need to Know* can be used by the school nurse or another qualified health care professional to train school personnel; it is available in ADA's online store at http://store.diabetes.org.

DIABETES CAMPS

One of the best places for peer support for the child with diabetes is a summer camping program or weekend retreat. Diabetes camps expose the child to other children with diabetes in a nonthreatening way. The focus of the camp will vary from an educational agenda to a purely recreational one. Children will often learn to give their first injections or may try a new injection site at camp. Both the American Camping Association and the ADA maintain lists of recommended camps for children with diabetes.

TRANSFERRING CARE TO THE CHILD

Parents must maintain a role in their child's care through adolescence. But that role changes from caregiver to coach as the child matures. Gradually, the child will need to take over his or her own care. The speed of the transfer and the skills to be transferred will vary with each child. Tips to keep in mind when transferring care to the child are included in Table 26.7.

Generally, school-aged children are ready to begin drawing and injecting insulin. Older school children and adolescents have the math skills necessary to make insulin dose decisions (15,46,47).

ADOLESCENT ISSUES

For the adolescent with diabetes, there are unique and complicating factors. Puberty creates an insulin-resistant state in the adolescent, making glycemic

Table 26.7 Transferring Responsibility of Diabetes Care to the Child

- Consider each child individually.
  - Is the child ready and eager to assume self-care?
  - What is motivating the child to take on self-care tasks?
  - Does the child have the physical dexterity and cognitive ability to take on the self-care task?
- Consider the parents' assessment of the child's readiness.
- Assess the parents' willingness to "let go."
  - How comfortable is the parent in allowing mistakes?
  - How much supervision will the parent continue to provide?
- Transfer care in small, manageable steps.
- Expect lapses in self-care, at any age.
  - The parent still has an important role in supervision and guidance.

control more challenging (48). On the other hand, chronic, suboptimal glycemic control can delay puberty. The teen's self-esteem and body image can be affected by the diagnosis of diabetes and its daily demands. The seemingly constant attention to food, nutrition, and blood glucose may contribute to eating disorders in some teens. Omitting insulin doses to control weight is common (49). Also, normal developmental phases, which may include experimentation with drugs, smoking, or alcohol, can be particularly risky for the adolescent with diabetes.

In addition, at a time when the young person is seeking differentiation and independence, parents may feel more overprotective and concerned (50). When parents most need to understand what is happening with the teen's diabetes management, communication may be the most strained. Parents are often not prepared for their changing role from caretaker to coach and supporter.

Adolescents with diabetes may also suffer from depression or diabetes burnout. Sometimes the signs of these problems are mistaken for typical adolescent behavior. Depression, for example, is two to three times more prevalent in youth with diabetes than in their nondiabetic peers (51). Depression in the adolescent may display as withdrawal, dramatic changes in sleeping or eating patterns, lack of goals, or suicidal ideation. Further clinical evaluation and management is needed for the teen with depression.

Diabetes burnout in the adolescent, however, may appear as feelings of failure or hopelessness, omission of insulin injections or blood glucose monitoring, or loss of motivation (52). These teens typically have high A1C values and suboptimal self-care behavior. Management for these adolescents may include more flexible, less complex insulin regimens, such as the use of commercially premixed insulin pens twice a day. Other strategies include setting realistic goals for self-care behavior, acknowledging the teen's feelings, and reinforcing the adolescent's efforts at self-care. Helping parents provide further guidance and support is also important. Teaching the teen social skills, problem-solving skills, effective communication, and stress-management skills can increase the young person's self-efficacy and sense of control (53,54). Referral for behavioral health services may be beneficial.

TRANSITION TO ADULT CARE

When the adolescent approaches adulthood, he or she will transition from pediatric to adult diabetes care. Many young adults will make this change between 17 and 20 years of age. Such transitions can be fraught with problems. The adolescent/young adult may still be living at home with some parental input or may be dealing with the stress of school, choosing a career, and evolving personal relationships. Poor transition to adult care may result in years of unsupervised medical management and limited complication prevention (55,56). In addition to the adolescent's concerns, parents may be anxious about moving to a more formal, less supportive environment that encourages the teen's independence. Health care professionals themselves who only treat adults may fail to appreciate the anxiety that this transition can present. The health care professional should help the family through this transition by introducing the topic in early adolescence and by aiding in gradually transferring care and independence to the emerging young adult.

SUMMARY

The challenges posed by diabetes during childhood require the nurse to find creative solutions based on knowledge of normal growth and development. Such innovative strategies will help the growing child and adolescent emerge with the emotional and technical skills necessary for a lifetime of successful diabetes self-care. Nurses play a key role in the support of children with diabetes and their families by providing support and appropriate resources, including referral to child specialists, diabetes camps, and other local resources. Establishing healthy lifestyle behaviors as a child will carry into adulthood.

REFERENCES

1. Kaufman F: Type 2 diabetes in children and youth: a new epidemic. *J Pediatr Endocrinol Metab* 15 (Suppl. 2):737–744, 2002

2. Rosenbloom A, Silverstein J: *Type 2 Diabetes in Children and Adolescents: A Guide to Diagnosis, Epidemiology, Pathogenesis, Prevention, and Treatment.* Alexandria, VA, American Diabetes Association, 2003

3. Rewers M, Norris J, Kretowski A: Epidemiology of type 1 diabetes. In *Type 1 Diabetes: Molecular, Cellular, and Clinical Immunology.* Online edition 3.0. Eisenbarth G, Ed. Available from http://www.uchsc.edu/misc/diabetes/books/type1/type1.html. Accessed 26 February 2009

4. Lombardo F, Valenzise M, Wasniewska M, Messina M, Ruggeri C, et al.: Two-year prospective evaluation of the factors affecting honeymoon frequency and duration in children with insulin dependent diabetes mellitus: the key-role of age at diagnosis. *Diabetes Nutr Metab* 15:246–251, 2002

5. Abdul-Rasoul M, Habib H, Al-Khouly M: 'The honeymoon phase' in children with type 1 diabetes mellitus: frequency, duration, and influential factors. *Pediatric Diabetes* 7:101–107, 2006

6. Franzese A, Iorio R, Buono M, Mascolo M, Mozzillo E: Mauriac syndrome still exists. *Diabetes Res Clin Pract* 54:219–221, 2000

7. Silverstein J, Deeb L, Klingensmith G, Grey M, Copeland K, et al.: Care of children and adolescents with type 1 diabetes. *Diabetes Care* 28:186–212, 2005

8. Schreiner B: Disorders of pancreatic hormone secretion: diabetes mellitus. In *Wong's Nursing Care of Infants and Children*. 7th ed. Wong D, Hockenberry M, Eds. St. Louis, MO, Mosby, 2002

9. Hoffman R: Eating disorders in adolescents with type 1 diabetes: a closer look at a complicated condition. *Postgrad Med* 109:67–69, 73–74, 2001

10. Kelly S, Howe C, Hendler J, Lipman T: Disordered eating behaviors in youth with type 1 diabetes. *Diabetes Educ* 34:572–583, 2005

11. Brosnan C, Upchurch S, Schreiner B: Type 2 diabetes in children and adolescents: an emerging disease. *J Pediatr Health Care* 15:187–193, 2001

12. Crespo C, Smit E, Troriano R, Cartlett S, Macera C, Andersen R: Television watching, energy intake and obesity in US children: results from the Third National Health and Nutrition Examination Survey, 1984–1994. *Arch Pediatr Adolesc Med* 155:360–365, 2001

13. Dennison B, Erb T, Jenkins P: Television viewing and television in bedroom associated with overweight risk among low-income preschool children. *Pediatrics* 109:1028–1035, 2002

14. Banion C, Valentine V: Type 1 diabetes throughout the life span. In *The Art and Science of Diabetes Self-Management Education*. Mensing C, Ed. Chicago, American Association of Diabetes Educators, 2006

15. Helgeson VS, Reynolds KA, Siminerio L, Escobar O, Becker D: Parent and adolescent distribution of responsibility for diabetes self-care: links to health outcomes. *J Pediatr Psychol* 33:497–508, 2008

16. Litton J, Rice A, Friedman N, Oden J, Lee M, Freemark M: Insulin pump therapy in toddlers and preschool children with type 1 diabetes mellitus. *J Pediatr* 141:490–495, 2002

17. Jones K, Arslanian S, Peterokova V, Park J, Tomlinson M: Effect of metformin in pediatric patients with type 2 diabetes: a randomized controlled trial. *Diabetes Care* 25:89–94, 2002

18. Jungheim K, Koschinsky T: Glucose monitoring at the arm: risky delays of hypoglycemia and hyperglycemia detection. *Diabetes Care* 25:956–960, 2002

19. Ellison J, Stegmann J, Colner S, Michael R, Sharma M, et al.: Rapid changes in postprandial blood glucose produce concentration differences at finger, forearm, and thigh sampling sites. *Diabetes Care* 25:961–964, 2002

20. American Diabetes Association: Diabetes care in the school and day care setting (Position Statement). *Diabetes Care* 28 (Suppl. 1):S43–S49, 2005

21. National Diabetes Education Program: *Helping the Student with Diabetes Succeed: A Guide for School Personnel.* Bethesda, MD, U.S. Department of Heath and Human Services, 2003

22. Streisand R, Swift E, Wickmark T, Chen R, Holmes C: Pediatric parenting stress among parents of children with type 1 diabetes: the role of self-efficacy, responsibility, and fear. *J Pediatr Psychol* 30:513–521, 2005

23. Loy V: *Real Life Parenting of Kids with Diabetes.* Alexandria, VA, American Diabetes Association, 2001

24. Sullivan-Bolyai S, Deatrick J, Gruppuso P, Tamborlane W, Grey M: Constant vigilance: mothers' work parenting young children with type 1 diabetes. *J Pediatr Nurs* 18:21–29, 2003

25. Rewers A, Chase P, Mackenzie T, Walravens P, Roback M, et al.: Predictors of acute complications in children with type 1 diabetes. *JAMA* 287:2511–2518, 2002

26. Children Network (DirecNet) Study Group: Impaired overnight counterregulatory hormone responses to spontaneous hypoglycemia in children with type 1 diabetes. *Pediatric Diabetes* 8:199–205, 2007

27. The Diabetes Control and Complications Trial/Epidemiology of Diabetes Interventions and Complications (DCCT/EDIC) Study Research Group: Long-term effect of diabetes and its treatment on cognitive function. *N Engl J Med* 356:1842–1852, 2007

28. Daneman D: Diabetes-related mortality: a pediatrician's view (Editorial). *Diabetes Care* 24:801–802, 2001

29. Kaufman F, Austin J, Neinstein A, Jeng L, Halvorson M, et al.: Nocturnal hypoglycemia detected with the continuous glucose monitoring system in pediatric patients with type 1 diabetes. *J Pediatr* 141:625–630, 2002

30. Wysocki T, Harris M, Mauras N, Fox L, Taylor A, et al.: Absence of adverse effects of severe hypoglycemia on cognitive function in school-aged children with diabetes over 18 months. *Diabetes Care* 26:1100–1105, 2003

31. Clarke W, Cox D, Gonder-Frederick L, Kovatchev B: Hypoglycemia and the decision to drive a motor vehicle by persons with diabetes. *JAMA* 282:750–754, 1999

32. Haymond M, Schreiner B: Use of mini-dose glucagon in children with impending hypoglycemia. *Diabetes Care* 24:643–645, 2001

33. Eli Lilly: Glucagon for injection [package insert]. Indianapolis, IN, 18 Feb 2005

34. Bismuth E, Laffel L: Can we prevent diabetic ketoacidosis in children? *Pediatr Diabetes* 6:24–33, 2007

35. Szadkowska A, Pietrzak I, Mianowska B, Bodalska-Lipińska J, Keenan H, et al.: Insulin sensitivity in type 1 diabetic children and adolescents. *Diabet Med* 25:282–288, 2008

36. Glaser N, Barnett P, McCaslin I, Nelson D, Trainor J, et al.: Risk factors for cerebral edema in children with diabetic ketoacidosis. *N Engl J Med* 344:264–269, 2001

37. Skinner T: Recurrent diabetic ketoacidosis: causes, prevention and management. *Horm Res* 57 (Suppl. 1):78–80, 2002

38. Donoghue K, Fairchild J, Craig M, Chan A, Hing S, et al.: Do all prepubertal years of diabetes duration contribute equally to diabetes complications? *Diabetes Care* 26:1224–1229, 2003

39. Goran M, Beall G, Cruz M: Obesity and risk of type 2 diabetes and cardiovascular disease in children and adolescents. *J Clin Endocrinol Metab* 88:1417–1427, 2003

40. Lowes L, Gregory J, Line P: Newly diagnosed childhood diabetes: a psychosocial transition for parents? *Adv Nurs* 50:253–261, 2005

41. Barker J, Barriga K, Yu L, Miao D, Erlich H, et al.: Prediction of autoantibody positivity and progression to type 1 diabetes: Diabetes Autoimmunity Study in the Young (DAISY). *J Clin Endocrinol Metab* 89:3896–3902, 2004

42. Anderson B, Rubin R: *Practical Psychology for Diabetes Clinicians.* 2nd ed. Alexandria, VA, American Diabetes Association, 2002

43. Anderson B, Vangsness L, Connell A, Butler D, Goebel-Fabbri A, Laffel L: Family conflict, adherence, and glycaemic control in youth with short duration type 1 diabetes. *Diabet Med* 19:635–642, 2002

44. Thompson S, Auslander W, White N: Influence of family structure on health among youths with diabetes. *Health Soc Work* 26:7–14, 2001

45. Kaufman F: Diabetes at school: what a child's health care team needs to know about the federal disability law (Commentary). *Clinical Diabetes* 20:91–92, 2002

46. Schilling L, Knafl K, Grey M: Changing patterns of self-management in youth with type I diabetes. *J Pediatr Nurs* 21:412–424, 2006

47. Wysocki T: *The Ten Keys to Helping Your Child Grow Up with Diabetes.* 2nd ed. Alexandria, VA, American Diabetes Association, 2004

48. Hamilton J, Daneman D: Deteriorating diabetes control during adolescence: physiological or psychosocial? *J Pediatr Endocrinol Metab* 15:115–126, 2002

49. Neumark-Sztainer D, Patterson J, Mellin A, Ackard D, Utter J, et al.: Weight control practices and disordered eating behaviors among adolescent females and males with type 1 diabetes: associations with sociodemographics, weight concerns, familial factors, and metabolic outcomes. *Diabetes Care* 25:1289–1296, 2002

50. Hanna K, Guthrie D: Adolescents' behavioral autonomy related to diabetes management and adolescent activities/rules. *Diabetes Educ* 29:283–291, 2003

51. Grey M, Whittemore R, Tamborlane W: Depression in type 1 diabetes in children: natural history and correlates. *J Psychosom Res* 53:907–911, 2002

52. Polonsky W: *Diabetes Burnout: What to Do When You Can't Take It Anymore* (book and audiotape). Alexandria, VA, American Diabetes Association, 1999

53. Grey M, Boland E, Davidson M, Li J, Tamborlane W: Coping skills training for youth with diabetes mellitus has long-lasting effects on metabolic control and quality of life. *J Pediatr* 137:107–113, 2000

54. Grey M, Davidson M, Boland E, Tamborlane W: Clinical and psychosocial factors associated with achievement of treatment goals in adolescents with diabetes mellitus. *J Adolesc Health* 28:377–385, 2001

55. Fleming E, Carter B, Gillibrand W: The transition of adolescents with diabetes from the children's health care service into the adult health care service: a review of the literature. *J Clin Nurs* 11:560–567, 2002

56. Weissberg-Benchell J, Wolpert H, Anderson BJ: transitioning from pediatric to adult care: a new approach to the post-adolescent young person with type 1 diabetes. *Diabetes Care* 30:2441–2446, 2007

Ms. Schreiner is a senior clinical education specialist with Amylin Pharmaceuticals, Inc., and a co-investigator with the TODAY study of type 2 diabetes in children.

27. Diabetes in the Elderly

Barbara Kocurek, PharmD, BCPS, CDE

In 1889, Otto von Bismarck of Germany set the arbitrary age of 65 years as the criterion necessary to receive benefits from a social security system. The U.S. adopted this age for its own social security system in 1935, and our definition of "elderly" was born.

In 2006, there were 37.3 million people, or 12.4% of the U.S. population, aged 65 years or older. It is projected that by 2030, this number will increase to 71.5 million people, or ~20% of the U.S. population (1). Age is a risk factor for developing diabetes, and the elderly now represent an increasingly larger portion of people newly diagnosed with diabetes (2). With the rising costs of health care, lack of prescription coverage, and lower economic status of many older Americans, diabetes in the elderly will be an important health care concern throughout the 21st century (3). Undiagnosed and untreated diabetes is more common in the elderly than in any other age-group (4). One-half of older individuals with diabetes are unaware of their illness, which may be related to physiological changes that occur with aging, such as the increase in renal threshold for glucose (3).

CLINICAL PRACTICE GUIDELINES

In 2003, the American Geriatrics Society published "Guidelines for Improving the Care of the Older Person with Diabetes Mellitus." These guidelines provide comprehensive information regarding the elderly and diabetes care and are included in Table 27.1 (5). The American Diabetes Association Clinical Practice Recommendations set the standards of care for patients with diabetes, including recommendations for older adults. These recommendations are listed in Table 27.2 (6).

Table 27.1 American Geriatrics Society Principles for the Care of the Elderly Adult with Diabetes

Aspirin	■ The older adult with diabetes who is not on other anticoagulant therapy and does not have any contraindications to aspirin should be offered daily aspirin therapy (81–325 mg/day).
Smoking	■ The older adult who has diabetes and smokes should be assessed for willingness to quit and should be offered counseling and pharmacological interventions to assist with smoking cessation.
Hypertension	■ If an older adult has diabetes and requires medical therapy for hypertension, the target blood pressure should be <140/80 mmHg if tolerated. Epidemiologic evidence shows that lowering blood pressure to <130/80 mmHg may provide further benefit. ■ Because older adults may have decreased tolerance for blood pressure reduction, hypertension should be treated gradually to avoid complications. ■ The older adult with diabetes and hypertension should be offered pharmacological and behavioral interventions to lower blood pressure within 3 months if systolic blood pressure is 140–160 mmHg or diastolic blood pressure is 90–100 mmHg or within 1 month if blood pressure is >160/100 mmHg.
Medication	■ The older adult with diabetes who is on an angiotensin-converting enzyme inhibitor or angiotensin receptor blocker should have renal function and serum potassium levels monitored within 1–2 weeks of initiation of therapy, with each dose increase, and at least annually. ■ The older adult with diabetes on a thiazide or loop diuretic should have his or her electrolytes checked within 1–2 weeks of initiation of therapy or increase in dosage and at least annually.
Glycemic control General *recommendations*	■ For older individuals, target A1C level should be individualized. A reasonable goal for A1C in relatively healthy adults with good functional status is <7%. For frail older individuals with a life expectancy of <5 years and others for whom the risks of intensive glycemic control appear to outweigh the benefits, a less stringent target of 8% is appropriate.
Monitoring	■ The older adult who has diabetes and whose individual targets are not being met should have A1C levels measured at least every 6 months. For individuals with stable A1C levels over several years, an annual measurement may be appropriate. ■ For the older adult with diabetes, a schedule for self-monitoring of blood glucose should be considered, depending on the individual's functional and cognitive abilities.

Table 27.1 American Geriatrics Society Principles for the Care of the Elderly Adult with Diabetes (*Continued*)

	■ The management plan for the older adult with diabetes who has severe or frequent hypoglycemic episodes should be evaluated. The patient should be offered referral to a diabetes educator or endocrinologist, and the patient and caregivers should have more frequent contacts with the health care team (e.g., physicians, certified diabetes educators, pharmacists, nurse case manager) while therapy is being adjusted.
Medications	■ If an older adult is prescribed an oral antidiabetic agent, chlorpropamide should not be used.
	■ Metformin is contraindicated when serum creatinine levels are ≥1.5 mg/dl in men and ≥1.4 mg/dl in women or in anyone with decreased creatinine clearance because of increased risk of lactic acidosis.
	■ The older adult with diabetes who is taking metformin should have serum creatinine measured at least annually and with any increase in dose. Individuals ≥80 years of age or those who have reduced muscle mass need a timed urine collection for measurement of creatinine clearance.
Lipids	■ For the older adult with diabetes who has dyslipidemia, efforts should be made to correct the lipid abnormalities, if feasible.
	■ The older adult with diabetes and an elevated LDL cholesterol level should be managed according to the severity of elevation.
	• ≤100 mg/dl: Lipid status should be rechecked at least every 2 years.
	• 100–129 mg/dl: Medical nutrition therapy and increased physical activity are recommended, lipid status should be checked at least annually, and response to therapy should be monitored. If an LDL ≤100 mg/dl is not achieved in 6 months, then pharmacological therapy should be initiated, if feasible.
	• ≥130 mg/dl: Pharmacological therapy is required in addition to lifestyle modification, lipid status should be checked at least annually, and response to therapy should be monitored.
	■ The older adult with diabetes who is newly prescribed or has had a dosage increase in niacin or a statin should have his or her alanine aminotransferase level measured within 12 weeks.
	■ The older adult with diabetes who is taking a fibrate should have an annual evaluation of liver enzymes.
Eye care	■ The older adult with new-onset diabetes should have an initial screening dilated eye examination performed by an eye care specialist with fundoscopic training.

(*continued*)

Table 27.1 American Geriatrics Society Principles for the Care of the Elderly Adult with Diabetes (*Continued*)

	■ The older adult with diabetes who is at high risk for eye disease (symptoms of eye disease present; evidence of retinopathy, glaucoma, or cataracts on an initial dilated eye examination or subsequent examinations during the prior 2 years; A1C ≥8%; type 1 diabetes; or blood pressure ≥140/80 mmHg) should have a dilated eye examination at least every 2 years.
Foot care	■ The older adult with diabetes should have a foot examination at least annually to evaluate skin integrity and check for bone deformity, sensation loss, or decreased perfusion. Examinations should be performed more frequently if there is positive evidence for any of these criteria.
Nephropathy	■ A test for the presence of microalbumin should be performed at the time of diagnosis in patients with type 2 diabetes. After the initial screening and in the absence of previously demonstrated macro- or microalbuminuria, a test for the presence of microalbumin should be performed annually.
Diabetes education	■ Individuals with diabetes and, if appropriate, family members and caregivers should be given written and verbal information about hypo- and hyperglycemia at diagnosis, with reassessment and reinforcement periodically as needed. Such documentation should include the following: • precipitating factors • prevention • symptoms and monitoring • treatment • when to notify a member of the health care team ■ The monitoring technique of the older adult with diabetes who self-monitors blood glucose levels should be routinely reviewed. ■ The older adult with diabetes should be evaluated regularly for level of physical activity and should be informed about the benefits of exercise and available resources for becoming more active. ■ The older adult with diabetes should be evaluated regularly for diet and nutritional status, and, if appropriate, referral for culturally appropriate medical nutrition therapy should be offered. Particular attention should be focused on the intake of high-cholesterol foods, the appropriate intake of carbohydrates, and the potential benefits of weight reduction. ■ The older adult with diabetes and any caregiver should receive education about the purpose of any medication, how to take it, common side effects, and important adverse reactions. All medications should be reviewed, and education should be periodically reinforced as needed.

Table 27.1 American Geriatrics Society Principles for the Care of the Elderly Adult with Diabetes (*Continued*)

	■ Education should be provided regarding the risk factors for foot ulcers and amputation. Physical ability to provide proper foot care should be evaluated, with periodic reassessment and reinforcement as needed.
Depression	■ The older adult with diabetes is at increased risk of major depression and should be screened for depression during the initial evaluation period (first 3 months) and when there is any unexplained decline in clinical status. ■ Any new onset or recurrence of depression should be referred for treatment. If the patient presents a danger to him- or herself or to others, an emergency evaluation is warranted. ■ The older adult who has received therapy for depression should be evaluated for improvement in target symptoms within 6 weeks of the initiation of therapy.
Polypharmacy (see chapter 23)	■ The older adult with diabetes should be advised to maintain an updated medication list for review by the clinician. ■ The medication list of an older adult with diabetes who presents with depression, falls, cognitive impairment, or urinary incontinence requires review.
Cognitive impairment	■ Use a standardized screening instrument at the initial visit and with any significant decline in clinical status. Increased difficulty with self-care should be considered a change in clinical status. ■ Referrals should be made to the neurology department if there is evidence of cognitive impairment.
Urinary incontinence	■ Evaluation for symptoms of urinary incontinence should be performed during annual screening and referred to the urology department if needed.
Injurious falls	■ The older adult who has diabetes should be asked about falls. ■ If an older adult presents with evidence of falls, the clinician should document a basic falls evaluation, including an assessment of injuries and examination of potentially reversible causes of the falls (e.g., medications, environmental factors).
Pain	The older adult who has diabetes should be assessed during the initial evaluation period for evidence of persistent pain.

Adapted from Brown et al. (5).

Table 27.2 American Diabetes Association Recommendations for Older Adults

- Older adults who are functional, cognitively intact, and have significant life expectancy should receive diabetes treatment using goals developed for younger adults.
- Glycemic goals for older adults not meeting the above criteria may be relaxed using individual criteria, but hyperglycemia leading to symptoms or risk of acute hyperglycemic complications should be avoided in all patients.
- Other cardiovascular risk factors should be treated in older adults with consideration of the timeframe of benefit and the individual patient. Treatment of hypertension is indicated in virtually all older adults, and lipid and aspirin therapy may benefit those with life expectancy at least equal to the timeframe of primary or secondary prevention trials.
- Screening for diabetic complications should be individualized in older adults, but particular attention should be paid to complications that would lead to functional impairment.

Adapted from the American Diabetes Association (6).

SPECIAL CONSIDERATIONS IN THE ELDERLY

Successful care of older individuals with diabetes requires an understanding of the effects of the aging process in general as well as issues specific to the disease in this population. While glycemic targets should not be automatically raised in the elderly, the risks and benefits of glycated hemoglobin A1c (A1C) levels <7% should be considered. It may be safer for certain elderly individuals (e.g., those who are frail, live alone, are unable to recognize signs and symptoms of hypoglycemia) to aim for A1C levels over 7%.

Cognitive dysfunction has been associated with poor diabetes control in the elderly. This can affect the ability to effectively perform diabetes self-management (7) and can be a safety issue. It is important to screen for cognitive dysfunction in this population. Sources of support may also be needed in terms of reminders to eat or take medications and should be assessed.

One of the concerns with achieving tight blood glucose control in the elderly is the risk of hypoglycemia. It has been suggested that the elderly are, in general, less able to detect signs of hypoglycemia and are particularly at risk for this acute complication (8). Until recently, many health care professionals believed that blood glucose levels should be higher in the elderly than in the general adult population. This has been supported by the fear that the elderly are more susceptible to oral agent–induced hypoglycemia and less sensitive to the warning signs of hypoglycemia (8). However, findings from the U.K. Prospective Diabetes Study showed that severe hypoglycemia among individuals with type 2 diabetes is a rare event (9). Tighter blood glucose control can be considered in the elderly, especially because there are several oral diabetes medications on the market that have lower incidences of hypoglycemia. If severe or frequent hypoglycemic events do occur in an individual, the causes should be investigated and corrected. This

Table 27.3 Special Considerations for Antidiabetic Medication Use in the Elderly

α-Glucosidase inhibitors: Use with caution in patients with gastrointestinal disease; the adverse effects may be troublesome.

Biguanide: Contraindicated in patients with elevated serum creatinine (men ≥1.5 mg/dl and women ≥1.4 mg/dl). A baseline creatinine measurement should be obtained before starting therapy and when a possible change in renal function has occurred.

DPP4 Inhibitors: Dosage adjustment needed in renal dysfunction

Incretin Mimetics: none known at this time

Sulfonylureas: Increased risk of hypoglycemia

Thiazolidinediones: Use with caution in patients with congestive heart failure. Thiazolidinediones can cause fluid retention and weight gain in individuals with a history of cardiac disease, chronic obstructive pulmonary disease, or liver disease. Liver enzymes should be obtained before starting therapy and periodically thereafter.

Insulins: Administration requires technical skill, visual acuity, and willingness to use.
Adapted from Odegard et al. (10).

may be an indication to change to an oral agent with a low or lower risk of hypoglycemia.

The choice of antidiabetic medication in an elderly individual depends on several factors, including renal and liver function and the ability to purchase medications and adhere to the regimen. In general, medications should be started at the lowest dose and titrated gradually until blood glucose goals are achieved. The short-acting insulin secretagogues, such as repaglinide and nateglinide, may be a good choice for the elderly because they carry a lower risk of hypoglycemia than sulfonylureas. However, adherence may be an issue because of premeal dosing, which usually requires medication doses three times a day. Insulin use should be considered in an elderly individual who is unable to take oral agents or has an A1C level above target (>7%). Use of insulin requires good visual and motor skills as well as the ability to learn and perform accurate and safe administration. Specific cautions regarding antidiabetic medications in the elderly are listed in Table 27.3 (10).

Advanced age can create special challenges in medical nutrition therapy. Food preferences may change, and food consumption may decrease as age-related changes in taste and olfaction occur (4). The social and economic issues facing some elderly people may force them into poor eating habits, such as choosing to eat more canned foods, frozen foods, or fast foods. An assessment of current eating habits, as well as dentition and swallowing ability, should be conducted to establish a realistic, individualized meal plan. Older adults with diabetes in long-term care facilities are often underweight (11). Even if being overweight is a contributing factor to diabetes, weight loss should be carefully considered because a restrictive diet in older adults may lead to nutrient deficits (11). The goal of medical nutrition therapy in the elderly with diabetes is to meet their nutritional needs and keep blood glucose, blood pressure, and blood lipids as close to normal as possible. Emphasis should be placed on the timing of meals as well as consistency in the amount eaten at each meal.

Table 27.4 Physiological Changes that Occur with Aging

Neurological	■ Decrease in auditory acuity ■ Decreased ability to taste sweet, sour, and bitter foods (ability to taste salty foods unchanged) ■ Generalized decreased sensation, including response to pain ■ Decrease in thirst response
Ophthalmologic	■ Decrease in lens transparency and presbyopia
Body composition	■ Decreased lean body mass and increased body fat ■ Decrease in extracellular fluid volume, plasma volume, and total body water
Gastrointestinal	■ Decrease in saliva production ■ Delays in transit time ■ Achlorhydria
Hepatic	■ Decreased liver size and weight ■ Decreased phase I (oxidative) metabolism
Renal	■ Decrease in glomerular filtration rate ■ Decreased renal blood flow
Endocrine	■ Hypothyroidism occurs secondary to atrophy of the thyroid gland ■ Decreased glucose-stimulated insulin release

The benefits of physical activity should be discussed. An individual's exercise plan should be based on activity preferences and physical limitations, such as visual impairment and neuropathy. Cardiac status should be monitored, a treadmill test should be performed, and any symptoms suggestive of cardiac decompensation must be assessed before an exercise program is initiated and then periodically thereafter. It may be appropriate to recommend the use of stationary bikes, walking, water aerobics, or exercise videos, such as the Armchair Fitness series.

The elderly are more prone to the effects of polypharmacy, defined as the use of medications that are not clinically indicated (12). Physiological changes that occur with aging (Table 27.4) can affect how medications are handled by the body and increase susceptibility to adverse drug reactions and interactions. Chapter 23 discusses strategies for dealing with polypharmacy in individuals with diabetes.

SUMMARY

Nurses play a pivotal role in advocating for the elderly. Effective diabetes education gives patients the knowledge and skills needed to manage their diabetes successfully. The capacity to learn and integrate new information remains intact throughout the life cycle, although age-related changes can affect this process (4). The nurse should perform an individualized learning-needs assessment, and educational strategies should be adjusted accordingly. A properly paced, stepwise method of teaching, with the provision of practical information focused on maintaining independence and quality of life, is an effective approach for older adults (4,13).

Treatment of elderly patients with diabetes is challenging because of the multiple comorbidities, social factors, and opportunities for polypharmacy. Their care requires a team approach (3). Multidisciplinary programs, particularly those involving family members caring for the patient, have been shown to result in improved adherence to therapy and better blood glucose control (3).

PRACTICAL POINT

Goals of Diabetes Care in the Elderly (5)

- Control of hyperglycemia and its symptoms
- Prevention, evaluation, and treatment of macro- and microvascular complications
- Self-management through education
- Maintenance or improvement of general health status

REFERENCES

1. Administration on Aging web site. Available from http://www.aoa.gov/prof/statistics/statistics.aspx. Accessed 26 February 2009

2. Selvin ES, Coresh J, Brancati FL: The burden and treatment of diabetes in elderly individuals in the U.S. *Diabetes Care* 29:2415–2410, 2006

3. Meneilly GS, Tessier D: Diabetes in elderly adults. *J Gerontol* 56:M5–M13, 2001

4. American Association of Diabetes Educators: Special considerations for the education and management of older adults with diabetes (Position Statement). *Diabetes Educ* 29:93–96, 2003

5. Brown AF, Mangione CM, Saliba D, Sarkisian CA: Guidelines for improving the care of the older person with diabetes mellitus. *J Am Geriatr Soc* 51 (Suppl. 5):S265–S280, 2003

6. American Diabetes Association: Standards of medical care in diabetes—2009. Diabetes Care 32:S13–S61, 2009

7. Munchi M, Grande L, Hays M, Ayres D, Suhl E, et al.: Cognitive dysfunction is associated with poor diabetes control in older adults. *Diabetes Care* 29:1794–1799, 2006

8. Benjamin EM: Case study: glycemic control in the elderly: risk and benefits. *Clinical Diabetes* 20:118–122, 2002

9. U.K. Prospective Diabetes Study Group: Intensive blood glucose control with sulphonylureas or insulin compared with conventional treatment and risk of complications in patients with type 2 diabetes (UKPDS 33). *Lancet* 352: 837–853, 1998

10. Odegard PS, Setter SM, Neumiller JJ: considerations for the pharmacologic treatment of diabetes in older adults. *Diabetes Spectrum* 20:239–247, 2007

11. Yen PK: Treating diabetes with diet. *Geriatr Nurs* 23:175–176, 2002

12. Good CB: Polypharmacy in elderly patients with diabetes. *Diabetes Spectrum* 15:240–248, 2002

13. Suhl ES, Bonsignore P: Diabetes self-management education for older adults: general principles and practical application. *Diabetes Spectrum* 19:234–240, 2006

Dr. Kocurek is the Diabetes Education Coordinator at Baylor Health Care Diabetes Services, Irving, TX.

DISEASES AND TREATMENTS
THAT AFFECT DIABETES

28. Glucocorticoid Use in Diabetes

Marjorie Cypress, PHD, MSN, RN, C-ANP, CDE

Glucocorticoids are used for many different conditions and may be prescribed in a variety of ways. They can cause significant hyperglycemia and uncontrolled diabetes in individuals with known diabetes and can cause steroid-induced diabetes in individuals with risk factors for developing type 2 diabetes. Because glucocorticoids are used for treating numerous chronic illnesses and conditions, it is not uncommon to encounter patients with severe hyperglycemia due to their use. Glucocorticoids (whether administered intravenously, by injection, or orally) increase glucose levels, particularly postprandial glucose levels, through insulin resistance and increased gluconeogenesis and glycogenolysis. The typical pattern when glucocorticoids are taken in the morning is elevated postprandial glucose levels that tend to normalize overnight. Thus, there may be risk of hyperglycemia and overnight hypoglycemia.

Treatment of resultant hyperglycemia depends on the type of glucocorticoid used; the route, amount, dosage schedule, and duration of therapy; and an individual's prior diagnosis, level of control, and use of diabetes medications. Table 28.1 shows the various glucocorticoid preparations and their durations of action. The goal of treating steroid-induced hyperglycemia is to prevent diabetic ketoacidosis or hyperglycemic hyperosmolar nonketotic syndrome and to avoid hypoglycemia while doing so.

In patients with known diabetes, insulin is almost always indicated for treating severe hyperglycemia from glucocorticoid therapy. Although there are some reports of using oral insulin secretagogues effectively (1), generally this will be ineffective in controlling hyperglycemia (2). These medications may not selectively target postprandial glucose levels and may even precipitate hypoglycemia in patients with poor appetites, who may miss a meal. Shorter-acting insulin secretagogues may be useful because they are taken before a meal. Several practitioners have advocated relaxing glycemic goals during short-term steroid therapy because

Table 28.1 Glucocorticoid Preparations and Durations of Action

Drug	Duration (h)
Cortisone acetate	6–10
Hydrocortisone	6–10
Prednisone	16–20
Methylprednisone	16–20
Dexamethasone	24–30

PRACTICAL POINT

When glucocorticoid doses are changed, insulin requirements change at the same time. The insulin dose will need to be increased or decreased as the glucocorticoid dose is increased or decreased. Patients must be instructed in frequent blood glucose monitoring to prevent episodes of severe hyperglycemia or hypoglycemia.

---

of the difficulty in managing glucose levels in both hospitalized and outpatient treatment so that fasting glucose levels are 120–140 mg/dl and 2-h postprandial levels are <200 mg/dl (3).

Some studies have observed better outcomes when blood glucose levels in hospital are kept between 80 and 110 mg/dl; however, the risk for hypoglycemia is such that the American Diabetes Association recommends glycemic targets in hospitalized patients of <126 mg/dl fasting and <180–200 mg/dl for all other values (4). In hospitalized patients already under significant stress from illness, intravenous glucocorticoids can raise glucose levels dangerously high, to >400–500 mg/dl. In the case of a 24-h intravenous glucocorticoid, insulin treatment should consist of a basal insulin as well as regular or rapid-acting insulin before meals or every 4–6 h if the patient is on an NPO order. Treating hyperglycemia with only short- or rapid-acting insulin will not maintain stable glucose levels because basal insulin is needed. As the steroid dose is reduced, insulin requirements are decreased. It is essential to closely monitor blood glucose levels so that insulin doses can also be decreased to avoid the risk of hypoglycemia.

Some patients receive glucocorticoid injections into joints or epidurally. These injections can increase glucose levels substantially in people with diabetes for the first few days, but glucose levels tend to decrease after a week or so (5,6). Insulin dosages may need to be increased 50% or more immediately and then slowly decreased over the next 5–10 days. Rapid-acting insulin is a choice for managing the resultant short-term severe hyperglycemia. It is important that patients be advised that these steroid injections into joints can cause increased blood glucose levels and that more frequent blood glucose monitoring is warranted. In individuals with a high risk for diabetes, a steroid injection into the joint can cause impaired glucose tolerance and progress to overt diabetes. These individuals should be counseled and monitored for symptoms of polyuria, polydipsia, polyphagia, and hyperglycemia.

For patients with type 2 diabetes controlled by diet or in patients without a prior history of diabetes, an oral agent such as glyburide may be effective in keeping blood glucose levels close to normal. It will probably become necessary to withdraw the oral agent as the blood glucose levels decrease. In this case, patients will need to be taught how to self-monitor blood glucose to be alert to changes in blood glucose levels.

When people with diabetes are treated with eye drops that contain steroids, the glucose levels may increase, particularly in those with poorly controlled diabetes, but will normalize (or come back to baseline) after the eye drops are discontinued. Therapy may need to be changed during that time (7).

Patients with cancer who are treated with chemotherapy are frequently given dexamethasone injections to control symptoms of nausea. In the person with diabetes, this may increase glucose levels for 2–3 days, requiring increased insulin dosages at the time of the steroid injection (8).

Many patients are discharged from the hospital during oral glucocorticoid therapy or are treated as outpatients with a steroid taper. Others may be on an alternate-day steroid treatment regimen. This makes glucose control more difficult. Frequent self-monitoring of blood glucose is essential because glucose levels can fluctuate widely during treatment. For patients on a short-term glucocorticoid (1–2 weeks), daily contact with the health care practitioner may be necessary to help titrate the insulin doses.

In patients whose diabetes is usually managed with insulin, it is not uncommon for their requirements to be increased by two to three times or more. However, with tapering doses of oral glucocorticoids, insulin requirements begin to return to normal, and hypoglycemia becomes a major risk. For patients who were previously treated with oral agents or are diet controlled and who are new to insulin during the course of glucocorticoid therapy, short- or rapid-acting insulin before meals may be a safe and appropriate therapy. Insulin algorithms can be prescribed based on blood glucose monitoring, and patients can be taught to regulate their own insulin doses based on home blood glucose readings. If long-term steroid therapy is indicated (≥4 weeks), basal or intermediate-acting insulin is often necessary to manage blood glucose levels. The most important issue for patients on

Diabetes and Glucocorticoids

1. Insulin is the most effective therapy.
2. Glucose levels tend to increase throughout the day and normalize overnight.
3. Primary effect is postprandial, making preprandial short- or rapid-acting insulin important.
4. Give basal or intermediate-acting insulin in the morning, and titrate based on the following morning's blood glucose level.
5. Target glucose levels: <126 mg/dl fasting and <180–200 mg/dl postprandial in hospital and 70–130 mg/dl preprandial and <180 mg/dl postprandial outpatient (4).

Adapted from Oyer et al. (8).

insulin and a glucocorticoid is education about the necessity of frequent blood glucose monitoring and the risks of hyperglycemia and hypoglycemia.

Special caution must be exercised in designing insulin regimens during glucocorticoid therapy. The most common oral glucocorticoid used in the outpatient setting is prednisone, which has a duration of action of 16–20 h. If given once daily in the morning, blood glucose levels will tend to be normal or even somewhat low in the morning (fasting), but increase during the day so that predinner and bedtime glucose levels can be very high. Using morning NPH insulin may help lower late-afternoon hyperglycemia. However, the use of an evening NPH dose can cause hypoglycemia as the effects of prednisone wear off and insulin resistance decreases, causing insulin requirements to be drastically reduced. In this case, NPH and short- or rapid-acting insulin in the morning and short- or rapid-acting insulin before lunch and before dinner may be a safe and effective insulin regimen that will avoid early-morning hypoglycemia. If the prednisone is taken twice daily, basal insulin once daily with preprandial short- or rapid-acting insulin may also be effective. Caution must be taken when prescribing any bedtime insulin, and using smaller doses to try to bring the glucose level into a more normal range will help in avoiding middle-of-the-night or early-morning hypoglycemia.

SUMMARY

Individualizing insulin regimens or the use of oral agents for people on glucocorticoid therapy is essential. Appetite, mealtimes, and timing of glucocorticoid treatment are all important considerations when developing a treatment regimen. Ideally, glucose control should be achieved before the initiation of glucocorticoid therapy, but this is rarely the case unless the treatment can be preplanned.

It is the role of the nurse to

- advise all individuals with diabetes that glucocorticoid therapy will result in hyperglycemia
- advise individuals that more frequent blood glucose monitoring will be necessary to avoid uncontrolled glucose levels
- advise them that insulin may be needed even for short-term therapy
- caution patients that insulin requirements will increase or decrease based on the dosage of the glucocorticoid
- advise individuals with no prior history of diabetes and high risk for diabetes of the possible increase in blood glucose levels related to glucocorticoid treatment and educate them regarding the signs and symptoms of hyperglycemia
- provide the telephone numbers of the health care professionals for the patient to contact in case of hyperglycemia or symptoms of hyperglycemia

REFERENCES

1. Willi SM, Kennedy A, Brant BP, Wallace P, Rogers NL, Garvey WT: Effective use of thiazolidinediones for the treatment of glucocorticoid-induced diabetes. *Diabetes Res Clin Pract* 58:87–96, 2002

2. Volgi JR, Baldwin D: Glucocorticoid therapy and diabetes management. *Nurs Clin North Am* 36:333–339, 2001

3. Braithwaite SS, Barr WG, Rahman A, Quddusi S: Managing diabetes during glucocorticoid therapy: how to avoid metabolic emergencies. *Postgrad Med* 104:163–166, 171, 175–176, 1998

4. American Diabetes Association: Standards of medical care in diabetes—2009. *Diabetes Care* 32:S13–S61, 2009

5. Wang AA, Hutchinson DT: The effect of corticosteroid injections for trigger finger on blood glucose levels in diabetic patients. *J Hand Surg* 31:979–981, 2006

6. Younes M, Nefat F, Touzi M, Hassen-Zrour S, Fendri Y, et al.: Systemic effects of epidural and intra-articular glucocorticoid injections in diabetic and non-diabetic patients. *Joint Bone Spine* 74:474–476, 2007

7. Bahar I, Rosenblat I, Erenberg M, Eldar I, Gaton D, et al.: Effect of dexamethasone eyedrops on blood glucose profiles. *Curr Eye Res* 32:739–742, 2007

8. Oyer DS, Shah A, Bettenhausen S: How to manage steroid diabetes in the patient with cancer. *J Support Oncol* 4:479–483, 2006

Dr. Cypress is an Adult Nurse Practitioner and Certified Diabetes Educator in Albuquerque, NM.

29. Cystic Fibrosis–Related Diabetes

GERALYN SPOLLETT, MSN, C-ANP, CDE

Cystic fibrosis (CF), one of the most common lethal genetic diseases in Caucasians, affects >30,000 Americans, with 1,000 children diagnosed each year (1). There is no cure for the disease, but with advances in research and treatment, people with CF are living longer. With the increase in survival, the number of patients with CF-related diabetes (CFRD) has also risen, becoming a leading comorbidity in this group. Approximately 40% of all adult CF patients develop diabetes (2). However, because many CF centers do not routinely screen for diabetes, the actual number of individuals with CF who are also affected by diabetes may be higher (3). CFRD occurs in ~40% of adults, 25% of adolescents, and 9% of children with CF (4).

CFRD is a distinct clinical entity. It shares component of both type 1 and type 2 diabetes. However, it differs from both type 1 and type 2 diabetes in that it is characterized by insulinopenia but ketoacidosis is extremely rare (3). Like type 2 diabetes, the onset is often insidious and can exist for 2–4 years before diagnosis. The initial deficiency is an impaired first-phase insulin response; as patients age, peak insulin response is delayed and less robust than normal (5). In CF, abnormal glucose tolerance is associated with progressive clinical deterioration (6). Research has shown that the rate of pulmonary decline is directly proportional to the magnitude of abnormal glucose tolerance and the degree of insulin deficiency (6). The diagnosis of diabetes in individuals with CF lowers survival rates. Only 25% of people with CFRD survive to 30 years of age, compared with a 60% survival rate to 30 years in individuals with CF and no diabetes (7).

CF affects the tissues that produce mucus secretions and alters the properties of that mucus so that it is no longer a protective substance but rather an obstructive, damaging one. Excessive, thick, sticky mucus blocks the airways, the gastrointestinal tract, the ducts of the pancreas, the bile ducts of the liver, and the male urogenital tract.

Chemical changes in the mucus proteins increase the viscosity and provide an environment ideal for bacterial growth. White blood cells are released to combat the infection but only result in complicating the problem. Genetic materials from dying white blood cells increase the stickiness of the mucus and initiate a cycle of further obstruction, infection, and inflammation.

The thick, sticky secretions can also clog the pancreatic ducts, damaging the pancreas in a variety of ways. A reduction in the amounts of pancreatic enzymes and bicarbonate alter the digestive and absorptive process. This insufficiency results in malnutrition and slowed growth and development. Stools become bulky and foul smelling. Eventually, blockage of the pancreatic ducts damages the β-cells, resulting in hyperglycemia. Fibrosis and fatty infiltrates disrupt the architecture of the islet cell and can result in islet destruction. Glucagon and pancreatic polypeptide secretion are reduced. Proinsulin levels are elevated, and first-phase insulin and C-peptide secretion in response to glucose are impaired. This results in delayed and diminished insulin secretion in response to oral stimuli (2). The pathophysiological changes associated with CF affect glucose metabolism. Malabsorption and abnormal intestinal transit time, glucagon deficiency, liver dysfunction, and increased caloric need to avoid malnutrition disrupt glucose control. Chronic systemic inflammation in CF significantly impacts multiple organ systems and contributes to the development of CF-related bone disease as well as CFRD (8). Systemic inflammatory processes, chronic and acute infections, and use of steroids increase insulin resistance and cause further deterioration in glucose stability.

DIAGNOSIS AND CLASSIFICATION OF CFRD

The 1998 Cystic Fibrosis–Related Diabetes (CFRD) Consensus Conference created classification and diagnosis criteria for CF patients with glucose abnormalities based on the oral glucose tolerance test (OGTT) (9). Four diagnostic categories were formed: normal glucose tolerance, impaired glucose tolerance, CFRD without fasting hyperglycemia, and CRFD with fasting hyperglycemia (Table 29.1). The separation of individuals with CFRD who were with or without fasting hyperglycemia is unique to CF and was largely done to track epidemiological data for future treatment decisions (2).

Table 29.1 Glucose Tolerance Categories in CF in Response to OGTT

Category	FPG (mg/dl)	2-h PG (mg/dl)
NGT	<126	<140
IGT	<126	140–199
CFRD without FH	<126	≥200
CFRD with FH	≥126	OGTT unnecessary

FH, fasting hyperglycemia; IGT, impaired glucose tolerance; NGT, normal glucose tolerance; OGTT, oral glucose tolerance test; PG, plasma glucose.

Adapted from Brunzell and Schwarzenberg (19).

PRACTICAL POINT

Screening for CFRD

If the patient's fasting plasma glucose (FPG) level is ≥126 mg/dl (7 mmol/l), then it must be repeated, or a casual glucose level should be drawn on the following day to confirm the diagnosis. If on the next day the follow-up FPG measurement is ≥126 mg/dl (7 mmol/l) or the casual glucose level ≥200 mg/dl (11.1 mmol/l), then the diagnosis of diabetes is confirmed. An FPG level <126 mg/dl (7 mmol/l) indicates that a standard OGTT should be performed.

The CFRD Consensus Conference committee recommended that a fasting plasma glucose (FPG) level be obtained annually in all patients ≥14 years of age. The most common age of onset is 18–21 years. Diabetes screening should be done whenever symptoms suggestive of hyperglycemia are present: polydipsia, polyuria, weight loss, alterations in growth patterns or puberty progression, unexplained pulmonary function decline, or increased infections. During steroid therapy or at the onset of pregnancy or pulmonary exacerbations, cautious monitoring for diabetes symptoms should be increased. Glycated hemoglobin A1c (A1C) testing is not used for diagnosis because it can be falsely low in this population. An elevated level may indicate the presence of hyperglycemia, but a normal A1C value does not exclude the diagnosis of diabetes. The rapid turnover rate of red blood cells in CF patients makes diagnosis through the A1C test unreliable.

Screening for CFRD has become more stringent in Europe, where an annual OGTT in patients age 10 or older is recommended (10). This recommendation is based on the evidence that CFRD can be present when fasting glucose is normal. By restricting OGTT orders to those patients with impaired fasting glucose, patients with other glucose abnormalities may not be appropriately screened and may remain undiagnosed for a longer period of time (10). Since pulmonary decline correlates with the extent of glucose intolerance, early diagnosis and insulin treatment can help reverse pulmonary deficits (11). Not only does insulin enhance the nutritional state, it can improve or stabilize pulmonary function, on average delaying decline in FEV1 by 34 months (12).

TREATMENT

In general, insulin is the treatment of choice for CFRD with fasting hyperglycemia. Depending on the level of β-cell impairment, bolus meal coverage with rapid-acting insulin may be all that is required (13). Carbohydrate counting and the use of an insulin-to-carbohydrate ratio system provide the flexible coverage needed in CFRD. Since undernutrition secondary to high energy requirements is a major problem in CF, weight maintenance is critical for these patients; therefore, caloric and carbohydrate restrictions seen in the treatment of diabetes are not part of the care regimen. An outline of medical nutrition therapy recommendations for CFRD compared with type 1/type 2 diabetes illustrates the differences in approach

Table 29.2 Medical Nutrition Therapy for Type 1/Type 2 Diabetes Versus for CFRD

	Type 1/Type 2 Diabetes	CFRD
Calories	Calculated for maintenance, growth, or reduction diets	120–150% RDA
Carbohydrate	Individualized	Individualized
Fat	Individualized; often <30% of total calories, <10% saturated fat, ≤10% of calories from polyunsaturated fat	40% of calories; no restriction on type of fat
Protein	10–20% of total calories; reduction to 0.8 g/kg with nephropathy	10–20% of total calories; no reduction with nephropathy*
Sodium	<2,400 mg/day	>4,000 mg/day
Vitamins/ minerals	No supplementation unless deficiency noted	Routine supplementation of vitamins A, D, E, K, and multivitamin

Adapted from Brunzell and Schwarzenberg (19).

*This is the recommendation of the consensus conference. In practice, a patient with severe nephropathy would require protein restriction to prevent azotemia. RDA, recommended daily allowance.

(Table 29.2). Achieving a balance of adequate nutrition for the increased metabolic needs of the person with CF and supporting the use of these calories through a matched insulin regimen is necessary for the health and survival of these patients. Basal insulin, such as an evening dose of an intermediate-acting insulin or a long-acting insulin, is frequently needed to achieve euglycemic levels and improve nutritional status. In a recent study, insulin glargine improved fasting plasma glucose without hypoglycemia and had a nonsignificant trend toward weight gain (14). Insulin pump therapy offers the patient more flexibility in dietary intake and improves glucose management (15).

The use of most oral agents is not recommended in the treatment of CFRD. Metformin and the thiazolidinediones rely on clearance mechanisms that are compromised in CF. The increased potential for liver toxicity with thiazolidinediones in CF restricts their use. α-Glucosidase inhibitors affect intestinal absorption patterns in an already altered gastrointestinal tract. The side effects of

---

PRACTICAL POINT

Goals of Treatment

The goals of CFRD treatment are to maintain optimum nutrition, reduce hyperglycemia, avoid hypoglycemia, and support the patient in adjusting to CFRD management.

the α-glucosidase inhibitors, such as nausea, flatulence, and diarrhea, may negatively affect the nutritional status of these patients. Sulfonylureas have been used but are also problematic. Higher rates of hypoglycemia have been observed before achievement of therapeutic glycemic ranges. Glyburide, 50% of which is eliminated in the bile, is not recommended because of the difficulty in drug excretion through bile ducts clogged due to CF (16).

In patients with CFRD without fasting hyperglycemia, repaglinide has been studied with some positive effect. In comparison with insulin lispro, repaglinide did not normalize glucose excursions postprandially as well as the insulin did. The investigators reported that suboptimal doses may have altered the results and that further studies were needed (13).

In CFRD, patients using insulin should be seen by a diabetes team on a quarterly basis. Blood glucose targets are the same as for all other forms of diabetes and follow the recommendations set forth by the American Diabetes Association (17). A1C testing and self-monitoring of blood glucose are prescribed based on management strategies and are also used in adjusting therapy.

Patients with CFRD are living longer with their disease. Microvascular complications, such as retinopathy and nephropathy, have been reported in CFRD and appear to be related to duration of disease and level of glycemic control (18). Therefore, annual retinopathy and microalbumin screenings should be initiated at diagnosis (16). The prevalence and severity of microvascular complications may be lower in CFRD because most patients have some degree of endogenous insulin secretion and hyperglycemic excursions are less severe (18). Patients with CFRD are usually thin and have normal lipid and blood pressure levels, reducing the risks of macrovascular complications.

Patients with CFRD without fasting hyperglycemia are carefully monitored for any changes in glucose metabolism. Glucose levels are maintained through a regulation of meal timing to spread carbohydrate and calories throughout the day, thus reducing glucose excursions. Insulin therapy becomes necessary if nutritional status changes and weight is no longer maintained or if there is a decline in pulmonary function (19). Reducing consumption of regular sodas or other sweetened beverages may also help control glucose excursions. It is important to remember that food substitutions for any alteration in caloric level must be made to avoid weight loss. Helping the patient choose more nutritious replacements for the sweetened beverages is essential for the treatment of both diabetes and CF. Protein intake should be ~15–20% of the daily diet. Fat and sodium restrictions usually prescribed for individuals with diabetes are not appropriate in CFRD. These patients are frequently depleted of sodium and may require supplementation. Despite the use of pancreatic enzymes, fat malabsorption is a common component of the clinical picture. Caloric needs take precedence, with the current fat recommendation being 40% of total calories per day.

For individuals with CF and impaired glucose tolerance, the usual recommendations for increased exercise and weight loss to address glucose intolerance are not implemented because they can adversely affect health status. Medical nutrition therapy focuses on healthy eating and meal/snack timing. Exercise, although helpful for CF patients, should not be used as a weight loss mechanism. Individuals who choose to exercise need to replace spent calories to avoid a negative energy balance. Appropriate glucose monitoring and the use of a portable carbohydrate snack to prevent hypoglycemia are important parts of this regimen. Yearly screening with an OGTT and self-monitoring of blood glucose performed during periods of infection and stress are necessary to therapeutically respond to glucose alterations.

Preconception and pregnancy care in CFRD follow the standard guidelines for glucose control. Weight maintenance takes on more significance in light of the nutritional needs of pregnancy and the caloric needs of CF. Referral to a dietitian is imperative for counseling and education to achieve positive outcomes. As with all diabetes-affected pregnancies, insulin requirements will change and the patient will need to remain in close contact with her health care providers. However, alterations in pulmonary function and its effect on both glucose control and fetal health make good communication among all members of the health care team vital.

SUMMARY

Adequate nutrition and glucose control are important components of therapy in all individuals with diabetes. However, in people with CFRD, the consequences of not meeting these basic requirements of diabetes care are life-threatening. Coordination of care between the diabetes and CF health care teams is imperative for positive outcomes. Patient education and support in managing two serious chronic diseases will help the patient maintain function and increase longevity. Without proper glycemic control, the patient's nutritional status declines and weight loss occurs. Assisting the patient in analyzing glucose levels and injecting the appropriate amount of premeal insulin requires an understanding of food and insulin action. Diabetes education plays a vital role in the health maintenance of people with CFRD. Literature is available from the American Diabetes Association, and the Cystic Fibrosis Foundation has educational literature and an informative web site (www.cff.org) to assist both patients and health care providers in remaining current on CF treatment protocols and lifestyle interventions.

REFERENCES

1. National Institute of Diabetes and Digestive and Kidney Diseases: Cystic fibrosis research directions [Internet], 1998. Available from http://www. niddk. nih.gov/health/endo/pubs/cystic/cystic.htm. Accessed 30 December 2003 (NIH publ. no. 97-4200)

2. Moran A: Diagnosis, screening, and management of cystic fibrosis-related diabetes. *Curr Diabetes Rep* 2:111–115, 2002

3. Allen H, Gay AC, Klingensmith GJ, Hamman RF: Identification and treatment of cystic fibrosis-related diabetes. *Diabetes Care* 21:943–948, 1998

4. Moran A, Doherty L, Wang X, Thomas W: Abnormal glucose metabolism in cystic fibrosis. *J Pediatr* 133:10–16, 1998

5. Hardin DS: A review of the management of two common clinical problems found in patients with cystic fibrosis: cystic fibrosis related diabetes and poor growth. *Horm Res* 68 (Suppl. 5):113–116, 2007

6. Milla CE, Warwick WJ, Moran A: Trends in pulmonary function in cystic fibrosis patients correlate with the degree of glucose intolerance at baseline. *Am J Respir Crit Care Med* 162:891–895, 2000

7. Finkelstein SM, Wielinski CL, Elliott GR, Warwick WJ, Barbosa J, et al.: Diabetes mellitus associated with cystic fibrosis. *J Pediatr* 112:373–377, 1988

8. Elborn JS: How can we prevent multisystem complications of cystic fibrosis? *Semin Respir Crit Care Med* 28:303–311, 2007

9. Moran A, Hardin D, Rodman D, Allen HF, Beall RJ, et al.: Diagnosis, screening and management of cystic fibrosis related diabetes mellitus: a consensus conference report. *Diabetes Res Clin Pract* 45:61–73, 1999

10. Mueller-Brandes C, Holl RW, Nastoll M, Ballmann M: New criteria for impaired fasting glucose and screening for diabetes in cystic fibrosis. *Eur Respir J* 25:715–717, 2005

11. Lanng S, Thosteinsson B, Nerup J, Koch C: Diabetes mellitus in cystic fibrosis: effect of insulin therapy on lung function and infection. *Acta Paediatr* 83:849–853, 1994

12. Mohan K, Israel KL, Miller H, Grainger R, Ledson MJ, Walshaw MJ: Long term effect of insulin treatment in cystic fibrosis related diabetes. *Respiration* 76:181–186, 2008

13. Moran A, Phillips J, Milla C: Insulin and glucose excursion following premeal insulin lispro or repaglinide in cystic fibrosis-related diabetes. *Diabetes Care* 24:1706–1710, 2001

14. Grover P, Thomas W, Moran A: Glargine vs NPH insulin in cystic fibrosis related diabetes. *J Cyst Fibros* 7:134–136, 2008

15. Sulli N, Bertasi S, Zullo S, Shashaj B: Use of continuous subcutaneous insulin infusion in patients with cystic fibrosis-related diabetes: three case reports. *J Cyst Fibros* 6:237–240, 2007

16. Hardin DS, Moran A: Diabetes mellitus in cystic fibrosis. *Endocrinol Metab Clin North Am* 28:787–799, 1999

17. American Diabetes Association: Standards of medical care in diabetes—2009 (Position Statement). *Diabetes Care* 32 (Suppl. 1):S13–S61, 2009

18. Schwarzenberg SJ, Thomas W, Olsen TW, Grover T, Walk D, Milla C, Moran A: Microvascular complications in cystic fibrosis-related diabetes. *Diabetes Care* 30:1056–1061, 2007

19. Brunzell C, Schwarzenberg SJ: Cystic fibrosis-related diabetes and abnormal glucose tolerance: overview and medical nutrition therapy. *Diabetes Spectrum* 15:124–127, 2002

Ms. Spollett is an Adult Nurse Practitioner at Yale Diabetes Center, New Haven, CT.

30. Endocrinopathies and Other Disorders

Marjorie Cypress, PHD, MSN, RN, C-ANP, CDE, and
Geralyn Spollett, MSN, C-ANP, CDE

Diabetes can be associated with other endocrine diseases through a shared etiological mechanism. There are three ways in which this can occur:

- In type 1 diabetes, an autoimmune process that destroys β-cells may also affect other endocrine cells, leading to adrenal, gonadal, thyroid, or parathyroid disease.
- β-Cell function may be disrupted through an infiltrative process that also damages other endocrine tissue.
- Insulin resistance and associated hyperinsulinemia may be at the root of the associated endocrinopathy (1).

The effects of the "other" endocrine diseases may cause a destabilization of diabetes control, resulting in either hypoglycemia or hyperglycemia. Most of these disorders are related to pituitary adenomas that secrete excessive amounts of counterregulatory hormones or to the administration of exogenous hormone therapy. The main endocrinopathies associated with diabetes or glucose intolerance are acromegaly, Cushing's syndrome, pheochromocytoma, and glucagonoma (2). Autoimmune diseases associated with diabetes include thyroid disease, Addison's disease, celiac disease, and pernicious anemia. Other diseases that are sometimes associated with diabetes or result in unstable diabetes control include fatty liver disease and cystic fibrosis (see chapter 29).

ENDOCRINOPATHIES

ACROMEGALY

Acromegaly is a condition caused by excess growth hormone, usually caused by a pituitary microadenoma. Growth hormone is diabetogenic because of its effects on peripheral insulin resistance and hepatic glucose production. The incidence of diabetes in acromegaly is estimated to be 13–32%, and the incidence of glucose intolerance in acromegaly is 60%. People who receive exogenous growth hormone (e.g., children with short stature) can also develop glucose intolerance or overt type 2 diabetes and can suffer the microvascular and neuropathic complications often associated with chronic suboptimally controlled diabetes (2).

Signs and symptoms of acromegaly in adults include excessive growth of hands and feet (with rapid increase in shoe and glove size), protruding jaw, enlarged tongue, coarse facial features, fatigue, weakness, acanthosis nigricans, hypertension, weakness, excessive growth of skin tags, and headaches (3). Sleep apnea is also noted to be very common in people with acromegaly (4).

Laboratory findings may include elevated serum growth hormone levels at fasting and after oral glucose. In healthy individuals, glucose will suppress growth hormone, but in those with acromegaly, growth hormone levels will increase (5). Other laboratory findings include elevated prolactin levels and elevated blood glucose levels. Magnetic resonance imaging (MRI) of the head may reveal a pituitary tumor in 90% of cases. Treatment consists of surgical excision of the tumor and has varying effects on glucose metabolism.

CUSHING'S SYNDROME

Cushing's syndrome is the result of excessive cortisol secondary to either exogenous therapy or an endogenous cortisol-secreting pituitary adenoma, which may be either benign or malignant. High cortisol levels can cause increased insulin resistance, increased gluconeogenesis, and decreased peripheral glucose uptake, which subsequently leads to glucose intolerance or overt type 2 diabetes. Many of the features of Cushing's syndrome closely resemble those associated with cardiometabolic risk. Because some of the conditions of the metabolic syndrome are reversible with treatment, it is important to evaluate patients to distinguish those who may have Cushing's syndrome versus those with possible pseudo Cushing's syndrome. If Cushing's is suspected, there should be a thorough workup looking for a tumor if no other cause can be found. If a tumor is found, surgery may be an option.

The clinical picture of an individual with Cushing's syndrome includes truncal obesity, hypertension, glucose intolerance, facial rounding (typical moon face), osteoporosis, abdominal striae, hirsutism, acanthosis nigricans, depression or emotional lability, and menstrual irregularity (2,3,6). Individuals with Cushing's syndrome may go on to develop atherosclerosis and cardiovascular disease (CVD), which are often associated with insulin resistance and conditions associated with cardiometabolic risk. It is not clear to what extent Cushing's syndrome is common or uncommon. There is belief that Cushing's syndrome may be more common than previously thought because it often resembles the metabolic syndrome and further evaluation may not be performed. In addition, its features are similar to those of polycystic ovary syndrome, and the diagnoses of polycystic ovary syndrome or Cushing's syndrome can be mistaken for each other.

Laboratory evaluation is somewhat problematic in that several tests can have false-negative or some false-positive results. A current recommended laboratory evaluation, which appears to be more specific and reliable, is evening salivary cortisol level (6). Because cortisol levels peak in the early morning hours, an evening level should be lower. Other more commonly used tests include a 24-h urine-free cortisol level. This test should include a urine creatinine level to help evaluate whether the urine collection was properly done (normal urine creatinine in 24 h is ~1 g and should not fluctuate more than 10%). The overnight dexamethasone suppression test involves administration of 1 mg dexamethasone at 11:00 p.m., with serum levels of cortisol drawn in the morning. In Cushing's syndrome, the cortisol level fails to be suppressed. This test, although commonly performed, can also have false-positive results, and questionable test results should be referred to an endocrinologist (6). Further evaluation may include an MRI to look for a pituitary tumor. Treatment focuses on surgical excision of the adenoma, which can result in a reversal of the metabolic abnormalities.

Pseudo Cushing's syndrome presents with some of the same clinical features with mildly elevated urinary free cortisol and sometimes an abnormal dexamethasone suppression that corrects with treatment of the underlying condition. Hypercortisolism has been seen in alcoholism, depression and obesity. Several studies have found relationships between high cortisol profiles (although still in the normal range) and elevated fasting blood glucose, postprandial blood glucose, A1C levels, and blood pressure. Whether the elevated cortisol levels are a result of chronic stress of hyperglycemia or enhanced HPA axis activity with type 2 diabetes is unknown. However, when the hyperglycemia and/or weight loss are treated, the clinical features of Cushing's diminish (7,8).

PHEOCHROMOCYTOMA

A pheochromocytoma is an adenoma that secretes excessive amounts of the catecholamines epinephrine, norepinephrine, and dopamine. Catecholamines are normally secreted in response to hypoglycemia and counter the effects of insulin by increasing glucose production through glycogenolysis. Therefore, the symptoms associated with glucose intolerance and symptoms of hypoglycemia are present and include headache, excessive diaphoresis, and palpitations.

Laboratory evaluation is conducted through urine catecholamine levels. Symptoms are controlled through α- and β-blockade, but resolution of pheochromocytoma is accomplished only through tumor removal (2).

GLUCAGONOMA

A glucagonoma is an often-malignant tumor that secretes excessive amounts of the hormone glucagon. The resulting glucose intolerance is the result of increased gluconeogenesis and glycogenolysis. Other associated symptoms are weight loss, glossitis, rash, and anemia (2). Treatment may consist of somatostatin therapy or surgical removal of the tumor.

HYPOGONADISM/LOW TESTOSTERONE IN MEN WITH DIABETES

Men with type 2 diabetes have higher rates of testosterone deficiency than those without diabetes. Some studies have found that 33–42% of men with diabetes have low testosterone (9,10) as measured by free testosterone levels. Other studies have demonstrated a strong association between conditions associated with the metabolic syndrome (i.e., insulin resistance, dyslipidemia, visceral obesity, and glucose intolerance) (11). In short term studies, replacement therapy has demonstrated improvements in insulin sensitivity, visceral obesity, and lipids (11).

Clinical symptoms of low testosterone include a decrease or loss of libido, decreased strength of erections, fatigue, decreased physical strength, and mood changes. Androgen Deficiency in the Aging Male (12) is a short questionnaire that assesses the clinical symptoms associated with low testosterone. Biochemical evaluations generally consist of free testosterone, and sex hormone–binding globulin, although FSH and LH are sometimes used to differentiate between a primary or secondary hypogonadism. Testosterone levels should be done in the morning, since testosterone is secreted in a circadian rhythm with peak levels in the morning.

Treating low testosterone with replacement therapy may consist of injections, patches, gels, mucoadhesive material applied to the teeth, or oral tablets. Each has its risks and benefits and should be discussed with a health care professional familiar with these therapies.

Unfortunately, some health professionals and patients are reluctant to discuss issues related to sex and erections. Nurses should be aware of the high prevalence of low testosterone among men with type 2 diabetes. Explaining how common these symptoms are among men with type 2 diabetes can make it easier to ask patients if they are experiencing any of these symptoms. Nurses should refer patients for evaluation and treatment.

NONALCOHOLIC FATTY LIVER DISEASE

Although nonalcoholic fatty liver disease (NAFLD) does not result in diabetes, it is mentioned here because it often coexists and is associated with other cardiometabolic risk factors, such as truncal obesity, type 2 diabetes, hyperlipidemia, and insulin resistance in adults and children (13,14). NAFLD is a common explanation for abnormal or elevated aminotransferase levels in up to 90% of cases once other causes of liver disease are excluded (13). Damage from NAFLD ranges from mild steatosis and hepatitis to cirrhosis and end-stage liver disease, but because this is a newly recognized condition, its natural history and progression require further study (15).

There are no obvious symptoms of NAFLD other than elevated liver function tests., although some studies have found normal ALT levels in a large number of patients with NAFLD (16). Evaluation may include ultrasound, computed tomography, or MRI to rule out other liver pathology.

NAFLD has been found to be very common in people with type 2 diabetes and is associated with a higher prevalence of cardiovascular disease, including coronary

PRACTICAL POINT

Managing people with diabetes involves not only attention to blood glucose, blood pressure, and lipid control, but also awareness of other endocrine diseases that can be associated with diabetes. Nurses and other health care professionals need to maintain a high index of suspicion when treating patients with diabetes, as many of the other endocrine diseases can present with mild symptoms. A thorough review of symptoms can help with early detection and treatment for some of these problems.

heart disease, peripheral vascular disease, and cerebrovascular disease (16). People who have abnormal liver function tests, are overweight or obese, and have known diabetes or multiple risk factors for the metabolic syndrome and type 2 diabetes should be encouraged to lose weight and exercise because weight loss has been associated with improved liver function tests. Blood glucose and lipid control has also been effective in improving liver function tests and fatty liver. There is some evidence that insulin sensitizers, such as metformin, thiazolidinediones, and gemfibrozil, have positive effects on normalizing liver function tests (15).

AUTOIMMUNE DISEASES ASSOCIATED WITH TYPE 1 DIABETES

Autoimmune-mediated (type 1) diabetes is associated with other autoimmune diseases, most notably thyroid disease, celiac disease, Addison's disease, and pernicious anemia. Often present in autoimmune-mediated diabetes, along with islet cell antibodies, are anti-thyroid peroxidase, adrenal, and anti-gastric parietal autoantibodies.

DIABETES AND THYROID DISEASE

The prevalence of thyroid disease in individuals with diabetes is much higher than in the general population (see also "Thyroid Disease and Diabetes," a patient handout in RESOURCES). Although there are no statistics for the U.S. population, a study conducted in Scotland showed that of the 13.4% of people diagnosed with thyroid disease, the highest incidence (31.4%) was found in women with type 1 diabetes and the lowest (6.8%) in men with type 2 diabetes, suggesting that those with type 1 diabetes are more susceptible to thyroid disease. In this group, the most common thyroid dysfunction was subclinical hypothyroidism (17).

Hyperthyroidism. In type 1 diabetes, Graves' disease is the most common autoimmune thyroid disease leading to hyperthyroidism. Most often diagnosed in young women, this thyroid disease has clear links to the HLA (human leukocyte antigen) markers. Thyrotoxicosis disrupts glucose control by causing an increase in glucose absorption, utilization, and production. The increased production of thyroid hormone and its subsequent effect on metabolism results in accelerated gluconeogenesis by the liver and an increase in peripheral tissue uptake of glucose.

The increased glucose production and disposal stimulated by the thyroid hormones occurs independent of insulin levels. In addition to these mechanisms, thyroid hormone can also cause insulin resistance and promote an increase in insulin clearance rates. To compensate for the lack of circulating insulin, more insulin must be secreted. In previously undiagnosed patients, hyperthyroidism may unmask impaired glucose tolerance and diabetes.

For patients with type 1 diabetes with undiagnosed hyperthyroidism, the rapid disposal of insulin results in hyperglycemia and can lead to ketoacidosis. Because this is a life-threatening acute complication, the importance of screening for thyroid disease in type 1 diabetes cannot be underestimated. Conversely, if a patient has thyrotoxicosis, a screening test for latent diabetes should be done.

The presentation of clinical signs and symptoms of hyperthyroid disease (see the box "Symptoms of Hyperthyroidism") warrants thyroid function evaluation. The thyroid-stimulating hormone (TSH) blood test is the best way to determine thyroid function. If the levels of TSH are suppressed, then the amount of thyroid hormone being produced is excessive, indicating a hyperthyroid state. A free thyroxine index or free T4 level will help determine the extent of the hyperthyroid problem. If the laboratory results do not match the clinical presentation, further workup by an endocrinologist may be necessary to determine the cause for the hyperthyroidism and subsequent treatment.

In Graves' disease, therapeutic options include ablation by radioactive iodine, surgical removal of the gland, or medical control with propylthiouracil (PTU) or methimazole. If the patient has tachycardia or tremors, the use of β-adrenergic blocking agents can ameliorate these symptoms, but may also decrease the patient's ability to recognize hypoglycemia and impair the counterregulatory response to hypoglycemia (1).

Lymphocytic thyroiditis, another cause of hyperthyroidism in young, usually postpartum, women, can spontaneously revert to hypothyroidism. Although the disease usually resolves, a percentage of women have permanent hypothyroidism. Careful monitoring of thyroid function must be done throughout the disease process to determine appropriate treatment and make the necessary adjustments in therapy. The changeable course of this condition further complicates diabetes control.

During the initial phases of treatment for hyperthyroidism, insulin needs are still increased, but as the patient becomes euthyroid, or in some cases hypothyroid, previous medication dosages may be excessive. Frequent self-monitoring of blood glucose and a flexible insulin regimen may be the best course of action to compensate for fluctuations in the insulin requirement.

Hypothyroidism. In hypothyroidism concomitant with diabetes, the most common cause is an autoimmune thyroid dysfunction, Hashimoto's disease. It occurs in

Symptoms of Hyperthyroidism

Tremor
Increased sweating
Heat intolerance
Nervousness and anxiety
Irritability
Muscle weakness
Palpitations and tachycardia
Fatigue
Hyperdefecation
Weight loss

type 1 diabetes but also has an increased prevalence in type 2 diabetes unrelated to autoimmunity factors.

Hypothyroidism slows the absorption of glucose from the gastrointestinal tract, reduces glucose uptake by the peripheral tissues, and decreases gluconeogenesis. In response to prolonged insulin half-life, endogenous insulin secretion may be reduced. Although these changes in glucose metabolism may not produce clinical symptoms in a person without diabetes, they have a substantial impact on glucose control in the person with diabetes. Overall glucose control deteriorates, and episodes of hypoglycemia increase. As with hyperthyroidism, TSH is the most accurate method to evaluate primary hypothyroidism. The level of TSH will be elevated in response to the decrease in thyroid hormone production. Most hypothyroidism is related to primary thyroid failure. However, in some instances, the hypothalamus or pituitary gland will be the cause of the hypothyroidism, and in such cases, the TSH may not be elevated. Further evaluation by an endocrinologist is needed to determine the cause. Regardless of etiology, the presenting clinical picture for hypothyroidism remains consistent. As hypothyroidism resolves with treatment, an increase in insulin dosage will be needed to meet the increased metabolic need (18).

Treatment for hypothyroidism relies on the replacement of L-thyroxine. The usual dose of levothyroxine is 75–125 µg. In elderly patients and those at risk for atherosclerotic heart disease, the initial dose should be reduced to 50 µg. Further adjustments in therapy are made based on the results of TSH testing done every 6–8 weeks. CVD is prevalent in type 2 diabetes; therefore, these therapeutic guidelines should be considered in patients with diabetes.

Dyslipidemia is prevalent in hypothyroidism. As thyroid function approaches normal levels, the lipid profile will also improve. However, with the persistence of unrecognized hypothyroidism or untreated subclinical hypothyroidism, the risk of CVD increases (19). Many patients with type 2 diabetes have features of the metabolic syndrome, with dyslipidemias that are slow to respond to treatment. If the underlying cause is hypothyroidism and it is not treated, there will be limited clinical improvement in lipid levels. This underlines the need for annual screening for thyroid disease in the diabetes population.

Nursing implications. The destabilization of glucose control in thyroid disease requires an intensification of diabetes management, particularly self-monitoring of blood glucose and adjustments in medication therapy. Nursing must focus on maintaining a continuity of care and coordination of therapies. Patient education regarding the interface of thyroid disease and diabetes and the ways to distinguish between the causes of clinical symptoms (for example, hypoglycemia versus hyperthyroidism) is a nursing priority (see "Thyroid Disease and Diabetes" in RESOURCES).

Symptoms of Hypothyroidism

Dry, coarse skin and hair
Cold intolerance
Hoarseness
Facial edema
Slow speech and mentation
Poor concentration
Constipation
Weight gain
Lower-extremity edema
Depression
Weakness and lethargy
Fatigue

> ### PRACTICAL POINT
>
> Thyroid disease is frequently seen in individuals with both type 1 and type 2 diabetes. Thyroid function tests should be performed annually on all people with diabetes or if the patient presents with symptoms suggestive of thyroid disease. Those already diagnosed with thyroid disease need to be monitored periodically by lab tests and physical examination. It is important that nurses advise patients of the potential for other medical and psychological complications when thyroid levels are not adequately controlled.

CELIAC DISEASE IN TYPE 1 DIABETES

Celiac disease is an often overlooked and underdiagnosed problem associated with type 1 diabetes. The symptoms may mimic other gastrointestinal problems and may be misdiagnosed. First noted in the late 1960s, celiac disease associated with type 1 diabetes has a prevalence rate of ~4–6% (20). Celiac disease has also been noted in other organ-specific autoimmune conditions, such as thyroid disease and Addison's disease (21).

Pathophysiology of celiac disease. A genetically mediated disease of the small bowel, celiac disease may present in infancy and early childhood and then again later in life (>60 years of age). It is most commonly seen in people of European descent and has a 95% genetic predisposition. Viral exposures may trigger an immune response in individuals predisposed to the disease, resulting in the onset of active disease.

In celiac disease, also known as gluten-sensitive enteropathy, there is an abnormal T-cell response against gliadin, a part of wheat gluten and prolamins (derived from barley, rye, and possibly oats). The production of proinflammatory cytokines results in an immune reaction to gluten, the storage protein of wheat. This inflammatory environment causes an immune deregulation and loss of tolerance that activates CD8+ T-cells and B-cells in the intestinal epithelium (22). The resulting pathophysiology affects the functioning of the villi of the small intestine and limits its ability to absorb nutrients. This inability to digest certain carbohydrates results in osmotic diarrhea, hypersecretion due to crypt hyperplasia, and dysmotility due to an inflammatory reaction (23).

The usual clinical presentation is that of chronic diarrhea and failure to thrive. Weight loss, muscle tenderness, and signs of immunological illnesses, such as atopic dermatitis and alopecia, may also be present. A papular/vesicular rash, dermatitis herpetiformis, may appear on the base of the scalp and on the elbows, knees, and trunk. Extreme itching and burning characterize the rash. Less typical presentations may include iron-deficiency anemia, osteoporosis/osteopenia, arthritis, alteration in teeth enamel, short stature, chronic hepatitis, or neurological problems. Although some patients have profound symptoms, such as abdominal cramping, flatulence, and violent diarrhea, many others are unaware of the problem or are asymptomatic. Symptomatic patients find that once a gluten-free diet is followed for a period of time, they notice a reduction in gastrointestinal symptoms, improved general health, and an increase in energy and well-being.

Diabetes and the effect of celiac disease. Two studies that focused on the effect of celiac disease on blood glucose control found little disruption in control. Acerini et al. (24) found no difference in metabolic control, as measured by hemoglobin A1c, in type 1 diabetes patients with or without celiac disease. No statistically significant change in insulin requirement was found. However, it was reported that after starting a gluten-free diet, some celiac patients had an increased incidence of morning hypoglycemia. The second study, by Kaukinen et al. (25), found no difference in metabolic control in diabetes with the initiation of treatment for celiac disease.

Before diagnosis and treatment, patients with celiac disease have hypoglycemic episodes and reduced insulin needs that are assumed to be related to the malabsorptive state. Over time, treatment with a gluten-free diet can help reduce the incidence of hypoglycemia. Therefore, Schwarzenberg and Brunzell (26) recommend closely monitoring insulin needs and blood glucose control during the early phase of treatment with a gluten-free diet, when changes in nutritional status may influence metabolic control.

Diagnosis of celiac disease. In people with a family predisposition to the disease, serological testing, used as a screening tool, may help discover atypical or silent celiac disease. Currently, most investigators advocate a profile of three antibody assays: *1)* anti-gliadin IgG, *2)* anti-gliadin IgA, and *3)* either anti-endomysial or an anti-tissue transglutaminase assay (26). If the results of all three assays are positive or the patient has symptoms but negative results, he or she should be referred to a gastroenterologist. It is important to note that a positive serological test alone is not sufficient for diagnosis. A small-bowel biopsy is necessary to confirm the diagnosis. Although there are no guidelines for continued screening of the at-risk population, many centers have adopted yearly testing for the first 3 years of diagnosed diabetes, then screening every 3–5 years thereafter or whenever symptoms develop (26).

Many affected patients have subclinical disease. Children in particular can benefit from early diagnosis and treatment. Undiagnosed celiac disease contributes to growth failure, low bone density, and potential neurological abnormalities. Freemark and colleagues (27) speculate that the treatment of celiac disease in type 1 diabetes could reduce the risk of developing other autoimmune diseases, such as Graves' or Addison's disease or non-Hodgkin's lymphoma of the small bowel (27). Although screening of children has potential issues—invasive testing with risks and psychological burdens—research has shown that the prevalence of celiac disease in children proven by biopsy is relatively high, with children who were <4 years of age at onset of type 1 diabetes at highest risk (28).

Treatment of celiac disease. The current recommendation for treatment is that a gluten-free diet be maintained for life. The most important reason to adhere strictly to the diet is to reduce the risk of small-bowel lymphoma associated with celiac disease. As nutritional status improves, patients note a positive change in energy. The malabsorptive state associated with celiac disease deprives the patient of important minerals, vitamins, and micronutrients. Adherence to the diet improves the absorption of these important nutrients and can reverse anemia, osteopenia, and other symptoms of vitamin deficiencies, such as cheilosis and neurological symptoms. After a period of time on the gluten-free diet, some patients become exquisitely sensitive to the smallest amounts of gluten, whereas others may find they can tolerate small amounts without experiencing diarrhea or cramping.

Despite the reduction of symptoms in response to gluten ingestion, the harmful effects of eating foods containing gluten have been demonstrated by small-bowel biopsies showing ongoing mucosal damage.

The gluten-free diet. Maintaining a gluten-free diet is difficult but not impossible. Obvious sources of gluten and prolamins, such as bread, processed cheese, and various wheat-based snack foods, are easily recognized and avoided (Tables 30.1 and 30.2). However, gluten is used as a thickener, emulsifier, binder, or stabilizer in many products. Oats, amaranth, and buckwheat (29) currently appear on the list of gluten-free foods, but there is still controversy over whether these foods are safe in large amounts over time. Even certain ground spices may contain gluten products. Other sources of prolamins, such as grain alcohol, postage stamps, cosmetics, lip balms, and mouthwashes, should also be avoided. Patients must be encouraged to read the labels on all foods because sometimes ingredients on previously "safe" foods change. Foods that are gluten free may be contaminated in transport or by the cooking process. Restaurant eating can be particularly difficult, and the person with celiac disease must learn to ask many questions regarding food preparation and possible kitchen contamination by gluten foods.

The addition of a gluten-free diet to the medical nutrition therapy recommended for diabetes presents a challenge and may be perceived as an additional burden. Referral to a registered dietitian can help educate and support the patient through this adaptive process. Patients who count carbohydrates need to know that gluten-free products may not contain the same number of carbohydrates as other starch products and that the digestion and glucose response may be quite

---

Table 30.1 Starches, Grains, and Other Foods Appropriate for a Gluten-Free Diet

- Amaranth,* arrowroot, whole-bean flour, buckwheat,* corn, cornstarch, cornmeal, flax, millet,* nut flours, oats,* oat bran,* oat gum,* pea flour, potato, sweet potato and yam, potato flour, potato starch, quinoa,* rice and wild rice, rice bran, rice flour, sago, sorghum, soy, tapioca, teff*
- Fresh, frozen, or canned unprocessed fruits and vegetables
- Fresh meats, poultry, seafood, fish, game, eggs, some processed meats with gluten-free ingredients, tofu, dried peas, beans, and lentils
- Milk, yogurt, and cheese made with gluten-free ingredients
- Oils, tree nuts, seeds, natural peanut butter, and salad dressings and spreads with gluten-free ingredients
- Honey, sugar, pure maple syrup, corn syrup, jams, jellies, candy, and ice cream with gluten-free ingredients
- Pure spices and herbs, salt, wheat-free soy sauce, vinegar with gluten-free ingredients
- Coffee ground from whole beans, brewed tea, carbonated beverages, some root beer

This is only a partial listing. Patients are encouraged to read all labels and to seek comprehensive food and additive lists from celiac organizations and the American Dietetic Association. *Recommendations about acceptability are inconsistent. Many physicians restrict these grains for the first 6 months after diagnosis or until patients are in full remission. Adapted from Schwarzenberg and Brunzell (26).

Table 30.2 Grains and Other Foods/Ingredients Not Appropriate for a Gluten-Free Diet

- Barley, bran, bulgur, couscous, durum flour, farina, graham flour, hydrolyzed plant protein (HPP), hydrolyzed vegetable protein (HVP), kamut, malt, malt extract, malt flavoring, malt syrup, semolina, rye, spelt (dinkel), triticale, wheat, wheat bran, wheat germ, wheat starch
- Imported foods that are labeled "gluten-free" but may contain wheat starch*
- Processed meats and luncheon meats containing HVP or HPP, breaded meats, meats with sauces or gravies, casseroles
- Fruits and vegetables with sauces, breading, or thickeners
- Flavored milk, yogurt, processed cheese, and spreads made with gluten-containing ingredients
- Canned soups, soup mixes, bouillon, miso
- Candy, snack foods, desserts, frozen yogurt, and ice cream with gluten-containing ingredients
- Ground spices, condiments, and soy sauce with gluten-containing ingredients
- Margarine, salad dressing, and dips with gluten-containing ingredients
- Instant coffee, instant tea, instant cocoa mixes, some root beer, grain alcohol

This is only a partial listing. Patients are encouraged to read all labels and to seek comprehensive food and additive lists from celiac organizations and the American Dietetic Association. *Foods produced in the U.S. or Canada and labeled "gluten-free" do not contain gluten or wheat starch. Adapted from Schwarzenberg and Brunzell (26).

different. Joining a support group or becoming active in celiac disease educational organizations will give the patient access to current information.

Psychosocial issues. Having celiac disease in addition to type 1 diabetes may present additional stress because of the nature of the symptoms, increased dietary restrictions, and serious consequences if untreated. Because the disease may go unrecognized for a long period, individuals who have multiple, recurring gastrointestinal complaints may be labeled as difficult patients. In addition, following a gluten-free diet is difficult in social situations where food is a focus. Patients may feel uncomfortable and isolated. While dietary education of the individual and family is central to the treatment, emotional support from the health care team is equally important in treating this disease.

Nursing implications. Like diabetes, celiac disease is a chronic condition that requires ongoing patient self-management. Assisting the patient in achieving positive outcomes in the management of both diseases is a challenge for the nurse. To

PRACTICAL POINT

Celiac disease is often missed as a diagnosis, and its symptoms are often attributed to other gastrointestinal diseases or poor adherence to the treatment regimen. Patients can become frustrated with their health care team and health care system. It is important that nurses be aware of the symptoms of this not-uncommon disease and promote early detection.

be successful at managing both conditions, the patient must have a working knowledge of diabetes and the rudiments of medical nutrition therapy as well as a sophisticated understanding of the gluten-free diet and how it interacts with glucose control issues such as hypoglycemia. Working as a team, the nurse and dietitian can educate the patient in the initial dietary changes and support the lifelong process of adaptation and readjustment.

ADDISON'S DISEASE

In Addison's disease, autoimmune destruction of the adrenal glands results in adrenal insufficiency and the absence of cortisol. Because Addison's disease can be effectively treated if diagnosed early, it is important to quickly evaluate for this disease to avoid fatalities. Clinical symptoms include weight loss; hyperpigmentation of the neck, elbows, and fingers; fatigability; muscle weakness; dehydration; increased craving for salt; and malaise. The risk of Addison's disease is 1 in 250 in individuals with immune-mediated type 1 diabetes. Therefore, individuals with immune-mediated type 1 diabetes plus the presence of thyroid autoantibodies should be tested for the presence of adrenal 21-hydroxylase autoantibodies (30). Another laboratory evaluation for Addison's disease is the adrenocorticotropic hormone cortisol-stimulation test, in which adrenocorticotropic hormone is administered intravenously and a cortisol level is drawn both 30 and 60 min later. If there is no response, the diagnosis of adrenocortical insufficiency, or Addison's disease, is made. The treatment is lifelong and consists of oral hydrocortisone.

PERNICIOUS ANEMIA

Another autoimmune disease associated with type 1 diabetes is anemia. Both iron deficiency anemia and pernicious anemia can be autoimmune mediated by parietal cell antibodies. The presence of antibodies to thyroid peroxidase and anti-gastric parietal cell antibodies and anti-adrenal antibodies is four to five times as frequent in individuals with type 1 diabetes as in the nondiabetic population. In a study of individuals with type 1 diabetes, 20.9% were found to be parietal cell antibody-positive; of those, 15.4% had iron deficiency anemia and 10.5% had pernicious anemia (31). Parietal cell antibodies can inhibit the secretion of the intrinsic factor necessary for the absorption of vitamin B12, leading to latent and eventually overt pernicious anemia. If laboratory tests indicate a deficiency of this vitamin, treatment typically consists of monthly injections of vitamin B12, though some elderly patients with gastric atrophy receive oral supplements in addition to the monthly injections.

SUMMARY

Many diseases can affect the level of glucose control that a person with diabetes achieves. These diseases cannot be overlooked in the treatment of diabetes. The metabolic changes that occur with the various disease states can make self-management of diabetes more difficult. Individuals who are coping with one or more chronic diseases will need nurses to provide additional patient education and psychological support to achieve positive outcomes.

REFERENCES

1. Ober K: Polyendocrine syndromes. In *Medical Management of Diabetes Mellitus*. Leahy J, Clark N, Cefalu W, Eds. New York, Marcel Dekker, 2000, p. 699–717

2. Berelowitz M, Kourides IA: Diabetes mellitus secondary to other endocrine disorders. In *Diabetes Mellitus: A Fundamental and Clinical Text*. 2nd ed. Philadelphia, Lippincott Williams & Wilkins, 2000, p. 588–594

3. Levin NA, Greer KE: Cutaneous manifestations of endocrine disorders. *Dermatol Nurs* 13:185–186, 189–196, 201–202, 2001

4. Grunstein RR, Ho KY, Sullivan CE: Sleep apnea in acromegaly. *Ann Intern Med* 115:527–532, 1991

5. Samuels MH: Growth hormone-secreting pituitary tumors. In *Endocrine Secrets*. 3rd ed. McDermott MT, Ed. Philadelphia, Hanley & Belfus, 2002, p. 189–193

6. Raff H, Findling JW: A physiologic approach to the diagnosis of the Cushing syndrome. *Ann Intern Med* 138:980–991, 2003

7. Oltmanns KM, Dodt B, Schwtes B, Raspe HH, Schweiger U, et al.: Cortisol correlates with metabolic disturbances in a population study of type 2 diabetic patients. *Eur J Endocrinol* 154:325–331, 2006

8. Chiodini I, Torlontano M, Scillitani A, Arosio M, Bacci S, et al.: Association of subclinical hypercortisolism with type 2 diabetes mellitus: a case control study in hospitalized patients. *Eur J Endocrinol* 153:837–844, 2005

9. Dhindsa S, Prabhakars S, Sethi M, Bandyopadhyay A, Dandona P: Frequent occurrence of hypogonatropic hypogonadism in type 2 diabetes. *J Clin Endocrinol Metab* 89:5462–5468, 2004

10. Kapoor D, Aldred H, Clerk C, Channer KS, Jones TH: Clinical and biochemical assessment of hypogonadism in men with type 2 diabetes. *Diabetes Care* 30:911–917, 2007

11. Kapoor D, Jones TH: Androgen deficiency as a predictor of metabolic syndrome in aging men. *Drugs Aging* 25:357–369, 2008

12. Morley JE, Charlton E, Patrick P, Kaiser FE, Cadeau P, et al.: Validation of a screening questionnaire for androgen deficiency in aging males. *Metabolism* 49:1239–1242, 2000

13. Angulo P: Nonalcoholic fatty liver disease. *N Engl J Med* 346:1221–1231, 2002

14. Jorgensen RA: Nonalcoholic fatty liver disease. *Gastroenterol Nurs* 26:150–155, 2003

15. Reid BM, Sanyal AJ: Evaluation and management of non-alcoholic steato-hepatitis. *Eur J Gastroenterol Hepatol* 16:1117–1122, 2004

16. Targher G, Bertolini L, Padovani R, Rodella S, Tessari R, et al.: Prevalence of nonalcoholic fatty liver disease and its association with cardiovascular disease among type 2 diabetic patients. *Diabetes Care* 30:1212–1218, 2007

17. Perros P, McCrimmon R, Shaw G, Frier B: Frequency of thyroid dysfunction in diabetic patients: value of annual screening. *Diabet Med* 7:622–627, 1995

18. Johnson J, Duick DS: Diabetes and thyroid disease: a likely combination. *Diabetes Spectrum* 15:140–142, 2002

19. Cooper D: Subclinical hyperthyroidism. *N Engl J Med* 345:260–265, 2001

20. Cronin CC, Feighery A, Ferriss JB, Liddy C, Shanahan F, Feighery C: High prevalence of celiac disease among patients with insulin-dependent (type 1) diabetes mellitus. *Am J Gastroenterol* 92:2210–2212, 1997

21. Eisenbarth GS, Gottlieb PA: Autoimmune polyendocrine syndromes. *N Engl J Med* 350:2068–2079, 2004

22. Waldron-Lynch F, O'Loughlin A, Dunne F: Gluten and glucose management in type 1 diabetes. *Br J Diabetes Vasc Dis* 8:67–71, 2008

23. Alsace NH, Maradiegue AH: Gastrointestinal health. In *Adult Primary Care*. Meredith PV, Horan NM, Eds. Philadelphia, W. B. Saunders, 2000, p. 414–418

24. Acerini CL, Ahmed MI, Ross KM, Sullivan PB, Bird G, Dunger DB: Coeliac disease in children and adolescents with IDDM: clinical characteristics and response to gluten-free diet. *Diabet Med* 15:38–44, 1998

25. Kaukinen K, Salmi J, Lahtela J, Siljamaki-Ojansuu U, Koivisto AM, et al.: No effect of gluten-free diet on the metabolic control of type 1 diabetes in patients with diabetes and celiac disease: retrospective and controlled prospective survey (Letter). *Diabetes Care* 22:1747–1748, 1999

26. Schwarzenberg SJ, Brunzell C: Type 1 diabetes and celiac disease: overview and medical nutrition therapy. *Diabetes Spectrum* 15:197–201, 2002

27. Freemark M, Levitsk LL: Screening for celiac disease in children with type 1 diabetes. *Diabetes Care* 26:1932–1939, 2003

28. Ceritti F, Beuno G, Chiarelli F, Lorini R, Meschi F, et al.: Younger age at onset and sex predict celiac disease in children and adolescents with type 1 diabetes: and Italian multicenter study. *Diabetes Care* 27:1294–1298, 2004

29. Thompson T: Case problem: questions regarding the acceptability of buck-wheat, amaranth, quinoa, and oats from a patient with celiac disease (Case Report). *J Am Diet Assoc* 101:586–587, 2001

30. Kukreja A, Balducci-Silano PL, Maclaren NK: Association between immune-mediated (type 1) diabetes mellitus and other autoimmune diseases. In *Diabetes Mellitus: A Fundamental and Clinical Text.* 2nd ed. LeRoith D, Taylor S, Olefsky JM, Eds. Philadelphia, Lippincott Williams & Wilkins, 2000, p. 410–419

31. De Block CE, De Leeuw IH, van Gaal LF, the Belgium Diabetes Registry: High prevalence of manifestations of gastric autoimmunity in parietal cell antibody-positive type 1 (insulin dependent) diabetic patients. *J Clin Endocrinol Metab* 84:4062–4067, 1999

Dr. Cypress is an Adult Nurse Practitioner and Certified Diabetes Educator in Albuquerque, NM. Ms. Spollett is an Adult Nurse Practitioner and Associate Director at Yale Diabetes Center, New Haven, CT.

31. Clinical Challenges in Caring for Patients with Diabetes and Cancer

Helen M. Psarakis, RN, APRN-BC

D iabetes and cancer are two diagnoses that individually overwhelm both patients and clinicians. Approximately 8–18% of people with cancer have diabetes (1). Together, these two diseases can pose formidable challenges to clinicians caring for this patient population. Unfortunately, our knowledge of this topic is limited by insufficient evidence to determine how best to manage diabetes while simultaneously treating cancer. This chapter seeks to review some of the most common problems encountered by clinicians caring for these patients.

CANCER SCREENING AND PREVENTION

Several studies published within the past decade demonstrate that patients with a chronic disease, such as diabetes, are less likely to receive preventive services, such as cancer screenings, than their counterparts without diabetes (2–5). One study concluded that patients with complex chronic diseases are 32% less likely to receive routine mammogram screening despite the fact that they see primary care and specialty physicians more frequently than their counterparts without diabetes (6). The discrepancy could not be explained by differences in comorbidity, income, age, access to care, or use of estrogen therapy. Instead, it was attributed to time constraints during office visits for complex chronic disease care, perceptions of decreased life expectancy among both patients and health care providers, and sociocultural barriers to health education. This should serve as a reminder for clinicians to question patients about their primary health care as routinely as they screen for diabetes complications.

This trend of decreased prevention services is disturbing given the evidence to suggest that insulin resistance and diabetes are linked to higher incidences of some cancers. Researchers hypothesize that exposure to hyperglycemia, elevated insulin

---

PRACTICAL POINT

Primary health screenings should not be overlooked in patients with diabetes. Routine screenings such as colonoscopy and mammograms are as important as diabetes complications screening tests.

---

concentrations, and the growth-promoting effects of insulin-like growth factor 1 may stimulate the development or progression of cancer. People with type 2 diabetes are at higher risk for developing breast, pancreatic, liver, kidney, endometrial, and colon cancers. Patients with type 1 diabetes are more likely to develop cervical and stomach cancers.

Several studies have also demonstrated that patients with diabetes and cancer have a poorer prognosis than those without diabetes. Diabetes and hyperglycemia are associated with higher infection rates, shorter remission periods, and shorter median survival times, as well as higher mortality rates from cancer (7–10).

CANCER TREATMENT: DIABETES AND CHEMOTHERAPEUTIC AGENTS

Patients with diabetes may present unique challenges to clinicians making cancer treatment decisions. Patients with longstanding diabetes or a history of poorly controlled diabetes may present for cancer treatment with preexisting renal, cardiac, or neuropathic complications. Several chemotherapeutic agents are known to cause or exacerbate these conditions. For example, cisplatin is known to cause renal insufficiency, and the anthracyclines may cause cardiotoxicity. Cisplatin, paclitaxel, and vincristine may be neurotoxic. Unfortunately, many of these side effects from chemotherapeutic agents are permanent.

Successful cancer treatment usually requires that at least 85% of the chemotherapeutic dose be given. Patients with diabetes must be carefully monitored before initiation of and during chemotherapy. Treatment decisions must be based on the patient's clinical picture, but always with the knowledge that any alterations in dose, timing of administration, or substitution of an alternate chemotherapeutic agent may compromise outcomes by lowering the treatment response rate and shortening survival (10).

CANCER TREATMENT: GLUCOCORTICOIDS

The use of glucocorticoids in patients with preexisting diabetes typically wreaks havoc on postprandial glycemic control (see chapter 28). Unfortunately, glucocorticoids are routinely used in many cancer treatment protocols. Glucocorticoid treatment for cancer patients usually consists of short-term therapy at a high dose. Lower dose steroids are also used to prevent chemotherapy-induced nausea and vomiting. All patients with cancer should be screened for diabetes before initiating glucocorticoid therapy and routinely monitored thereafter. These medications

Risk Factors for Steroid-Induced Diabetes

Family history of diabetes
Previous diagnosis of gestational diabetes
Advanced age
Obesity
High-dose steroid treatment

raise blood glucose through increased insulin resistance, gluconeogenesis, and glycogenolysis and decreased insulin production and secretion.

It is also common for patients to be diagnosed with diabetes while receiving glucocorticoid therapy. A family history of diabetes, a personal history of gestational diabetes, increased age, obesity, and high doses of steroids are the strongest predictors for glucocorticoid-induced diabetes (11). See chapter 28 for recommendations on management of hyperglycemia.

TUBE FEEDING AND TOTAL PARENTERAL NUTRITION

Tube feeding and total parenteral nutrition (TPN) are frequently used in oncology to supplement or replace a regular diet for patients who cannot sustain their usual intake of nutritional requirements. Hyperglycemia is a frequent complication from both of these forms of nutrition. It may be exacerbated by coexisting infection, use of steroids, and physiological responses to the stress of severe illness. Hyperglycemia can lead to dehydration, diabetic ketoacidosis (DKA), or hyperosmolar hyperglycemic state (HHS) if left untreated.

Adding regular insulin to the TPN solution can help control blood glucose levels. Initial doses are usually 1 unit per 10 g of carbohydrate. The dose should be titrated daily until glycemic control is attained. Using a lower carbohydrate formula will help with glycemic control in enterally fed patients (12). In individuals with preexisting type 2 diabetes not previously on insulin, 77% of the patients required insulin to control glycemia during TPN. Doses in this group averaged 100 ± 8 units/day (13).

These patients may also benefit from the use of basal insulin. The type of basal insulin used depends on the duration of the tube feeding. Some clinicians prefer glargine/detemir for continuous tube feeding. However, NPH given two or three times per day may work as well and allow for a quicker titration of the insulin dose. One program is successfully using a protocol of Humulin 70/30 (NPH/regular) given every 8 hours. The starting dose calculation varies based on renal/hepatic/cardiac dysfunction, obesity, open wounds/infection, or steroid therapy. NPH and Humulin 70/30 also offer an easier transition from continuous to timed or bolus tube feedings because a dose can be eliminated when the feedings are discontinued.

Patients receiving tube feeding or TPN should have their blood glucose monitored every 4–6 h. Short- or rapid-acting insulin dosed according to an algorithm may be given every 4–6 h to correct for any hyperglycemia (14–16). Hypoglycemia is likely to occur if TPN is stopped abruptly. Gradually decreasing the insulin infusion rate at least 1 h before discontinuing TPN reduces the risk of hypoglycemia (16). Extra caution should be used when changing from continuous to bolus feedings in the setting of long-acting basal insulin. Timing the change when the basal insulin action nears its end will help alleviate hypoglycemia.

NAUSEA AND VOMITING

Nausea and vomiting are common adverse drug reactions in some chemotherapy regimens. These reactions can occur in anticipation of therapy, acutely during or within 24 h of the therapy, or persistently over an extended period of time after therapy. Breakthrough nausea and vomiting may occur despite prophylactic treatment.

All patients should be screened for a history of nausea and vomiting before initiation of any chemotherapy. The history should include nausea and vomiting related to motion sickness, anesthesia, pregnancy, and any previous chemotherapy treatments. It should also include the frequency, severity, and duration of episodes, as well as the effect of nausea and vomiting on the patient's ability to eat and drink. Document all previous treatments for nausea and vomiting, including medications, doses, frequency, and effectiveness of the therapy.

Always consider the differential diagnoses for nausea and vomiting. These diagnoses include but are not limited to metabolic abnormalities (including DKA and HHS), bowel obstruction, infection, hepatic dysfunction, increased intracranial pressure, medication interactions, and radiation therapy.

Before initiating any chemotherapy regimen, consider the emetogenic potential of any agent or combination of agents in conjunction with the patient's history of nausea and vomiting and pre-treat the patient accordingly. Tables 31.1 and 2, created by Yale New Haven Hospital's Oncology Nursing and Pharmocology Services, rank chemotherapy agents in order of those most likely to induce emesis in adult and pediatric patients along with the appropriate antiemetic treatment. Patients with diabetes should be assessed frequently for nausea and vomiting, hydration status, ability to eat and drink, and glycemic control. Encourage patients to eat small, frequent meals, while avoiding sweet, fatty, salty, or spicy foods that may increase the severity of nausea and vomiting. Treat any breakthrough nausea immediately. Consider increasing the frequency of blood glucose monitoring for any patient with nausea and vomiting or a decreased tolerance to food and drink, especially if a steroid is used to manage emesis.

Adjust antihyperglycemic medication doses accordingly. Consider using a short-acting secretagogue (nateglinide or repaglinide) instead of a sulfonylurea (glimepiride, glipizide, glyburide) for postprandial glycemic control. Advantages include dosing intervals that can be timed with meals or withheld when patients are unable or unwilling to eat. Nateglinide and repaglinide are also much quicker to peak and have a shorter half-life than the sulfonylureas (Table 31.3). Rapid-acting insulins, such as aspart, glulisine, and lispro, have similar advantages to the nonsulfonylurea secretagogues but can also be dosed immediately following a meal. Rapid-acting insulin is also easier to titrate to precisely cover the amount of carbohydrate consumed during meals, thus affording patients more flexibility in food selections and portion sizes.

Table 31.1 Yale New Haven Hospital Guidelines for the Control of Chemotherapy-Induced Emesis in Adult Patients

Emetogenic Level	Frequency of Emesis	Chemotherapy Agent	Antiemetic Dose and Schedule
5	>90%	Carmustine >250 mg/m^2 Cisplatin ≥50 mg/m^2 Cychlophosphamide >1,500 mg/m^2 Dacarbazine Dactinomcin Mechlorethamine Streptozocin Any agent used at myeloablative doses	Ondansetron, 8 mg intravenously + Dexamethasone 20 mg intravenously, pretreatment + At 8–12 hours after treatment or at bedtime, give: Prochlorperaxine, 10 mg intravenously or by mouth *or* Metoclopramide, 20–40 mg intravenously or by mouth Lorazepam 0.5–1.0 mg intravenously or by mouth may be given pre- or post-treatment if needed
4	60–90%	Carboplatin Carmustine ≤250 mg/m^2 Cisplatin <50 mg/m^2 Cychlophosphamide >750–1,500 mg/m^2 Cytarabine >1 g/m^2 Doxorubicin >60 mg/m^2 Ifosfamide >1,000 mg/m^2 Irinotecan Melphalan intravenously Methotrexate >1,000 mg/m^2 Oxaliplatin Procarbazine (by mouth)[a]	Ondansetron 8 mg intravenously + Dexamethasone 20 mg intravenously, pretreatment + At 8–12 hours after treatment or at bedtime, give: Prochlorperaxine 10 mg intravenously or by mouth *or* Metoclopramide 20–40 mg intravenously or by mouth Lorazepam 0.5–1.0 mg intravenously or by mouth may be given pre- or post-treatment if needed
3	30–60%	Cyclophosphamide ≤750 mg/m^2 Cyclophosphamide by mouth[a] Doxorubicin 20–60 mg/m^2 Epirubicin ≤90 mg/m^2 Gemcitabine Hexamethylmelamine by mouth[a]	Ondansetron 8 mg intravenously, pretreatment + Dexamethasone 10–20 mg intravenously, pretreatment

(continued)

Table 31.1 Yale New Haven Hospital Guidelines for the Control of Chemotherapy-Induced Emesis in Adult Patients (*continued*)

Emetogenic Level	Frequency of Emesis	Chemotherapy Agent	Antiemetic Dose and Schedule
		Idarubicin Ifosfamide ≤1000 mg/m² Lomustine by mouth Methotrexate 250–1,000 mg/m² Mitoxantrone	
2	10–30%	Docetaxel Etoposide 5-Fluorouracil <1,000 mg/m² Liposomal doxorubicin Methotrexate >50–249 mg/m² Mitomycin Paclitaxel Teniposide Thiotepa Topotecan	Dexamethasone 4–8 mg intravenously or by mouth, pretreatment
1	<10%	Asparaginase Bleomycin Busulfan po Chlorambucil po 2-Chlorodeoxyadenosine Fludarabine Hydroxyurea Methotrexate ≤ 50 mg/m² Melphalan PO 6-Mercaptopurine Tamoxifen 6-Thioguanine Vinblastine Vincristine Vinorelbine	No routine pretreatment recommended

The most highly emetogenic agent in the combination should be identified, and the contribution of other agents should be considered using the following rules: *1)* Level 1 agents do not contribute to the emetogenicity of a given regimen; *2)* adding one or more Level 2 agents increases the emetogenicity of the combination by one level greater than the most emetogenic agent in the combination; *3)* adding Level 3 and Level 4 agents increases the emetogenicity of the combination by one level per agent.

ªOral chemotherapeutic agents that are highly emetogenic at high doses may be less emetogenic in lower doses given over a longer period (e.g., 2 weeks). Oral procarbazine and cyclophosphamide are usually given in combination chemotherapy regimens that include a moderate dose of corticosteroid (prednisone), which can serve as a sufficient antiemetic. On the other hand, the combination of moderate-risk emetogenic drugs can result in high emetogenic potential and should be treated accordingly.

ᵇAlthough given orally, lomustine is highly emetogenic and should be treated with the listed pre-medication.

From Yale New Haven Hospital: Nausea and vomiting related to cancer chemotherapy. In *Clinical Practice Manual*. New Haven, CT, Yale New Haven Hospital, 2005

Table 31.2 Yale New Haven Hospital Guidelines for the Control of Chemotherapy-Induced Emesis in Pediatric Patients

Emetogenic Level	Frequency of Emesis	Chemotherapy Agent	Antiemetic Dose and Schedule
High	>90 %	Busulfan intravenously Carmustine Cisplatin >75 mg/m² Cisplatin <75 mg/m²* Cyclophosphamide ≥1,250 mg/m² Dacarbazine ≥500 mg/m² Ifosfamide/ Carboplatin or Cisplatin/Etoposide (ICE) Lomustine >60 mg/ m² Melphalan intravenously Methotrexate ≥10,000 mg/m² Mitoxantrone >15 mg/m² Any agent used at myeloablative doses	Ondansetron, 0.15 mg/kg intravenously or by mouth 30 min pre-chemotherapy, then every 4 h for two additional doses (alternatively, ondansetron, 0.45 mg/ kg 30 min pre-chemotherapy for one dose daily) + Dexamethasone, 8 mg/m² intravenously or by mouth pre-chemotherapy, then 4 mg/m² intravenously or by mouth every 6 h. Repeat on each day of chemotherapy. *Consider ondansetron as above plus dexamethasone pre-chemotherapy only. For breakthrough nausea and vomiting, consider the following agents: Diphenhydramine 0.5 mg/kg intravenously (may increase to 1 mg/ kg, to a maximum 50 mg/dose) + Promethazine, 0.5 mg/kg intravenously (maximum 25 mg/dose) every 6 h as needed *or* Chlorpromazine, 0.55 mg/kg Intravenously or by mouth (maximum 40 mg/dose), may repeat every 4–6 h *or* Lorazepam, 0.05 mg/kg intravenously (maximum 3 mg/dose), may repeat every 8–12 h *or* Dexamethasone, 5–10 mg/m² Intravenously or by mouth, may repeat every 12 h as needed If one or more of these agents fails, consider a single dose of ondansetron, 0.15 mg/kg intravenously. For delayed nausea and vomiting associated with cisplatin or

(continued)

Table 31.2 Yale New Haven Hospital Guidelines for the Control of Chemotherapy-Induced Emesis in Pediatric Patients (*continued*)

Emetogenic Level	Frequency of Emesis	Chemotherapy Agent	Antiemetic Dose and Schedule
			cyclophosphamide, consider treatment with one of the following 12–24 h post-chemotherapy: chlorpromazine, lorazepam, ondansetron.
Moderate	30–60%	Carboplatin Cyclophosphamide intravenously <1,250 mg/m² Cytarabine ≥1 g/m² Dactinomycin Daunorubicin Doxorubicin Idarubicin Ifosfamide Methotrexate 250–10,000 mg/m² Mitoxantrone ≤15 mg/m²	Ondansetron, 0.15 mg/kg intravenously or by mouth 30 min pre-chemotherapy, then every 4 h for two additional doses (alternatively, ondansetron, 0.45 mg/kg 30 min pre-chemotherapy for one dose daily) Add as needed dexamethasone (8 mg/m²) pre-chemotherapy, then 4 mg/m² every 6 h if ondansetron alone fails
Low	10–30%	Cytarabine <1 g/m² Etoposide Fluorouacil <1,000 mg/m² Paclitaxel Teniposide Topotecan	Dexamethasone, 5–10 mg/m² intravenously or by mouth pre-chemotherapy *or* Ondansetron, 0.15 mg/kg intravenously or by mouth pre-chemotherapy
Low	<10%	Androgens Asparaginase Bleomycin Cladribine Corticosteroids Cyclophosphamide by mouth Hydroxyurea Mercaptopurine Methotrexate ≤250 mg/m² Thioguanine by mouth Vinblastine Vincristine	No antiemetic prophylaxis necessary

*In multiple agent regimens, the most highly emetogenic agent should be identified. Very low level (< 10%) agents do not contribute to emetogenicity of combination regimens.

Adding one or more low-level (10–30%) agent(s) increases emetogenicity of the combination by one level more than the most emetogenic agent.

From Yale New Haven Hospital: Nausea and vomiting related to cancer chemotherapy. In *Clinical Practice Manual*. New Haven, CT, Yale New Haven Hospital, 2005.

Table 31.3. Comparison of Sulfonylureas and Nonsulfonylurea Secretagogues

Agent	Dose (mg)	Dose Interval	Peak (h)	Half-life (h)	Duration (h)
Glyburide	2.5, 5	Daily, twice daily	4	10	12–24
Micronized Glyburide	1.5, 3, 6	Daily, twice daily	2	4	12–24
Glipizide	5, 10	Daily, twice daily	1–3	2–4	12–24
Glipizide – GITS	2.5, 5, 10	Daily	6–12	n/a	24
Glimepiride	1, 2, 4	Daily	2–3	9	24
Nateglinide	60, 120	Three times daily with meals	0.3	1	4
Repaglinide	0.5, 1, 2	Three or four times daily with meals	1	1	4–6

Adapted from Inzucchi (21).

BLOOD GLUCOSE MANAGEMENT DURING END-OF-LIFE CARE

Glycemic control goals may become less stringent but should not be ignored during end-of-life care. Some patients may desire tight glycemic control as a means of exerting some degree of control over an otherwise untenable medical situation. Insulin and oral hypoglycemic agents should still be used in "comfort care" or "palliative care" patients because the signs and symptoms of uncontrolled hyperglycemia decrease quality of life. A blood glucose goal of <200 mg/dl minimizes the risk of polyuria, polydipsia, electrolyte imbalance, and dehydration and may be a realistic goal for some patients. Clinicians should elicit patients' opinions and adhere to their wishes when making treatment decisions. These decisions should be reevaluated and revised with each significant change in patients' clinical status and always within the context of the patients' overall goals.

SUMMARY

Overall, the treatment of and therapies for diabetes in the setting of cancer present a major challenge for clinicians. Maintaining adequate glucose control reduces the incidence of infection in at-risk patients with cancer. Sustaining adequate nutrition and providing appropriate calories for patients receiving chemotherapy demands careful glucose control with whatever therapy improves the clinical situation. Having an understanding of the complexities of both diseases is necessary to achieve the best outcomes.

REFERENCES

1. Ko C, Chaudhry S: The need for a multidisciplinary approach to cancer care. *J Surg Res* 105:53–57, 2002

2. Beckman T, Cuddihy R, Scheitel S, Naessens J, Killian J, Pankratz V: Screening mammogram utilization in women with diabetes. *Diabetes Care* 24:2049–2053, 2001

3. Kief C, Funkhouser E, Fouad M, May D: Chronic disease as a barrier to breast and cervical cancer screening. *J Gen Intern Med* 13:357–365, 1998

4. Fontana S, Baumann L, Helberg C, Love R: The delivery of preventive services in primary care practices according to chronic disease status. *Am J Public Health* 87:1190–1196, 1997

5. Redelmeier D, Tan S, Booth G: The treatment of unrelated disorders in patients with chronic medical diseases. *N Eng J Med* 338:1516–1520, 1998

6. Lipscombe L, Hux J, Booth G: Reduced screening mammography among women with diabetes. *Arch Intern Med* 165:2090–2095, 2005

7. Bloomgarden Z: Diabetes and cancer. *Diabetes Care* 24:780–781, 2001

8. Bloomgarden Z: Second World Congress on the Insulin Resistance Syndrome. *Diabetes Care* 28:1821–1830, 2005

9. Balkau B, Kahn H, Courbon D, Eschwege E, Ducimetiere P: Hyperinsulinemia predicts fatal liver cancer but is inversely associated with fatal cancer at some other sites. *Diabetes Care* 24:843–849, 2001

10. Richardson L, Pollack L: Influence of type 2 diabetes on the development, treatment and outcomes of cancer. *Nat Clin Pract Oncol* 2:48–53, 2005

11. Clement S, Braithwaite SS, Magee M, Ahmann A, Smith EP, Schafer RG, Hirsch IB: Management of diabetes and hyperglycemia in hospitals. *Diabetes Care* 27:553–591, 2004

12. Hirsch IB, Paauw DS: Diabetes management in special situations. *Endocrinol Metab Clin North Am* 26:631–645, 1997

13. Clement S, Braithwaite SS, Magee MF, Ahmann A, Smith EP, et al.: Management of diabetes and hyperglycemia in hospitals. *Diabetes Care* 27:553–591, 2004

14. Leahy J: Insulin management of diabetic patients on general medical and surgical floors. In *Improving Inpatient Diabetes Care: A Call to Action Conference*. Jacksonville, FL, American College of Endocrinology and American Association of Clinical Endocrinologists, and Alexandria, VA, American Diabetes Association, 2006, p. 145–149

15. Lyman B: Metabolic complications associated with parenteral nutrition. *J Infusion Nurs* 25:36–44, 2002

16. McMahon M, Rizza R: Concise review for primary-care physicians: nutrition support in hospitalized patients with diabetes mellitus. *Mayo Clin Proc* 71:587–594, 1996

17. Inzucchi SE: *Diabetes Facts and Guidelines 2008*. New Haven, CT, Yale University School of Medicine, 2008

Ms. Psarakis is a diabetes clinical nurse specialist at Yale New Haven Hospital in New Haven, Conn.

DIABETES CARE
IN COMMUNITY SETTINGS

32. Diabetes Care in the Inpatient Setting

Jane Jeffrie Seley, MPH, MSN, GNP, BC-ADM, CDE

Until recently, tight glycemic control in acutely ill patients was of little concern to many health care professionals. A paradigm shift is occurring as a growing body of knowledge continues to show a relationship between hyperglycemia and poor outcomes in hospitalized patients (1). Organizations such as the American Diabetes Association (2,3), the American Association of Clinical Endocrinologists (3), and the Joint Commission (4) have made inpatient diabetes management a priority and have offered recommendations to help health care providers achieve lower glycemic targets.

The diabetes epidemic is evident in both the outpatient and inpatient settings. In 2002 alone, close to 5 million hospital discharges in the U.S. had diabetes listed as a diagnosis, with an estimated cost of $40 billion. It is during hospitalization that many patients learn that they have diabetes. It is estimated that 12–25% of hospitalized adults have preexisting or newly diagnosed diabetes at the time of discharge (2). Hospitalized patients with hyperglycemia may have previously diagnosed diabetes, previously undiagnosed diabetes, or stress-related hyperglycemia secondary to the acute illness or medications.

Controlling blood glucose during hospitalization in patients with known diabetes is particularly challenging, since there are often disruptions in meals and mealtimes, food choices, medication taking, physical activity, and sleep-and-wake cycle. Patients who routinely self-manage their diabetes are suddenly placed in a position where their care is done by others, taking away their independence. The fluctuations of glucose levels during an acute illness are often frightening to someone who has maintained good glycemic control. Health care professionals should be sensitive to these issues when caring for patients with preexisting diabetes. The challenge of overseeing this comprehensive care and facilitating a safe discharge plan is often the role of the nurse (5). In the inpatient setting, nurses are key providers of self-management education.

THE CASE FOR GLUCOSE CONTROL

Optimal glucose control can prevent infection, support healing, and promote patient well-being. In addition, it can reduce mortality and morbidity (6). Improved glycemic control has proven to be beneficial in studies in diverse populations, such as post–acute myocardial infarction (MI), cardiac-surgery, and critically ill patients in a surgical intensive care unit. In the Diabetes Mellitus, Insulin Glucose Infusion in Acute Myocardial Infarction (DIGAMI) study, patients had a 29% reduction in mortality 1 year after having received intravenous insulin in the first 24 h post MI and multiple injections of subcutaneous insulin for the next 3 months (6). Furnary et al. (7) achieved a 66% reduction in mortality with mean blood glucose levels of <150 mg/dl using intravenous insulin as compared with prior use of subcutaneous injections in cardiac surgery patients. Van den Berghe et al. (8) reduced mortality by 34% and sepsis by 46% in a surgical intensive care unit by lowering blood glucose levels to <110 mg/dl. In a retrospective chart review of general medicine and surgery patients, Umpierrez et al. (9) found that patients with "new" hyperglycemia and patients with known diabetes had 18-fold and 2.7-fold increased mortality risks, respectively, if the blood glucose levels exceeded >126 mg/dl fasting or >200 mg/dl at least twice during hospitalization. This evidence has shifted the pendulum to the current focus on stricter glycemic targets in acute care.

Trauma patients with diabetes also present a challenging balance between management of critical injuries and maintenance of glycemic control. One study found that even patients with mild hyperglycemia (>135 mg/dl [>7.5 mmol/l]) with or without diagnosed diabetes have significantly longer hospital stays, infection morbidity (e.g., urinary tract infections, wound infections, pneumonia, bacteremia), longer intensive care unit stays, and increased mortality compared with normoglycemic patients (8,10). Intensive glucose control requires close monitoring and proper intervention by the team to improve patient outcomes.

When choosing more aggressive critical care and noncritical care targets, each institution has to consider the culture and current practice. Barriers such as fear of hypoglycemia and lack of understanding of basal/bolus insulin therapy are real concerns and must be addressed (11). Conservative targets may be established initially and then modified as staff become educated and competent in carrying out order sets and protocols. The American Diabetes Association recommends a blood glucose <140 mg/dl in critical care patients, with the ultimate goal of as close to 110 mg/dl as possible. The blood glucose goal for non–critically ill patients is currently <126 mg/dl fasting and <180–200 mg/dl at all other times (12).

Glycemic control protocols or order sets may make it easier to achieve targets. These may include bedside or point-of-care blood glucose levels, initial insulin dosages, scheduled insulin doses administered in relation to meals, and orders for nursing staff of when to hold insulin or call the physician (13). Hospital routines, products, and protocols should be reviewed on an ongoing basis to evaluate whether they may conflict with diabetes management best practices. It is therefore important that hospital staff be knowledgeable about strategies to improve glycemic control while avoiding acute complications.

THE NURSE'S ROLE

Nurses may have several roles in the care of the hospitalized patient. They may be part of a team that develops policies and protocols for the care of inpatients with diabetes and hyperglycemia or be responsible for educating other nursing staff, and they are frequently the bedside nurse who is the first to identify patient needs and is responsible for care and education of the patient.

TEAM APPROACH TO INPATIENT MANAGEMENT

While there are many strategies that can be implemented to improve diabetes care in the hospital setting, the most accepted is a system-wide approach with the creation of an interdisciplinary team to seek opportunities and solutions to improve diabetes care (2–4). The team should be made up of all disciplines and departments that provide routine care to patients with diabetes, e.g., endocrinologist, certified diabetes educator, nurses such as a clinical nurse specialist or manager, nurse educator and/or bedside nurse, pharmacist, dietitian, social worker or case manager, point-of-care testing administrator, data analyst, and house staff. The team responsibilities include review of evidence and published protocols, adoption of standards, and formation of protocols and established outcomes.

ASSESSING THE PATIENT

Management of the hospitalized patient with diabetes can be challenging, with shortened inpatient stays and complex medication regimens coupled with comorbidities and diabetes-related chronic complications. Regardless of the reason for admission, it is essential to identify suboptimally controlled diabetes and acute hyperglycemia at the time of hospital admission and to implement therapy to improve glycemia (2). Table 32.1 identifies key information that should be obtained on admission (14).

The nurse should seek opportunities to improve diabetes self-care behaviors and treatments, particularly if suboptimal glycemic control is the underlying cause for hospitalization. Patients with ineffective or suboptimal home regimens, as evidenced by hemoglobin A1c (A1C) values >7% and frequently 8–12% or higher, experience increased counterregulatory hormones, resulting in increased insulin resistance and marked hyperglycemia. Careful monitoring of blood glucose levels and appropriate interventions to meet target goals for glycemic levels can help promote optimal outcomes. Diabetes knowledge and performance of self-care, including coping skills, need to be determined.

HOSPITAL GLUCOSE MONITORING

A1C testing and regular glucose monitoring are recommended for all patients with or at risk of hyperglycemia (9,15). A1C can be used to evaluate diabetes control prior to or at admission in people with previously diagnosed diabetes and to determine whether a patient with "new" hyperglycemia actually has undiagnosed diabetes (9).

Table 32.1 Baseline Diabetes Assessment

I. Initial Questions
A. Type of diabetes
B. Duration of diabetes
C. Primary care physician (PCP)
D. Primary diabetes physician, if different from PCP

II. Medical Nutrition Assessment
A. Diet prescription
B. Estimated compliance
C. Weight change in past 6 months

III. Physical Activity

IV. Medications Taken
A. Insulin (type, amount, and frequency)
B. Diabetes medications
C. Other prescription medications
D. Over the counter

V. Assessment of Control
A. Type of meter/strips
B. Frequency of monitoring
C. Results of home monitoring, if available
D. A1C frequency, date of last test, and results, if available
E. Ketones

VI. Acute Symptoms of Diabetes
A. Hyperglycemia
  1. Thirst
  2. Frequent urination
  3. Urination during night
  4. Yeast infection
  5. History of diabetic ketoacidosis
  6. Blurred vision
B. Hypoglycemia
  1. Episodes of sweating, shaking, pounding heart, headache, and/or confusion
  2. Frequency, timing, symptoms, and treatment

VII. Reproductive Assessment
A. Preconception
B. Pregnancy
C. Menopause

VIII. Substance Abuse
A. Tobacco
B. Alcohol
C. Other

IX. Barriers to Care
A. Internal
  1. Hearing or sight impairment
  2. Cognitive dysfunction
  3. Language/literacy
  4. Physical impairment
B. External
  1. Financial
  2. Transportation
  3. Family/significant other status

X. Chronic Complications/ Comorbidities
A. Neuromuscular/psychiatric
  1. Pain and/or numbness
  2. Depression
  3. Unusual mood dysfunction
  4. Dizziness
B. Eye
  1. Last dilated eye exam
  2. History of diabetic eye disease
C. Kidney/bladder
  1. History of protein in urine
  2. Kidney disease
D. Cardiovascular
  1. Hypertension
  2. Shortness of breath
  3. Smoking
  4. Chest pain
  5. Dyslipidemia
  6. Obesity
  7. Family history
E. Infections
  1. Recurrent infections
  2. Immunizations (flu and pneumonia)
F. Foot and limb
  1. Numbness
  2. Foot ulcers
  3. Amputations

Goals for Blood Glucose Levels in Hospital

Critically ill patients: Blood glucose levels should be kept as close to 110 mg/dl as possible and generally <140 mg/dl. These patients require an intravenous insulin protocol that has demonstrated efficacy and safety in achieving the desired glucose range without increasing risk for severe hypoglycemia.

Non–critically ill patients: There is no clear evidence for specific blood glucose goals. Cohort data suggest that outcomes are better in hospitalized patients with fasting glucose <126 mg/dl and all random glucoses <180–200 mg/dl (if safe to achieve). Insulin is the preferred drug to treat hyperglycemia in most cases.

Scheduled preprandial insulin doses should be appropriately timed in relation to meals and adjusted according to point-of-care glucose levels. Sliding-scale insulin regimens are ineffective as monotherapy and are not recommended.

Using correction-dose or supplemental insulin to correct premeal hyperglycemia in addition to prandial and basal insulin is recommended.

From the American Diabetes Association (12).

During hospitalization, timing of blood glucose monitoring, also known as point-of-care glucose monitoring, needs to match the patient's nutritional intake and medication management for optimal glycemic control. Patients that are on NPO orders often have orders for blood glucose monitoring every 4–6 h or more often if unstable or on an insulin drip (16). Patients who require enteral feedings and parenteral nutrition usually require blood glucose monitoring every 4–6 h or as ordered. For the individual who is consuming regular meals, a 2-h postprandial test will be necessary to achieve the stated goal to keep the blood glucose level <180 mg/dl (<10 mmol/l) at all times. Premeal or pre-insulin dose blood glucose monitoring may be necessary to determine an appropriate correctional insulin dose. Short- or rapid-acting insulin is given before or with the meal, respectively, based on eating patterns.

Specific patient situations may warrant closer monitoring, such as hourly blood glucose monitoring when initiating and titrating intravenous insulin. According to Clement et al. (2), once a patient's insulin drip rate has stabilized and the glycemic target has been achieved, the frequency of blood glucose monitoring can be reduced to every 2–3 h. Patients with prolonged hypoglycemia secondary to sulfonylurea use, especially those sulfonylureas with long half-lives such as chlorpropamide, glimepiride, and glyburide, require more intensive monitoring and may need an intravenous dextrose infusion. Nurses should watch for signs and symptoms of hypoglycemia and monitor patients more frequently when there are changes made in medications that impact glycemia, such as glucocorticoids, anti-hyperglycemic agents, and insulin. Nurses need to be aware of conditions and medications that may lead to inaccurate blood glucose readings, such as peritoneal dialysate that contains maltose, which can cause false-positive glucose elevations.

Nurses can play an important role in bedside blood glucose monitoring by assessing the equipment used, accuracy, and patient comfort. Required blood sample size and choice of lancet are key areas to evaluate when considering comfort. When they are able, patients should be involved in obtaining their own fingerstick sample, applying the blood to the test strip, and evaluating the result as a learning opportunity. Although the home equipment may not be the same, these skills will be important once the patient resumes self-management at home.

Some patients will bring their glucose meters into the hospital. This provides an opportunity for validating the meter's accuracy and the patient's proficiency. In acute-care settings, an individual's use of a personal meter must be addressed in the organization's policies and procedures. The hospital meter should be used for all treatment and charting, since quality control is done on the hospital meter daily and the results are utilized for surveillance. Patients can use their own meters if they want to know their glucose levels between hospital checks, but the nurse should confirm an abnormal value with the hospital meter before acting on the glucose reading.

The data collected from blood glucose monitoring on each hospital unit provide an opportunity for performance improvement by evaluating incidences of hypoglycemia and hyperglycemia by patient type, location, and regimen. This form of glucometrics, or standardized measures of glycemia, can guide the development, evaluation, and revision of protocols (17). Progress toward achieving glycemic targets unit by unit can be tracked, and interventions can be targeted.

Regulatory and licensing agencies mandate that hospitals and other facilities must have quality assurance programs for blood glucose monitoring (18). Correlation studies comparing bedside results with laboratory values are essential elements of the quality assurance process (19). Accuracy of blood glucose monitoring is an essential component in ensuring that treatment decisions are appropriate for optimal glycemic targets.

NUTRITION

Goals of therapy include providing adequate calories to meet the increased nutritional needs of the acutely ill while balancing metabolic control, including glucose, lipids, and blood pressure. Diabetes control is interrupted by adjustments in nutrition orders, such as NPO, clear liquids only, and parenteral or enteral feedings that are necessary for the treatment of other conditions. Medication adjustments need to match the altered intake to avoid acute complications, most notably hypoglycemia. Patients must be carefully monitored for glucose fluctuations resulting from changes in their meal plans.

As in the outpatient setting, consistent carbohydrate meal planning is recommended. Although this presents a loss of flexibility for the patient, offering the same amount of carbohydrates on each meal tray provides a way to easily match the prandial insulin dose to a known amount of carbohydrate (2,3). In order to provide consistent carbohydrates, a number of system changes may be needed. The hospital menus may need to be examined to calculate the carbohydrate content of foods. Carbohydrate-friendly menus should clearly identify which foods contain carbohydrate to the nearest half serving or number of grams and identify how many servings or total grams of carbohydrate the patient is offered for the meal. This allows the patient to order the correct amount of carbohydrate, thus avoiding the disappointment when the tray comes up and items have been arbitrarily deleted because the patient selected more than the meal plan provides. This type of menu becomes a learning tool for teaching carbohydrate counting and practicing the skill with each meal tray.

Hospital routines often lead to a mismatch of when the blood glucose is checked, the insulin is given, and the meal is consumed. Streamlining this can vastly improve glycemic control. One hospital (anecdotally) was able to reduce morning hypoglycemia by restricting the timing of the fasting blood glucose to after 7:00 a.m. and expediting the meal tray delivery so that patients with diabetes got their breakfast first. Patients are rarely, if ever, taught to check their blood glucose values and administer insulin 30 min prior to a meal. Rapid-acting insulin needs to be given as near to the consumption of the meal as possible. Frequently in hospitals, insulin is given and the meal is delayed or insulin is given long after the meal is consumed, leading to problems with hypoglycemia or hyperglycemia. Rapid-acting insulin analogs allow for the flexibility of giving the insulin before or just after the start of the meal. It is helpful to deliver the meal trays first to patients on consistent-carbohydrate meal plans to give the nurse ample time to plan and coordinate the timing of monitoring, medication, and meals.

Many providers mistakenly believe that the cardiac diet includes a restriction in carbohydrates and neglect to order the diabetes meal plan. It is up to the nurse to ensure that the patient is receiving the best meal plan for the primary diagnosis and all comorbidities. The nurse and the dietitian should assist the patient and/or their family in meal selection to maintain a consistent amount of carbohydrate as the patient progresses from NPO to liquids, soft foods, and regular diet. Patients on clear or full liquid diets should receive ~200 g of carbohydrates throughout the day divided into equal amounts and snack times (20). Options for substitutions from preprinted hospital menus give patients added choices and reduce the chance that the meal will not be eaten.

Parenteral and enteral feedings require special monitoring, careful nutrition formula selection, and diabetes medication adjustment. If the gastrointestinal tract is intact, enteral feeding is the preferred route (21). The duration of the need for parenteral or enteral feeding will drive the formula selection. It is necessary that the formula provide adequate nutrition along with acceptable glucose control and blood lipid concentrations. Insulin is generally delivered according to calculated protocols, and necessary adjustments are made regularly. Protocol examples are available at http://www.hospitalmedicine.org/ResourceRoomRedesign/html/12Clinical_Tools/04_Insulin_OrdersIV.cfm (22).

Insulin pump users and other patients who follow an intensive insulin management regimen may be more comfortable with a hospital's regular meal plan so they can choose from a wider variety of foods and calculate their own mealtime insulin dose using insulin-to-carbohydrate ratio.

Gastroparesis, or delayed gastric emptying, presents a challenge to match the timing of the insulin to the breakdown of the meal to maintain glucose control. Hyperglycemia alone can cause delayed gastric emptying (23). It is important to include the dietitian and the patient in meal planning to identify optimal foods to decrease the impact of gastroparesis on glucose control.

MEDICATION MANAGEMENT

Regardless of whether the patient has type 1 or type 2 diabetes, maintaining glycemic control is a primary goal and a determinant in achieving positive health outcomes. The primary consideration in caring for patients with type 1 diabetes is adequate insulin replacement. Individuals with type 1 diabetes require basal insulin and multiple-dose injections of rapid-acting insulin with meals. Even if patients are not eating, they will require basal insulin either as glargine, levemir, NPH injections or continuous intravenous infusion, and they may require rapid-acting insulin to correct the hyperglycemia produced in response to stress or illness.

In the hospital, oral antihyperglycemic agents are often discontinued because they lack the flexibility and efficacy needed in an acute-care setting and can present additional problems. Oral antihyperglycemic agents should be avoided during hospitalization and should be held until close to or after discharge (2,3). For example, a long-acting sulfonylurea can promote hypoglycemia if a meal is delayed or the patient eats poorly. Biguanides, such as metformin, and thiazolidinediones are not recommended in times of impaired renal and hepatic function and fluid changes. Metformin must be discontinued on the day of any surgical procedure and not reinitiated for at least 48 h after the procedure (see chapter 5). Because metformin is metabolized by the kidney, adequate perfusion must be present for the drug to clear the system properly. Any procedure that may interfere with the clearing of the medication may allow it to build up in the system and puts the patient at risk for developing lactic acidosis, a sometimes fatal complication. Near normal (50% or better) renal function, as determined by laboratory assessment, must be established before reinitiating metformin. In addition, it is not uncommon for patients to have insurmountable insulin requirements during acute illness that require exogenous insulin therapy to accommodate the need.

INSULIN THERAPY

Aggressive initiation and intensification of insulin therapy is often required to achieve glycemic targets in acutely ill patients (Table 32.2). The patient's A1C, current glycemia, weight, renal function, oral intake, and medications should all be taken into consideration. Hospital intensive insulin management often requires both basal and nutritional insulin to cover metabolic needs and the carbohydrate in meals or enteral or parenteral nutrition, as well as supplemental insulin based on a formula to correct for glycemic excursions.

There is no evidence that traditional sliding-scale regimens are an effective method for maintaining optimal glucose control in the hospital. In fact, when used alone, sliding scales may actually promote hyperglycemia (24). Short-term use of supplemental/correctional insulin may be appropriate to correct hyperglycemia. Scheduled nutritional and supplemental/correctional insulin doses should be evaluated daily and adjusted to compensate for patterns of hyperglycemia or hypoglycemia.

Many studies that have shown improved outcomes in critical care have used insulin drip protocols to get to goal safer and sooner than with subcutaneous insulin (6–8). Many of these protocols are available on the infonet at no charge

Table 32.2 Inpatient Management of the Patient with Diabetes

- Step 1: Discontinue oral antidiabetic agents if using this insulin protocol
  - Target inpatient blood glucose levels: 80–130 mg/dl
  - Consider a medicine consult and don't forget to order diabetes education
- Step 2: Calculate the estimated total daily dosage of insulin
- Step 3: Determine the distribution of the total daily dosage
  - If patient is eating or receiving bolus tube feeds
  - If patient is receiving continuous enteral nutrition
  - If patient is NPO or taking clear liquids only
- Step 4: Reevaluate and adjust the total daily dosage based on the glycemic control of the previous 24 h

From the Society of Hospital Medicine Glycemic Control Taskforce (22).

(25,26). Several protocols exist and have been published, but studies comparing these protocols do not exist. In addition, there are several computerized programs for sale to assist the nurse in titrating the insulin drip rate based on current blood glucose level and rate of change from the last reading (14,27). Less aggressive insulin drip protocols are gaining in popularity to be used in non–critical care areas where hourly glucose measurements are unrealistic.

The development of algorithms, protocols, and order sets will guide the less experienced provider in achieving targets in a timely fashion with less hypoglycemia (2,3). Standing order sets for supplemental insulin and intravenous insulin drip protocols ensure that all providers aim for ideal goals as patients deal with the glucose level variations common during hospitalization. Scheduled basal and prandial insulin is the method of choice for subcutaneous insulin therapy (2,3). Correctional insulin can be combined with prandial insulin; however, separating the orders may allow the nurse more flexibility to assess whether or not the patient is eating and which insulins should be given each time. This method of management will become simpler and more seamless as more facilities adopt electronic medical record systems. For example, an electronic medical record program can allow for initiation of weight-based subcutaneous basal insulin that also considers expected insulin sensitivity (e.g., sensitive, average, resistant). Nurses need opportunities to learn about intravenous insulin management and the tools available to reduce the level of work that can be associated with intravenous insulin management.

TRANSITIONING FROM INTRAVENOUS INSULIN DRIPS TO SUBCUTANEOUS INSULIN

Once a patient's condition begins to stabilize and he or she is starting to eat, intravenous insulin is no longer necessary. If not planned and implemented carefully, the transition from intravenous to subcutaneous insulin not only can cause a major disruption in glucose control, but can also trigger diabetic ketoacidosis (DKA) in individuals with type 1 diabetes. Basal insulin should be given subcutaneously at least 2 h before the insulin drip is discontinued. One option would be to discontinue the insulin drip just before a meal so that rapid-acting insulin can be given. Careful monitoring of blood glucose levels is necessary during the transition to prevent hypoglycemia or hyperglycemia.

The nurse's role in inpatient diabetes management should include proactive attention to whether or not glycemic targets are reached and maintained. For example, bedside nurses can be empowered to identify patients who are above predetermined glycemic targets for their unit and notify prescribers to initiate or intensify insulin therapy (28).

Since diabetes is frequently diagnosed during hospitalization and acute illness increases the likelihood that insulin will be required, many patients with diabetes go home on insulin for the first time. From the moment a patient starts receiving insulin, the nurse should begin teaching insulin administration. This may start simply with the patient learning to self-inject. Too often, this is overlooked and the patient is given a rushed lesson moments before discharge with no opportunity for practice. Should the patient go home not requiring insulin, he or she will gain confidence in being capable of safe administration when the time comes. For patients with preexisting diabetes, hospitalization is an excellent opportunity to evaluate prior treatment regimens and modify them if necessary.

PRACTICAL POINT

Nurses have a vital role in assisting patients to discover ways to eat healthy and maintain diabetes control. There are many opportunities for patient teaching in hospitals. Meal and snack adjustments, interrupted meals, changes in meal timing, alternate feedings, and hypoglycemia treatment, all of which occur in the hospital setting, provide opportunities for patient education. Every hospital nurse must be comfortable with the principles of good nutrition and healthy food choices so that patient questions can become a teachable moment (see chapter 3 for more about healthy lifestyle choices).

MANAGEMENT OF PATIENTS USING INSULIN PUMPS

More individuals are using continuous subcutaneous insulin infusion (CSII) therapy (insulin pump therapy), so having patients presenting to the hospital on insulin pumps is no longer that unusual. Hospital staff must be prepared to ensure that glucose control is maintained. If staff nurses are not educated in CSII management, a consultation with the diabetes specialist or diabetes management team should be obtained. Staff nurses should be instructed in assessing the infusion site for infection, know how to verify if a bolus was administered, and know how to disconnect the insulin pump if necessary. (For more information, see chapter 24.) Because not all staff nurses are familiar with CSII management, it is in the best interest of the patient that the hospital support a policy allowing the patient or family to maintain pump therapy. However, if the patient or family is unable to support CSII safely, the health care provider may change the patient to an alternative method of insulin delivery (Table 32.3). Because maintaining good metabolic control plays a critical role in achieving positive health outcomes, the insulin delivery method that best accomplishes this goal should be supported by the patient's care team. In some cases, maintaining pump therapy may not be feasible and the hospital will need to have a written protocol that allows for the conversion to another method of insulin delivery.

MANAGEMENT OF HYPOGLYCEMIA

Treating hypoglycemia in the hospitalized patient with diabetes is a nursing intervention. All hospitals should have protocols for treating hypoglycemia. These protocols should indicate the glucose level at which treatment is initiated and the type and amount of glucose to be administered to patients who are able to take oral treatment. In case the patient is unable to take oral treatment for hypoglycemia, indications for the use of glucagon and intravenous dextrose should be clearly stated in the guidelines. Certain circumstances may require that the attending or resident physician be notified if the glucose level does not respond to the prescribed treatment (see also chapter 7).

In hospitalized patients receiving intensive therapy for glycemic control, prevention of hypoglycemia should be an important goal. Hypoglycemia can often be anticipated and should be prevented by measures other than undertreatment of hyperglycemia (28). Hypoglycemia is normally preceded by a preventable triggering event, which usually includes a sudden change in caloric intake, transportation off ward, alteration in total parenteral nutrition or enteral feedings, or continuous venovenous hemodialysis (28). Additionally, patients who are receiving

Table 32.3 Sample Insulin Pump Policy

POLICY/PROCEDURE		
SUBJECT: Insulin Pumps	NUMBER: M30-11	PAGE: 1 OF: 1
ORIG. 6/98	REVISED: 1/00	REVIEWED: 10/02
PREPARED BY INTERDISCIPLINARY POLICY/PROCEDURE COMMITTEE		
APPROVED BY PCMH PRESIDENT APPROVED BY VICE PRESIDENT, PATIENT CARE SERVICES		
When a patient is admitted with an insulin pump, the patient and his/her physician assume responsibility for the pump. If the patient is a pediatric patient, he or she, the parent, and physician assume responsibility for the pump. Nurses observe and document the patient's response to therapy, but they do not make any adjustment in the dose/rate of the pump.		
If the patient becomes incapacitated and cannot manage the pump, the physician will order that administration of insulin by pump be discontinued. Further orders for management of the patient will be written by the physician.		

Reprinted with permission from Pitt County Memorial Hospital.

Myocardial Infarction

The landmark DIGAMI study demonstrated the effect glucose control has on improved outcomes for previously diagnosed and undiagnosed patients with diabetes (6). In patients with myocardial infarction, early aggressive intervention with intravenous insulin administered when glucose levels were >198 mg/dl (>11 mmol/l), followed by subcutaneous insulin therapy four times a day for 3 months, resulted in a 30% reduction in mortality at 1 year, an average 28% reduction at 3.5 years in patients with known diabetes, and a 51% reduction in those not previously diagnosed with diabetes. Better glycemic control improved the survival rates of patients with diabetes who had a myocardial infarction.

medications for hyperglycemia and have certain diseases or conditions, such as renal insufficiency, advanced age, malnutrition, liver disease, sepsis, shock, pregnancy, total parenteral nutrition, burns, congestive heart failure, stroke, hypoglycemia unawareness, tapering steroids, alcoholism, or polypharmacy, may be predisposed to hypoglycemic events.

During oral treatment, once the customary amount of glucose (15–20 g) is administered, the nurse usually must remain with the patient or provide close observation and assess the response to treatment. Blood glucose monitoring should be performed 15–20 min after treatment. If the resulting glucose level has not returned to the target range (>70 mg/dl [3.8 mmol/l]), then treatment should be repeated (see Fig. 32.1). At the resolution of the hypoglycemic episode, the nurse should document the initial blood glucose levels and symptoms experienced by the patient, the treatment, and the follow-up blood glucose monitoring results.

An episode of hypoglycemia should involve an evaluation of what caused the hypoglycemia. This is a good time for nurses to teach patients how to recognize, prevent, and appropriately treat hypoglycemia.

PATIENT EDUCATION

The nurse is pivotal in the implementation of the education plan, which must begin early in the admission to prepare the patient for self-care at home. In addition, the nurse can help facilitate outpatient follow up. Whether a short stay, less than 24 h, or an inpatient admission, the opportunity to provide diabetes education, review, and reinforcement must not be missed.

Bedside nurses have the most opportunity to provide diabetes self-management training in "survival skills." Survival skills generally include self-monitoring of blood glucose, meal planning, medication taking, and hypoglycemia treatment and prevention (2,29). Whenever possible, the nurse should include patients by having them participate in the glucose monitoring and insulin administration.

Washington
Hospital Center   *MedStar Health*

Checked; ___   Transcribed; ___   Scanned; ___
Date/Time   Name   Date/Time   Name   Date/Time   Name   Date/Time   Name

Standardized Subcutaneous Insulin Orders

All orders to be carried out unless crossed out.
Prescriber: Check all boxes & specify insulin doses that apply.
Unit clerk, enter: "Standardized subcutaneous insulin orders, see standardized subcutaneous insulin flowsheet" on kardex. (Text in parentheses is informational and does not need to be transcribed onto kardex.)

1. **Diagnosis:** □ Uncontrolled or □ Controlled; □ with complications; □ Diabetes Type: □ 1, □ 2, □ gestational, or □ diabetes secondary to other cause, specify _____ ; or □ Stress/Situational Hyperglycemia.
2. **Blood glucose target range:** 80–180 mg/dl or specify □ _____ – _____ mg/dl
3. **Diet:** □ Consistent carbohydrate with Crystal Lite products. No juice.
4. □ **Draw glycohemoglobin A1C with next blood draw** (if not already drawn during this admit).
5. **Discontinue all previous insulin orders.**
6. **For transition from insulin drip to subcutaneous insulin: STOP INSULIN DRIP** <u>after</u> first subcutaneous dose of Novolog® given; or □ 45 minutes after first dose of regular; or □ 2 hours after first dose of NPH or Lantus given alone.

7. **HYPOGLYCEMIA TREATMENT: For FSBG < 60 mg/dL or** □ **FSBG < _____ mg/dl**

   A) If patient <u>can take PO</u>, give 15 grams of fast acting carbohydrate such as:
   8 oz milk (skim preferred) or 4 oz apple juice or orange juice or regular soda.

   B) If pateint <u>cannot take PO</u>, give (check as applicable):
   □ Dextrose 50% 12.5 grams (25 ml) IV push OR □ Glucagon IM 1 mg if no IV access and insert IV.

   C) Recheck FSBG every 20 minutes until:
   FSBG □ ≥ 90 mg/dl or □ ≥ _____ mg/dl;
   If repeat FSBG < 90 mg/dl, repeat treatment as in A) or B) above

   D) **Call MD/NP if 2 serial FSBG < 60 mg/dL or** □ **< _____ mg/dl, and/or change in mental status**

   E) **If FSBG ≤ 40 mg/dl,** repeat FSBG with bedside monitor to cconfirm value;
   Treat as in steps A-C above, and
   If pateint does not have symptoms of low blood glucose, send STAT serum glucose to confirm value was low.

8. **IF patient made PRE-OP or NPO for procedure, call MD/HO/NP/PA for insulin doses for:**

   A) **NIGHT BEFORE** (Suggest 20% reduction in NPH/ glargine (Lantus®) and
   B) **AM of procedure** (Suggest reducing AM NPH by 50% or glargine (Lantus®) by 20% and HOLD other scheduled insulins)

   FSBG and insulins orders should be reviewed and modified at least once daily, or more frequency as needed.

			PRINT NAME	
DATE	TIME	PRESCRIBER'S SIGNATURE	PRESCRIBER'S #	PAGER OR PHONE

PREPRINTED PRESCRIBERS ORDERS

Place LABEL precisely
in this space

P&T: 0302 (2/2006)

FORM 1168   REV. 08/02/02

FIGURE 32.1 Sample standardized hospital insulin orders. From the Society of Hospital Medicine Glycemic Control Taskforce (22).

Survival Skills for Patients in the Hospital

- A general understanding of the key components of the disease and its treatment
- The ability to take medications and injections accurately
- A basic ability to eat consistently with needs
- The ability to self-test and understand the results at a basic level
- The ability to recognize and treat hypoglycemia when applicable
- Sometimes, the ability to perform foot self-exams and other screenings for complications
- Key follow-up contact information and appointments for follow-up
- Education for acute illness

From Nettles (29).

Nurses should abandon the practice of performing portions of these skills away from the bedside, where the patient cannot observe the technique. Patients who have a more challenging treatment regimen may benefit from consultation with a diabetes care team while in the hospital.

Menu selection and identifying carbohydrates and portion sizes on the meal tray provide opportunities to practice skills. The hospitalization may provide the patient's only opportunity to meet with a dietitian. A referral to the dietitian for assessment and instruction should be considered.

PATIENTS WITH KNOWN DIABETES

Patients who have been self-managing their diabetes at home are often frustrated when they are admitted to the hospital and find they can take better care of their diabetes than the hospital staff. It is therefore important that hospital staff be knowledgeable about strategies to improve glycemic control and respect the patient's ability to self-manage while avoiding acute complications.

For the previously diagnosed patient, nurses must assess the current level of knowledge regarding diabetes management. Only through evaluation of the patient's current knowledge can the nurse review, reinforce, and observe self-management skills. It is important to assess each patient's learning needs and prior diabetes knowledge as early in the admission as possible and to set mutual goals (2). Early assessment will provide opportunities to identify any barriers and identify available resources, such as a visiting nurse or a family member who can be taught skills needed for home care. One should not assume that the patient is performing a skill correctly just because he or she has been doing it for years. With cognitive and physical changes, especially in the elderly, and increasingly complex regimens, the patient's ability to perform self-care may have changed over time.

PATIENTS NEW TO INSULIN

The patient with newly diagnosed type 1 diabetes and some patients with type 2 diabetes will need to begin insulin therapy while hospitalized. Although individuals with newly diagnosed type 2 diabetes do not depend on exogenous insulin for survival, because of the progressive nature of the disease, many of these individuals have decreased insulin production and require insulin for adequate blood glucose control, especially during times of stress and illness. Patients must be informed that the change to insulin is not a failure on their part and occurs because of the exhaustion of β-cell function.

At times, although not ideal, the educational process must begin in the intensive care unit. Once the patient is stabilized, the remaining time spent in the hospital may be brief. Therefore, the nurse must be alert to the patient's progress and begin demonstrating insulin administration and self-monitoring of blood glucose as soon as the patient is able to participate. If family members are available, they should be included in these education sessions to support and assist the patient in this period of adjustment. The educational focus is on the survival skills needed to make the transition to the home setting. Home care referral may be needed to continue and reinforce diabetes self-management skills. All patients should be referred for outpatient diabetes self-management education. Diabetes self-management education is an ongoing process, and survival skills are only the beginning of what is needed by the patient to effectively manage diabetes at home and throughout life.

When teaching patients about insulin administration, the goal is for the patient to understand and successfully demonstrate the following skills, with validation by the nurse:

- Insulin storage and injection preparation
  Onset, peak, and duration of insulin(s)
  Injection site selection and correct injection technique
  Needle safety
  Recognition of and how to treat hypoglycemia

See chapter 4 for more on insulin administration.

Since patients are likely to be under increased stress and to be fatigued secondary to hospitalization, it is best to keep education sessions short (10). The focus should be on providing the immediate skills and knowledge that the patient needs to go home safely. Short, easy-to-read materials should be made available in multiple languages to reinforce education and ensure consistency from educator

Discharge Planning

Discharge planning anticipates what the patient will need to continue diabetes self-management at home and must be initiated early in admission. When needs are anticipated early, patients and their families are better informed and more confident about how they will care for themselves at home. The nurse needs to coordinate with interdisciplinary team members in planning care, teaching and reinforcing skills, and connecting with community resources for self-management support after discharge. Financial assistance, links to diabetes services and community resources, and evaluation of an existing support system minimize barriers and promote successful diabetes self-management.

to educator. Simple one-page handouts available on the hospital infonet help ensure that patients receive the same consistent information across settings from inpatient to outpatient.

NEWLY DIAGNOSED TYPE 2 DIABETES AND PRE-DIABETES

It is important that the hospitalized patient with newly diagnosed type 2 diabetes or pre-diabetes have an understanding of the seriousness of the new diagnosis and the importance of follow up with a health care provider. The nurse should facilitate scheduling outpatient follow up after discharge and provide the patient with the positive message that making healthy lifestyle choices now may affect the progression of their disease.

Diabetes educators should be available as a resource to guide the education, working collaboratively with the bedside nurse and other members of the team. Documentation is important to facilitate communication between the team members to insure that each team member knows the status of the patient's education plan and whether specific goals are being met.

PATIENT CONCERNS

Patients accustomed to managing their diabetes in their own way find it difficult to relinquish control and trust the health care team to take over. Patients can be adamant about when and how much insulin should be given, how often glucose should be monitored, and exactly what should be on their meal plan at every meal. The best way for nurses to take advantage of the expertise that the patient brings to his or her diabetes management is to make the patient a central part of the health care team and facilitate and accommodate the patient's wishes as much as possible. When it is not possible to accommodate the patient's wishes, an understanding attitude and detailed explanations about why the care is being managed the way it is will assist the patient in accepting the treatment plan.

Patients who struggle with taking care of their diabetes present a different opportunity. A hospitalization may be a good time to talk to patients about their concerns regarding diabetes. Open communication may allow the nurse to assist the patient in identifying barriers that may be preventing optimal self-care. Lack of finances may be preventing adherence to a medication regimen or appropriate monitoring of blood glucose in the home setting. A referral to social services may be necessary. A consultation with a diabetes educator and/or dietitian may be helpful, but should not replace the opportunity for nurse/patient interaction at the bedside. Education with every medication administration, discussion of glucose readings, careful explanation of all tests and lab results, assistance with food choices from a menu, and solicitation of support from family and friends can all send the message that diabetes control is important and possible.

SPECIAL CONSIDERATIONS FOR SURGICAL PATIENTS

During their lifetimes, many patients with diabetes will require surgery. Regardless of whether the surgery is related to diabetes, managing diabetes during the pre-, intra-, and postoperative periods presents a challenge (see also "Diabetes and Surgery," a patient handout in RESOURCES). Several studies indicate that suboptimal diabetes control increases lengths of stay and rates of infection (30–32). The stress of surgery itself upsets glucose control, increasing the secretion of counterregulatory hormones, inhibiting the release of endogenous insulin, and possibly resulting in ketogenesis (33). Interruption of the patient's usual management adds to this problem. Depending on the type of surgery, nutritional intake can be different from normal intake for short to extended periods. In addition, the surgical team may not be familiar with the patient's presurgery management and fail to reinitiate the treatment regimen. Long-term cardiac, renal, and neuropathic diabetes complications can put the patient at greater risk of postoperative complications. For all of these reasons, diabetes status must be carefully assessed and glucose control maintained during each hospitalization for surgery.

Whether surgery is a planned one or an emergency procedure, the decision regarding how to maintain glucose control depends on the type of diabetes, the type of surgery, and the length of time before the patient will be able to return to the preoperative diabetes treatment plan. For example,

- For same-day, short-stay surgery, major changes are not usually required.
- Most CSII patients do not remove the pump or change their basal rates.
- Whenever possible, surgery should be scheduled early in the day to reduce the effect on the patient's treatment plan.
- Medication management would be similar to the management used for the inpatient, except metformin, which should always be discontinued (see "Medication Management" in this chapter and see chapter 5).

Patients on insulin should continue their long- or intermediate-acting insulin the day before surgery. Patients may be individually advised to lower their bedtime NPH, evening glargine, or detemir dose the day prior to the admission. On the morning of surgery, one-half to two-thirds of the usual dose of long- or intermediate-acting insulin is given and blood glucose is monitored every 2 h. A slow glucose infusion (100–125 ml/h of 5% dextrose) is given to prevent hypoglycemia, and hyperglycemia can be treated with small doses of regular insulin every 4–6 h or rapid-acting insulin every 2 h at ~0.05–0.1 units/kg. In individuals with type 2 diabetes who are not managed with insulin, oral agents should be discontinued at least 24 h before surgery if possible and insulin should be administered if blood glucose levels are >180 mg/dl (>10.0 mmol/l).

Management of diabetes during an outpatient procedure, or day surgery, may be accomplished with intravenous or subcutaneous insulin in patients with type 1 or type 2 diabetes. Insulin should be used in patients with type 2 diabetes if blood glucose levels are >180 mg/dl (10.0 mmol/l). When individuals are discharged, directions should be given for frequent blood glucose monitoring with an algorithm for supplemental short- or rapid-acting insulin to be administered. Patients with type 2 diabetes who can resume their previous management should do so, but they may require supplemental short- or rapid-acting insulin to treat stress-related hyperglycemia. Instruction should be given to call the health care provider if blood glucose levels are >250 mg/dl (13.9 mmol/l) (34).

STAFF EDUCATION

Staff education is a key component to a successful glycemic control program (1). Staff education and the development of protocols will help providers achieve glucose targets. Standardized order sets using the "right" insulin in safe dosages help direct less experienced providers away from ordering sliding scale coverage (2,12). All health care professionals who care for patients with diabetes should receive management updates on an ongoing basis. This includes physicians, physician assistants, nurse practitioners, nurses, dietitians, pharmacists, and case managers (4). Diabetes educators can work with nurse educators to develop staff competencies, curricula, teaching checklists, and handouts to improve the nurse's knowledge and confidence level in educating patients with diabetes. To accommodate the needs of the busy nurse, educational opportunities should be offered in a variety of ways, such as unit-based classes, continuing education programs, staff orientation, self-learning modules, including web-based programs, grand rounds, and mentoring programs. The availability of supplies, such as home blood glucose meters and demonstration insulin pens, on units will facilitate patient teaching.

DISCHARGE PLANNING AND CARE MANAGEMENT

The prospect of diabetes self-management can be overwhelming to the patient contemplating discharge, especially when the patient has other conditions to address. It is important to link the patient to outside resources to continue care. The Case Management Society of America offers some helpful guidelines on its website (http://www.cmsa.org) (35). Nurses need to collaborate with case managers, home care coordinators and social workers to create a safe discharge plan. The diabetes management plan and the patient's ability to perform self-care need to be communicated to the next provider to smooth the transition from inpatient to outpatient (4).

SUMMARY

Because ~7.8% of the U.S. population has diabetes and an estimated 57 million have pre-diabetes, hospital nurses in all units need to be proficient in caring for people with diabetes and hyperglycemia (36). Nurses must be familiar with the basic elements of care as well as the protocols necessary for acute care management.

Specific management protocols, order sets, treatment algorithms for insulin drips, hypoglycemia, and hyperglycemic crises, either DKA or hyperglycemic hyperosmolar syndrome, and clinical pathways should be developed and implemented by institutions to guide the best practice for caring for the hospitalized patient with diabetes (37). With adequate training, all units can be prepared to administer intravenous insulin (15,38). The need for intravenous insulin should never be the criterion for transfer to a higher level of care. When diabetes management is seen as an integral part of the treatment of other acute medical problems, outcomes are improved and hospital stays are shortened (15). Studies provide supporting evidence about the importance of glycemic control during acute illness, and this valuable research must be incorporated into clinical practice to improve outcomes and quality of life for patients with diabetes.

Patient education should be looked upon as part of the responsibilities of the hospital nurse and incorporated into regular, routine patient care. It should not create an additional burden to the busy nurse if it is performed as part of daily care. Inpatient diabetes management is a team effort. Nurses are important members of the team, with many opportunities to improve glycemic control and care in general.

REFERENCES

1. Abourizk NN, Vora CK, Verma PK: Inpatient diabetology: the new frontier. *J Gen Intern Med* 19:466–471, 2004

2. Clement S, Braithwaite SS, Magee MF, Ahmann A, Smith EP, et al.: Management of diabetes and hyperglycemia in hospitals (Technical Review). *Diabetes Care* 27:553–591, 2004

3. The ACE/ADA Task Force on Inpatient Diabetes: American College of Endocrinology and American Diabetes Association consensus statement on inpatient diabetes and glycemic control: a call to action. *Diabetes Care* 29:1955–1962, 2006

4. Joint Commission: Management of the patient with diabetes in the inpatient setting [Internet]. Available at http://www.jointcommission.org/NR/rdonlyres/1F9B67C2-72A6-4DC3-A047-15BEB394FE3C/0/diabetes_addendum.pdf. Accessed 2 March 2009

5. Peeples M, Seley JJ: Diabetes care: the need for change. *AJN* 107:13–19, 2006

6. Malmberg K, the DIGAMI (Diabetes Mellitus, Insulin Glucose Infusion in Acute Myocardial Infarction) Study Group: Prospective randomised study of intensive insulin treatment on long term survival after acute myocardial infarction in patients with diabetes mellitus. *BMJ* 314:1512–1515, 1997

7. Furnary AP, Gao G, Grunkemeier GL, Wu Y, Zerr KJ, et al.: Continuous insulin infusion reduces mortality in patients with diabetes undergoing coronary artery bypass grafting. *J Thorac Cardiovasc Surg* 125:1007–1021, 2003

8. Van den Berghe G, Wouters P, Weekers F, Verwaest C, Bruyninckx F, et al.: Intensive insulin therapy in the critically ill patients. *N Engl J Med* 345:1359–1367, 2001

9. Umpierrez GE, Isaacs SD, Bazargan N, You X, Thaler LM, Kitabchi AE: Hyperglycemia: an independent marker of inhospital mortality in patients with undiagnosed diabetes. *J Clin Endocrinol Metab* 87:978–982, 2002

10. Yendamuri S, Fulda GJ, Tinkoff GH: Admission hyperglycemia as a prognostic indicator in trauma. *J Trauma* 55:33–38, 2003

11. Cook CB, Jameson KA, Hartsell ZC, Boyle ME, Leonhardi BJ, et al.: Beliefs about hospital diabetes and perceived barriers to glucose management among inpatient midlevel practitioners. *Diabetes Educ* 34:75–83, 2008

12. American Diabetes Association: Standards of medical care in diabetes—2009. *Diabetes Care* 32 (Suppl. 1):S13–S61, 2009

13. Reynolds LR, Cook AM, Lewis DA, Colliver MC, Legg SS, et al.: An institutional process to improve inpatient glycemic control. *Qual Manage Health Care* 16:239–249, 2007

14. American Healthways: *Inpatient Management Guidelines for People with Diabetes*. Nashville, TN, American Healthways, 2003

15. Levetan CS, Magee MF: Hospital management of diabetes. *Endocrinol Metab Clin* 29:745–770, 2000

16. Estrada CA, Young JA, Nifong LW, Chitwood WR: Outcomes and perioperative hyperglycemia in patients with or without diabetes mellitus undergoing coronary artery bypass grafting. *Ann Thorac Surg* 75:1392–1399, 2003

17. Kosiborod M, Inzucchi SE, Krumholz HM, Xiao L, Jones PG, et al.: Glucometrics in patients hospitalized with acute myocardial infarction: defining the optimal outcomes-based measure of risk. *Circulation* 117:1018–1027, 2008

18. Walker EA: Quality assurance for blood monitoring. *Nurs Clin North Am* 28:61–70, 1993

19. Peragallo-Dittko V: Monitoring. In *A Core Curriculum for Diabetes Education*. 5th ed. Franz MJ, Ed. Chicago, American Association of Diabetes Educators, 2003, p. 189–209

20. American Diabetes Association: Nutrition recommendations and interventions for diabetes. Diabetes Care 31:S61–S78, 2008

21. Coulston AM: Enteral nutrition in patients with diabetes mellitus. *Curr Opin Clin Nutr Metab Care* 3:11–15, 2000

22. Society of Hospital Medicine Glycemic Control Taskforce: Workbook for Improvement: Improving Glycemic Control, Preventing Hypoglycemia, and Optimizing Care of the Inpatient with Hyperglycemia and Diabetes [Internet], 2007. Available from http://www.hospitalmedicine.org. Accessed 3 March 2009

23. Rayner CK, Samson M, Jones KL, Horowitz M: Relationships of upper gastrointestinal motor and sensory function with glycemic control. *Diabetes Care* 24:371–381, 2001

24. Queale W, Seidler A, Brancatti F: Glycemic control and sliding scale insulin use in medical inpatients with diabetes mellitus. *Arch Intern Med* 157:545–551, 1997

25. Furnary AP, Wu Y, Bookin SO: Effect of hyperglycemia and continuous intravenous insulin infusions on outcomes of cardiac surgical procedures: The Portland Diabetic Project. *Endocr Pract* 10 (Suppl. 2):21–33, 2004

26. Goldberg PA, Siegel MD, Sherwin RS, Halickman JI, Lee M, et al.: Implementation of a safe and effective insulin infusion protocol in a medical intensive care unit. *Diabetes Care* 27:461–467, 2004

27. Davidson PC, Steed RD, Bode BW: Glucommander, a computer-directed intravenous insulin system shown to be safe, simple and effective in 120,618 h of operation. *Diabetes Care* 28:2418–2423, 2005

28. Braithwaite S, Buie M, Thompson C, Baldwin D, Oertel M, et al.: Hospital hypoglycemia: not only treatment but also prevention. *Endocr Pract* 10 (Suppl. 2):88–99, 2004

29. Nettles A: Patient education in the hospital. *Diabetes Spectrum* 18:44–48, 2005

30. Sadhu AR, Ang AC, Ingram-Drake LA, Martinez DS, Hsueh WA, Ettner SL: Economic benefits of intensive insulin therapy in critically ill patients: the targeted insulin therapy to improve hospital outcomes (TRIUMPH) project. *Diabetes Care* 31:1556–1561, 2008

31. Schaberg DS, Norwood JM: Case study: infections in diabetes mellitus. *Diabetes Spectrum* 25:37–40, 2002

32. Golden SH, Peart-Vigilance C, Kao WH, Brancati FL: Perioperative glycemic control and the risk of infectious complications in a cohort of adults with diabetes. *Diabetes Care* 22:1408–1414, 1999

33. Jacober SJ, Sowers JR: Management of diabetes in patients undergoing surgery. *Pract Diabetol* 20:7–14, 2001

34. Marks JB: Perioperative management of diabetes. *Am Fam Phys* 67:93–100, 2003

35. Case Management Society of America: Case Management Adherence Guidelines [Internet]. Available from http://www.cmsa.org/Individual/Education/CaseManagementAdherenceGuidelines/tabid/253/Default.aspx. Accessed 3 March 2009

36. Centers for Disease Control and Prevention: National Diabetes Fact Sheet, 2007 [Internet]. Available from http://www.cdc.gov/diabetes/pubs/pdf/ndfs_2007.pdf. Accessed 3 March 2009

37. Quevedo S, Sullivan E, Kington R, Rogers W: Improving diabetes care in the hospital using guideline-directed orders. *Diabetes Spectrum* 14:226–233, 2001

38. Metchick LN, Petit WA, Inzucchi SE: Inpatient management of diabetes. *Am J Med* 113:317–323, 2002

Ms. Seley is a Diabetes Nurse Practitioner and Certified Diabetes Educator on the Diabetes Team at New York Presbyterian-Weill Cornell Medical Center in New York City.

Sylvia English, MS, RN, CDE, and Sandra Young, MSN, BCRN contributed to this chapter for the prior edition.

33. Role of the Office Nurse in Diabetes Management

Kathy J. Berkowitz, APRN, BC, FNP, CDE

O ver the past 20 years, the responsibility for the care of patients with diabetes has shifted away from hospitals and toward primary care (1,2). Currently, physician office visits constitute the largest and most widely used segment of the American health care system. Diabetes was listed as the primary diagnosis for 25.5 million office-based physician visits in 2005. The number of visits made by adults 18 years and over with diabetes has increased by 53% since 1995. The patient is seen during office visits by a physician 96% of the time and/or by a registered or licensed practical nurse 28% of the time. The overall mean time spent with a physician is 20 min; visits lasting 16–30 min have increased by 20% since 1995 (3). Expenditures for visits attributable to diabetes were $10 billion in 2007 (4).

Significant opportunities exist for nurses in ambulatory care, as the emphasis in health care has shifted from acute episodic care to prevention and health maintenance. Nurses in ambulatory care historically have been underused (5). Shifting the care of patients with complex disease states to physician offices has changed and expanded ambulatory nursing practice (6). Furthermore, patient education activities have extended beyond treatment preparation instructions to include the culturally sensitive counseling of individuals and their families on lifestyle changes that prevent or mediate chronic disease.

Although the dimensions of ambulatory nursing intervention have expanded, response to the encounter primarily remains with the patient; acceptance of and implementation of health care regimens are determined by the patient. Thus, to appropriately counsel the patient with diabetes, the nurse in an ambulatory care setting needs to be competent in use of technology, critical thinking, and evaluative skills, as well as the implementation of effective interpersonal, culturally sensitive communication and interventions (7).

MEDICAL OFFICE PRACTICE

Today, in an ambulatory setting, a nurse's function includes a diverse set of roles oriented toward implementing collaborative practice, managing continuity of care, and using other nursing staff to triage patients and provide clinically complex care. Previously, nursing functions in small-office settings were minimal, usually involving such things as administering injections and assisting with procedures. However, as physicians began to create large specialty-group practices, organized nursing services began to emerge that focused on the ability to respond to knowledgeable, service-oriented clients and to assist physicians in practice management (8).

ROLES AND COMPETENCIES

Nursing competency is determined by the individual nurse's education, knowledge, certification, experience, and abilities. Each nurse is responsible for identifying appropriate practice parameters within a state's nurse practice act, professional code and professional practice standards, and employer policies for performing activities or functions in accordance with the nurse's own educational level and competence. In addition to clinical core competencies, the office nurse must demonstrate role-based competencies related to the management and coordination of patient care, supervision of unlicensed assisting personnel, management of relationships with clients and families, documentation of care provided, and support of office operations (7).

The nurse's role becomes a strong source of continuity. In specialty-practice settings, such as a diabetes clinic, nurses will often work with patients and their families over extended periods while engaging in patient teaching, follow-up activities, and monitoring outcomes. They will continue to assist patients in accessing care throughout health care networks. Increasingly they will be making clients aware of their rights and will negotiate on the patient's behalf when the patient is not well served (7).

TEAM RELATIONSHIPS

In partnership with the patient, nursing practice occurs within the context of a multidisciplinary team comprised of other licensed professionals, technicians, and unlicensed assisting personnel. In office settings, nurses typically work much more closely and continuously with physicians and other health care providers.

The nursing role within the ambulatory care team is limited only by the nurse's willingness to perform, levels of knowledge and competency, time constraints, and ability to negotiate the role with the team. In cases where more than one provider is able to meet patient needs, responsibilities for care will require negotiation. Areas of potential role overlap include determining which discipline performs screening assessments and who documents data regarding past history, medications, allergies, and response to treatment. As attempts to develop cost-effective delivery models occur, health care teams are being reconfigured so provider levels meet the needs of the patient without unnecessary duplication and without compromising outcomes (7). For example, nurse-managed health maintenance organizations and nurse-run clinics may be able to manage populations with diabetes more effectively and efficiently (9–15).

One factor frequently identified by office nurses is the unique collaborative relationship between the nurse and the physician. This role requires that the nurse demonstrate the ability to communicate effectively. The nurse becomes a conduit between the patient, who is self-managing his or her diabetes daily, and the physician, who may be directing care without having seen the patient, helping the two parties make decisions based on what may have been identified in a telephone assessment. Telephone communication with nurses has been shown to positively affect patient satisfaction and patient perception of easy access (16).

IMPROVING PATIENT CARE

In the U.S., many adults with diabetes are receiving suboptimal care, and empirical data suggest that compliance with diabetes clinical practice recommendations is inadequate in primary care (17,18). There is growing evidence that enhancing the role of the nurse in the family physician's office can save lives and money (19).

High-quality diabetes care consists of a combination of factors: a knowledgeable staff, an involved patient empowered to improve his or her care, and an office practice system designed to help the care process. Practice systems have been identified as the richest area of improved care for most medical office practices. Most approaches have been multidisciplinary, but often the primary staff member responsible for delivering intervention and monitoring guidelines has been a nurse (20–22).

Comprehensive diabetes care using a prioritized record-keeping system, such as diabetes care checklists, can help identify the important tasks that need to be performed during each office visit (23). The office nurse can serve a vital role in assisting in the development of these improved practice systems. Preplanning for office visits can increase the quality of patient encounters and prevent excessive follow-up work (Tables 33.1 and 33.2).

Table 33.1 Maximizing Care at Office Visits

- Identify patients with diabetes.
- Contact patients with reminder letters for appointments and list specific tests to be completed before the visit, e.g., glycated hemoglobin A1c, lipids.
- Encourage patients to be involved in their own care: get them to think about what they hope to accomplish and identify areas in which they may need assistance before the visit.
- Facilitate the use of standardized assessment tools, encounter forms, and diabetes flow sheets to ensure that key standards of care are not overlooked.
- Facilitate the use of technology, e.g., uploading blood glucose data to the Internet, faxing records, etc.

Table 33.2 Facilitating ADA Standards of Diabetes Care

- Ensure collection of and record results of key laboratory tests.
- Measure and record blood pressure and weight at each visit.
- Have the patient remove his or her shoes and socks for a foot examination.
- Coordinate and document referrals for nutrition counseling and self-management training.
- Coordinate and document annual referrals to an eye care specialist, dental care professional, or other health care professionals as appropriate.
- Administer/document annual flu vaccination and one-time pneumococcal vaccination.
- Monitor smoking status/cessation referral.

From ADA (26).

PATIENT EDUCATION

Diabetes self-management education is the key to successful diabetes management. The office nurse can play a significant role in empowering patients to accept their disease and take responsibility for their health. Diabetes self-management training must start at the time of diagnosis with the initiation of survival-skills training and continue throughout the health care relationship. The depth of education offered to the patient in the office setting will be determined by the knowledge and skills of the nurse. Teaching opportunities generally occur at the time of the individual visit, but sometimes several patients with similar learning needs may be offered a class in the waiting room or another identified space. Group visits can provide beneficial discussions and support while improving efficiency. Referral to a dietitian, diabetes self-management training program, or certified diabetes educator is recommended. However, office nurses trained in diabetes self-management education have been shown to be beneficial in community clinics where patients would not attend diabetes self-management training outside the clinic or community (24).

The office nurse can play a vital role in promoting self-care and helping empower patients by encouraging and supporting diabetes self-management and behavior change, providing regular follow-up, demonstrating and allowing the opportunity for patients to practice skills, using practical aids to help support behavior change (such as reminders to take medications), involving the family or signifi-

---

PRACTICAL POINT

Key Assessment Questions (see also chapter 17)
- What is your goal for this visit?
- What is the most difficult issue for you in managing your diabetes?
- Are you willing to do something about it?
- What changes would you suggest to make things better?

Survival Skills Education

- Basic nutrition guidelines
- Healthy eating habits
- Role of physical activity
- Monitoring glycemic control
- Record keeping of blood glucose levels
- Medication administration and side effects
- Symptoms of and treatment for hyperglycemia and hypoglycemia
- Sick-day management
- Skin/dental care
- Emergency phone numbers and when to call for help
- Community resources/support

cant other in patient education, and helping patients to simplify their self-care (25).

SUMMARY

Nurses in the office setting have a unique opportunity to improve patient care by helping individuals with diabetes and their families adjust to the disease and advised lifestyle changes and by identifying support systems and resources within the community.

REFERENCES

1. Goyder EC, McNally PG, Drucquer M, Spiers N, Botha JL: Shifting of care for diabetes from secondary to primary care 1990–5: review of general practices. *BMJ* 316:1505–1506, 1998

2. Ho M, Marger M, Beart J, Yip I, Shekelle P: Is the quality of diabetes care better in a diabetes clinic or in a general medicine clinic? *Diabetes Care* 20:472–475, 1997

3. Cherry DK, Burt CW, Woodwell DA, Rechsteiner E: *National Ambulatory Medical Care Survey: 2005 Summary: Advance Data #387, June 29, 2007.* Hyattsville, MD, U.S. Department of Health and Human Services, Centers for Disease Control and Prevention, National Center for Health Statistics, 2007

4. American Diabetes Association: Economic costs of diabetes in the U.S. in 2007. *Diabetes Care* 31:596–615, 2008

5. Marszelak E: Ambulatory nursing: at the crossroads? *Nurs Health Care* 1:254–255, 1980

6. Curran C: An interview with Linda D'Angelo. *Nurs Econ* 13:193–196, 1995

7. American Academy of Ambulatory Care Nursing, American Nurses Association: *Nursing in Ambulatory Care*. Silver Spring, MD, American Nurses Publishing, 1997

8. Moore M, Geving A: Nursing's role in the ambulatory care setting. *Med Group Manage J* 37:18–24, 1990

9. Aubert R, Herman W, Waters J, Moore W, Sutton D, et al.: Nurse case management to improve glycemic control in diabetes patients in a health maintenance organization. *Ann Intern Med* 129:605–612, 1998

10. Wagner E, Grothaus L, Sandhu N, Galvin M, McGregor M, et al.: Chronic care clinics for diabetes in primary care. *Diabetes Care* 24:695–700, 2001

11. Pine D, Madlon-Kay D, Sauser M: Effectiveness of a nurse-based intervention in a community practice on patients' dietary fat intake and total serum cholesterol level. *Arch Fam Med* 6:129–134, 1997

12. Denver E, Barnard M, Woolfson R, Earle K: Management of uncontrolled hypertension in a nurse-led clinic compared with conventional care for patients with type 2 diabetes. *Diabetes Care* 26:2256–2260, 2003

13. Taylor C, Miller N, Reilly K, Greenwald G, Cunning D, et al.: Evaluation of a nurse-care management system to improve outcomes in patients with complicated diabetes. *Diabetes Care* 26:1058–1063, 2003

14. New J, Mason J, Freemantle N, Teasdale S, Wong L, et al.: Specialist nurse-led intervention to treat and control hypertension and hyperlipidemia in diabetes (SPLINT). *Diabetes Care* 26:2250–2255, 2003

15. Davidson M: Effect of nurse-directed diabetes care in a minority population. *Diabetes Care* 26:2281–2287, 2003

16. Mastal M, Bulgar J, Chinault L, Donaghue J, Klein M, Kraynak M, Lusk E, McNamara M, Pray M, Roberts B, Zopp L: Functions and Outcomes of Advice Nursing Practice (unpublished research study). Kaiser Permanente Mid-Atlantic States Region, 1993

17. Saaddine J, Engelgau M, Beckles G, Gregg E, Thompson T, Narayan K: A diabetes report card for the United States: quality of care in the 1990s. *Ann Intern Med* 136:565–571, 2002

18. Renders C, Valk G, Griffin S, Wagner E, Eijk Van J, Assendelft W: Interventions to improve the management of diabetes in primary care, outpatient, and community settings: a systematic review. *Diabetes Care* 24:1821–1833, 2001

19. O'Connor P: Improving diabetes care: organize your office, intensify your care. *J Am Board Fam Pract* 14:320–322, 2001

20. White B: Making diabetes checkups more fruitful. *Fam Pract Manag* 7:51–52, 2000

21. Glasgow R: Translating research to practice. *Diabetes Care* 26:2451–2456, 2003

22. Cohen S: Potential barriers to diabetes care. *Diabetes Care* 6:499–500, 1983

23. Reith P: Comprehensive diabetes care in the office. *Clinical Diabetes* 11:109–114, 1993

24. Weiler DM, Tirrel L: Office nurse educators: improving diabetes self management for the Latino population in the clinic setting. *Hisp Health Care Int* 5:21–26, 2007

25. Capaldi B: Patient empowerment in diabetes. *Practice Nursing* 19:14–19, 2008

26. American Diabetes Association: Standards of medical care in diabetes—2009 (Position Statement). *Diabetes Care* 32 (Suppl. 1):S13–S61, 2009

Ms. Berkowitz is Senior Medical Science Liaison, Medical Affairs, Amylin Pharmaceuticals, Inc., San Diego, CA.

34. Role of the Home Health Care Nurse

CARYL ANN O'REILLY, RN, MBA, CDE

T he home health care nurse is an increasingly important member of the health care team. Patients are discharged from hospitals and rehabilitation centers early in the episode of care and require more sophisticated nursing intervention at home. The home health care nurse acts as liaison among members of the health care team, the patient, the family, and caregivers. Often, as the only professional who has a complete overview of the patient's medical regimen, the home care nurse takes on responsibility for the coordination of care.

The role of the home health care nurse in diabetes care can be critical in preventing acute and even some chronic complications. Often, the patient has other comorbidities, resulting in complex care that includes medical, social, and emotional issues. This may include an assessment of educational needs of the patient and caregivers in weight management; general nutrition; insulin management; sick-day guidelines; foot care; risks of smoking; recognition, treatment, and prevention of hyperglycemia and hypoglycemia; physical activity; medication management; and complication screening (1). Failure to provide this kind of care can result in re-hospitalizations or emergency room visits.

NURSING ASSESSMENT

When patients are referred to home care agencies for acute episodes of care, the tool often used to determine patient needs is the Outcome and Assessment Information Set (OASIS) (2). If used correctly, OASIS can give important information about the patient's deficits and illuminate the patient's specific needs from skilled nursing. There are three domains—clinical, functional, and service—that provide essential information, such as patient history and integumentary, respiratory,

Table 34.1 Initial Patient Assessment

Area of Observation	Risk
Age	■ Mental status • Confusion • Depression • Loneliness ■ Dehydration ■ Neuropathy ■ Urinary tract infection (UTI) ■ Falls
Incontinence	■ UTI ■ Skin breakdown ■ Falls ■ Embarrassment
Visual deficit	■ Medication errors ■ Falls ■ Inability to test blood glucose
Polypharmacy	■ Drug interactions ■ Multiple physicians ■ Expense ■ Timing and action of medications ■ Hypo-/hyperglycemia

elimination, and emotional/behavioral status. Additionally, living arrangements, support system, therapy needs related to activities of daily living (ADL) and independent activities of daily living (IADL), medication management, and equipment management are addressed. Patients may not always give accurate information, particularly when related to incontinence and vision. Understating patient status will lead to reduced payment for services as well as under-serving of the patient. OASIS may be required when care is initiated, interrupted, and resumed; when the patient is discharged; and when there is a significant change in health status. Managed care insurers often authorize only one or two nursing visits for assessment and teaching. Accurately identifying and documenting patient status can be the catalyst for patients to receive the care necessary to return to optimal health and functional status. OASIS provides standardized information, tracks patient outcomes, and is valuable for data collection and research potential.

The initial assessment of a patient should include the observations found in Table 34.1. Risks identified can then be evaluated and incorporated into the care plan for each patient.

AGE

Age is an important factor in patient assessment. More than 50% of people newly diagnosed with diabetes are over the age of 65, and most patients referred to home care are between the ages of 65 and 85 years (3). Age-related changes in the body can alter clinical presentation. With increased age, symptoms of hyperglycemia, such as polyuria, polydipsia, and polyphagia, may be absent. After congestive heart failure, diabetes is ranked second as the primary diagnosis at entry into home care, and it is the top diagnosis if primary and secondary diagnoses are combined.

Seniors may exhibit cognitive impairment, but this has to be evaluated carefully. Hyperglycemia, dehydration, and hypoglycemia can profoundly affect cognitive function. This may result in limitations in ADLs, undiagnosed depression, and social isolation. Normalizing blood glucose levels may restore a patient's ability to communicate and participate more fully in diabetes self-management. Too hasty a judgment by the home care nurse may overlook important, yet subtle, alterations in mental and emotional status. The mechanism associated with diabetes and cognitive impairment is unclear, but may be related to episodes of hypoglycemia.

DEHYDRATION

Dehydration is a serious complication of diabetes. Seniors lose moisture through thinning dermal layers. They do not sense thirst until they are already significantly dehydrated and may choose not to drink water because of fear of incontinence or nocturnal polyuria. Dehydration alone can increase the blood glucose level as well as medication concentrations in the blood. Also, renal threshold increases with age, compounding the problem. Patients should be encouraged to drink 48 oz water daily as long as there are no contraindications, such as heart failure. Having a filled water bottle available, with cuing by the family or caregiver, may be helpful. Identifying the potential for dehydration, instructing the patient and/or caregiver in identifying and treating dehydration, and observing the response to this instruction should be documented in the patient record.

NEUROPATHIES

Nerve damage occurs in 50% of individuals with diabetes age >60 years. Autonomic neuropathies may be difficult to detect but can have various manifestations, e.g., abnormal heart rate or orthostatic hypotension, that can be life-threatening indicators (see chapter 14). It is advisable to obtain a blood pressure reading while the patient is sitting, followed by a standing reading, if the patient indicates dizziness or lightheadedness on standing. Although there is no cure for this form of neuropathy, detection and preventive measures, such as wearing compression stockings and dangling the legs before standing, can prevent serious outcomes. Hypoglycemia unawareness can result from impaired glucose counterregulation and may be a hidden cause of falls. Patients with symptomatic autonomic neuropathy have a threefold greater 5-year mortality rate than diabetes patients without autonomic neuropathy (4).

Alternating bouts of constipation followed by explosive diarrhea and gastroparesis are two common forms of gastrointestinal autonomic neuropathy. They impinge on quality of life and make glucose management difficult. There are pharmacological options available to the physician; therefore, it is important that the nurse document findings and communicate these with the primary care provider.

Bladder dysfunction and urinary tract infection (UTI) are related to both diabetic neuropathy and aging. Diabetic cystopathy is chronic, predisposing patients to UTIs. It is insidious, with the only early sign being increased intervals between times of urination. This leads to enlarged bladder, atonic musculature, and incomplete emptying (5). These factors increase the probability of a UTI. The usual signs and symptoms of a UTI are frequently absent in patients with diabetes, and the diagnosis may be missed. If a urinalysis is performed, a UTI can be suspected if the nitrites are positive, regardless of the presence of leukocytes. A UTI should be suspected if blood glucose levels are elevated and other possible explanations are exhausted. Patients may complain of back pain, pressure in the lower abdomen, or dribbling of urine or may say they just do not feel well. A strong urine odor or signs of incontinence, such as a urine-stained chair pad or wet socks and shoes, may be recognized. Incontinence increases the risk of UTIs, falls, embarrassment, and social isolation. Bladder training should be considered. A consult with urology may be needed to assess the need for other interventions.

Peripheral neuropathy may cause pain or numbness in the lower extremities and make it difficult for the patient to determine where the foot is in relation to the floor. Intrinsic weakness of the small muscles of the foot can alter joint mobility and affect foot mechanics (6). Patients with neuropathy develop gait abnormalities and problems with balance, which increase the risk for falling. When gait abnormality is observed, a physical therapy consultation for evaluation and recommendation should be initiated.

FOOT CARE

Nurses should inspect patients' feet at every visit. Podiatric intervention can be beneficial for providing patients with orthotic footwear for off-loading pressure. Medicare provides benefits to covered individuals for routine podiatric care and therapeutic footwear. A comprehensive nursing foot examination is an important part of the initial patient assessment and should be repeated at each recertification period to evaluate the progression of diabetic foot complications and promote early detection of vascular and nerve complications of the lower extremities. This should include a visual inspection of the feet that includes assessment of color, temperature, pulses, and hair growth. A monofilament test for detecting the insensate foot is also extremely valuable and should be incorporated into the examination if possible (see chapter 15).

Primary sites for repetitive stress injuries are the metatarsal heads and the great toe. Patients who are bed bound are at risk for pressure ulcers of the heel, which are second only to sacral pressure ulcers in prevalence (6). Heels should be protected at all times from pressure that prevents vascular perfusion, which leads to ischemia and tissue death. Limb loss is more likely to occur with a heel ulcer than with a forefoot ulcer, and functional disability is also more profound (6).

EYE CARE

Visual deficits should be considered if the patient has had diabetes for ≥5 years. Many patients are able to disguise the fact that they are visually impaired when they are in their own environment. Patients frequently associate loss of vision with loss of independence and will avoid its discovery as long as possible. However, it is this compromised vision that leads to errors in medication, falls, and functional deficits (see chapter 10).

The home care nurse is in the position to assess patients' visual acuity by asking them to read small print, such as a medication label or phone book. Visiting nurses should also observe the patient checking blood glucose levels to assure that a proper technique is being used. If vision is impaired, the patient may benefit from adaptive equipment to assist with blood glucose monitoring and insulin administration. If impairment is significant, the patient may be eligible for referral to a low-vision center and for services through the state's Commission for the Blind. Refer the patient to a local agency, such as The Lighthouse, which works with the Commission to provide patient ADL and mobility training (see RESOURCES for more information).

MEDICATION MANAGEMENT

The nurse is in the unique position of being able to identify all of the medications the patient is taking. This may require an investigative approach, however. Patients often have several physicians (podiatrist, optometrist, etc.), each of whom may be prescribing medications. Patients generally assume that each provider communicates with the others regarding medications. Patients also take a variety of over-the-counter medications and herbal supplements that may have adverse interactions with prescribed medications. Have the patient or caregiver compile a complete list of medications and supplements that are being taken. In some cases, it is best that the nurse compose this list, examining the medications and their bottles and verifying medication adherence. This list should be taken to each health care provider visit and included in the patient's chart. Another copy should be readily available in the event that the patient requires hospitalization or emergency care.

Medication adherence is a major factor in achieving optimal diabetes control. Patients with diabetes have multiple comorbidities, each requiring one or more pharmacological agents as treatment. Cost may be a barrier to adherence. Ask patients whether they are able to afford their medications. Most patients on fixed incomes have difficulty with the costs of medication. Sometimes, they will not let the physician know that they cannot afford the medication but will share this information with the nurse. Another barrier to adherence is a lack of knowledge about the timing of medications. Ask patients what kind of insulin they are taking. Frequently, they will know the brand name but not the type of insulin. There is a general lack of understanding about the time at which certain medications should be taken and why that timing is important. Using "teach back," in which the patient tells you what he understood you to say, can reinforce the learning and identify misunderstandings.

Adherence is not necessarily a matter of whether a patient will do what is medically indicated, but whether they have the knowledge, cognitive skills, finances, and physical ability to do what is indicated. For patients with difficulty, the nurse can help enhance adherence in a number of ways, by putting together a pill box, for instance, or by writing out instructions for taking medications.

NUTRITION

Meal planning and good nutrition are the cornerstones of optimal diabetes control. The home care nurse, however, should guard against being the "diet police." This has a negative effect on the patient and can be very unproductive. Understand that as the coordinator of care, the home care nurse assesses the patient's status, identifies problems, and one hopes, leaves the patient with important "take-away" lifetime self-management skills, even though there is only a brief period of interaction with the patient. Rather than trying to change years of eating habits, it is more productive to identify one or two nutrition deficits that can be altered in the short term. For example, many individuals with diabetes continue to drink sugared soda or large amounts of juice or milk. Working with patients toward modifying this habit can have dramatic effects on blood glucose control, which may encourage them to consider additional changes. Referral to a diabetes self-management education program or a nutrition program for ongoing nutrition counseling is important.

COMMUNICATION/NEW TECHNOLOGIES

The coordinator of care has the opportunity and responsibility for 360-degree communication. Changes in status, positive and negative, should be documented and communicated to the patient, physician, therapist, home health aide, or other health care team member. This ongoing dialogue keeps the team focused on the plan of care and promotes desired outcomes. Telehealth, interactive health care services provided over technologies such as videoconferencing, the Internet, streaming media, and satellite and wireless communications, has been used in rural and inner city communities and is also entering the realm of home care nursing (7). Telehealth that includes telemonitoring and phone monitoring has been shown to reduce hospitalizations among patients with diabetes (8). Although it is used infrequently (primarily for diabetes and chronic care), it has demonstrated improvements in patient outcomes and is being recommended as a best practice for the home care industry to reduce unplanned and/or preventable hospitalizations in the U.S. (9). Changes in communication strategies and technology in the treatment of diabetes are revolutionizing the possibilities and role for the home care nurse.

PRACTICAL POINT

Documentation Is a Priority
All aspects of nursing assessment and interventions should be carefully documented, including a patient's response to a procedure. Any changes noted should be documented, the patient and/or caregiver should be notified, and a written report should be sent to the physician. Documentation allows consistent levels of care to be provided and ensures that the patient's health care team is always aware of any issues arising during treatment.

SUMMARY

Home care nurses are in a position to be the first-line professionals to assess and identify problems that physicians and other health care professionals may never see or recognize. By conducting a diabetes-specific assessment, home care nurses can act as advocates for people with diabetes as they detect, intervene, and facilitate care. It is important for home care nurses to communicate their findings to the health care team and ensure that follow up has occurred, that interventions are effective, and that the message to the patient from all professionals is consistent and understood.

REFERENCES

1. Beacham T, Williams PR, Askew R, Walker J, Schenk L, May M: Insulin management: a guide for the home health nurse. *Home Healthc Nurse* 26:421–428, 2008

2. Centers for Medicare and Medicaid Services: Oasis overview [Internet], 2005. Available from http://www.cms.hhs.gov/oasis. Accessed 8 April 2008

3. Visiting Nurse Service of New York: Center for Home Care Policy and Research web site. Available from http://www.vnsny.org/research/homecare.html. Accessed 8 April 2008

4. Vinik A, Erbas T, Stansberry K: Gastrointestinal, genitourinary and neurovascular disturbances in diabetes. *Diabetes Rev* 7:358–378, 1999

5. Vinik A, Erbas T, Pfeifer M, Feldman M, Feldman E, Stevens M, Russell J: Diabetic autonomic neuropathy. In: Porte D Jr, Sherwin RS, Baron A, eds. *Ellenberg & Rifkin's Diabetes Mellitus*. 6th ed. New York, NY: McGraw-Hill, 2003, 789–804

6. National Diabetes Education Program: *Feet Can Last A Lifetime: Revised Kit*. Bethesda, MD, National Diabetes Education Program, 2002

7. U.S. Department of Health and Human Services, Health Resources and Services Administration: Telehealth [Internet]. Available from http://www.hrsa.gov/telehealth/. Accessed 3 March 2009

8. Peterson-Sjrok K: Reducing acute care hospitalizations and emergent care use through home health disease management: one agency's success story. *Home Healthc Nurse* 25:622–627, 2007

9. Briggs Corporation, NAHC, and Fazzi Associates: *Briggs National Quality Improvement/Hospitalization Reduction Study*. Des Moines, IA, Briggs Corporation, 2006

Ms. O'Reilly is a Diabetes Clinical Nurse Specialist at the Visiting Nurse Service of New York, Staten Island, NY.

35. Diabetes Care in Long-Term Care Facilities

Belinda P. Childs, ARNP, MN, CDE, BC-ADM

It is estimated that one in every three people in the U.S. will reside in a long-term care facility sometime during their life. Although only 11% of our population is currently >65 years of age, that figure is expected to grow to >20% by 2020 (1). Twenty percent of the population over age 65 has diabetes (2,3). When considering the aging of the population, the increased life expectancy, and the increase in diabetes prevalence, long-term care facilities will play an even larger role in providing care for the individual with diabetes. The nurse's role as advocate, care provider, and educator of staff, patient, and family will be pivotal.

The 2004 National Nursing Home Survey collected cross-sectional data showing that 24.6% of the 11,939 nursing home residents aged 65 years had diabetes as a primary admission and/or current diagnosis. This survey represented 1.32 million individuals. Diabetes was present in 22.5 and 35.6% of white and nonwhite residents, respectively. Residents with diabetes were admitted more often from acute-care hospitals (42.5 vs. 35.3%), were more likely to have a length of stay ≥100 days (22.6 vs. 20.1%), and took more medications (10.3 vs. 8.4) than residents without diabetes. The residents with diabetes had 39% higher odds of having emergency department visits in the previous 90 days at the time of the survey and 56% higher odds of having a pressure ulcer. In the U.S. in 2004, one in four nursing home residents aged 65 years had diabetes (2).

Compared with residents without diabetes, residents with diabetes show greater limitations in activities of daily living in terms of their ability to bathe (91.9 vs. 88.7% for diabetes versus no diabetes, respectively), dress (82.4 vs. 78.5%), perform toileting activities (72.9 vs. 68.6%), transfer from bed to chair (70.0 vs. 65.8%), walk (76.1 vs. 71.1%), and control bowel movements (48.4 vs. 44%). The two groups were similar in having difficulty feeding (35%) and controlling urine (42%). Nursing home residents with diabetes were considered more limited in the activities of daily living than the general population with diabetes (2).

UNDIAGNOSED DIABETES IN THE NURSING HOME

Nearly 6 million Americans have undiagnosed diabetes. Type 1 and type 2 diabetes can be diagnosed at any age. The polyuria of hyperglycemia in an incontinent patient may be overlooked. The polydipsia of hyperglycemia may not be recognized because of decreased thirst sensation in elderly patients. The signs and symptoms of hyperglycemia may go unnoticed. It is important to be alert to the potential for newly diagnosed diabetes in the nursing home setting.

The care of the resident with diabetes is complicated by the number of chronic conditions, their limitations in daily living activities, and specific management issues related to diabetes that differ from routine nursing home care (4). In addition, providing quality care is hampered by staff shortages, staff turnover, poor pay, and lack of education and educational materials on diabetes for residents and staff in the nursing home setting.

Diabetes care in the nursing home is carried out primarily by vocational or licensed practical nurses, medication aides, and nurse's aides. The nurse is responsible for coordination of care and development of care plans for the residents. All staff should have some knowledge of standards of diabetes care. The team approach to the delivery of care improves the quality of care.

CLINICAL IMPLICATIONS

Diabetes care areas that need special attention include glycemic control, diabetes medications, medication interactions, glucose monitoring, medical nutrition therapy (including hydration), acute and chronic complications of diabetes, and self-management education and empowerment of the individual with diabetes (Table 35.1).

GLYCEMIC CONTROL

Appropriate target blood glucose levels for this population remain controversial. The American Diabetes Association (ADA) notes that "less stringent treatment goals may be appropriate for adults with limited life expectancies or advanced vascular disease.... Severe or frequent hypoglycemia is an indication for the modification of treatment regimens, including setting higher glycemic goals" (3).

However, the increased risk for dehydration, infection, and acute complications; greater sensitivity to pain; urinary incontinence; and decreased visual acuity and cognition may occur as a result of elevated glucose levels. Target levels designed to control hyperglycemia and prevent symptoms and acute complications are appropriate. The health care team should take all these factors into consideration when setting target levels for glucose control. Medical treatment options are improving, allowing for safer management of glucose levels. If one regimen is not achieving the identified glucose targets, then alternative medication strategies are indicated.

Table 35.1 Considerations for Nurses Providing Diabetes Care in Nursing Homes

Diabetes Issues	Key Considerations
Diabetes medications	
■ Oral agents	■ Is the oral diabetes medication given on time, before the meal, or with food? ■ What are the side effects? Are lab results and signs and symptoms observed routinely?
■ Insulin	■ Is the type of insulin to be given with or before the meal? ■ Is the insulin being stored properly? ■ Is a new bottle of insulin opened every 28 days? ■ Is there an injection site rotation plan? Is there a way to document? ■ Is the injection subcutaneous?
Medication interactions	■ Review medication list after a hospitalization. Confirm if medications have been dropped that they were not to be restarted on return to the facility. ■ Review for potential interactions of medications.
Medical nutrition therapy	■ Provide adequate calories, prevent malnutrition. ■ Consult the dietitian if problems exist. ■ Regular diet is acceptable with consistent carbohydrates in meals and snacks. ■ Obtain blood glucose levels 2 h after meals to determine the effect of foods. ■ Fats do not need to be restricted in the older population. ■ Consider the individual.
Acute complications of diabetes	■ Observe for signs of DKA, HHS, LA, hypoglycemia. ■ Contact the health care provider immediately with signs of DKA, HHS, or LA. ■ Protocols for treatment of hyperglycemia and hypoglycemia are valuable. ■ Be cautious not to overtreat hypoglycemia. ■ Recheck blood glucose 15–20 min after treatment; repeat treatment if needed. ■ Try to problem solve why acute complication occurred in order to decrease the risk of a recurrence.
Chronic complications of diabetes	■ Follow the ADA Standards of Medical Care in Diabetes (4) to reduce risks for blindness, strokes, and amputations.
Foot and skin care	■ Daily inspection for individuals who cannot inspect their own feet ■ Weekly nurse examination of feet ■ Careful skin care, prevention of ulcers and skin tears ■ Referral to podiatrist for foot care/footwear ■ The resident should always wear shoes and socks whether walking or in a wheelchair.
Empowerment/ self-care	■ Respect the individual's history of living with diabetes. ■ Provide choices whenever possible. ■ Include the family in care.

DKA, diabetic ketoacidosis; HHS, hyperglycemic hyperosmolar syndrome; LA, lactic acidosis.

DIABETES MEDICATION

Key considerations with medication include appropriate timing of the diabetes medications and monitoring for side effects. Most long-term care residents will be on insulin, oral agents, or a combination (4). It is important to properly administer the medication(s). Time constraints make the administration of multiple medications to residents a challenge for the nurse who must administer medications to several patients in a timely fashion. Inappropriate administration of diabetes medication can mean the difference between hypoglycemia, euglycemia, and hyperglycemia. Inconsistent timing of medication, especially insulin, can also lead to variable patterns in blood glucose levels. The health care provider who reviews the blood glucose records must be astute in asking the right questions before making dosage adjustments. The health care provider and long-term care staff should also consider the timing of snacks. Note the insulin action table in chapter 4 when considering times for snacks, glucose testing, and increased activity. A person should match snacks with the peak of the insulin and avoid increased activity (such as physical therapy) during these peaks. If activity is increased, then monitoring blood glucose levels and, if required, providing an extra snack might be appropriate.

A well-trained health care provider must know the ins and outs of insulin therapy before making dose adjustments. For example, a 70/30 NPH/regular insulin formulation administered after breakfast and supper may lead to high postprandial blood glucose levels but low preprandial levels. The corrective action is not adjusting the dose of 70/30 NPH/regular but ensuring careful administration ≥15 min (preferably 30 min) before the meal. Moreover, a different formulation may also be appropriate. Usually, the doctor is called on for dose adjustments.

Storage and administration of insulin should be reviewed. Injection sites should be rotated, and hypertrophied or scarred areas should not be used for administering insulin. Attention should be given to the technique of insulin administration. A nurse may inadvertently administer the insulin in the muscle in a lean individual, which will cause the insulin to peak sooner, placing the patient at risk for hypoglycemia and reducing its duration of action. Routine insulin should be administered subcutaneously. Insulin bottles should be dated and discarded when they have exceeded the usage limit, which is typically 28 days (5,6).

It is important to monitor for potential side effects from antihyperglycemic oral agents. If a resident on thiazolidinediones develops edema or increasing congestive heart failure or if the resident has an increase in serum creatinine level and he or she is on metformin, the health care provider should be notified. Renal function may deteriorate with age, making this an important consideration in medication use and dosage. Chapter 5 reviews the potential side effects of oral agents and recommended monitoring techniques.

MEDICATION INTERACTIONS

Polypharmacy can be an issue for individuals with diabetes. Control of the multiple complications requires treatment with multiple medications. Chapter 23 discusses the issues of polypharmacy.

Diligent review of medications and observation by the nurse can prevent a resident from experiencing serious side effects. If a resident returns to the facility after a hospitalization, a careful review of medications should occur. Compare the medication list before hospitalization and the discharge list on return to the facility. Medications may have been discontinued during the hospitalization that should have been restarted on return to the nursing home facility, e.g., medications for pain, sleeping, or antiplatelet therapy. Do not assume that just because a medication is not on the discharge list that it was discontinued. It may have been overlooked. Verify the orders with the health care provider.

GLUCOSE MONITORING

To achieve optimal glycemic control, glucose monitoring is important, regardless of the location of care. Glucose monitoring is necessary to determine the effects of food and medication as well as activity, stress, and illness. Glucose monitoring can be important in determining whether the resident's symptoms are related to hyperglycemia or hypoglycemia. It is an important tool in the management of the resident with diabetes. Chapter 6 is an excellent resource on self-management of diabetes.

MEDICAL NUTRITION THERAPY

According to the ADA nutrition recommendations, providing adequate nutrition is a primary concern for residents of long-term care facilities (7). Prevention of malnourishment and malnutrition are key considerations. Experience has shown that residents eat better if they are given less-restrictive meal plans. According to the guidelines, it is appropriate to serve residents regular menus with consistent amounts of carbohydrates at each meal and snacks. The caveat of this recommendation is that there must be consistent amounts of carbohydrates such that the same amount is given each day and distributed throughout the three meals and snacks in a consistent manner. Glucose monitoring and notation of foods eaten will assist in adjusting medication to control blood glucose levels.

Glucose Monitoring

Important considerations for glucose monitoring for the staff in the nursing home:
1. Wash hands in warm water to make sure there is no sucrose on the hands and to improve circulation.
2. Using alcohol is not advised because elderly patients have dry skin and alcohol increases dryness.
3. When obtaining blood from the finger, drop the resident's hand to the side to improve blood flow before sticking the finger.
4. Use the sides of the finger rather than the tips to prevent tenderness.
5. Try not to squeeze the finger (squeezing leads to bruising and soreness).
6. If you suspect hypoglycemia or hyperglycemia, test the patient's blood glucose level for verification.

Other Key Nutrition Considerations

1. Fat restriction is generally not needed in this population.
2. Residents on pureed or softened foods should receive adequate calories for nutrition.
3. Adequate hydration is also essential in the nursing home environment.

Two other aspects of poor nutrition need to be mentioned: *1*) eating meals alone discourages appetite and *2*) dentition issues may deter patients from eating protein foods or raw fruits and vegetables that are difficult to chew. Since eating is generally a social behavior, appetite can increase when patients eat in a common dining room or have companionship while eating. Spending time with the patient during a meal can help the nurse cue in on the patient's food preferences in type and preparation style. Substitutions can then be made that will encourage nutritional balance.

Consultation with a dietitian is essential, and individual needs and preferences should be considered when developing a nutritional plan. If the dietitian suggests changes in daily intake, the health care provider should be notified of these changes. If the individual's appetite, quantity of food, or types of food change, increased glucose monitoring should occur, and the health care provider should be notified; the antihyperglycemic medication may need to be adjusted.

ACUTE COMPLICATIONS OF DIABETES

Hyperglycemia, including diabetic ketoacidosis, hyperglycemic hyperosmolar syndrome, and hypoglycemia are the most common acute complications of diabetes. The symptoms and management of these acute complications are addressed in chapter 7. It is most important to try to prevent acute complications by recognizing symptoms and identifying the problem early so that treatment can be initiated as soon as possible.

The long-term care population is at increased risk for lactic acidosis. Lactic acidosis results from inadequate oxygen delivery or utilization in individuals with serious underlying disease. The accumulation of lactic acid indicates that the balance between lactate production and utilization has been disturbed. Metformin has been associated with lactic acidosis and primarily occurs in patients with renal insufficiency and/or other concomitant conditions associated with poor renal perfusion or hypoxia. These conditions include congestive heart failure, chronic obstructive pulmonary disease, and age >80 years (8). Nausea and vomiting and failure to offer adequate fluids may lead to dehydration and subsequently to lactic acidosis. An individual's health status may change, necessitating a reevaluation of their medication and safety issues.

Lactic acidosis will be difficult to differentiate from the other forms of critical illnesses. Conscious monitoring and notifying the health care provider of any changes in hydration, oxygen perfusion, and mental orientation may prevent an acute crisis from occurring in the nursing home.

CHRONIC COMPLICATIONS OF DIABETES

Even though the prevention of diabetes complications may not seem as important in this population, maintaining function to enhance quality of life is imperative. Screening for long-term complications is recommended so that problems can be detected and treated early. The ADA guidelines recommend that screening should be individualized, with particular attention to those complications that can develop over short periods of time and/or would significantly impair one's functional status (3). An annual dilated eye examination may contribute to the prevention of blindness. Assessing visual acuity and fitting with proper eyewear may prevent falls, increase quality of life, and reduce sensory deprivations. Management of hypertension reduces the incidence of strokes and kidney disease. Decreased quality of life and its associated cost of care underscores the need to provide preventive care for this population, regardless of age (4).

FOOT AND SKIN CARE

Early recognition and management of independent risk factors for foot ulcers and amputations can prevent or delay the onset of adverse outcomes (9). Individuals with diabetes are taught to do daily foot examinations, and it would seem appropriate that this recommendation be carried out in the nursing home. If the individual is unable to perform this exam, then the nursing home staff should conduct a visual inspection daily. The nurse should do a complete examination on a weekly basis (10). Many facilities have access to podiatric services and should recommend that all individuals with diabetes receive these services, particularly for nail care. Evaluation for appropriate footwear should be done by a professional. The individual should always wear shoes when walking or when riding in a wheelchair to prevent foot injuries; this is especially critical for those with sensory loss.

Prevention and management of other skin ulcers and tears is also critical. Skin yeast infections are common in this population (11). Red rashy areas in the skinfolds or groin, especially if the resident is incontinent, may indicate yeast infections. In the nursing home survey, nearly 14% and 9.4% of diabetic and nondiabetic residents had a pressure ulcer at the time of the survey, yielding 56% higher odds of ulceration among residents with diabetes (2). Keeping the skin of long-term-care residents dry and turning the bedridden frequently is imperative for skin preservation.

EMPOWERMENT AND SELF-MANAGEMENT

Nursing home residents are usually not responsible for the majority of their care. However, they can benefit from simple and new information. They deserve the opportunity to learn about their disease and have control over procedures whenever possible.

It is important for the caregiver to recognize that residents may have lived with diabetes for many years. It is important to listen to residents. They may have successfully managed this disease for years. Or this may be a new diagnosis, and they may not understand the medications, the glucose testing, or the symptoms of hypoglycemia. Allow them the opportunity to have some control over what and when they eat and over their medications, within reason. For example, the individual may direct the timing, location, and administration of the insulin injection. Encourage residents to be as physically active as they are able, and assess physical activity areas for safety. Include the family in the treatment plan and listen to them. They may have insight into the resident's likes and dislikes. Older individuals with diabetes should be screened for depression and cognitive impairment (12).

SUMMARY

Long-term care residents are a special population in a special setting. This setting offers an opportunity to provide quality diabetes care. Not only will the individual's quality of life improve, but mortality, morbidity, and medical care costs will decrease (13). It is important to provide regular opportunities for continuing education for the staff. Nurses should guide the development and implementation of protocols for care, following the standards of care, and ensure that a trained staff is providing daily care for the individual with diabetes living in a nursing home/long-term care facility.

REFERENCES

1. Mayfield JA, Deb P, Potter DEB: Diabetes and long term care. In *Diabetes in America*. 2nd ed. Harris MI, Cowie CC, Stern MP, Boyko EJ, Reiber GE, Bennett PH, Eds. Washington, DC, U.S. Govt. Printing Office, 1995, p. 571–590 (NIH publ. no. 95-1468)

2. Resnick HE, Heineman J, Stone R, Shorr RI: Diabetes in US nursing homes, 2004. *Diabetes Care* 31:287–288, 2008

3. American Diabetes Association: Standards of medical care in diabetes—2009 (Position Statement). *Diabetes Care* 32 (Suppl. 1):S13–S61, 2009

4. Funnell MM: Care of the nursing home resident with diabetes. *Clin Geriatr Med* 15:413–422, 1999

5. Aventis: Insulin glargine (Lantus) [package insert]. Bridgewater, NJ, Aventis

6. Grajower MM, Fraser CG, Holcombe JH, Daugherty ML, Harris WC, et al.: How long should insulin be used once a vial is started? (Commentary). *Diabetes Care* 26:2665–2669, 2003

7. American Diabetes Association: Diabetes nutrition recommendations for health care institutions (Position Statement). *Diabetes Care* 31 (Suppl. 1):S61–S78, 2008

8. Clement SC: Lactic acidosis. In *Therapy for Diabetes Mellitus and Related Disorders*. 4th ed. Lebovitz HE, Ed. Alexandria, VA, American Diabetes Association, 2004, p. 100–105

9. American Diabetes Association: Preventive foot care in diabetes (Position Statement). *Diabetes Care* 27 (Suppl. 1):S63–S64, 2004

10. American Diabetes Association/American Association of Diabetes Educators: Guidelines for diabetes care in skilled nursing facilities. In *Guidelines for Diabetes Care*. New York, American Diabetes Association, 1981, p. 40–44

11. American Diabetes Association: Skin complications [Internet]. Available from http://www.diabetes.org/for-parents-and-kids/what-is-diabetes/skin-complications.jsp. Accessed 6 March 2009

12. American Geriatrics Society: New guidelines for improving the care of the older person with diabetes mellitus [Internet], 2008. Available from http://www.americangeriatrics.org/education/diabetes_executive_summ.shtml. Accessed 10 October 2008

13. Morley JE, Kaiser FE: Unique aspects of diabetes mellitus in the elderly. *Clin Geriatr Med* 6:693–701, 1990

Ms. Childs is a Diabetes Nurse Specialist at Mid-America Diabetes Associates, Wichita, KS.

RESOURCES

Introduction

Providing comprehensive, up-to-date diabetes care and education is a challenge for the health care provider today. Keeping up with the latest treatments, standards of care, technology, and support programs available can seem overwhelming. The purpose of this section is to provide tools and resources that will be useful in your practice.

The mission of the American Diabetes Association (ADA) is to prevent and cure diabetes and improve the lives of all people affected by diabetes, and its motto is "cure, care, commitment." In addition to research, the ADA is committed to providing access to current information for health care professionals and individuals with diabetes and their families. One way that the ADA carries out this mission is through its web site (http://www.diabetes.org). This web site provides access to the annually updated (every January) ADA Clinical Practice Recommendations, which has been referred to extensively in this book. It is available as an annual supplement to the journal *Diabetes Care* and in its entirety on the ADA web site at http://professional.diabetes.org/CPR_search.aspx and http://care.diabetesjournals.org. The ADA position statement Standards of Medical Care in Diabetes, updated each year as part of the Clinical Practice Recommendations, provides the latest guidelines for the care of people with diabetes.

Another invaluable resource available in its entirety from the ADA is the Resource Guide published in *Diabetes Forecast*. This resource is published in December of each year and is available online (http://www.forecast.diabetes.org). The guide covers such vital information as insulin delivery systems, blood glucose meters and data management systems, products for treating low blood glucose, wound gels and prescription lotions, medical identification products, and manufacturers and exclusive distributors. Products change so frequently that studying this resource will keep the health care provider up to date on the most advanced information on technology and new therapies. Pharmaceutical companies are an excellent resource for patient education materials, and most have web sites that provide patient and professional information. Pharmaceutical representatives can also frequently provide materials without charge. Addresses and web information are available through the Resource Guide. Any portion of the ADA Clinical Practice Recommendations and the Resource Guide can be reprinted with proper reference.

The ADA has an extensive list of publications for professionals and individuals with diabetes and their families. This list is accessible online (http://store.diabetes.org) or by calling 1-800-DIABETES.

Numerous other organizations are listed in the RESOURCES section of this book, including other not-for-profit organizations. Many, including the ADA, provide information in Spanish. Most have information for professionals and the public. Some have information that can be printed for patient use. Government agencies are included, too. The National Diabetes Education Program, National Diabetes Information Clearinghouse, and Centers for Disease Control and Prevention all have information for professionals and the public that can be printed out and shared with patients.

Resources for special populations have been listed, including those relevant for senior citizens, young people, and people with disabilities and for weight management. A web site that may identify resources for medication for your low-income or uninsured patients is also listed.

A listing of professional journals and patient-oriented magazines is provided. *Diabetes Spectrum, Clinical Diabetes, Diabetes Care,* and *Diabetes* are all publications of the ADA. *Diabetes Spectrum* translates diabetes research into practice, and its readership consists primarily of nurses, dietitians, psychologists, nurse practitioners, physician's assistants, and other health care professionals. *Clinical Diabetes* is mainly directed toward primary care physicians. *Diabetes* and *Diabetes Care* present the latest in basic and clinical diabetes research, respectively.

Access to information on how to become a certified diabetes educator (CDE), to obtain certification through American Nurses Credentialing Center (BC-ADM), and to become a recognized diabetes education program is included.

Several Patient Information Sheets that were previously published in *Diabetes Spectrum* or *Clinical Diabetes* are included in this RESOURCES section. They were selected because they are topics that are not frequently available in other education materials. An updated listing of antihyperglycemic agents excluding insulins, antihypertensive agents, and antilipidemic agents has been included to complete this resource guide.

Education is critical if patients are going to understand and follow treatment protocols and develop healthier lifestyle habits. A sample list of educational objectives from the ADA-published educational curriculum, *Life With Diabetes,* is included to help identify the important elements of a complete educational program. This is only an example. The final curriculum can be customized to meet the needs of individual programs.

The use of resources is invaluable for patients and professionals alike. Knowledge is the key to understanding and improving quality of care.

Organizations and Government Agencies

These organizations and government agencies have been identified to provide additional information and to provide updated information on a number of topics. Most of these organizations provide information for both health professionals (including education) and the public. Those that do not have been indicated.

FOR HEALTH PROFESSIONALS

Organizations

American Association of Clinical Endocrinologists
245 Riverside Ave., Suite 200
Jacksonville, FL 32202
Phone: 904-353-7878
www.aace.com

American Association of Diabetes Educators
200 W. Madison St.
Suite 800
Chicago, IL 60606
Phone: 800-338-3633
www.diabeteseducator.org

American Celiac Society
P.O. Box 23455
New Orleans, LA 70183
Phone: 504-737-3293
www.americanceliacsociety.org

American Council on Exercise
(no educational materials)
4851 Paramount Dr.
San Diego, CA 92123
Phone: 888-825-3636
www.acefitness.org

American Dental Association
211 East Chicago Ave.
Chicago, IL 60611-2678
Phone: 312-440-2500
www.ada.org

American Diabetes Association
1701 N. Beauregard St.
Alexandria, VA 22311
Phone: 800-342-2383
www.diabetes.org

American Dietetic Association
120 S. Riverside Plaza
Suite 2000
Chicago, IL 60606-6995
Phone: 800-877-1600
www.eatright.org

American Heart Association
National Center
7272 Greenville Ave.
Dallas, TX 75231
Phone: 800-242-8721
www.americanheart.org

American Podiatric Medical Association
9312 Old Georgetown Rd.
Bethesda, MD 20814
Phone: 800-ASK-APMA
www.apma.org

American Stroke Association
National Center
7272 Greenville Ave.
Dallas, TX 75231
Phone: 888-478-7653
www.strokeassociation.org

Celiac Sprue Association
P.O. Box 31700
Omaha, NE 68131-0700
Phone: 877-CSA-4CSA
www.csaceliacs.org

Cystic Fibrosis Foundation
6931 Arlington Rd.
Bethesda, MD 20814
Phone: 800-344-4823
www.cff.org

Diabetes Exercise and Sports Association
10216 Taylorville Rd.
Suite 900
Louisville, KY 40299
Phone: 800-898-4322
www.diabetes-exercise.org

Juvenile Diabetes Research Foundation International
120 Wall St.
New York, NY 10005-4001
Phone: 800-533-2873
www.jdrf.org

Mental Health America (formerly National Mental Health Association)
2000 N. Beauregard St., 6th Floor
Alexandria, VA 22311
Phone: 800-969-6642
www.nmha.org

National Kidney Foundation
30 E. 33rd St.
New York, NY 10016
Phone: 800-622-9010
www.kidney.org

National Mental Health Association
2000 N. Beauregard St., 6th Floor
Alexandria, VA 22311
Phone: 800-969-6642
www.nmha.org

Government Agencies

Centers for Disease Control and Prevention, Division of Diabetes Translation
4770 Buford Highway NE
Mail stop K-10
Atlanta, GA 30341-3717
Phone: 800-232-4636
www.cdc.gov/diabetes

Indian Health Services, Division of Diabetes Treatment and Prevention
5300 Homestead Road
Albuquerque, NM 87110
Phone: 505-248-4182
www.ihs.gov/medicalprograms/diabetes

National Diabetes Education Program
One Diabetes Way
Bethesda, MD 20814-9692
Phone: 888-693-6337
www.ndep.nih.gov

National Diabetes Information Clearinghouse
1 Information Way
Bethesda, MD 20892-3560
Phone: 800-860-8747
www.diabetes.niddk.nih.gov

National Eye Institute
Information Office
2020 Vision Place
Bethesda, MD 20892-3655
Phone: 301-496-5248
www.nei.nih.gov

National Institute of Diabetes and Digestive and Kidney Diseases
National Institutes of Health
Building 31, Rm. 9A06
31 Center Dr., MSC 2560
Bethesda, MD 20892-2560
www2.niddk.nih.gov

U.S. Department of Health and Human Services
200 Independence Ave. SW
Washington, DC 20201
www.hhs.gov

FOR THE PERSON WITH DIABETES

Senior Citizens

AARP
601 E St. NW
Washington, DC 20049
Phone: 888-687-2277
www.aarp.org

National Association of Area Agencies on Aging
1730 Rhode Island Ave. NW
Suite 1200
Washington, DC 20036
Phone: 202-872-0888
www.n4a.org

National Institute on Aging
Building 31, Room 5C27
31 Center Dr. MSC 2292
Bethesda, MD 20892
Phone: 800-222-2225
www.nia.nih.gov

Young People

American Diabetes Association Youth Zone
1701 N. Beauregard St.
Alexandria, VA 22311
Phone: 800-342-2383
www.diabetes.org/youthzone/youth-zone.jsp

American School Health Association
7263 State Route 43
P.O. Box 708
Kent, OH 44240
Phone: 330-678-1601
www.ashaweb.org

Children with Diabetes, Inc.
8216 Princeton-Glendale Rd.
PMB 200
West Chester, OH 45069-1675
www.childrenwithdiabetes.com

Centers for Disease Control and Prevention, Division of Adolescent and School Health
1600 Clifton Rd.
Atlanta, GA 30333
Phone: 800-323-4636
www.cdc.gov/HealthyYouth/index.htm

National Association of School Nurses
8484 Georgia Ave.
Suite 420
Silver Spring, MD 20910
Phone: 866-627-6767
www.nasn.org

National Education Association Health Information Network
1201 16th St. NW
Suite 216
Washington, DC 20036-3290
Phone: 202-822-7570
www.neahin.org

Resources for Low-Income and Uninsured Patients

Partnership for Prescription Assistance
PhRMA
1100 15th St. NW
Washington, DC 20005
Phone: 888-477-2669
www.helpingpatients.org
www.pparx.org
(single point of access for more than
  475 public and private patient
  assistance programs)

For Ethnic and Racial Minorities

National Center on Minority Health and Health Disparities
National Institutes of Health
6707 Democracy Blvd.
Suite 800
Bethesda, MD 20892-5465
Phone: 301-402-1366
www.ncmhd.nih.gov

Office of Minority Health
Centers for Disease Control and Prevention
1600 Clifton Rd.
Atlanta, GA 30333
Phone: 800-311-3435
www.cdc.gov/omh

Weight Management

The Obesity Society
8630 Fenton St.
Suite 814
Silver Spring, MD 20910
Phone: 301-563-6526
www.obesity.org

Federal Trade Commission
Consumer Information
Health: Weight Loss and Fitness
600 Pennsylvania Ave. NW
Washington, DC 20580
Phone: 202-326-2222
www.ftc.gov/bcp/menus/consumer/
health/weight.shtm

Shape Up America
www.shapeup.org
Weight Control Information Network
National Institute of Diabetes and Digestive and Kidney Diseases
1 WIN Way
Bethesda, MD 20892-3665
Phone: 877-946-4627
www.niddk.nih.gov/health/nutrit/win.
htm

Weight-Loss Web sites

American Diabetes Association
"Weight Loss Matters" Tip Sheets
http://www.diabetes.org/weightloss-
and-exercise/weightloss/monthly-
tip-sheets.jsp

Federal Trade Commission
Consumer Information Guidance
Documents: Diet, Health & Fitness
www.ftc.gov/bcp/menus/resources/
guidance/health.shtm
(brochures on many health topics,
including exercise and weight loss)

Partnership for Healthy Weight Management
www.consumer.gov/weightloss/bmi.htm
(Find out your body mass index to learn
whether you weigh too much.)

People with Disabilities

American Foundation for the Blind
11 Penn Plaza
Suite 300
New York, NY 10001
Phone: 800-232-5463
www.afb.org

Lighthouse International
The Sol and Lillian Goldman Bldg.
111 E. 59th St.
New York, NY 10022-1202
Phone: 800-829-0500
www.lighthouse.org

National Federation for the Blind
1800 Johnson St.
Baltimore, MD 21230
Phone: 410-659-9314
www.nfb.org

Amputee Coalition of America
900 E. Hill Ave.
Suite 205
Knoxville, TN 37915-2566
Phone: 888-267-5669
www.amputee-coalition.org

National Center on Physical Activity and Disability
1640 W. Roosevelt Rd.
Chicago, IL 60608-6904
Phone: 800-900-8086
www.ncpad.org

Identification

MedicAlert Foundation International
2323 Colorado Ave.
Turlock, CA 95382
Phone: 888-633-4298
www.medicalert.org

Publications

Clinical Diabetes
This quarterly journal is dedicated to improving diabetes care in primary care settings. It provides concise, clinically relevant articles on diabetes management, including pharmacological management, exercise and diet, medical legal issues, and health care delivery.

American Diabetes Association
Membership/Subscription Services
1701 N Beauregard St.
Alexandria, VA 22311
Phone: 800-232-3472 ext. 2343
http://clinical.diabetesjournals.org

Diabetes
This professional journal of original, basic research in diabetes includes articles on all aspects of laboratory, animal, and human research relating to the physiology and pathophysiology of diabetes.

American Diabetes Association
Membership/Subscription Services
1701 N Beauregard St.
Alexandria, VA 22311
Phone: 800-232-3472 ext. 2343
http://diabetes.diabetesjournals.org

Diabetes Care
The world's highest circulation and most-cited journal of clinical diabetes research, including reviews, commentaries, and original articles covering clinical care, education, and nutrition, epidemiology and health services, emerging technologies and treatments, pathophysiology and complications, and pre-diabetes.

American Diabetes Association
Membership/Subscription Services
1701 N Beauregard St.
Alexandria, VA 22311
Phone: 800-232-3472 ext. 2343
http://care.diabetesjournals.org

Diabetes Spectrum
The health care professional's tool for translating new diabetes research into clinical practice. Articles cover medical management, patient education, nutrition and behavioral science, exercise, and other topics.

American Diabetes Association
Membership/Subscription Services
1701 N Beauregard St.
Alexandria, VA 22311
Phone: 800-232-3472 ext. 2343
http://spectrum.diabetesjournals.org

For People with Diabetes

Diabetes Forecast
The most widely circulated magazine for people with diabetes for over 50 years, covering advances in research and treatment, healthy diet, exercise, fitness, and advocacy. Includes the Annual Resource Guide.

American Diabetes Association
Membership Center
P.O. Box 363
Mount Morris, IL 61054-0363
Phone: 800-806-7801
www.forecast.diabetes.org

BOOKS

For Health Professionals
The American Diabetes Association offers numerous professional publications covering a variety of pertinent topics from clinical treatment protocols to educational curriculum to patient handouts. A sample of professional books includes:

ADA Medical Management Series
Therapy for Diabetes Mellitus and Related Disorders, 5th edition (2009)
ISBN: 978-1-58040-325-5
Medical Management of Type 1 Diabetes, 5th edition (2008)
　　ISBN: 978-1-58040-309-2

Medical Management of Type 2 Diabetes, 6th edition (2008)
　　ISBN: 978-1-58040-310-8
Medical Management of Pregnancy Complicated by Diabetes, 4th edition (2009)
　　ISBN: 978-1-58040-232-3
Intensive Diabetes Management, 4th edition (2009)
　　ISBN: 978-1-58040-328-X
ADA/PDR Medications for the Treatment of Diabetes (2008)
　　ISBN: 978-1-56363-734-6

For People with Diabetes
The American Diabetes Association offers a variety of books to help people with diabetes cope the disease and related disorders. For cookbooks and self-help guides contact the association at http://store.diabetes.org. Examples include:

The Ultimate Diabetes Meal Planner
　　ISBN: 978-1-58040-299-6
Your First Year with Diabetes: What to Do, Month by Month
　　ISBN: 978-1-58040-301-6
Real-Life Guide to Diabetes: Practical Answers to Your Diabetes Problems
　　ISBN: 978-1-58040-314-6
Diabetes 911: How to Handle Everyday Emergencies
　　ISBN: 978-1-58040-300-9

Certification Programs

Education Recognition Program

American Diabetes Association
1701 N Beauregard St.
Alexandria, VA 22311
Phone: 888-232-0822
http://professional.diabetes.org/
recognition.aspx

**Board Certified in Advanced
Diabetes Management
(BC-ADM), RN, RD, Pharmacist
American Nurses Credentialing
Center**
8515 Georgia Ave.
Suite 400
Silver Spring, MD 20910-3492
Phone: 800-284-2378
http://www.nursecredentialing.org

**Certified Diabetes Educator (CDE)
National Certification Board for
Diabetes Educators (NCBDE)**
330 E. Algonquin Rd.
Suite 4
Arlington Heights, IL 60005
Phone: 847-228-9795
http://www.ncbde.org

Forms

Patient Education Tools

Online Depression Screening Test: http://psych.med.nyu.edu/patient-care/
depression-screening-test

Stress Management Tools

We all have stress. Finding ways to relieve stress and relax will make us healthier and happier. Ask yourself some simple questions.

What do you do when you feel stressed? _____

What do you do to relax? _____
(Some people like to listen to music, read a book, or talk with a friend.)

There are a number of stress-management skills that you can learn and make part of your life to reduce feelings of stress.

DIRECT APPROACH	INDIRECT APPROACH
Positive Self-Talk: Telling oneself that there is hope. Seeing challenges, not defeat. Preparing oneself for success through positive input, positive affirmations, and reframing negative thoughts.	*Exercise:* Using regular, aerobic exercise to decrease the effect of stress on the body.
Communication Skills: Being able to use "I" messages. Being able to actively listen. Using "both-win" approaches to negotiation.	*Relaxation* *Progressive Relaxation:* Deep muscle relaxation by alternatively tensing and relaxing groups of muscles.
Assertiveness Training: Being able to say "no." Being able to ask questions of others, especially your medical team. Being able to express your feelings.	*Deep breathing (diaphragmatic breathing):* Abdominal rises and falls with respirations. The upper body does not move.
Time Management: Learning to be more organized and efficient through good decision making and goal setting.	*Meditating:* Trance-like state where noncritical focus is maintained one thought at a time.

DIRECT APPROACH	INDIRECT APPROACH
Priority Setting: Making conscious choices.	*Biofeedback:* Getting visual, audible, or tactile information about various body functions, such as heart rate, muscle tension, and hand temperature, in order to learn control over that body function.
Thought Stopping: Learning not to be consumed by concerns and worries. Stopping habitual negative thought patterns.	
	Nutrition: Learning to eat healthy foods that maximize the body's energy.
Refuting Irrational Ideas: Learning to identify and refute unrealistic expectations and ideas that may have one overreacting to a situation.	*Sleep:* Prioritizing adequate sleep and developing good sleep patterns.

Adapted from Guthrie DW, Rhiley DS: *Care and Control of Your Diabetes.* Wichita, KS, Via Christi Regional Medical Center, Diabetes Treatment and Research Center, 2002.

PATIENT INFORMATION SHEETS

Take Charge of Your Diabetes
Making Time for Diabetes Care in a Woman's Busy Life
Taking Many Medications
Is an Insulin Pump Right for Your Child and Family?
A Step-by-Step Approach to Complementary Therapies
Diabetes and Eating Disorders
For Great Diabetes Care, Remember Your ABCs!
How Can We Help You?
Keeping Medicine Costs Under Control
Be Prepared: Sick Day Management
Diabetes in the Hospital: Taking Charge
Diabetes and Surgery
Thyroid Disease and Diabetes
Guidelines for Using Vitamin, Mineral, and Herbal Supplements
Leaving Home for Life on Your Own

Take Charge of Your Diabetes

The most important person in your diabetes care is **you.** Your diabetes health care team members may be the best, but they aren't there all day to advise you. At home, at work, or at play, you are in charge.

Teamwork
Your health care team are experts on diabetes, but you are the expert on you. It takes all of you to adapt diabetes care to your life and to adapt your life to diabetes care.

Learn about diabetes. If you are new to diabetes, ask your health care provider to refer you to a diabetes education program and dietitian. Even if you have had diabetes for a while, diabetes education can bring your knowledge up to date and help you with any problems that you may be having.

Tell your health care provider what your goals are. Ask for your provider's opinion. If your goals are not the same, ask why. Then devise a plan for your diabetes care to achieve your goals. Do not agree to a plan that you are not able to or will not use. Speak up about what will and won't work for you.

Ask questions. Write down your questions before your visit so you won't forget them. Examples of things you may want to ask about are:
- side effects of and interactions between your medicines
- herbs and supplements
- referrals for an eye doctor or a foot doctor
- how to reduce your risk of heart disease and other diabetes complications
- how to cope with your emotional response to diabetes.

Don't be afraid to ask any question that is on your mind. Bring a notebook to jot down the answers. Or bring a friend or relative to take notes. If you need someone to translate from English into your language, bring an adult, not a child.

Make the most of your visit. The time you have with your provider is often short. Plan ahead of time what you want to accomplish during the visit. Are there issues or concerns that are affecting how you care for your diabetes? Are you facing barriers in meeting your goals? Are you struggling with your feelings about diabetes? What questions do you have? Make sure to bring up the one that is most important to you first.

Bring a list of the medications you take. Be ready to list any symptoms you have. Take off your shoes and socks when you get to the exam room so that your provider can look at your feet. Answer your health care provider's questions honestly and fully. At the end of the visit, repeat back instructions in different words to make sure you understand them.

Follow up. Don't assume if your provider's office doesn't call with test results that everything is okay. Always call to find out what your results are and ask about what they mean.

On Your Own

Set goals. Decide what you want to do and create a plan to reach your goal. Focus on what you need to do each week to reach your goal. Choose steps that are measurable and realistic. For example, start by walking 1,000 steps a day for three days a week and slowly work up to 10,000 steps a day.

Read up. Build on your diabetes education. You can find books about diabetes at your local library and bookstore. The American Diabetes Association and the National Institutes of Health websites (among others) give trustworthy information about diabetes.

Take care of yourself. Get all the check-ups and screening tests your health care team recommends. It's the best way to catch problems early when

treatment can do the most good.

Seek support. Find people to support you and to cheer you on. Seek out a friend or relative willing to listen to your concerns. A diabetes support group can be an emotional lifeline and a way to learn more about diabetes as well.

Keep good records. Records of your blood glucose levels, your doses of medications, side effects you have, and factors that may have affected your blood glucose levels will help you and your provider fine-tune your care. A logbook or computer record works better than scraps of paper or your meter memory to look for patterns.

Use reminders. Keep your meter at hand, not buried in a drawer or closet. Use timers, sticky notes, or other memory joggers to remind you to take your medicines or check your blood.

Stay motivated. Remind yourself of the benefits you hope to gain by reaching your goals. For example, you can watch your grandchildren grow up and be independent. Give yourself a positive message every day. Pat yourself on the back or reward yourself with a CD, book, time spent doing something you enjoy, or something meaningful to you. Recognize your efforts, not the results. And remember, diabetes care is all about you!

American Diabetes Association.

Cure • Care • Commitment®

Diabetes Spectrum/Patient Information

Making Time for Diabetes Care in a Woman's Busy Life

Women live diverse lives. But one constant for almost all women is too little time. Most women juggle many roles and duties. It's hard to squeeze everything in—doubly hard when you have a disease such as diabetes.

Reviewing how you spend your time can help you manage better. Some diabetes tasks need to be done every day:
- Testing your blood sugar
- Taking pills or insulin and determining how much to take and when to supplement
- Recording test results and medicine doses in your log
- Exercising

Here are ways to give your diabetes the daily attention it deserves:
- Don't feel guilty about making diabetes care a top goal. Staying healthy makes it easier to be a good employee, wife, mother, and daughter.
- Make diabetes care part of your everyday routine. You'll be more likely to exercise, for example, if you have a time set aside for it.
- Make daily to-do lists. Mark the most urgent activities.
- Use memory aids:
  ✔ Link testing and taking medicines to things you do every day at the same time, such as brushing your teeth.

  ✔ Keep your medicines and glucose meter near where you do these acts.
  ✔ Create rituals. Do things in the same order in the same place at the same time each day.
  ✔ Set a timer to remind you of your next blood test or medicine dose.
  ✔ Make a daily chart of tasks. Check off each medicine as you take it and each blood test as you do it.

Some diabetes tasks are done only when needed:
- Deciding what foods to buy, cook, and eat
- Reviewing your blood sugar records and food records
- Testing your urine for ketones
- Seeing your health care providers
- Getting lab work done
- Filling prescriptions and buying supplies
- Traveling to and from and waiting at the clinic, lab, and drugstore

Planning for these is much harder than fitting in daily tasks. They don't occur regularly. The time they require is less predictable. And many take hours instead of minutes.

Still, there are many ways to free up time for such tasks.

Start by setting personal, family, and career goals. Rank these by importance. You want to spend most of your time and effort on important goals. Then look at how you spend your time each week. Ask yourself:
- Are there ways you can spend your time more usefully? Do you watch TV shows that you don't really enjoy? Catch up on work or chores during that time instead.
- Are you using any time inefficiently? Do you go to the grocery twice a week instead of once? Planning ahead to avoid double effort can free up large blocks of time.

If you still have too little time:
- Delegate. If your husband or children have time to goof off, but you are always frantically busy, something is out of whack.
- Say "no" more often.
- Plan your schedule around your natural body clock. Do important tasks when you are most alert and energetic.
- Cut down health care visits by doubling up. Try to see the dietitian and have lab work done on the same day you visit your provider.

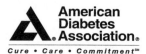

American Diabetes Association.

Cure • Care • Commitment™

Diabetes Spectrum 16:173, 2003

Taking Many Medications

Diabetes often goes hand-in-hand with other medical problems. Besides your diabetes medications, you may be taking medications for kidney disease, high cholesterol, or high blood pressure. Many people need three or more medications to get their blood pressure under control. Use of more than one medication to treat type 2 diabetes is becoming common, too. It's easy to be overwhelmed by so many medications.

Problems That Can Occur
Several problems can occur when you take many medications:
- They may interact.
- You may have side effects.
- You may have an overdose because two providers prescribe the same medication or medications in the same family.
- You may not be able to afford them.
- You may forget to take them or renew them.

The tips below can help.

Stay Safe
To avoid medications that interact or are from the same family, both you and your health care providers should know all the medications you take and what they are for.

Everyone who takes medicines should make a list of them and carry it at all times. This list should include for each medication:
- Its generic and brand names
- Its dose and how often you take it
- What it is for
- Who prescribed it
- When you started taking it

Also put on your list the supplements and over-the-counter medicines you take. These include vitamins, pain relievers, herbal products, laxatives, and food supplements.

Knowing both the generic and the brand name is vital. Some medications have many brand names. You need to know all the names to be sure that two doctors haven't prescribed the same medication.

When you go to any health care provider, take your list. Put all your current medicine containers in a bag and take that, too.

If your provider wants to prescribe a new medication, ask whether it is safe to take with your current medicines. When you fill a new prescription, ask your pharmacist the same question.

Fill all your prescriptions at the same pharmacy if you can. Get to know your pharmacist and discuss with him or her your concerns about the medications you are taking.

Take your medications as prescribed. If you don't, they may not have the desired effect. Be honest with your provider if you sometimes forget or skip doses. Otherwise, your provider may think the medication isn't working well for you. He or she may then increase your dose or add another medication, making your "medication burden" even heavier.

Once a year, review your treatment goals and medications with your primary care provider. Do you still need all your medications? Do the doses need adjustment? How about your daily schedule for taking your medications? Have any medications stopped working or started causing side effects? Can your regimen be made less expensive or easier to take?

Afford Your Medications

Health care providers do not always know the cost of the medications they prescribe. If you cannot afford your medicines, speak up! Your providers can help you, but only if they know there's a problem. For example:

- Some drugs are available in less expensive generic forms.
- Sometimes, an older, less expensive medication can be used instead of a newer more expensive one.
- Some medications can be bought more economically in a larger dose and cut in half.
- Your provider may have free samples.
- Your provider can help you apply to a drug company's prescription assistance program.

• Improving your diet, being more active, and making other behavior changes can sometimes cut the amount of medications you need for certain problems, such as high blood pressure, diabetes, and high cholesterol.

Remember To Take Your Medications

Your medications do you no good if you do not take them. If you often forget, talk to your doctor. He or she may be able to change your dosing schedule or switch you to a long-acting once-a-day form. The less often you need to take medications, the less likely you are to miss a dose.

Know why you need each medication and what will happen if you don't take it. You may then be less inclined to "forget" a medication on purpose.

Setting up a routine helps a lot:
- Make taking your medications a habit. Take your medications at the same times

and in the same place each day.
- Link medication taking to daily routines, such as at mealtimes, at bedtime, or when brushing your teeth. Check with your pharmacist for the best time of day to take any given medication if you aren't sure.
- Use kitchen timers or a multi-alarm watch to alert you that it's time for your medications.
- If your health care provider approves, get a week-long medication organizer with three or four compartments for each day. Once a week, refill the organizer.
- Keep a wall calendar. Each time you renew prescriptions, write it on the calendar. Also mark the day you need to renew again.
- Renew prescriptions at regular intervals. Then, if you forget to renew on time or an emergency comes up, you still have enough on hand.

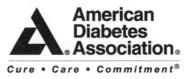

American Diabetes Association

Cure • Care • Commitment®

Diabetes Spectrum/Patient Information

Is an Insulin Pump Right for Your Child and Family?

Insulin pump therapy can help people with type 1 diabetes. Pumps deliver insulin in a way that resembles the body's own release of insulin. They can improve blood sugar control, make low blood sugar (hypoglycemia) less of a problem, and lessen the risk of diabetic ketoacidosis. But pump use in children, especially very young children, is controversial. If you are considering an insulin pump for your child, read on.

How Pumps Work

Insulin pumps are about the size of a pager. They are attached to the body by a needle placed under the skin. They can remain in place for 2–3 days at a time. Pump therapy delivers rapid- or short-acting insulin continuously through the needle. The continuous insulin is called the basal rate.

In addition to providing basal insulin throughout the day, pumps are programmed to give additional insulin (bolus doses) with each meal and snack. Older children or the parents of younger children must test the blood sugar four to eight times a day to check the pump's effectiveness, adjust mealtime boluses, and correct high blood sugar levels.

So What's Not to Like?

Pumps can improve diabetes control and give children more flexibility, but very young children cannot manage their own pump use. Even older kids need a good deal of help from parents. Therefore, pump therapy requires a knowledgeable parent or caregiver to be on hand 24 hours a day, 7 days a week to help with blood sugar tests, determine mealtime insulin needs, adjust pump settings, and troubleshoot any problems.

Consider These Questions

Is your child

- willing to wear the pump?
- able to tolerate the needle-insertion process?

As your child's main caregiver, do you

- fully understand basal-bolus insulin therapy?
- know how to count carbohydrate or use some other insulin-to-food ratio?
- know how to correct for high or low blood sugar levels?
- know how to change insulin doses for changes in exercise, sick days, travel, or other special situations?
- understand how to measure ketones and what to do if they are present?

- feel sure that you can operate an insulin pump?
- have the time to care for your child's diabetes every day?
- have partnerships with school personnel and other caregivers who are willing and able to work with a pump?

Does your diabetes care team

- include a doctor, a diabetes nurse educator, a registered dietitian, a mental health professional, and other health care professionals?
- have experience using insulin pumps with young children?
- offer 24-hour telephone contact for patients who use insulin pumps?

Still Interested?

Good. Pump therapy may be a good fit for your child and family. Before making a final decision, sit down with your child's diabetes health care providers. Weigh the pros and cons for your own family situation. Consider wearing a pump yourself and having your child wear one for a few days to see what it's like. Find out all you can so that you and your child can make an informed choice.

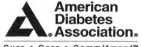

American Diabetes Association®

Cure • Care • Commitment™

A Step-by-Step Approach to Complementary Therapies

Often, the greatest levels of health and well-being can be reached when people have an integrative medical care team that is trained not only in the latest treatments and technologies, but also in how to create a healing environment for the mind, body, and spirit. Integrative care includes the best of standard medical care and complementary therapies as well as patients' full involvement in mind, body, and spirit.

The following steps can help you safely integrate complementary therapies into your health care plan.

Step 1. Identify the symptom you hope to improve.
Start a symptom diary. Record what your symptoms are, when they occur, and what makes them better or worse. For example, if you have periodic shooting pain in your legs, an entry in your symptom diary might read, "Shooting leg pain three times this evening. On a scale of 1 to 10, this pain was an 8."

Step 2. Identify possible complementary therapies.
Collect information about complementary therapies you may want to try. Discuss them with your medical team.

Ask your standard health care team:
- Is this treatment dangerous? Does it cause any side effects?
- Is it safe to combine this with my current medical treatments?
- What should I ask when I meet with possible complementary care providers?
- What type of follow-up should I schedule with you if I use this therapy?

Step 3. Interview potential complementary therapy providers.
Expect that it will take some time and effort to find the right provider for you.

Ask potential complementary care providers.
- What do you think is causing my symptoms?
- What treatment do you recommend? What benefits can I expect from it?
- Are there any dangers or concerns associated with this treatment?
- Is it safe to combine this treatment with my current medical treatments?
- How and when will we decide whether it is working?
- What is the cost? Will my insurance pay for it? Can you help me look into this?
- What is your training? Are you licensed or certified? How do I contact the licensing agency?
- Do you need information from my medical team about my medical history and current treatments?
- Will you follow-up with my doctor about your recommendations?

Step 4. Choose a complementary therapy provider and begin treatment.
You may wish to consult your medical team before selecting a complementary care provider. Continue to keep your symptom diary as you begin complementary therapy. For example, you may record, "Reiki session on Saturday. I feel a sense of well-being and peacefulness. I felt shooting pain in my legs three times tonight, but it was less painful—a 5 on a scale of 1 to 10."

Step 5. Follow-up regularly with your complementary and standard care providers.
Review your symptom diary and the effects of the complementary treatment. Report any side effects to both your complementary and standard care providers.

To learn more about complementary and alternative therapies, contact the National Center for Complementary and Alternative Medicine (NCCAM, formerly the National Institutes of Health Office of Alternative Medicine) at 800-531-1794 or visit the NCCAM website http://altmed.od.nih.gov

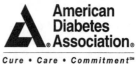

American Diabetes Association.

Cure • Care • Commitment℠

Diabetes and Eating Disorders

Eating disorders are common in teenaged girls and young women. They are rarely seen in boys and men. Girls and young women with type 1 diabetes have about twice the risk of developing eating disorders as their peers without diabetes. This may be because of the weight changes that can occur with insulin therapy and good metabolic control and the extra attention people with diabetes must pay to what they eat.

The two main eating disorders are anorexia nervosa and bulimia nervosa. People with anorexia restrict their food intake to stay thin. Their perceptions of their body are often distorted. People with bulimia repeatedly eat excessive amounts of food and then induce vomiting or take laxatives to purge the food from their body.

The most common features of eating disorders in girls and young women with type 1 diabetes are:
• dissatisfaction with their body weight and shape and desire to be thinner;
• dieting or manipulation of insulin doses to control weight; and,
• binge eating.

Researchers estimate that 10–20 percent of girls in their mid-teen years and 30–40 percent of late teenaged girls and young adult women with diabetes skip or alter insulin doses to control their weight. In people with diabetes, eating disorders can lead to poor metabolic control and repeated hospitalizations for dangerously high or low blood sugar. Chronic poor blood sugar control leads to long-term complications, such as eye, kidney, and nerve damage.

Early Warning Signs
• Extremely high A1C test results
• Frequent bouts of and hospitalizations for poor blood sugar control
• Anxiety about or avoidance of being weighed
• Frequent requests to switch meal-planning approaches
• Frequent severe low blood sugar
• Widely fluctuating blood sugar levels without obvious reason
• Delay in puberty or sexual maturation or irregular or no menses
• Binging with food or alcohol at least twice a week for 3 months
• Exercise more than is necessary to stay fit
• Severe family stress

If you think that you or a loved one has an eating disorder, talk to your diabetes health care providers. They will recommend a mental health counselor who will work with the diabetes team to help you and your family deal with this problem. It is important to be nonjudgmental and supportive. It is also extremely important to seek evaluation and treatment.

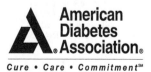

Diabetes Spectrum 14:106, 2002

For Great Diabetes Care, Remember Your ABCs!

Taking good care of your diabetes can be complex and confusing. This handy list will make remembering all the steps you need to take as easy as A B C D E F G H I!

A is for A1C.
The A1C ("A-one-C") test—short for hemoglobin A_{1c}—measures your average blood glucose (sugar) over the past 3 months.
Suggested target: Below 7
How often: At least twice a year

A is also for albuminuria.
Albuminuria means protein in the urine. A test that measures your urine microalbumin-to-creatinine ratio can detect kidney disease very early, when it can usually be stopped. This can prevent dialysis or kidney transplantation later on.
Suggested target: Below 30
How often: At least once a year

And, finally, A is for aspirin.
Taking low-dose aspirin every day can help prevent heart attacks and strokes. Children and young adults with no history of heart disease should not take aspirin without a doctor's order, nor should some older adults. Check with your doctor before starting daily aspirin.

B is for blood pressure.
High blood pressure makes your heart work too hard and can cause damage to your kidneys and eyes.
Suggested target: Below 130/80
How often: At every visit

C is for cholesterol.
Bad cholesterol, or LDL, builds up and clogs your arteries, leading to heart attacks and strokes.
Suggested LDL target: Below 100
How often: At least once a year

D is for diabetes education.
Help your doctor help you. The more you know about how food, exercise, and medicines affect your diabetes control, the better you and your doctor can work together to make any needed changes.
Suggested resources: Dietitians, nurse diabetes educators
How often: Ongoing

E is for eye exam.
Regular eye exams can catch diabetic eye disease early enough to prevent eventual blindness.
How often: At least once a year

F is for foot care
Keep an eye on your feet. If you have nerve disease and can't feel your feet, your feet can't tell you when something is wrong.

How often: Check your feet daily. Remind your doctor to check them at every visit. Get an extensive foot exam once a year.

G is for glucose (sugar) monitoring.
If you know when your blood sugar level is too high or too low, you'll know better how to treat it.
How often: Decide with your doctor.

H is for staying healthy.
For people with diabetes, getting the flu or pneumonia can lead to serious complications. Avoid them by getting vaccinated.
How often: Flu vaccine, every year; pneumonia, at least once.

I is for identifying special medical needs.
Complications are complicated. As they occur, your doctor may need to send you to various specialists. Voicing your health concerns at every visit can help your doctor spot trouble and get any extra help you need quickly.
How often: When needed

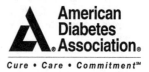

American Diabetes Association

Cure • Care • Commitment^{SM}

How Can We Help You?

Having a chronic illness such as diabetes can affect just about every aspect of your life. Consequently, many different problems can get in the way of your efforts to control your diabetes. Perhaps you have other illnesses or physical problems that make it hard for you to deal with your diabetes. Maybe the demanding nature of diabetes has left you feeling overwhelmed, sad, or even angry.

The good news is that your health care team can help you find ways to overcome many of the obstacles you may be facing. But they need your help to figure out exactly what types of help you may need. Here's a list of questions to ask yourself before your next visit to your health care provider to help pinpoint any problem areas you may want to discuss with your diabetes team.

Knowledge

- Do you know enough about your diabetes?

- Do you know all the members of your diabetes team?

- Are you always able to speak with and understand members of your diabetes team?

- Who or what do you believe is responsible for the cause, treatment, and progress of your diabetes?

Health and Physical Issues

- Do you have other health problems that affect your diabetes?

- Are you happy with the way your diabetes medications are working?

Stress, Feelings, and Attitudes

- Are you willing to look after your diabetes?

- Do you feel you are able to look after your own diabetes?

- Would you look after your diabetes more if you felt worse?

- What is more important than looking after your diabetes?

- Do you or your diabetes team have enough time for your diabetes?

- Are you worried, afraid, or ashamed of your diabetes?

- Are you willing to look after your diabetes fully from today?

Access

- Can you get to your diabetes team easily?

- Would you prefer your diabetes service to be closer?

- Do you have all the services you need?

- Are you happy with how these services are provided?

- Have you been unhappy with any members of the diabetes team?

- Are you happy with your diabetes education and care?

- Do you feel comfortable talking with your diabetes team?

Support

- Do you feel pressure from others not to look after your diabetes?

- Do you feel that others are holding your diabetes against you?

- Is your family helping you look after your diabetes?

- Do family demands stop you from looking after your diabetes?

Society

- Can you afford to have diabetes?

- Is there enough support for you in the community or at work?

- Should the public bear more financial responsibility for your care?

- Do people other than your family need to know more about diabetes?

There are no right or wrong answers to these questions. But there are resources to help you improve your diabetes care if you are not getting the care you need. Talk to your health care provider or call your local American Diabetes Association for more information.

Keeping Medicine Costs Under Control

The high price of medicines and supplies weighs heavily on people with diabetes. The burden can be overwhelming when you use several medicines. Here's how you can lighten the load.

Everyday Cost Cutters
- When you need an over-the-counter medicine, consider a generic instead of the name brand. Generic versions contain the same active agents but cost less. To find generic versions of a name-brand product, compare ingredient labels. Look for the same active ingredient in the same strength. Your pharmacist can help.
- Keep receipts for medical expenses, including prescription costs your insurance doesn't cover. When these are large relative to your income, some can be deducted from your income taxes.
- Scan drugstore ads for coupons.
- Check out your insurance coverage. Some health plans cover medicines. Some let you order prescriptions by mail for a reduced co-payment. If you order insulin through the mail, be sure it will be protected from getting too hot or too cold.
- Call several pharmacies to find out which one is cheapest for all your medicines put together. (For safety's sake, buy all of your medicines at one place.) If you can, check prices at online pharmacies, too.
- Limit your use of supplements and herbs to those your provider recommends. Few have been proven to have any benefit. Yet they can cost as much as—or more than—medicines proven to be safe and to work.

Working With Providers
Your diabetes team can help if you let them know how you are concerned about costs.
- Ask whether adopting good health habits could cut your prescription costs. For example, exercising, quitting smoking, and limiting salt are cheaper than buying medicines to treat high blood pressure.
- Don't pressure your doctor for medicines you see in TV ads. New and heavily advertised products often cost the most.
- On the other hand, new medicines can sometimes save you money. For example, you may be taking products B and C to treat side effects of product A. If you switch from product A to new product D with milder side effects, you might be able to stop using products B and C.
- When your health care provider suggests a new medicine, ask whether there's a cheaper alternative. Providers don't always take cost into account when choosing treatments.
- Tell your provider or pharmacist you'd like to use generic medicines whenever possible.
- Check whether your insurance company has a formulary (a list of preferred products with reduced co-payments). If so, give a copy to your provider.
- Each year, review all of your medicines with your provider. Some you may no longer need. Others may now be available in cheaper generic or over-the-counter versions.
- When starting a new medicine, ask for free samples. That way, if the side effects are bad or the product doesn't work well for you, you haven't bought an entire bottle.

Specials for Seniors
- Check with your local pharmacies to see whether any offer a senior discount card.
- If your grocery or drugstore gives seniors a discount on a certain day, buy your over-the-counter products that day.
- The American Association of Retired Persons has a pharmacy service. You can get medicines and vitamins at a discount at local pharmacies or by mail.

Programs for the Needy
Programs for people with low incomes vary. Ask your diabetes team what your area has. If they don't know, talk to a social worker or your local public health or social services department.
- Some drug companies have "pharmacy assistance programs." These provide medicines for free or at a reduced price to people with low incomes.
- Some cities have free clinics or public health clinics.
- Some states have special programs to help people afford their prescriptions. These are often for low-income elderly or disabled people.

Shauna S. Roberts, PhD, is a science and medical writer in New Orleans, La.

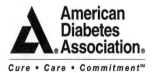

American Diabetes Association

Cure • Care • Commitment™

Diabetes Spectrum/Patient Information

Be Prepared: Sick Day Management

Planning ahead can help you stay in control of your blood sugar levels during illness. Being prepared can prevent a hospitalization or emergency room visit.

Complete this checklist of "things to do" with your doctor or diabetes educator *before* you get sick. Review it once a year for changes.

❑ Know to keep taking your insulin or diabetes medications unless

_____

_____

Adjust your insulin by

_____

_____

❑ Plan to maintain a meal plan containing 150 grams of carbohydrates. Have on hand for illness the following foods, which contain 15 grams of carbohydrates each in the amounts shown.

- apple juice (1/2 cup)
- regular soda (1/2 cup)
- regular gelatin (1/2 cup)
- crackers (6 squares)

- bouillon (no calories)
- sports drink (1 cup)
- other: _____

❑ Know when to monitor your blood glucose.

_____
_____
_____
_____

❑ Know when to monitor your urine ketones:
- When blood sugar level is greater than
  _____.
- Regardless of blood sugar level, when vomiting or experiencing diarrhea.

Remember to check the bottle of ketone test strips for an expiration date.

❑ Know when to call your doctor or diabetes educator:
- If your blood sugar level is greater than_____
- If your ketones are _____for more than _____hours or if you

do not urinate for more than _____hours
- If vomiting lasts longer than _____hours
- If you are dehydrated. Signs of dehydration include dry tongue and difficulty breathing.
- If surgery or a test is planned that will prevent you from eating normally
- Any time you have a question or concern about your blood sugar level

❑ Know who to call during illness or an emergency:

Doctor_____

Daytime phone:
_____

Evening/Weekend:
_____

Diabetes educator
_____

Daytime phone:
_____

Evening/Weekend:
_____

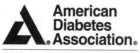

American Diabetes Association®

Cure • Care • Commitment℠

Diabetes in the Hospital: Taking Charge

Going into the hospital? Knowing what to expect and how to prepare can make it easier.

First, find out the basics. You may be in the hospital for a short-stay surgery or test, a planned surgery, an illness, or a diabetes complication. Ask questions. Why does your doctor think you need to be in the hospital? Are there other options? What risks are there? Will you need someone to care for you at home? If you are having a procedure, you may wish to see another doctor for a second opinion. How long will you be there? If you do not understand the answers, ask again.

Before You Go
Talk to your doctor about handling your own diabetes care in the hospital. If you tend to stay in good control, your doctor may allow you to test your own blood glucose and take your own insulin or pills. If so, your doctor should put a self-management order in your hospital chart that says what you will do yourself.

If you can, also talk to the surgeon and other providers involved in your care. Tell each about your diabetes and other health problems. Ask whether and when you should stop taking your medicines. Ask how and by whom your blood glucose will be controlled during and after surgery. If you have a diabetes doctor or team, you have the right to ask that they manage your diabetes in the hospital.

Contact your health insurance company. Make sure your doctors and hospital accept your insurance. Find out how to get your treatment covered and what you will have to pay.

If you smoke, quit or cut down.

> ## Good diabetes control in the hospital is vital.

Remember to pack and put your name on:
- Slippers
- A copy of your meal plan
- Your medical history
- A list of the drugs you take (prescription and over-the-counter)
- A pocket carbohydrate guide to help you choose meals
- If you are on a insulin pump, take enough supplies for a daily site change.

Ask about taking your glucose meter, monitoring supplies, and drugs. Usually, the hospital will ask you to use their supplies. When you feel up to it, you may ask to take over monitoring fingersticks, injections, and diabetes management.

Find out what to expect after the procedure or treatment. Talk to your doctor and to others who have had the same treatment to help you prepare. For example, if you learn you should not drive for a week after you go home, stock up on food before you go.

At the Hospital
Good diabetes control in the hospital is vital. High blood

glucose levels slow healing and increase your risk of infection. The American Diabetes Association recommends that blood glucose should be less than 180 mg/dl for people in the hospital or having surgery. For some, the goal is less than 110 mg/dl.

But good control in the hospital is hard for several reasons:

- Stress can raise blood glucose levels.
- Treatments may affect your blood glucose level.
- It may be hard to stick to your meal plan when you don't feel well or have few food options.
- Going for tests may make your meals, shots, or glucose tests late.
- Some hospitals let blood glucose levels get too high on purpose to prevent potentially harmful lows.
- Many hospitals dose insulin by the "sliding-scale" method, which can cause wild swings in blood glucose levels.

To make things easier:

- Ask that your meal plan be given to the hospital dietit-

ian. If you can, talk to the dietitian about how to adapt it for your stay.

- Know that the hospital may change the doses of your diabetes drugs or put you on new drugs. You may be given

Speaking up in the hospital is important.

Ask questions.

Be prepared.

an insulin drip or injections to aid in your healing and recovery.

- Changes in what you eat, the stress of illness or surgery, and the healing process can change the amount of drugs or insulin you need.
- If you're not in charge of your own diabetes care, call

the nurse if your meal comes before your diabetes pills or insulin. Also, call if you've taken your medicine but your meal doesn't arrive.

- When you are admitted, tell the nurses what your usual symptoms are for high and low blood glucose.
- Keep glucose tablets close by in case your meal is late. Report symptoms of low blood glucose right away.
- If you are in pain, taking pain medicine, or not thinking clearly, ask family or friends to watch out for your diabetes care.
- Before going home, get written instructions for any changes in your usual medicines, meal plan, glucose testing, or exercise.
- If you are worried about caring for yourself at home, ask the nurse early on for help finding support.

Speaking up in the hospital is important. Ask questions. Be prepared. If you are concerned about your diabetes care, talk to your doctor, the nurse in charge, or your diabetes team.

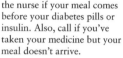

American Diabetes Association.

Cure • Care • Commitment®

1/05

Diabetes Spectrum 18:49–50, 2005

Diabetes and Surgery

The prospect of surgery can make anyone feel worried and fearful. However, careful planning, especially for people with diabetes, can help you make your operation as safe as possible and your recovery period less stressful.

The key is to start planning well before your surgery date. This "to do" list can help you cover all the bases before your operation.

1. Meet with your primary care doctor or endocrinologist. Work with your doctor to develop a plan for getting your blood sugar in the best possible control several weeks before you have surgery. Having good control of your blood sugar will lessen the chance of high blood sugar (hyperglycemia) or low blood sugar (hypoglycemia) reactions during your operation. Good blood sugar control also makes infections less likely and promotes healing.

Your doctor may also want to do a complete medical history and physical examination and other tests before your surgery.

2. Talk to your anesthesiologist. This is the doctor who is responsible for monitoring your diabetes while your surgeon is performing the operation. Tell the anesthesiologist about your medical history, including details about your diabetes. Be sure to include your current medication regimen and any diabetes-related complications you have.

You may also want to discuss different types of anesthesia. Some procedures can be done with local or spinal anesthesia, allowing you to remain awake during the procedure. In such cases, recovery time is often shorter.

Other procedures require general anesthesia, which puts you to sleep during your operation. More careful monitoring of your diabetes is required during the procedure and after you undergo general anesthesia.

3. Schedule your surgery for the early morning. Try to get the first morning time slot in the operating room. There will be less of a chance for high or low blood sugar reactions while you are waiting for your operation and are unable to eat.

4. Talk to your doctor in advance about how you will manage your diabetes immediately after your operation. After surgery, you may need to adjust your medication or insulin doses based on your blood sugar level. Ask your doctor how you should manage your diabetes so that you can prepare in advance.

5. Get a temporary disabled parking permit, if necessary. If you are having orthopedic surgery or another operation that will make it hard for you to walk during recovery, go to your local Department of Motor Vehicles and request the appropriate paperwork. Ask your doctor to sign it in advance so that you can get your temporary permit before your operation.

6. Fill any new prescriptions before your surgery. Ask your doctor and surgeon whether you will need any pain medication or other prescriptions after your operation. These may include antinausea pills, laxatives, or other drugs. Ask for the prescriptions in advance, so you can have the medications ready when you need them.

7. Find out how long you will need to recover. If you will not be eating for an extended period of time, you and your doctor will need to change your diabetes care regimen. Also, you may need to make arrangements with your workplace for an extended recovery time.

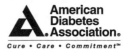

Diabetes Spectrum/Patient Information

Thyroid Disease and Diabetes

Diabetes and thyroid disease are both endocrine, or hormone, problems. When thyroid disease occurs in someone with diabetes, it can make blood glucose control more difficult.

The thyroid is a butterfly-shaped gland in your lower neck just beneath your skin. It regulates your body's metabolism, the processes of using and storing energy, by releasing a substance called thyroid hormone. If it produces too much thyroid hormone, your metabolism quickens (hyperthyroidism), too little and your body functions slow down (hypothyroidism).

Hyperthyroidism Symptoms
- Pounding heart
- Quick pulse
- Increased sweating
- Weight loss despite normal or increased appetite
- Shortness of breath when exercising
- Diarrhea
- Muscle weakness or tremors
- Trouble concentrating

- Change in menstrual periods
- Thick skin on the knees, elbows, and shins

Hypothyroidism Symptoms
- Fatigue
- Sluggishness
- Depression
- Feeling of being cold even when others feel warm
- Constipation
- Weight gain unrelated to increase in eating
- Low blood pressure
- Slow pulse

Effects on Diabetes
Hyperthyroidism. When your metabolism quickens, your medicines go through your body quicker. Your blood glucose level may rise because your usual dosage does not stay in your body long enough to control it.

Hyperthyroidism and low blood glucose can be hard to tell apart. If you are sweating and having tremors from hyperthyroidism, you may think you have low blood glucose and eat extra food, causing your blood glucose to rise. Using your glucose meter to

verify low blood glucose levels can help you avoid this problem.

Hypothyroidism. When your metabolism slows, your blood glucose level may drop because your diabetes medicine doesn't pass through your body as quickly as usual and so stays active longer. In hypothyroidism, it is often necessary to reduce your dose of diabetes medicines to prevent low blood glucose.

If You Think You Have Thyroid Disease
Tell your health care provider about any symptoms you have. A physical exam and simple blood tests can identify hyper- or hypothyroidism.

If you have hyperthyroidism, medicines and other treatments can help slow your metabolism by controlling the release of thyroid hormone. If you have hypothyroidism, your health care provider can prescribe thyroid hormone pills to speed up your metabolism. You will need follow-up blood tests every few months to adjust your dosage of thyroid hormone.

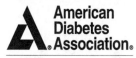

American Diabetes Association®

Cure • Care • Commitment℠

Diabetes Spectrum 15:143, 2002

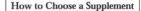

Guidelines for Using Vitamin, Mineral, and Herbal Supplements

- **Learn about the supplements you are interested in taking.** Know the name, amounts, and effects of products you use.

- **Discuss supplements with your doctor.** Tell your health care provider about all of the medicines, herbal products, and supplements you take.

- **Keep records.** Record the doses, date started, and side effects of any supplement you use. Note your blood sugar levels while using the supplement and the effects of the supplement. Did it work?

- **Know what benefits to expect.** Long-term use of most supplements is not recommended. If a supplement is not working, stop taking it.

- **Add only one new product at a time.** It is easier to track effects if you take only one supplement at a time. If you use more than one or a combination formula, check labels to ensure that you do not exceed total dosage guidelines for individual substances.

- **Carefully follow dosage guidelines on labels.** To be cautious, start with a half dose, working up to a full dose over a week or more. Do not take greater amounts than recommended.

- **Do not combine supplements and prescription drugs without your doctor's knowledge.** Many supplements can change the way medicines work. In some cases, serious side effects can occur.

- **Never stop taking a prescribed drug without your doctor's knowledge.** Many supplements are unproven. They are not a substitute for prescription drugs you may be using.

- **Stop using supplements and contact your doctor if you notice bad side effects.** Side effects from supplements can be very serious.

- **Do not use supplements if you are pregnant or nursing or give them to young children.** The effects of many of these products on fetuses and children are not known.

- **Stop using all supplements (or check with your doctor) before surgery, anesthesia, and other medical procedures.** Several herbs can decrease the body's ability to form blood clots and could be dangerous. Others can alter the effects of anesthesia or lead to seizures.

- **Store capsules and tablets in a cool dark place at home.** Fresh herbs can be frozen in airtight containers; capsules and tablets should not be frozen.

How to Choose a Supplement

- Look for nationally known food and supplement companies.

- Look for products that have recognized symbols of quality, such as the USP, NF, TruLabel, or ConsumerLabs symbol.

- Avoid foreign products unless quality is known. Foreign products, especially those from China and India, are more likely to have dangerous contaminants.

- Avoid companies that make sensational claims or have misleading labeling.

- Look for products that have standardized extracts. Labels should clearly identify the quantities of active ingredients.

- Look for products that have an expiration date.

- Look for products that provide a toll-free customer service phone number. Call and ask if their products undergo outside testing or if there are any published studies supporting their use.

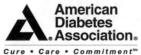

American Diabetes Association®

Cure • Care • Commitment℠

Leaving Home For Life On Your Own

The year after high school graduation is full of changes. You may face diabetes challenges whether you go to college or enter the work world.

Start Off Right

Before leaving home, you should be ready to manage all of your diabetes care. You need to get your skills down pat while your family and diabetes team can help.

Make a list of your diabetes supplies. You will need to buy these regularly to keep from running out.

Talk with your diabetes educator to help you plan how to fit diabetes care into your new life.

If you don't have a medical ID bracelet or necklace, buy one, and wear it.

Prepare For A Doctor's Visit

If you don't move away, your new insurance may allow you to keep your current diabetes care team. Find out from your parents:

- Phone numbers for your team members
- How often you should see each one

- How far ahead you need to schedule visits
- What you should take to visits

If you go away to school, set up a visit with the student health center to discuss your diabetes. Take a copy of your medical records, a list of your drugs, and your treatment plan. Find out what services (including flu, meningitis, and hepatitis shots) student health provides and their cost. Ask how you should get rid of sharps. If its diabetes services are scanty, ask your former diabetes team to help you find other diabetes care in your college town. If student health is not open around the clock, find out where to get urgent care during off-hours.

As long as you are a student, your parents' health insurance will probably cover your care and prescriptions, including supplies. If you use a mail order service, you will need to communicate with your parents and the prescription service to make sure you have enough supplies at school. You should identify a pharmacy where you are going to school.

Obtain prescriptions from your diabetes team to take to a pharmacy near your school as a backup in an emergency (i.e. you drop your last bottle of insulin.)

If you are moving away for a job, talk to your diabetes team before you go. Ask for suggestions for diabetes care providers and educators in your new town. Get extra copies of your medical records in case you don't click with the first doctor or educator you try. Make finding a new health care team a top priority.

Drink Safely

Social life among your peers may center on drinking. You should know that alcohol puts you at risk for low blood glucose levels for 6 to 36 hours. Alcohol can make it hard to tell that your blood glucose levels are dropping too low (hypoglycemia).

You may choose not to drink. If so, seek out events that do not involve drinking. For example, join a club or take part in volunteer work or your local church, synagogue, or mosque.

If you do drink:
- Eat before and while drinking.
- Set limits ahead of time, and stop drinking when you reach them.
- If your diabetes is not in good control, skip drinking.
- Drink only with people you trust and who know what to do if you have hypoglycemia.
- Test your blood glucose levels while drinking and carefully for at least 24 hours after drinking alcohol.

Prepare For Sick Days
Take your sick-day plan with you. If you do not have a sick-day plan, work with your health care team to create one before you leave home. It should include what drugs to take when you are sick, how to adjust your insulin, and a list of the symptoms that should prompt you to call your doctor.

You will need to keep on hand sick-day foods. These include regular and sugar-free caffeine-free soft drinks, regular and sugar-free pudding and gelatin mixes, juice, instant soup mix, and crackers. You'll also need to have ketone strips and a thermometer. You may wish to stock up on cold remedies as well.

When you are not feeling well, test your blood glucose and urine ketone levels at least every 3–4 hours.

You should try to eat. If your stomach rebels, try light foods such as crackers, chicken soup, and sugared soda. Every hour, try to eat something with about 15 grams of carbohydrates and drink a cup of fluid. Take your insulin unless your doctor tells you otherwise.

Tell Friends
For safety's sake, tell your roommate(s), resident advisor, neighbor(s), co-workers, or new friends you have diabetes. Your life could be at risk if you had hypoglycemia and your roommate did not know what to do.

You should explain to key people what hypoglycemia is, what its symptoms are, and what they should do. All should know to call 911 if they find you unconscious or cannot wake you. You should also ask some people to learn how to give you a glucagon shot.

If you are an athlete, your coach and teammates need to know about your diabetes and how to treat hypoglycemia.

Learn More
- Tips for College Students:
  http://www.childrensdiabetesfdn.com/educ/college.htm
- Countdown to College:
  ✓ http://www.diabetes.org/all-about-diabetes/diabetes-news/enews-archive/04-08-04.jsp
  ✓ http://www.diabetes.org/all-about-diabetes/diabetes-news/enews-archive/05-06-04.jsp
  ✓ http://www.diabetes.org/all-about-diabetes/diabetes-news/enews-archive/08-05-04.jsp
- Getting Ready for College:
  http://www.diabetesselfmanagement.com/print.cfm?aid=1224

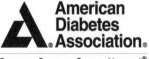

American Diabetes Association®

Cure • Care • Commitment®

EDUCATIONAL OBJECTIVES

Sample Educational Objectives

The following sample illustrates how one program cross-referenced their educational objectives to the curriculum content of *Life With Diabetes*. This documentation is not a requirement for programs applying for recognition. For Recognition requirements, please refer to the American Diabetes Association at http://professional.diabetes.org/recognition.aspx.

SAMPLE EDUCATIONAL OBJECTIVES

Learning and Skill Objectives	Outline	Learning and Skill Objectives	Outline
A. Overview/Understanding of Diabetes		2. Informs others of ways they can be supportive.	
1. States:	1	3. Identifies local sources for diabetes support.	16
a. excess glucose in blood due to too little insulin in relationship to body needs.		**D. Nutrition and Meal Planning**	
b. lifelong condition requiring treatment.		1. States:	3
c. which type of diabetes they have.		a. reasons for meal planning.	
		b. rationale for eating meals on time.	
B. Stress and Psychosocial Adjustment		c. rationale for eating bedtime snack.	
1. Identifies self as having diabetes.	2	d. rationale for reaching/ maintaining desirable weight.	3, 17
2. Identifies thoughts, feelings, and areas of concern about diabetes.		e. rationale for eating less fat.	3, 18
3. Identifies personal meaning of diabetes.		f. awareness of types of fat and effects of each.	18
4. Identifies effects of stress on blood glucose.	12	g. awareness of need to change diet with activity changes.	3, 7
5. Identifies one strategy for coping with stress/feelings related to diabetes.		2. Has a meal plan.	5
6. Identifies signs and symptoms of depression.		3. Is able to:	
7. Identifies personal diabetes care goals.	15	a. describe personal meal plan.	5, 19
		b. use meal plan to plan meals.	5, 19
C. Family and Social Support		c. use meal plan when eating away from home.	
1. Identifies desired level of support from family/friends.	2	d. identify behaviors that help control weight.	17

Learning and Skill Objectives	Outline
e. identify eating behaviors that help reduce risk of heart disease.	18
f. plan a sick-day diet.	11
g. explain how alcohol affects blood glucose.	
h. use product labels to choose foods that fit meal plan.	6
i. explain the benefits and cautions of a high-fiber diet.	18
j. plan eating/behavior changes that work toward personal goals.	15
4. Referral to a dietitian.	3

E. Exercise and Activity

1. States that exercise/activity lowers blood glucose.	7
2. Identifies personal exercise plan.	
3. Identifies when not to exercise.	
4. Describes exercise snack, if needed.	11
5. Identifies insulin adjustment for exercise if needed.	
6. Identifies monitoring needed for exercise.	

F. Medication

▪ **ORAL HYPOGLYCEMIC AGENTS**

1. States:	8
a. name and dose of agent.	
b. when to take.	
c. effect on blood glucose.	
d. side effects.	
e. precautions	

▪ **INSULIN**

1. States:	9
a. type(s) and dose to take.	
b. when to take.	
c. onset, peak, and duration.	

Learning and Skill Objectives	Outline
d. effect on blood glucose.	
e. when low blood glucose is most likely to occur.	11
f. insulin adjustment plan.	
g. how to store insulin.	9
2. Prepares and administers own insulin correctly.	
a. gently rolls insulin to mix.	
b. injects air into bottle.	
c. checks for/removes bubbles.	
d. draws up correct dose.	
e. disposes of syringes/ lancets correctly.	
3. Selects appropriate injection site.	
a. selects suitable sub-Q tissue.	
b. states rotation plan.	
4. If using intensive therapy, states:	9
a. benefits of intensive therapy.	
b. type of insulin that affects specific blood glucose levels.	
c. need for frequent blood glucose testing.	
d. personal insulin plan and blood glucose goals.	

G. Monitoring and Use of Results

▪ **BLOOD GLUCOSE**

1. Demonstrates ability to test blood glucose.	10
a. uses appropriate site to obtain blood samples.	
b. uses correct testing technique.	
c. accurately tests blood glucose.	
d. cares for meter and stores strips properly.	

Learning and Skill Objectives	Outline	Learning and Skill Objectives	Outline

2. States:
  a. need for monitoring.
  b. plan for monitoring blood glucose and record keeping at home.
  c. that normal blood glucose is 70–115 mg/dl.
  d. personal goal or target range.
  e. appropriate decisions to make about glucose regulation based on results.
  f. where to obtain glucose meters and supplies.
3. Defines A1C.
  a. states normal value.
  b. states personal goal.
	
	11
	
	10
		c. relationship of exercise to blood glucose.
		3. States benefits of improved glucose control.
		4. States risks of improved glucose control.
		5. Identifies treatment methods to improve glucose control.
			
			7, 11
			
			11, 14
			
			11

■ **URINE KETONE TESTING**
1. States purpose of urine ketone testing.
2. Tests urine ketones:
  a. if blood glucose >300 mg/dl.
  b. if ill or unable to eat.
  c. as otherwise prescribed.
3. Interprets test results correctly.
4. States proper action to take for ketonuria.
5. Stores strips properly.
	
	10
		■ **HYPOGLYCEMIA**
		1. States:
		  a. meaning and other names.
		  b. personal/common symptoms.
		    1) occurring while awake.
		    2) occurring while asleep.
		  c. causes and how to prevent.
		  d. when to contact health professional.
		  e. proper action to be taken to treat hypoglycemia.
		2. Family member/roommate is able to give glucagon.
		3. Wears/carries diabetes identification.
			
			11

H. Regulating Blood Glucose
■ **GLUCOSE CONTROL RELATIONSHIPS**
1. Identifies factors that influence blood glucose levels.
2. Identifies personal behaviors that influence blood glucose levels.
  a. relationship of food intake to blood glucose.
  b. relationship of diabetes medications to blood glucose.
	
	11
	
	4, 11
	
	8, 9, 11
		■ **HYPERGLYCEMIA**
		1. States:
		  a. meaning and other names.
		  b. personal common symptoms.
		  c. causes and how to prevent.
		  d. states proper action to take and when to contact provider.
		  e. relationship of ketoacidosis to high blood glucose.
		
		I. Personal Health Habits
		1. States:
		  a. body areas most susceptible to infection.
		  b. signs/symptoms of infection and treatment measures.
			
			11
			
			13

Learning and Skill Objectives	Outline	Learning and Skill Objectives	Outline
c. effects of smoking on circulation.		**L. Health Care Systems**	
d. need for foot care.		1. States importance of plans for regular health monitoring.	13
e. plan for personal foot care.		a. diabetes management.	
f. need for skin care.		b. ophthalmological exams.	
g. plan for personal skin care.		c. dental care.	
h. need for regular dental care.		d. regular physical exams.	
i. benefits of regular medical care.		e. other as indicated.	
		2. Identifies personal risk factors for complications/ health problems.	14
J. Long-Term Complications		3. States how to obtain driver's license and insurance, and employment rights.	16
1. States:	14	4. States awareness of community resources.	16
a. awareness of potential long-term complications and target organs.		5. States name(s) and phone number(s) of health professional(s) to contact.	
1) cardiovascular.		a. stop smoking.	
2) peripheral vascular.		b. weight control program.	
3) sensory neuropathy.		c. social worker.	
4) autonomic neuropathy.		d. visiting nurse/home health.	
5) retinopathy.		e. dietitian.	
6) nephropathy.		f. diabetes support group.	
b. symptoms indicating onset of complications and importance of early diagnosis.		g. education program.	
c. ways to prevent, delay, or detect complications.		h. other.	
d. common diabetes-related sexual concerns, dysfunctions, and treatment methods.	20	**M. Pregnancy**	
		1. Preconception.	
K. Problem-Solving and Behavior Change		a. states importance of normal blood glucose levels before pregnancy.	9
1. Identifies problem-solving strategies.	15	b. states need for thorough medical exam before pregnancy.	
2. Identifies personal long-term diabetes care goals.		2. Preexisting diabetes.	
3. Identifies personal short-term diabetes care goals.		a. identifies importance of frequent care for changing insulin/dietary needs.	
4. Identifies personal behavior-change goals.		3. Gestational diabetes.	
5. Identifies strategies to achieve goals.		a. defines as hyperglycemia related to hormonal changes during pregnancy.	

Learning and Skill Objectives	Outline	Learning and Skill Objectives	Outline
b. states importance of follow-up care after delivery.		h. how often to change equipment.	
4. Blood glucose control.		i. signs/symptoms/treatment of irritation/inflammation/infection.	
a. states need to maintain glucose levels in the target range throughout pregnancy.		j. what to do with the pump for the following activities: sleeping, sexual activities, bathing, swimming, sports, traveling.	
b. lists symptoms of hyperglycemia and when to call a physician.			
c. states symptoms of hypoglycemia and how to treat.		k. awareness of alarms and how to handle.	
5. Prenatal care.		l. hotline phone number for appropriate company.	
a. lists danger signs during pregnancy; when to call a physician.		m. how to obtain pump supplies.	
b. identifies tests to monitor health of mother and infant.		n. various ways the pump can be worn.	
		o. usual battery life	
N. Pump Therapy		2. Demonstrates ability to:	
1. States:	22	a. administer bolus dose three times.	
a. correct name of pump used.		b. change basal rate three times.	
b. correct type of insulin used.		c. change battery.	
c. advantages/disadvantages of pump therapy.		d. fill pump syringe/cartridge with insulin; place in pump.	
d. definition of *basal* and *bolus*; how they relate to normal body physiology.		e. attach tubing; check for secure connection.	22
e. that bolus insulin is given intermittently throughout the day based on:		f. prime tubing with insulin.	
1) meals.		g. select and prepare suitable infusion site.	
2) blood glucose levels at time bolus is given.		h. correctly insert infusion needle and secure.	
3) glucose values out of target range other than at meal times.		i. check pump for correct/current basal rate program.	
f. how pump will affect lifestyle.		j. program bolus dose based on blood glucose reading.	
g. proper equipment to be used.		k. activate pump to deliver bolus dose.	
		l. terminate bolus delivery once dose is activated.	

Learning and Skill Objectives	Outline	Learning and Skill Objectives	Outline
3. Able to recognize signs of possible pump malfunction, and steps to address: a. change site; administer bolus with syringe.		b. telephone pump manufacturer for technical help. c. monitor ketones for glucose over 240 mg/dl; respond appropriately.	

From American Diabetes Association: *Life with Diabetes: A Series of Teaching Outlines by the Michigan Diabetes Research and Training Center.* 4th ed. Funnell MM et al., Eds. Alexandria, VA, American Diabetes Association, 2009.

ORAL AGENTS

Trade Name	Generic name	When to Take	Doses	Side Effects

Secretagogues (Hypoglycemia Agents)—Stimulates the pancreas to produce more insulin

Sulfonylureas

Trade Name	Generic name	When to Take	Doses	Side Effects
Diabeta or Micronase	(Glyburide)	30 min before meals	1.25, 2.5, 5 mg Max: 20 mg	
Glynase	(Glyburide- press tab)	30 min before meals	1.5, 3, 6 mg Max: 12 mg	Low blood glucose (BG)- Hypoglycemia
Glucotrol	(Glipizide)	30 min before meals	5, 10 mg Max: 40 mg	Weight gain
Glucotrol XL	(Glipizide)	before or with meals	5, 10 mg Max: 20 mg	
Amaryl	(Glimepiride)	before or with meals	1, 2, 4 mg Max: 8 mg	

Meglitinides

Trade Name	Generic name	When to Take	Doses	Side Effects
Prandin	(Repaglinide)	5–30 min before meals	0.5, 1, 2 mg Max: 16 mg	Low BG Headaches
Starlix	(Nateglinide)	5–30 min before meals	120mg, 60mg	

Biguanides—Decrease hepatic glucose production

Glucophage	(Metformin) (Riomet-liquid)	Take with meals	500, 850, 1000 mg	Nausea, Diarrhea
Glucophage XR; Glumetza; Fortamet		500&1000 mg	Max: 2550 mg	Metallic Taste,
COMBINATION PILLS				Lactic Acidosis
Glucovance	(Glyburide/Metformin)	Take with meals	1.25/250; 2.5/500; 5/500 mg	(also hypoglycemia)
Metaglip	(Glipizide/Metformin)	Take with meals	2.5/250;5/500; 2.5/500	
Avandamet	(Rosiglitizone /Metformin)	Take with meals	1mg/500mg, 2/500, 4/500	
Acto*plus*met	(Pioglitazone/Metformin)	Take with meals	15mg/500mg; 15/850	
Avandaryl	(Avandia/Amaryl)	Take same time/d	4mg/1mg; 4/2; 4/4	
DuetAct	(Amaryl/Actos); JanuMet (Januvia/Metformin)			

Note: Stop if kidney dye study; check creatinine and liver function; need good oxygenation in body.

Alpha-glucosidase Inhibitors—Slows carbohydrate absorption in intestines

Precose	(Acarbose)	Take with first bite	25, 50, 100 mg Max: 300 mg	Nausea, Diarrhea Flatulence
Glyset	(Miglitol)	Take with first bite	25, 50, 100 mg Max: 300 mg	

Note: If low blood sugar, use honey or glucose gel/tablets; do not use table or brown sugar.

Thiazolidinediones (Insulin Sensitizer)—Improves peripheral insulin sensitivity

Actos	(Pioglitazone)	With or without meals	15, 30, mg Max: 45 mg	Possible liver dysfunction Possible anemia, edema, congestive heart failure, fractures
Avandia	(Rosiglitazone)	With or without meals	2, 4, 6, 8 mg (max)	Same as Actos + may increase risk of myocardial infarction (MI)

Note: May take 6 weeks to work best, need live function studies before starting and periodically thereafter, may decrease effectiveness of birth control

INCRETINS—Gliptins; for T2DM's on Secretagogue, Metformin, or TZD's

1. Byetta (exenatide injection) 5–10mcg 2x/d. Stimulates insulin release when BG increasing, regulates food release ~stomach, slows hepatic glucose release, ↑ satiety. Side effect: wt loss & ~nausea.
2. Januvia (oral agent)100mg 1x/d. Increases GLP1 (gut hormones) by stopping breakdown of internal GLP1. Increases insulin release and reduces hepatic glucose release. **MidAmerica Diabetes Associates** **Rev 3-09**

Prescribing Information for Antihypertensive Agents

GENERIC (BRAND)	FORM/ STRENGTH	DOSAGE	WARNINGS/PRECAUTIONS & CONTRAINDICATIONS	ADVERSE REACTIONS
ALPHA ANTAGONISTS				
Doxazosin mesylate (Cardura)	**Tab:** 1mg*, 2mg*, 4mg*, 8mg* *scored	***Adults:* HTN:** Initial: 1mg qd (am or pm). Monitor BP 2-6 hrs and 24 hrs after 1st dose. Titrate: Increase to 2mg qd then upwards as needed. Max: 16mg/day. **BPH:** Initial: 1mg qd (am or pm). Titrate: May double the dose every 1-2 weeks. Max: 8mg/day.	**W/P:** Monitor for orthostatic hypotension and syncope with 1st dose and dose increase. Caution with hepatic dysfunction. Rule out prostate cancer. Priapism (rare), leukopenia/neutropenia reported. **P/N:** Category C, caution with nursing.	Fatigue/malaise, hypotension, edema, dizziness, dyspnea, weight gain.
Prazosin HCl (Minipress)	**Cap:** 1mg, 2mg, 5mg	***Adults:*** Initial: 1mg bid-tid. Maint: 6-15mg/day in divided doses. Max: 40mg/day. **Concomitant Diuretic/ Antihypertensive:** Reduce to 1-2mg tid, then retitrate.	**W/P:** Syncope may occur, usually after initial dose or dose increase. Excessive postural hypotensive effects. Avoid driving for 24 hrs after 1st dose or dose increase. Always start on 1mg cap. False (+) for pheochromocytoma. **P/N:** Category C, caution in nursing.	Dizziness, headache, drowsiness, lack of energy, weakness, palpitations, nausea.
Terazosin HCl (Hytrin)	**Cap:** 1mg, 2mg, 5mg, 10mg	***Adults:* HTN:** Initial: 1mg hs, then slowly increase dose. Usual: 1-5mg/day. Max: 20mg/day. If response is substantially diminished at 24 hrs, may increase dose or give in 2 divided doses. **BPH:** Initial: 1mg qhs. Titrate: Increase stepwise as needed. Usual: 10mg/day. May increase to 20mg/day after 4-6 weeks. Max: 20mg/day. If discontinue for several days, restart at initial dose.	**W/P:** Monitor for orthostatic hypotension and syncope initially and with dose increase. Rule out prostate cancer. Priapism (rare) reported. Possibility of hemodilution. **P/N:** Category C, caution with nursing.	Asthenia, postural hypotension, headache, dizziness, dyspnea, nasal congestion/rhinitis, somnolence, impotence, blurred vision, palpitations, nausea, peripheral edema, priapism, thrombocytopenia, atrial fibrillation.
ALPHA ANTAGONIST COMBINATION				
Prazosin HCl/ Polythiazide (Minizide)	**Cap:** (Polythiazide-Prazosin) 0.5mg-1mg, 0.5mg-2mg, 0.5mg-5mg	***Adults:*** 1 cap bid-tid. Determine strength by individual component titration.	**BB:** Not for initial therapy of HTN. **W/P:** Syncope may occur, usually after initial dose or dose increase. Excessive postural hypotensive effects. Avoid driving for 24 hrs after 1st dose or dose increase. Always start on 1mg prazosin. Caution with severe renal disease, hepatic dysfunction, or progressive liver disease. Sensitivity reactions may occur with history of allergy or bronchial asthma. May exacerbate or activate SLE. Hyperuricemia, hypokalemia or frank gout may occur. Monitor electrolytes. May manifest latent DM. Enhanced effects in the post-sympathectomy patient. May decrease serum protein-bound iodine levels. False (+) for pheochromocytoma. **Contra:** Anuria, thiazide or sulfonamide sensitivity. **P/N:** Category C, not for use in nursing.	Dizziness, headache, drowsiness, lack of energy, weakness, palpitations, nausea, blood dyscrasias, rash.
ALPHA- AND BETA-BLOCKERS				
Carvedilol (Coreg, Coreg CR)	**Tab:** 3.125mg, 6.25mg, 12.5mg, 25mg; **Cap, Extended-Release:** 10mg, 20mg, 40mg, 80mg	***Adults:*** Individualize dose. Take with food. Monitor dose increases. Take extended-release capsules in am and swallow whole. **CHF: Tab:** Initial: 3.125mg bid for 2 weeks. Titrate: May double dose every 2 weeks as tolerated. Max: 50mg bid if >85kg. Reduce dose if HR <55 beats/min. **Cap, Extended-Release:** Initial: 10mg qd for 2 weeks. Titrate: May double dose every 2 weeks as tolerated. Max: 80mg/day. Reduce dose if HR <55 beats/min. **HTN: Tab:** Initial: 6.25mg bid for 7-14 days. Titrate: May double dose at 7-14 day intervals. Max: 50mg/day. **Cap, Extended-Release:** Initial: 20mg qd for 7-14 days. Titrate: May double dose every 7-14 days as tolerated. Max: 80mg/day. **LVD Post-MI: Tab:** Initial: 6.25mg bid for 3-10 days. Titrate: May double dose every	**W/P:** Avoid abrupt discontinuation; taper over 1-2 weeks. Hepatic injury reported; d/c and do not restart if develop hepatic injury. Hypotension and syncope reported, most commonly during up-titration period; avoid driving or hazardous tasks during initiation period. May mask hypoglycemia and hyperthyroidism. May potentiate insulin-induced hypoglycemia and delay recovery of serum glucose levels. Decrease dose if pulse <55 beats/min. Monitor renal function during uptitration with low BP (SBP <100mmHg), ischemic heart disease, diffuse vascular disease and/or renal insufficiency. Worsening heart failure or fluid retention may occur with uptitration. Caution in pheochromocytoma, peripheral vascular disease, major surgery with anesthesia, Prinzmetal's variant angina,	Bradycardia, fatigue, edema, hypotension, dizziness, headache, diarrhea, nausea, vomiting, hyperglycemia, weight increase, dyspnea, anemia, increased cough, arthralgia.

BB = black box warning; **W/P** = warnings/precautions; **Contra** = contraindications; **P/N** = pregnancy category rating and nursing considerations.

Prescribing Information for Antihypertensive Agents

GENERIC (BRAND)	FORM/ STRENGTH	DOSAGE	WARNINGS/PRECAUTIONS & CONTRAINDICATIONS	ADVERSE REACTIONS
ALPHA- AND BETA-BLOCKERS *(Cont.)*				
Carvedilol (Coreg, Coreg CR) *(Cont.)*		3-10 days to target of 25mg bid. May begin with 3.125mg bid and slow up-titration rate if clinically indicated. **Cap, Extended-Release:** Initial: 20mg qd for 3-10 days. Titrate: May double dose every 3-10 days to target of 80mg qd.	and bronchospastic disease. Effectiveness of carvedilol in patients younger than 18 years of age has not been established. **Contra:** Bronchial asthma or related bronchospastic conditions, 2nd- or 3rd-degree AV block, sick sinus syndrome, severe bradycardia (without permanent pacemaker), cardiogenic shock, decompensated heart failure requiring IV inotropic therapy, severe hepatic impairment. **P/N:** Category C, not for use in nursing.	
Labetalol HCl (Trandate)	**Tab:** 100mg*, 200mg*, 300mg* *scored	**Adults:** PO: Initial: 100mg bid. Titrate: May increase by 100mg bid every 2-3 days. Maint: 200-400mg bid. **Severe HTN:** 1200-2400mg/day given bid-tid. Titrate: Do not increase by more than 200mg bid. **Elderly:** Initial: 100mg bid. Titrate: May increase by 100mg bid. Maint: 100-200mg bid.	**W/P:** Caution with hepatic dysfunction. Avoid abrupt withdrawal; may exacerbate ischemic heart disease. Caution with latent cardiac insufficiency, may exacerbate cardiac failure, reduce sinus HR, and slow AV conduction. Avoid in overt CHF. Avoid with bronchospastic disease. Paradoxical HTN in pheochromocytoma reported. D/C prior to surgery. Caution with DM; may mask symptoms of hypoglycemia. **Contra:** Bronchial asthma, overt cardiac failure, greater than first degree heart block, cardiogenic shock, severe bradycardia, other conditions associated with hypotension, history of obstructive airway disease. **P/N:** Category C, caution in nursing.	Dizziness, fatigue, nausea, vomiting, dyspepsia, paresthesia, nasal stuffiness, ejaculation failure, impotence, edema, dyspnea, headache, vertigo, postural hypotension, increased sweating.
ANGIOTENSIN CONVERTING ENZYME (ACE) INHIBITORS				
Benazepril HCl (Lotensin)	**Tab:** 5mg, 10mg, 20mg, 40mg	**Adults:** If possible, d/c diuretic 2-3 days prior to initiation of therapy. Initial: 10mg qd or 5mg with concomitant diuretic. Maint: 20-40mg/day given qd-bid. Resume diuretic if BP not controlled. Max: 80mg/day. **CrCl <30mL/min/1.73m²:** Initial: 5mg qd. Max: 40mg/day. **Pediatrics: ≥6 yrs:** Initial: 0.2mg/kg qd. Max: 0.6mg/kg.	**BB:** When used in pregnancy, ACE inhibitors can cause injury and even death to the developing fetus. D/C therapy when pregnancy detected. **W/P:** D/C if angioedema, jaundice, or if marked LFT elevation occurs. Risk of hyperkalemia with DM, renal dysfunction. Persistent nonproductive cough reported. Monitor WBCs in renal and collagen vascular disease. Anaphylactoid reactions reported. Fetal/neonatal morbidity and death reported. Monitor for hypotension in high risk patients (eg, surgery/anesthesia, prolonged diuretic therapy, heart failure, volume and/or salt depletion, etc). Caution with CHF, renal dysfunction, and renal artery stenosis. Less effective on BP in blacks and more reports of angioedema than nonblacks. **Contra:** History of ACE inhibitor-associated angioedema. **P/N:** Category D, not for use in nursing.	Cough, dizziness, headache, fatigue, somnolence, postural dizziness, nausea.
Captopril (Capoten)	**Tab:** 12.5mg*, 25mg*, 50mg*, 100mg* *scored	**Adults:** Take 1 hour before meals. **HTN:** If possible, d/c recent antihypertensive drug for 1 week prior to therapy. Initial: 25mg bid-tid. Titrate: May increase to 50mg bid-tid after 1-2 weeks. Usual: 25-150mg bid-tid. Max: 450mg/day. **CHF:** Initial: 25mg tid; 6.25-12.5mg tid with risk of hypotension or salt/volume depletion. Usual: 50-100mg tid. Max: 450mg/day. **Left Ventricular Dysfunction Post-MI:** Initial: 6.25mg single dose, then 12.5mg tid. Titrate: Increase to 25mg tid over next several days, then to 50mg tid over next several weeks. Usual: 50mg tid. **Diabetic Nephropathy:** 25mg tid. **Significant Renal Dysfunction:** Decrease initial dose and titrate slowly.	**BB:** ACE inhibitors can cause death/injury to developing fetus during 2nd and 3rd trimesters. Stop therapy if pregnancy detected. **W/P:** D/C if jaundice or marked LFT elevation occurs. Risk of hyperkalemia with DM, renal dysfunction. Persistent nonproductive cough, anaphylactoid reactions, neutropenia with myeloid hypoplasia reported. Fetal/neonatal morbidity and death reported. Monitor for hypotension in high-risk patients (surgery/ anesthesia, dialysis, heart failure, volume/ salt depletion, etc). Caution with CHF, renal dysfunction, renal artery stenosis, collagen vascular disease (especially with renal dysfunction). Monitor WBC before therapy, then every 2 weeks for 3 months, then periodically. Less effective on BP in blacks	Proteinuria, rash, hypotension, dysgeusia, cough, MI, CHF.

BB = black box warning; **W/P** = warnings/precautions; **Contra** = contraindications; **P/N** = pregnancy category rating and nursing considerations.

(Continued)

Prescribing Information for Antihypertensive Agents

GENERIC (BRAND)	FORM/ STRENGTH	DOSAGE	WARNINGS/PRECAUTIONS & CONTRAINDICATIONS	ADVERSE REACTIONS
Captopril (Capoten) *(Cont.)*			and more reports of angioedema than nonblacks. **Contra:** History of ACE inhibitor associated angioedema. **P/N:** Category C (1st trimester) and D (2nd and 3rd trimesters), not for use in nursing.	
Enalapril maleate (Vasotec)	**Tab:** 2.5mg*, 5mg*, 10mg, 20mg *scored	**Adults: HTN:** If possible, d/c diuretic 2-3 days prior to therapy. Initial: 5mg qd, 2.5mg qd with concomitant diuretic. Usual: 10-40mg/day given qd or bid. Resume diuretic if BP not controlled. CrCl ≤30mL/min: Initial: 2.5mg/day. **Dialysis:** 2.5mg/day on dialysis days. **Heart Failure:** Initial: 2.5mg/day. Usual: 2.5-20mg given bid. Max: 40mg/day. **Left Ventricular Dysfunction:** Initial: 2.5mg bid. Titrate: Increase to 20mg/ day. **Hyponatremia or SrCr 1.6mg/dL with Heart Failure:** Initial: 2.5mg qd. Titrate: Increase to 2.5mg bid, then 5mg bid. Max: 40mg/day. **Pediatrics: HTN: 1 month-16 yrs:** Initial: 0.08mg/kg (up to 5mg) qd. Titrate: Adjust according to response. Max: 0.58mg/kg/dose (or 40mg/dose). Avoid if GFR <30mL/min/ 1.73m2. (To prepare 200mL of 1mg/mL sus: Add 50mL of Bicitra®; to polyethylene terephthalate bottle with ten 20mg tabs and shake for at least 2 min. Let stand for 60 min, then shake again for 1 min. Add 150mL of Ora-Sweet SF™; and shake, then refrigerate. Can store up to 30 days.)	**BB:** ACE inhibitors can cause death/injury to developing fetus during 2nd and 3rd trimesters. Stop therapy if pregnancy detected. **W/P:** D/C if angioedema, jaundice, or if marked LFT elevation occurs. Risk of hyperkalemia with DM, renal dysfunction. Persistent nonproductive cough reported. Monitor WBCs in renal or collagen vascular disease. Anaphylactoid reactions reported. Fetal/neonatal morbidity and death reported. Monitor for hypotension in high-risk patients (heart failure, surgery/ anesthesia, hyponatremia, high-dose diuretic therapy, severe volume and/or salt depletion, etc). Caution with CHF, obstruction to left ventricle outflow tract, renal dysfunction, and renal artery stenosis. Less effective on BP in blacks and more reports of angioedema than nonblacks. Intestinal angioedema reported. **Contra:** History of ACE inhibitor associated angioedema and hereditary or idiopathic angioedema. **P/N:** Category C (1st trimester) and D (2nd and 3rd trimesters), not for use in nursing.	Fatigue, orthostatic effects, asthenia, diarrhea, nausea, headache, dizziness, cough, rash, hypotension, vomiting.
Enalaprilat (Vasotec I.V.)	**Inj:** 1.25mg/mL	**Adults:** Administer IV over 5 min. Usual: 1.25mg q6h for no longer than 48 hrs. Max: 20mg/day. **Concomitant Diuretic/ CrCl ≤30mL/min:** Initial: 0.625mg, may repeat after 1 hr. Maint: 1.25mg q6h. **Risk of Excessive Hypotension:** Initial: 0.625mg over 5 min to 1 hr. **PO/IV Conversion:** Give 5mg/day PO for 1.25mg IV q6h and 2.5mg/day PO for 0.625mg q6h IV.	**BB:** ACE inhibitors can cause death/injury to developing fetus during 2nd and 3rd trimesters. Stop therapy if pregnancy detected. **W/P:** D/C if angioedema, jaundice, or if marked LFT elevation occurs. Risk of hyperkalemia with DM, renal dysfunction. Persistent nonproductive cough reported. Monitor WBCs in renal or collagen vascular disease. Anaphylactoid reactions reported. Fetal/neonatal morbidity and death reported. Monitor for hypotension in high risk patients (heart failure, surgery/ anesthesia, hyponatremia, high dose diuretic therapy, severe volume and/or salt depletion, etc). Caution with CHF, obstruction to left ventricle outflow tract, renal dysfunction, and renal artery stenosis. Less effective on BP in blacks and more reports of angioedema than nonblacks. **Contra:** History of ACE inhibitor associated angioedema and hereditary or idiopathic angioedema. **P/N:** Category C (1st trimester) and D (2nd and 3rd trimesters), not for use in nursing.	Hypotension, headache, angioedema, myocardial infarction, fatigue, dizziness, fever, rash, constipation, cough.
Fosinopril sodium (Monopril)	**Tab:** 10mg*, 20mg, 40mg *scored	**Adults:** If possible, d/c diuretic 2-3 days before therapy. Initial: 10mg qd, monitor carefully if cannot d/c diuretic. Maint: 20-40mg/day. Resume diuretic if BP not controlled. Max: 80mg/day. **Heart Failure:** Initial: 10mg qd, 5mg with moderate to severe renal failure or vigorous diuresis. Titrate: Increase over several weeks. Maint: 20-40mg qd. Max: 40mg qd. **Elderly:** Start at low end of dosing range.	**BB:** ACE inhibitors can cause death/injury to developing fetus during 2nd and 3rd trimesters. Stop therapy if pregnancy detected. **W/P:** D/C if angioedema, jaundice, or if marked LFT elevation occur. Risk of hyperkalemia with DM, renal dysfunction. Persistent non-productive cough reported. Monitor WBCs in renal and collagen vascular disease. Anaphylactoid reactions reported. Fetal/neonatal morbidity and death reported. Monitor for hypotension in high-risk patients (heart failure, volume and/or salt depletion, surgery/anesthesia, etc). Less effective on BP in blacks and	Dizziness, cough, hypotension, musculoskeletal pain.

BB = black box warning; **W/P** = warnings/precautions; **Contra** = contraindications; **P/N** = pregnancy category rating and nursing considerations.

Prescribing Information for Antihypertensive Agents

GENERIC (BRAND)	FORM/ STRENGTH	DOSAGE	WARNINGS/PRECAUTIONS & CONTRAINDICATIONS	ADVERSE REACTIONS
ANGIOTENSIN CONVERTING ENZYME (ACE) INHIBITORS *(cont.)*				
Fosinopril sodium (Monopril) *(Cont.)*			more reports of angioedema than nonblacks. Caution with CHF, renal or hepatic dysfunction, renal artery stenosis. May cause false low measurement of serum digoxin level. **Contra:** History of ACE inhibitor associated angioedema. **P/N:** Category C (1st trimester) and D (2nd and 3rd trimesters), not for use in nursing.	
Lisinopril (Prinivil)	**Tab:** 5mg*, 10mg*, 20mg* *scored	***Adults: HTN:*** If possible, d/c diuretic 2-3 days prior to therapy. Initial: 10mg qd; 5mg qd with diuretic. Usual: 20-40mg qd. Resume diuretic if BP not controlled. Max: 80mg/day. **CrCl 10-30mL/min:** Initial: 5mg/day. Max: 40mg/day. **CrCl <10mL/ min:** Initial: 2.5mg/day. Max: 40mg/day. **Heart Failure:** Initial: 5mg qd. Usual: 5-20mg qd. **Hyponatremia or CrCl ≤30mL/ min:** Initial: 2.5mg qd. AMI: Initial: 5mg within 24 hrs, then 5mg after 24 hrs, then 10mg after 48 hrs, then daily. Use 2.5mg during first 3 days with low systolic BP. Maint: 10mg qd for 6 weeks, 2.5-5mg with hypotension. D/C with prolonged hypotension. **Elderly:** Caution with dose adjustment. ***Pediatrics:*** **≥6 yrs: HTN:** Initial: 0.07mg/kg qd (up to 5mg total). Adjust dose based on BP response. Max: 0.61mg/kg qd (40mg/day).	**BB:** ACE inhibitors can cause death/injury to developing fetus during 2nd and 3rd trimesters. Stop therapy if pregnancy detected. **W/P:** Intestinal/head/neck occurs. angioedema reported. D/C if angioedema, jaundice, or if marked LFT elevation Risk of hyperkalemia with DM, renal dysfunction. Persistent nonproductive cough reported. Monitor WBCs in renal and collagen vascular disease. Anaphylactoid reactions reported. Fetal/neonatal morbidity and death reported. Monitor for hypotension in high-risk patients (eg, heart failure with systolic BP <100mmHg, surgery/anesthesia, hyponatremia, high dose diuretic therapy, severe volume and/or salt depletion). Caution with renal artery stenosis, CHF, renal dysfunction, or if obstruction to left ventricle outflow tract. Less effective on BP in blacks and more reports of angioedema than nonblacks. Caution in hypoglycemia and leukopenia/neutropenia. Patients should report any indication of infection which may be sign of leukopenia/ neutropenia. **Contra:** History of ACE inhibitor-associated angioedema and hereditary or idiopathic angioedema. **P/N:** Category C (1st trimester) and D (2nd and 3rd trimesters), not for use in nursing.	Hypotension, diarrhea, headache, dizziness, cough, chest pain.
Lisinopril (Zestril)	**Tab:** 2.5mg, 5mg, 10mg, 20mg, 30mg, 40mg	***Adults: HTN:*** If possible, d/c diuretic 2-3 days prior to therapy. Initial: 10mg qd, 5mg qd with diuretic. Usual: 20-40mg qd. Resume diuretic if BP not controlled. Max: 80mg/day. **CrCl 10-30mL/min:** Initial: 5mg/day. Max: 40mg/day. CrCl <10mL/min: Initial: 2.5mg/day. Max: 40mg/ day. **Heart Failure:** Initial: 5mg qd. Usual: 5-40mg qd. May increase by 10mg every 2 weeks. Max: 40mg/day. **Hyponatremia or CrCl ≤30mL/min:** Initial: 2.5mg qd. AMI: Initial: 5mg within 24 hrs, then 5mg after 24 hrs, then 10mg after 48 hrs, then 10mg qd. Use 2.5mg during first 3 days with low SBP. Maint: 10mg qd for 6 weeks, 2.5-5mg with hypotension. D/C with prolonged hypotension. **Elderly:** Caution with dose adjustment. ***Pediatrics:*** **≥6 yrs: HTN:** Initial: 0.07mg/kg qd up to 5mg total. Dose adjust according to response. Max: 0.61mg/kg or 40mg.	**BB:** ACE inhibitors can cause death/injury to developing fetus during 2nd and 3rd trimesters. D/C if pregnancy is detected. **W/P:** D/C if angioedema, jaundice, or marked LFT elevation occur. Risk of hyperkalemia, hypoglycemia with DM, renal dysfunction. Persistent nonproductive cough reported. Monitor WBCs in renal and collagen vascular disease. Anaphylactoid reactions during membrane exposure reported. Fetal/neonatal morbidity and death reported. Monitor for hypotension in high-risk patients (heart failure with SBP <100mmHg, surgery/anesthesia, hyponatremia, high-dose diuretic therapy, severe volume and/or salt depletion, etc). Caution with CHF, aortic stenosis/ hypertrophic cardiomyopathy, renal dysfunction, and renal artery stenosis. Less effective on BP in blacks and more reports of angioedema than nonblacks. **Contra:** History of ACE inhibitor-associated angioedema, hereditary or idiopathic angioedema. **P/N:** Category C (1st trimester) and D (2nd and 3rd trimesters), not for use in nursing.	Hypotension, diarrhea, headache, dizziness, hyperkalemia, chest pain, cough, cutaneous pseudolymphoma.

BB = black box warning; W/P = warnings/precautions; **Contra** = contraindications; P/N = pregnancy category rating and nursing considerations.

(Continued)

Prescribing Information for Antihypertensive Agents

GENERIC (BRAND)	FORM/ STRENGTH	DOSAGE	WARNINGS/PRECAUTIONS & CONTRAINDICATIONS	ADVERSE REACTIONS
Moexipril HCl (Univasc)	**Tab:** 7.5mg*, 15mg* *scored	***Adults:*** If possible, d/c diuretic 2-3 days prior to therapy. Take 1 hr before meals. Initial: 7.5mg qd, 3.75mg with concomitant diuretic therapy. Maint: 7.5-30mg/day given qd-bid. Resume diuretic if BP not controlled. Max: 60mg/day. **CrCl ≤40mL/min:** Initial: 3.75mg qd. Max: 15mg/day.	**BB:** ACE inhibitors can cause death/injury to developing fetus during 2nd and 3rd trimesters. Stop therapy if pregnancy detected. **W/P:** D/C if angioedema, jaundice, or if marked LFT elevation occurs. Intestinal angioedema reported. Risk of hyperkalemia with DM, renal dysfunction. Persistent nonproductive cough reported. Monitor WBCs in renal and collagen vascular disease. Anaphylactoid reactions reported. Fetal/ neonatal morbidity and death reported. Monitor for hypotension in high risk patients (heart failure, surgery/anesthesia, prolonged diuretic therapy, volume and/or salt depletion, etc.). Caution with CHF, renal dysfunction, and renal artery stenosis. Less effective on BP in blacks and more reports of angioedema than nonblacks. **Contra:** History of ACE inhibitor-associated angioedema. **P/N:** Category C (1st trimester) and D (2nd and 3rd trimesters), not for use in nursing.	Cough, dizziness, diarrhea, flu syndrome, fatigue, pharyngitis, flushing, rash, myalgia.
Perindopril erbumine (Aceon)	**Tab:** 2mg*, 4mg*, 8mg* *scored	***Adults:* HTN:** If possible, d/c diuretic 2-3 days prior to therapy. Initial: 4mg qd; 2-4mg/day given qd-bid with concomitant diuretic. Maint: 4-8mg/day given qd-bid. Resume diuretic if BP not controlled. Max: 16mg/day. **Elderly (>65 yrs):** Initial: 4mg/ day given qd-bid. Max (usual): 8mg/day. **Renal Impairment: CrCl >30mL/min:** Initial: 2mg/day. Max: 8mg/day. **CAD:** Initial: 4mg qd for 2 weeks. Maint: 8mg qd. **Elderly (>70 yrs):** Initial: 2mg qd for 1 week. Titrate: 4mg qd for Week 2. Maint: 8mg qd.	**BB:** ACE inhibitors can cause death/injury to developing fetus during 2nd and 3rd trimesters. Stop therapy if pregnancy detected. **W/P:** D/C if angioedema, jaundice, or if marked LFT elevation occurs. Risk of hyperkalemia with DM, renal dysfunction. Persistent nonproductive cough reported. Monitor WBCs in renal and collagen vascular disease. Anaphylactoid reactions reported. Fetal/neonatal morbidity and death reported. Monitor for hypotension in high-risk patients (heart failure, surgery/ anesthesia, hyponatremia, prolonged diuretic therapy, or volume and/or salt depletion). Caution with CHF, renal dysfunction, and renal artery stenosis. Less effective on BP in blacks and more reports of angioedema than nonblacks. Avoid if CrCl <30mL/min. **Contra:** History of ACE inhibitor-associated angioedema. **P/N:** Category C (1st trimester) and D (2nd and 3rd trimesters), caution in nursing.	Cough, headache, asthenia, dizziness, diarrhea, edema, respiratory infection, lower extremity pain.
Quinapril HCl (Accupril)	**Tab:** 5mg*, 10mg, 20mg, 40mg *scored	***Adults:* HTN:** If possible, d/c diuretic 2-3 days prior to therapy. Initial: 10-20mg qd; 5mg qd with concomitant diuretic. Titrate at intervals of at least 2 weeks. Usual: 20-80mg/day given qd-bid. **CrCl >60mL/min:** Initial: 10mg/day. **CrCl 30-60mL/min:** Initial: 5mg/day. **CrCl 10-30mL/min:** Initial: 2.5mg/day. **Heart Failure:** Initial: 5mg bid. Titrate at weekly intervals. Usual: 10-20mg bid. **CrCl >30mL/min:** Initial: 5mg/day. **CrCl 10-30mL/min:** Initial: 2.5mg/day.	**BB:** ACE inhibitors can cause death/injury to developing fetus during 2nd and 3rd trimesters. Stop therapy if pregnancy detected. **W/P:** D/C if angioedema, jaundice, or if marked LFT elevation occurs. Risk of hyperkalemia with DM, renal dysfunction. Persistent nonproductive cough reported. Monitor WBCs in renal or collagen vascular disease. Anaphylactoid reactions reported. Fetal/neonatal morbidity and death reported. Monitor for hypotension in high risk patients (heart failure, surgery/anesthesia, hyponatremia, high-dose diuretic therapy, recent intensive diuresis, dialysis, or severe volume and/or salt depletion, etc). Caution with CHF, renal dysfunction, and renal artery stenosis. Less effective on BP in blacks and more reports of angioedema than nonblacks. **Contra:** History of ACE inhibitor-associated angioedema. **P/N:** Category C (1st trimester) and D (2nd and 3rd trimesters), not for use in nursing.	Fatigue, headache, dizziness, cough, nausea, vomiting, hypotension, chest pain.

BB = black box warning; **W/P** = warnings/precautions; **Contra** = contraindications; **P/N** = pregnancy category rating and nursing considerations.

Prescribing Information for Antihypertensive Agents

GENERIC (BRAND)	FORM/ STRENGTH	DOSAGE	WARNINGS/PRECAUTIONS & CONTRAINDICATIONS	ADVERSE REACTIONS
ANGIOTENSIN CONVERTING ENZYME (ACE) INHIBITORS *(Cont.)*				
Ramipril (Altace)	Cap: 1.25mg, 2.5mg, 5mg, 10mg	**Adults: HTN:** Initial: 2.5mg qd. Maint: 2.5-20mg/day given qd or bid. Add diuretic if BP not controlled. **CrCl <40mL/ min:** Initial: 1.25mg qd. Titrate/Max: 5mg/ day. **CHF Post-MI:** Initial: 2.5mg bid, 1.25mg bid if hypotensive. Titrate: Increase to 5mg bid. **CrCl <40mL/min:** Initial: 1.25mg qd. Titrate: May increase to 1.25mg bid. Max: 2.5mg bid. **Risk Reduction of MI, Stroke, Death (≥55 yrs):** Initial: 2.5mg qd for 1 week. Increase to 5mg qd for next 3 weeks. Maint: 10mg qd. Reduce or d/c diuretic if possible. **With Volume Depletion/Renal Artery Stenosis:** Initial: 1.25mg qd.	**BB:** ACE inhibitors can cause death/injury to developing fetus during 2nd and 3rd trimesters. Stop therapy if pregnancy detected. **W/P:** D/C if angioedema, jaundice, or if marked LFT elevation occurs. Risk of hyperkalemia with DM, renal dysfunction. Persistent nonproductive cough and anaphylactoid reactions reported. Monitor WBCs in renal and collagen vascular disease. Fetal/neonatal morbidity and death reported. Monitor for hypotension in high-risk patients (heart failure, surgery/anesthesia, hyponatremia, high dose diuretic therapy, recent intensive diuresis, dialysis, or severe volume and/or salt depletion, etc). Caution with CHF, renal dysfunction, severe liver cirrhosis and/or ascites, and renal artery stenosis. Less effective on BP in blacks and more reports of angioedema than nonblacks. May reduce RBCs, Hgb, WBCs or platelets. May cause agranulocytosis, pancytopenia, and bone marrow depression. **Contra:** History of ACE inhibitor-associated angioedema. **P/N:** Category C (1st trimester) and D (2nd and 3rd trimesters), not for use in nursing.	Hypotension, cough, dizziness, fatigue, angina, impotence, Stevens-Johnson syndrome.
Trandolapril (Mavik)	Tab: 1mg*, 2mg, 4mg *scored	**Adults: HTN:** If possible, d/c diuretic 2-3 days before therapy. Initial: 1mg qd in nonblack patients; 2mg qd in black patients; 0.5mg with concomitant diuretic. Titrate: Adjust at 1-week intervals. Usual: 2-4mg qd. Resume diuretic if not controlled. Max: 8mg/day. **Post-MI:** Initial: 1mg qd. Titrate: Increase to target dose of 4mg qd as tolerated. **CrCl <30mL/min/Hepatic Cirrhosis for HTN or Post-MI:** Initial: 0.5mg qd.	**BB:** ACE inhibitors can cause death/injury to developing fetus during 2nd and 3rd trimesters. Stop therapy if pregnancy detected. **W/P:** D/C if angioedema or jaundice occurs. Risk of hyperkalemia with DM, renal dysfunction. Persistent nonproductive cough reported. Monitor WBCs in renal impairment and/or collagen vascular disease. Anaphylactoid reactions reported. Fetal/neonatal morbidity and death reported. Monitor for hypotension in high-risk patients (heart failure, surgery/anesthesia, prolonged diuretic therapy, volume and/or salt depletion, etc). Caution with CHF, renal dysfunction, and renal artery stenosis. More reports of angioedema in blacks than nonblacks. **Contra:** History of ACE inhibitor-associated angioedema. **P/N:** Category C (1st trimester) and D (2nd and 3rd trimesters), not for use in nursing.	Cough, dizziness, hypotension, elevated asthenia, syncope, elevated BUN, elevated creatinine, myalgia, gastritis, hypocalcemia, hyperkalemia, dyspepsia.
ACE INHIBITOR COMBINATIONS				
Benazepril HCl/ Hydrochloro- thiazide (Lotensin HCT)	Tab: (Benazepril-HCTZ) 5mg-6.25mg*, 10mg-12.5mg*, 20mg-12.5mg*, 20mg-25mg* *scored	**Adults:** Initial (if not controlled on benazepril monotherapy): 10mg-12.5mg or 20mg-12.5mg. Titrate: May increase after 2-3 weeks. **Initial (if controlled on 25mg HCTZ/day with hypokalemia):** 5mg-6.25mg. **Replacement Therapy:** Substitute combination for titrated components.	**BB:** When used in pregnancy, ACE inhibitors can cause injury and even death to the developing fetus. D/C therapy when pregnancy detected. **W/P:** Avoid if CrCl ≤30mL/min/1.73m². D/C if angioedema, jaundice, or marked LFT elevation occur. Risk of hyperkalemia with DM, renal dysfunction. May cause persistent nonproductive cough, hypokalemia, hyperuricemia, hypomagnesemia, hypercalcemia, hypophosphatemia. Monitor WBCs in renal and collagen vascular disease. Anaphylactoid reactions reported. Fetal/ neonatal morbidity and death reported. Monitor for hypotension in high risk patients (eg, surgery/anesthesia, prolonged diuretic therapy, heart failure, volume and/or salt depletion, etc). Caution with	Cough, dizziness/postural dizziness, headache, fatigue.

BB = black box warning; W/P = warnings/precautions; **Contra** = contraindications; **P/N** = pregnancy category rating and nursing considerations.

(Continued)

Prescribing Information for Antihypertensive Agents

GENERIC (BRAND)	FORM/ STRENGTH	DOSAGE	WARNINGS/PRECAUTIONS & CONTRAINDICATIONS	ADVERSE REACTIONS
Benazepril HCl/ Hydrochloro- thiazide (Lotensin HCT) *(Cont.)*			CHF, renal dysfunction, and renal artery stenosis. More reports of angioedema in blacks than nonblacks. Monitor for fluid/ electrolyte imbalance. May increase cholesterol and TG levels. May exacerbate/ activate SLE. **Contra:** Anuria, sulfonamide hypersensitivity. **P/N:** Category D, not for use in nursing.	
Captopril/ Hydrochloro- thiazide (Capozide)	**Tab:** (Captopril- HCTZ) 25mg-15mg*, 25mg-25mg*, 50mg-15mg*, 50mg-25mg* *scored	***Adults:*** Initial: 25mg-15mg tab qd. Titrate: Adjust dose at 6-week intervals. Max: 150mg captopril/50mg HCTZ per day. **Replacement Therapy:** Substitute combination for titrated components. **Renal Impairment:** Decrease dose or increase interval. Take 1 hr before meals.	**BB:** ACE inhibitors can cause death/injury to developing fetus during 2nd and 3rd trimesters. Stop therapy if pregnancy detected. **W/P:** D/C if angioedema, jaundice, or if marked LFT elevation occurs. Risk of hyperkalemia with DM, renal dysfunction. Monitor WBCs in renal and collagen vascular disease. Fetal/neonatal morbidity and death reported. Monitor for hypotension in high-risk patients (eg, surgery/anesthesia, volume/salt depletion). Caution with renal or hepatic dysfunction. More reports of angioedema in blacks than nonblacks. May exacerbate or activate systemic lupus erythematosus. Monitor electrolytes. Hypercalcemia, hypomagnesemia, hyperuricemia may occur. With renal impairment, monitor WBCs and differential before therapy, every 2 weeks for 3 months, then periodically. Neutropenia with myeloid hypoplasia, persistent nonproductive cough, anaphylactoid reactions, proteinuria reported. **Contra:** History of ACE inhibitor-associated angioedema, anuria, sulfonamide hypersensitivity. **P/N:** Category C (1st trimester) and D (2nd and 3rd trimesters), not for use in nursing.	Cough, hypotension, rash, pruritus, fever, arthralgia, eosinophilia, dysgeusia, neutropenia/thrombo-cytopenia.
Enalapril maleate/ Hydrochloro- thiazide (Vaseretic)	**Tab:** (Enalapril-HCTZ) 5mg-12.5mg, 10mg-25mg	***Adults:*** **Initial (if not controlled with enalapril/HCTZ monotherapy):** 5mg-12.5mg tab or 10mg-25mg tab qd. Titrate: May increase after 2-3 weeks. Max: 20mg enalapril/50mg HCTZ per day. **Replacement Therapy:** Substitute combination for titrated components.	**BB:** ACE inhibitors can cause death/injury to developing fetus during 2nd and 3rd trimesters. Stop therapy if pregnancy detected. **W/P:** D/C if angioedema, jaundice, or if marked LFT elevation occurs. Risk of hyperkalemia with DM, renal dysfunction. Persistent nonproductive cough reported. Monitor WBCs in renal and collagen vascular disease. Anaphylactoid reactions reported. Fetal/ neonatal morbidity and death reported. Monitor for hypotension in high-risk patients (surgery/anesthesia, hyponatremia, severe volume/salt depletion, etc). Caution with CHF, renal or hepatic dysfunction, obstruction to left ventricle outflow tract, elderly, renal artery stenosis. More reports of angioedema in blacks than nonblacks. May exacerbate or activate SLE. Monitor serum electrolytes. Avoid if CrCl ≤30mL/ min/1.73m². May increase cholesterol, TG, uric acid levels, and blood glucose. Intestinal angioedema reported. **Contra:** History of ACE inhibitor-associated angioedema and hereditary or idiopathic angioedema. Anuria, sulfonamide hypersensitivity. **P/N:** Category C (1st trimester) and D (2nd and 3rd trimesters), not for use in nursing.	Dizziness, cough, fatigue, orthostatic effects, diarrhea, nausea, muscle cramps, asthenia, impotence.

BB = black box warning; W/P = warnings/precautions; **Contra** = contraindications; P/N = pregnancy category rating and nursing considerations.

Prescribing Information for Antihypertensive Agents

GENERIC (BRAND)	FORM/ STRENGTH	DOSAGE	WARNINGS/PRECAUTIONS & CONTRAINDICATIONS	ADVERSE REACTIONS
ACE INHIBITOR COMBINATIONS *(Cont.)*				
Fosinopril sodium/ Hydrochloro-thiazide (Monopril HCT)	**Tab:** (Fosinopril-HCTZ) 10mg-12.5mg, 20mg-12.5mg	***Adults:* Initial (if not controlled with fosinopril/HCTZ monotherapy):** 12.5mg-10mg tab or 12.5mg-20mg tab qd.	**BB:** ACE inhibitors can cause death/injury to developing fetus during 2nd and 3rd trimesters. Stop therapy if pregnancy detected. **W/P:** D/C if angioedema, jaundice or marked LFT elevation occurs. Risk of hyperkalemia with DM, renal dysfunction. Persistent nonproductive cough reported. Monitor WBCs in renal and collagen vascular disease. Anaphylactoid reactions reported. Fetal/neonatal morbidity and death reported. Monitor for hypotension in high-risk patients (eg, surgery/anesthesia, volume/salt depletion). Caution with CHF, renal or hepatic dysfunction. More reports of angioedema in blacks than nonblacks. May exacerbate or activate SLE. Monitor electrolytes. Avoid if CrCl ≤30mL/min/1.73m². May increase cholesterol, TG. Hypercalcemia, hypomagnesemia, hyperuricemia may occur. **Contra:** Anuria, sulfonamide hypersensitivity. **P/N:** Category C (1st trimester) and D (2nd and 3rd trimesters), not for use in nursing.	Headache, cough, fatigue, dizziness, upper respiratory infection, musculoskeletal pain.
Lisinopril/ Hydrochloro-thiazide (Prinzide, Zestoretic)	**Tab:** (Lisinopril-HCTZ) 10mg-12.5mg, 20mg-12.5mg, 20mg-25mg	***Adults:* Initial (If Not Controlled with Lisinopril/HCTZ monotherapy):** 10mg-12.5mg tab or 20mg-12.5mg tab daily. Titrate: May increase after 2-3 weeks. **Initial (If Controlled on 25mg HCTZ/Day with Hypokalemia):** 10mg-12.5mg tab. Replacement Therapy: Substitute combination for titrated components.	**BB:** ACE inhibitors can cause death/injury to developing fetus during 2nd and 3rd trimesters. Stop therapy if pregnancy detected. **W/P:** D/C if angioedema, jaundice, or marked LFT elevation occur. Risk of hyperkalemia with DM, renal dysfunction. Persistent nonproductive cough reported. Monitor WBCs in renal and collagen vascular disease. Anaphylactoid reactions during membrane exposure reported. Fetal/neonatal morbidity and death reported. Monitor for hypotension in high-risk patients (eg, surgery/anesthesia, volume/salt depletion). Caution with CHF, renal or hepatic dysfunction. More reports of angioedema in blacks than nonblacks. May exacerbate or activate SLE. Monitor electrolytes. Avoid if CrCl ≤30mL/min/1.7m². May increase cholesterol, TG. Hypercalcemia, hypomagnesemia, hyperuricemia may occur. Caution with left ventricle outflow obstruction. **Contra:** History of ACE inhibitor-associated angioedema, hereditary or idiopathic angioedema, anuria, sulfonamide hypersensitivity. **P/N:** Category C (1st trimester) and D (2nd and 3rd trimesters), not for use in nursing.	Dizziness, headache, cough, fatigue, orthostatic effects, diarrhea, nausea, muscle cramps, angioedema, cutaneous pseudolymphoma.
Moexipril HCl/ Hydrochloro-thiazide (Uniretic)	**Tab:** (Moexipril-HCTZ) 7.5mg-12.5mg*, 15mg-12.5mg*, 15mg-25mg* *scored	***Adults:* Initial (if not controlled on moexipril/HCTZ monotherapy):** Switch to 7.5mg-12.5mg tab, 15mg-12.5mg tab, or 15mg-25mg tab qd. Titrate: May increase after 2-3 weeks. **Initial (if controlled on 25mg HCTZ/day with hypokalemia):** 3.75mg-6.25mg (1/2 of 7.5mg-12.5mg tab). If excessive reduction with 7.5mg-12.5mg tab, may switch to 3.75mg-6.25mg. **Replacement Therapy:** Substitute combination for titrated components. Take 1 hr before meals.	**BB:** ACE inhibitors can cause death/injury to developing fetus during 2nd and 3rd trimesters. Stop therapy if pregnancy detected. **W/P:** D/C if angioedema, jaundice, or if marked LFT elevation occurs. Intestinal angioedema reported. Risk of hyperkalemia with DM, renal dysfunction. Persistent nonproductive cough reported. Monitor WBCs in renal and collagen vascular disease. Anaphylactoid reactions reported. Fetal/neonatal morbidity and death reported. Monitor for hypotension in high-risk patients (eg, surgery/anesthesia, volume/salt depletion). Caution in elderly, CHF, renal or hepatic dysfunction. More reports of angioedema in blacks than nonblacks. May exacerbate or activate SLE. Monitor	Cough, dizziness, fatigue.

BB = black box warning; **W/P** = warnings/precautions; **Contra** = contraindications; **P/N** = pregnancy category rating and nursing considerations.

(Continued)

Prescribing Information for Antihypertensive Agents

GENERIC (BRAND)	FORM/ STRENGTH	DOSAGE	WARNINGS/PRECAUTIONS & CONTRAINDICATIONS	ADVERSE REACTIONS
Moexipril HCl/ Hydrochloro- thiazide (Uniretic) (Cont.)			electrolytes. Avoid if CrCl ≤40mL/min/ 1.73m². May increase cholesterol, TG. Hypercalcemia, hypomagnesemia, hyperuricemia may occur. **Contra:** History of ACE inhibitor-associated angioedema, anuria, sulfonamide hypersensitivity. **P/N:** Category C (1st trimester) and D (2nd and 3rd trimesters), not for use in nursing.	
Quinapril HCl/ Hydrochloro- thiazide (Accuretic)	**Tab:** (Quinapril-HCTZ) 10mg-12.5mg*, 20mg-12.5mg*, 20mg-25mg* *scored	***Adults:*** **Initial (if not controlled on quinapril monotherapy):** 10mg-12.5mg or 20mg-12.5mg tab qd. Titrate: May increase after 2-3 weeks. **Initial (if controlled on HCTZ 25mg/day but significant K+ loss):** 10mg-12.5mg or 20mg-12.5mg tab qd. If previously treated with 20mg quinapril and 25mg HCTZ, may switch to 20mg-25mg tab qd.	**BB:** ACE inhibitors can cause death/injury to developing fetus during 2nd and 3rd trimesters. Stop therapy if pregnancy detected. **W/P:** D/C if angioedema, jaundice, or marked LFT elevation occurs. Risk of hyperkalemia with DM, renal dysfunction. Persistent nonproductive cough reported. Monitor WBCs in renal or collagen vascular disease. Anaphylactoid reactions reported. Fetal/neonatal morbidity and death reported. Monitor for hypotension in high-risk patients (heart failure, surgery/anesthesia, hyponatremia, severe volume/salt depletion, etc). Caution with CHF, renal or hepatic dysfunction, and renal artery stenosis. Less effective on BP in blacks and more reports of angioedema than nonblacks. May exacerbate or activate SLE. Monitor serum electrolytes. Avoid if CrCl ≤30mL/min/ 1.73m². May increase cholesterol, TG, and uric acid levels and decrease glucose tolerance. **Contra:** History of ACE inhibitor-associated angioedema, anuria, sulfonamide hypersensitivity. **P/N:** Category C (1st trimester) and D (2nd and 3rd trimesters), not for use in nursing.	Dizziness, headache, cough, myalgia.
ANGIOTENSIN RECEPTOR BLOCKERS (ARBs)				
Candesartan cilexetil (Atacand)	**Tab:** 4mg, 8mg, 16mg, 32mg	***Adults:*** **HTN: Monotherapy Without Volume Depletion:** Initial: 16mg qd. Usual: 8-32mg/day given qd-bid. May add diuretic if BP not controlled. **Intravascular Volume Depletion/Moderate Hepatic Impairment:** Lower initial dose. Initial: 4mg qd. Usual: 32mg qd. Titrate: Double dose every 2 weeks, as tolerated.	**BB:** Can cause death/injury to developing fetus during 2nd and 3rd trimesters. Stop therapy if pregnancy is detected. **W/P:** Can cause fetal injury/death. Correct volume or salt depletion before therapy or monitor closely. Changes in renal function may occur; caution with renal artery stenosis, CHF. Risk of hypotension; caution in major surgery and anesthesia, or when initiating therapy in heart failure. May cause hyperkalemia in heart failure patients; monitor serum potassium. **P/N:** Category C (1st trimester) and D (2nd and 3rd trimesters), not for use in nursing.	Back pain, dizziness, upper respiratory infection.
Eprosartan mesylate (Teveten)	**Tab:** 400mg, 600mg	***Adults:*** Initial: 600mg qd. Usual: 400-800mg/day, given qd-bid. **Moderate to Severe Renal Impairment:** Max: 600mg/day.	**BB:** Can cause death/injury to developing fetus during 2nd and 3rd trimesters. Stop therapy if pregnancy detected. **W/P:** Can cause fetal injury/death. Correct volume or salt depletion before therapy. Changes in renal function may occur; caution with renal artery stenosis, severe CHF. **P/N:** Category C (1st trimester) and D (2nd and 3rd trimesters), not for use in nursing.	Upper respiratory infection, rhinitis, pharyngitis, cough.
Irbesartan (Avapro)	**Tab:** 75mg, 150mg, 300mg	***Adults:*** **HTN:** Initial: 150mg qd. Titrate: May increase to 300mg qd. **Intravascular Volume/Salt Depletion:** Initial: 75mg qd. **Nephropathy:** Maint: 300mg qd. ***Pediatrics:*** **HTN:** ≥17 yrs: Initial: 150mg qd. Titrate: May increase to 300mg qd. **Intravascular Volume/Salt Depletion:** Initial: 75mg qd.	**BB:** Can cause death/injury to developing fetus during 2nd and 3rd trimesters. Stop therapy if pregnancy detected. **W/P:** Can cause fetal injury/death. Correct volume or salt depletion before therapy. Changes in renal function may occur; caution with renal artery stenosis, severe CHF. Angioedema reported. **P/N:** Category C (1st trimester) and D (2nd and 3rd trimesters), not for use in nursing.	Diarrhea, dyspepsia/ heartburn, musculoskeletal trauma, fatigue, upper respiratory infection.

BB = black box warning; **W/P** = warnings/precautions; **Contra** = contraindications; **P/N** = pregnancy category rating and nursing considerations.

Prescribing Information for Antihypertensive Agents

GENERIC (BRAND)	FORM/ STRENGTH	DOSAGE	WARNINGS/PRECAUTIONS & CONTRAINDICATIONS	ADVERSE REACTIONS
ANGIOTENSIN RECEPTOR BLOCKERS (ARBs) *(Cont.)*				
Losartan potassium (Cozaar)	**Tab:** 25mg, 50mg, 100mg	***Adults: HTN:*** Initial: 50mg qd. Usual: 25-100mg/day given qd-bid. **Intravascular Volume Depletion/Hepatic Impairment:** Initial: 25mg qd. **HTN with LVH:** Initial: 50mg qd. Add hydrochlorothiazide (HCTZ) 12.5mg qd and/or increase losartan to 100mg qd, followed by an increase in HCTZ to 25mg qd based on BP response. ***Nephropathy:*** Initial: 50 mg qd. Titrate: Increase to 100mg qd based on BP response. ***Pediatrics:*** ≥6 yrs: HTN: Initial: 0.7mg/kg qd (up to 50mg/day). Max: 1.4mg/kg/day (100mg/day).	**BB:** Can cause death/injury to developing fetus during 2nd and 3rd trimesters. Stop therapy if pregnancy detected. **W/P:** Can cause fetal injury/death. Correct volume or salt depletion before therapy. Changes in renal function may occur; caution with renal artery stenosis, severe CHF. Angioedema reported. Consider dose adjustment with hepatic dysfunction. **P/N:** Category C (1st trimester) and D (2nd and 3rd trimesters), not for use in nursing.	Dizziness, cough, upper respiratory infection, diarrhea.
Olmesartan medoxomil (Benicar)	**Tab:** 5mg, 20mg, 40mg	***Adults: Monotherapy Without Volume Depletion:*** Initial: 20mg qd. Titrate: May increase to 40mg qd after 2 weeks if needed. May add diuretic if BP not controlled. **Intravascular Volume Depletion** (eg, with diuretics, impaired renal function): Lower initial dose; monitor closely.	**BB:** Can cause death/injury to developing fetus during 2nd and 3rd trimesters. Stop therapy if pregnancy detected. **W/P:** Can cause fetal injury/death. Symptomatic hypotension may occur in volume- and/or salt-depleted patients; monitor closely. Changes in renal function may occur; caution with severe CHF. Increases in serum creatinine or BUN reported with renal artery stenosis. **P/N:** Category C (1st trimester) and D (2nd and 3rd trimesters), not for use in nursing.	Dizziness, transient hypotension, hyperkalemia.
Telmisartan (Micardis)	**Tab:** 20mg, 40mg*, 80mg* *scored	***Adults:*** Initial: 40mg qd. Usual: 20-80mg/day. May add diuretic if need additional BP reduction after 80mg/day.	**BB:** Can cause death/injury to developing fetus during 2nd and 3rd trimesters. Stop therapy if pregancy detected. **W/P:** Can cause fetal injury/death. Correct volume or salt depletion before therapy. Changes in renal function may occur; caution with renal artery stenosis, severe CHF. Closely monitor with biliary obstructive disorders or hepatic dysfunction. **P/N:** Category C (1st trimester) and D (2nd and 3rd trimesters), not for use in nursing.	Upper respiratory infection, back pain, sinusitis, diarrhea, bradycardia, eosinophilia, thrombocytopenia, increased uric acid, increased CPK, increased hepatic function/liver sweating, abnormal disorder, renal impairment failure, anemia, edema and cough.
Valsartan (Diovan)	**Tab:** 40mg*, 80mg, 160mg, 320mg *scored	***Adults: HTN: Monotherapy Without Volume Depletion:*** Initial: 80mg or 160mg qd. Titrate: May increase to 320mg qd or add diuretic (greater effect than increasing dose >80mg). **Hepatic/ Severe Renal Dysfunction:** Use with caution. **Heart Failure:** Initial: 40mg bid. Titrate: May increase to 80mg or 160mg bid (use highest dose tolerated). Max: 320mg/day in divided doses. **Post-MI:** Initial: 20mg bid. Titrate: May increase to 40mg bid within 7 days, with subsequent titrations up to 160mg bid. ***Pediatrics:*** 6-16 yrs: HTN: Initial: 1.3mg/kg qd (up to 40mg total). Adjust dose according to BP response. Max: 2.7mg/kg (up to 160mg) qd. Use of a sus recommended for children who cannot swallow tabs, or children for whom calculated dosage (mg/kg) does not correspond to available tab strengths. Adjust dose accordingly when switching dosage forms. **Hepatic/ Severe Renal Impairment:** Use with caution. Avoid use in pediatrics with GFR <30mL/min/1.73m².	**BB:** When used in pregnancy, drugs that act directly on the renin-angiotensin system can cause injury and even death to the developing fetus. D/C therapy when pregnancy is detected. **W/P:** Changes in renal function may occur; caution with renal artery stenosis, severe CHF. Caution with hepatic dysfunction, renal dysfunction, and obstructive biliary disorder. Risk of hypotension; caution when initiating therapy in heart failure or post-MI. Correct volume or salt depletion before therapy. Avoid use in pediatric patients with GFR <30mL/min/1.73m². May cause fetal harm when administered to pregnant women. **P/N:** Category D, not for use in nursing.	(HTN) Headache, dizziness, viral infection, fatigue, abdominal pain. (Heart Failure) dizziness, hypotension, diarrhea, arthralgia, fatigue, back pain, hyperkalemia. (Post-MI) hypotension, cough, increased blood creatinine.

BB = black box warning; **W/P** = warnings/precautions; **P/N** = pregnancy category rating and nursing considerations.

(Continued)

Prescribing Information for Antihypertensive Agents

GENERIC (BRAND)	FORM/ STRENGTH	DOSAGE	WARNINGS/PRECAUTIONS & CONTRAINDICATIONS	ADVERSE REACTIONS
ARBs COMBINATIONS				
Candesartan cilexetil/ Hydrochloro- thiazide (Atacand HCT)	**Tab:** (Candesartan-HCTZ) 16mg-12.5mg, 32mg-12.5mg	***Adults:*** Initial: If BP not controlled on HCTZ 25mg/day or controlled but serum K+ decreased: 16mg-12.5mg tab qd. If BP not controlled on 32mg candesartan/ day, give 32mg-12.5mg qd; may increase to 32mg-25mg qd.	**BB:** Can cause death/injury to developing fetus during 2nd and 3rd trimesters. Stop therapy if pregnancy detected. **W/P:** Can cause fetal injury/death. Correct volume or salt depletion before therapy. Caution with hepatic or renal dysfunction, renal artery stenosis, severe CHF, history of allergies, and asthma. May exacerbate or activate SLE. Monitor serum electrolytes. Avoid if CrCl ≤30mL/min. Hyperuricemia, hyperglycemia, hypokalemia, hypomagnesemia, hypercalcemia may occur. Enhanced effects in post-sympathectomy patient. May increase cholesterol and triglyceride levels. Risk of hypotension; caution in major surgery or anesthesia. **Contra:** Anuria, sulfonamide hypersensitivity. **P/N:** Category C (1st trimester) and D (2nd and 3rd trimesters), not for use in nursing.	Upper respiratory infection, back pain, influenza-like symptoms, dizziness, headache.
Eprosartan mesylate/ Hydrochloro- thiazide (Teveten HCT)	**Tab:** (Eprosartan-HCTZ) 600mg-12.5mg, 600mg-25mg	***Adults:*** Usual (Not Volume Depleted): 600mg-12.5mg qd. Titrate: May increase to 600mg-25mg qd if needed. **Renal Impairment:** Max: 600mg/day (eprosartan).	**BB:** Can cause death/injury to developing fetus during 2nd and 3rd trimesters. Stop therapy if pregnancy detected. **W/P:** Hypersensitivity reactions reported. Fetal/neonatal morbidity and death reported. Monitor for hypotension in volume/salt depletion. Caution with CHF, renal or hepatic dysfunction. May exacerbate or activate SLE. Monitor electrolytes periodically. Hypercalcemia, hypomagnesemia, hyperuricemia, hyperglycemia may occur. Enhanced effects in post-sympathectomy patient. **Contra:** Anuria, sulfonamide hypersensitivity. **P/N:** Category C (1st trimester) and D (2nd and 3rd trimesters), not for use in nursing.	Dizziness, headache, back pain, fatigue, myalgia, upper respiratory tract infection, sinusitis, viral infection.
Irbesartan/ Hydrochloro- thiazide (Avalide)	**Tab:** (Irbesartan-HCTZ) 150mg-12.5mg, 300mg-12.5mg, 300mg-25mg	***Adults:*** **Not controlled on Monotherapy:** 150mg/12.5mg qd. Titrate: May increase to 300mg/12.5mg, then 300mg/25mg qd if needed. **Intial Therapy:** Initiate with 150mg/12.5mg qd for 1 to 2 weeks. Titrate: As needed to maximum 300mg/25mg qd. **Replacement Therapy:** May substitute for titrated components. **Elderly:** Start at low end of dosing range. Avoid with CrCl ≤30mL/min.	**BB:** Can cause death/injury to developing fetus during 2nd and 3rd trimesters. Stop therapy if pregnancy detected. **W/P:** Can cause fetal injury/death when administered to pregnant women. Correct volume or salt depletion before therapy. Caution with hepatic or renal dysfunction, renal artery stenosis, severe CHF, history of allergies, elderly, and asthma. May exacerbate or activate SLE. Monitor serum electrolytes. Avoid if CrCl ≤30mL/min. Hyperuricemia, hyperglycemia, hypokalemia, hypomagnes-emia, and hypercalcemia may occur. Enhanced effects in post-sympathectomy patient. May increase cholesterol and TG levels. Caution in elderly. **Contra:** Anuria, sulfonamide hypersensitivity. **P/N:** Category D, not for use in nursing.	Dizziness, fatigue, influenza, edema, nausea, vomiting, fever, chills, flushing, HTN, pruritus, sexual dysfunction, diarrhea, anxiety, vision disturbance, pancreatitis, aplastic anemia.
Losartan potassium/ Hydrochloro- thiazide (Hyzaar)	**Tab:** (Losartan-HCTZ) 50mg-12.5mg, 100mg-12.5mg, 100mg-25mg	***Adults:*** **HTN:** If BP uncontrolled on losartan monotherapy, HCTZ alone or controlled with HCTZ 25mg/day but hypokalemic: 50mg-12.5mg tab qd. Titrate/Max: If uncontrolled after 3 weeks, increase to 2 tabs of 50mg-12.5mg qd or 1 tab of 100mg-25mg qd. If uncontrolled on losartan 100mg monotherapy, may switch to 100mg-12.5mg qd. **Severe HTN:** Initial: 50mg-12.5mg qd. Titrate/Max: If inadequate response after 2-4 weeks, increase to 1 tab of 100mg-25mg qd.	**BB:** Can cause death/injury to developing fetus during 2nd and 3rd trimesters. D/C if pregnancy detected. **W/P:** Can cause fetal injury/death. Correct volume or salt depletion before therapy. Caution with hepatic or renal dysfunction, renal artery stenosis, severe CHF, history of allergies, asthma. May exacerbate or activate SLE. Monitor serum electrolytes. Avoid if CrCl ≤30mL/min. Observe for signs of fluid or electrolyte imbalance. May precipitate hyperuricemia or gout.	Dizziness, upper respiratory infection, back pain, cough.

BB = black box warning; **W/P** = warnings/precautions; **Contra** = contraindications; **P/N** = pregnancy category rating and nursing considerations.

Prescribing Information for Antihypertensive Agents

GENERIC (BRAND)	FORM/ STRENGTH	DOSAGE	WARNINGS/PRECAUTIONS & CONTRAINDICATIONS	ADVERSE REACTIONS
ARBs COMBINATIONS *(Cont.)*				
Losartan potassium/ Hydrochloro-thiazide (Hyzaar) *(Cont.)*		**HTN With Left Ventricular Hypertrophy:** Initial: Losartan 50mg qd. If BP reduction inadequate, add HCTZ 12.5mg or substitute losartan/HCTZ 50-12.5. If additional BP reduction is needed, losartan 100mg and HCTZ 12.5mg or losartan/HCTZ 100-12.5 may be substituted, followed by losartan 100mg and HCTZ 25mg or losartan/HCTZ 100-25.	Enhanced effects in post-sympathectomy patient. May increase cholesterol, TG levels. Angioedema reported. Not recommended with hepatic dysfunction requiring losartan titration. **Contra:** Anuria, sulfonamide hypersensitivity. **P/N:** Category C (1st trimester) and D (2nd and 3rd trimesters), not for use in nursing.	
Olmesartan medoxomil/ Hydrochloro-thiazide (Benicar HCT)	**Tab:** (Olmesartan-HCTZ) 20mg-12.5mg, 40mg-12.5mg, 40mg-25mg	***Adults:*** If BP not controlled with olmesartan alone: Add HCTZ 12.5mg qd. May titrate to 25mg qd if BP uncontrolled after 2-4 weeks. If BP not controlled with HCTZ alone: Add olmesartan 20mg qd. May titrate to 40mg qd if BP uncontrolled after 2-4 weeks. **Intravascular Volume Depletion** (eg, with diuretics, impaired renal function): Lower initial dose; monitor closely. **Elderly:** Start at lower end of dosing range.	**BB:** Can cause death/injury to developing fetus during 2nd and 3rd trimesters. Stop therapy if pregnancy detected. **W/P:** Can cause fetal injury/death. Correct volume or salt depletion before therapy or monitor closely. Caution with hepatic or severe renal dysfunction, progressive liver disease, history of allergies or asthma, renal artery stenosis, severe CHF. Avoid if CrCl ≤30mL/min. May exacerbate or activate SLE. Monitor serum electrolytes. Hyperuricemia, hyperglycemia, hypercalcemia, hypomagnesemia may occur. May increase cholesterol and triglyceride levels. **Contra:** Sulfonamide hypersensitivity. **P/N:** Category C (1st trimester) and D (2nd and 3rd trimesters), not for use in nursing.	Dizziness, upper respiratory tract infection, hyperuricemia, nausea, asthenia, angioedema, vomiting, hyperkalemia, rhabdomyolysis, ARF, alopecia, urticaria.
Telmisartan/ Hydrochloro-thiazide (Micardis HCT)	**Tab:** (HCTZ-Telmisartan) 12.5mg-40mg, 12.5mg-80mg, 25mg-80mg	***Adults:*** If BP not controlled on 80mg telmisartan, or 25mg HCTZ/day, or controlled on 25mg HCTZ/day but serum K+ decreased, 80mg-12.5mg tab qd. Titrate/Max: If uncontrolled after 2-4 weeks, increase to 160mg-25mg. **Biliary Obstruction/Hepatic Dysfunction:** Initial: 40mg-12.5mg tab qd; monitor closely.	**BB:** Can cause death/injury to developing fetus during 2nd and 3rd trimesters. Stop therapy if pregnancy detected. **W/P:** Can cause fetal injury/death. Correct volume or salt depletion before therapy. Caution with hepatic or renal dysfunction, biliary obstructive disorders, renal artery stenosis, severe CHF, history of allergies, and asthma. May exacerbate or activate SLE. Monitor serum electrolytes. Avoid if CrCl ≤30mL/min. Hyperuricemia, hyperglycemia, hypokalemia, hypomagnesemia, hypercalcemia may occur. Enhanced effects in post-sympathectomy patient. May increase cholesterol and triglyceride levels. **Contra:** Anuria, sulfonamide hypersensitivity. **P/N:** Category C (1st trimester) and D (2nd and 3rd trimesters), not for use in nursing.	Dizziness, fatigue, sinusitis, upper respiratory infection, diarrhea, bradycardia, eosinophilia, thrombocytopenia, uric acid increased, abnormal hepatic function/liver disorder, renal impairment including acute renal failure, anemia, and increased CPK.
Valsartan/ Hydrochloro-thiazide (Diovan HCT)	**Tab:** (Valsartan-HCTZ) 80mg-12.5mg, 160mg-12.5mg, 160mg-25mg, 320mg-12.5mg, 320mg-25mg	***Adults:* Initial: Uncontrolled on Valsartan Monotherapy:** Switch to 80mg-12.5mg, 160mg-12.5mg, or 320mg-12.5mg qd. May increase dose if uncontrolled after 3-4 weeks. Max: 320mg-25mg/day. **Uncontrolled on 25mg HCTZ/day or Controlled on 25mg HCTZ/day with Hypokalemia:** Switch to 80mg-12.5mg or 160mg-12.5mg qd. May titrate if uncontrolled after 3-4 weeks. Max: 320mg-25mg/day. **CrCl ≤30mL/min:** Use not recommended.	**BB:** When used in pregnancy, drugs that act directly on the renin-angiotensin system can cause injuryand even death to the developing fetus. D/C therapy when pregnancy is detected. **W/P:** Correct volume or salt depletion before therapy. Caution with hepatic or renal dysfunction, biliary obstructive disorders, renal artery stenosis, severe CHF, history of allergies, and asthma. May exacerbate or activate SLE. Monitor serum electrolytes. Avoid if CrCl ≤30mL/min. Hyperuricemia, hyperglycemia, hypokalemia, hypomagnesemia, hypercalcemia may occur. Enhanced effects in post-sympathectomy patient. May increase cholesterol and triglyceride levels. May cause fetal and neonatal morbidity and death when given to pregnant women. **Contra:** Anuria, sulfonamide hypersensitivity. **P/N:** Category C (1st trimester) and D (2nd and 3rd trimesters), not for use in nursing.	Cough, headache, dizziness, fatigue, viral infection, pharyngitis, diarrhea.

BB = black box warning; **W/P** = warnings/precautions; **Contra** = contraindications; **P/N** = pregnancy category rating and nursing considerations.

(Continued)

Prescribing Information for Antihypertensive Agents

GENERIC (BRAND)	FORM/ STRENGTH	DOSAGE	WARNINGS/PRECAUTIONS & CONTRAINDICATIONS	ADVERSE REACTIONS
BETA-BLOCKERS (Nonselective)				
Nadolol (Corgard)	**Tab:** 20mg*, 40mg*, 80mg*, 120mg*, 160mg* *scored	***Adults: Angina Pectoris:*** Initial: 40mg qd. Titrate: Increase by 40-80mg every 3-7 days. Usual: 40-80mg qd. Max: 240mg/day. **HTN:** Initial: 40mg qd. Titrate: Increase by 40-80mg. Max: 320mg/day. **CrCl 31-50mL/min:** Dose q24-36h. **CrCl 10-30mL/min:** Dose q24-48h. **CrCl <10mL/min:** Dose q40-60h.	**W/P:** Caution in well-compensated cardiac failure, nonallergic bronchospasm, renal dysfunction. Exacerbation of ischemic heart disease with abrupt withdrawal. Withdrawal before surgery is controversial. May mask hyperthyroidism or hypoglycemia symptoms. Can cause cardiac failure. **Contra:** Bronchial asthma, sinus bradycardia and >1st-degree conduction block, cardiogenic shock, overt cardiac failure. **P/N:** Category C, not for use in nursing.	Bradycardia, peripheral vascular insufficiency, dizziness, fatigue.
Penbutolol sulfate (Levatol)	**Tab:** 20mg* *scored	***Adults:*** 20mg qd.	**W/P:** Caution with well-compensated heart failure, elderly, nonallergic bronchospasm, renal impairment. Can cause cardiac failure. Avoid abrupt withdrawal. Withdrawal before surgery is controversial. May mask hypoglycemia or hyperthyroidism symptoms. **Contra:** Cardiogenic shock, sinus bradycardia, 2nd- and 3rd-degree AV block, bronchial asthma. **P/N:** Category C, caution in nursing.	Diarrhea, nausea, dyspepsia, dizziness, fatigue, headache, insomnia, cough.
Pindolol*	**Tab:** 5mg, 10mg	***Adults:*** Initial: 5mg bid. Titrate: May increase by 10mg/day after 3-4 weeks. Max: 60mg/day.	**W/P:** Caution with well-compensated heart failure, nonallergic bronchospasm, renal or hepatic impairment. Can cause cardiac failure. Avoid abrupt withdrawal. Withdrawal before surgery is controversial. May mask hypoglycemia or hyperthyroidism symptoms. **Contra:** Bronchial asthma, overt cardiac failure, cardiogenic shock, 2nd- and 3rd-degree heart block, severe bradycardia. **P/N:** Category B, not for use in nursing.	Dizziness, fatigue, insomnia, nervousness, dyspnea, edema, joint pain, muscle cramps/pain.
Propranolol HCl (Inderal)	**Inj:** 1mg/mL; **Tab:** 10mg*, 20mg*, 40mg*, 60mg*, 80mg* *scored	***Adults: HTN: (Tab)*** Initial: 40mg bid. Titrate: Increase gradually. Maint: 120-240mg/day. **Angina: (Tab)** 80-320mg/day, given bid-qid. **Arrhythmia: (Inj)** 1-3mg IV at 1 mg/min. **(Tab)** 10-30mg tid-qid ac and qhs. **MI: (Tab)** 180-240mg/day, given bid-tid. **Migraine: (Tab)** Initial: 80mg/day in divided doses. Usual: 160-240mg/day in divided doses. **Tremor: (Tab)** Initial: 40mg bid. Maint: 120mg/day. Max: 320mg/day. **Hypertrophic Subaortic Stenosis: (Tab)** 20-40mg tid-qid, ac and qhs. **Pheochromocytoma: (Tab)** 60mg/day in divided doses for 3 days before surgery with β-blocker. **Inoperable Tumor: (Tab)** 30mg/day in divided doses. ***Pediatrics:*** HTN **(Tab):** Initial: 1mg/kg/day PO. Usual: 1-2mg/kg bid. Max: 16mg/kg/day.	**W/P:** Caution with well-compensated cardiac failure, nonallergic bronchospasm, Wolff-Parkinson-White (WPW) syndrome, hepatic or renal dysfunction. Withdrawal before surgery is controversial. May mask hypoglycemia or hyperthyroidism symptoms. Avoid abrupt discontinuation. May reduce IOP. Can cause cardiac failure. Both digitalis glycosides and β-blockers slow atrioventricular conduction and decrease HR. Concomitant use can increase risk of bradycardia. **Contra:** Cardiogenic shock, sinus bradycardia and >1st-degree block, bronchial asthma, CHF (unless failure is secondary to tachyarrhythmia treatable with propranolol). **P/N:** Category C, caution in nursing. Intrauterine growth retardation, small placenta, and congenital abnormalities have been reported in neonates whose mothers received propranolol during pregnancy. Neonates whose mothers received propranolol at parturition have exhibited bradycardia, hypoglycemia, and/or respiratory depression.	Bradycardia, CHF, hypotension, lightheaded ness, mental depression, nausea, vomiting, allergic reactions, agranulocytosis.
Propranolol HCl (Inderal LA)	**Cap, Extended-Release:** 60mg, 80mg, 120mg, 160mg	***Adults: HTN:*** Initial: 80mg qd. Maint: 120-160mg qd. **Angina:** Initial: 80mg qd. Titrate: Increase gradually every 3-7 days. Maint: 160mg qd. Max: 320mg/day. **Migraine:** Initial: 80mg qd. Maint: 160-240mg qd. Discontinue gradually if no response within 4-6 weeks. **Hypertrophic Subaortic Stenosis:** 80-160mg qd.	**W/P:** Caution with well-compensated cardiac failure, nonallergic bronchospasm, Wolff-Parkinson-White (WPW) syndrome, hepatic or renal dysfunction. Withdrawal before surgery is controversial. May mask hypoglycemia or hyperthyroidism symptoms. Avoid abrupt discontinuation. May reduce IOP. Can cause cardiac failure. Exacerbation of angina, in some cases	Bradycardia, CHF, hypotension, lightheadedness, mental depression, nausea, vomiting, allergic reactions, agranulocytosis, dry eyes, alopecia, SLE-like reactions, male impotence,

* Available only in generic form.
W/P = warnings/precautions; **Contra** = contraindications; **P/N** = pregnancy category rating and nursing considerations.

Prescribing Information for Antihypertensive Agents

GENERIC (BRAND)	FORM/ STRENGTH	DOSAGE	WARNINGS/PRECAUTIONS & CONTRAINDICATIONS	ADVERSE REACTIONS
BETA-BLOCKERS (Nonselective) *(Cont.)*				
Propranolol HCl (Inderal LA) *(Cont.)*			myocardial reported. D/C if these occured. Stevens-Johnson Syndrome, toxic epidermal necrolysis, exfoliative dermatitis, erythema multiforme, and urticaria reported. Hypoglycemia and postural hypotension reported. **Contra:** Cardiogenic shock, sinus bradycardia and >1st-degree block, bronchial asthma, CHF (unless failure is secondary to tachyarrhythmia treatable with propranolol). **P/N:** Category C, caution in nursing.	Peyronie's disease.
Propranolol HCl (InnoPran XL)	**Cap, Extended-Release:** 80mg, 120mg	**Adults:** Initial: 80mg qhs (approximately 10 PM) consistently either on empty stomach or with food. Titrate: Based on response may titrate to dose of 120mg.	**W/P:** Caution with well-compensated cardiac failure, nonallergic bronchospasm (eg, chronic bronchitis, emphysema), Wolff-Parkinson-White syndrome, hepatic or renal dysfunction or with history of severe anaphylactic reactions. Withdrawal before surgery is controversial. May mask hypoglycemia or hyperthyroidism symptoms. Avoid abrupt discontinuation. May reduce IOP. Can cause cardiac failure. Caution in patients with impaired hepatic or renal function. Not for treatment of hypertensive emrgencies. **Contra:** Cardiogenic shock, sinus bradycardia and >1st-degree block, bronchial asthma. **P/N:** Category C; caution in nursing.	Fatigue, dizziness (except vertigo), constipation.
Timolol Maleate*	**Tab:** 5mg, 10mg*, 20mg* *scored	**Adults: HTN:** Initial: 10mg bid. Maint: 20-40mg/day. Wait at least 7 days between dose increases. Max: 60mg/day given bid. **MI:** 10mg bid. **Migraine:** Initial: 10mg bid. Maint: 20mg qd. Max: 30mg/day in divided doses. May decrease to 10mg qd. D/C if inadequate response after 6-8 weeks with max dose.	**W/P:** Caution with well-compensated cardiac failure, DM, mild to moderate COPD, bronchospastic disease, dialysis, hepatic/renal impairment, or cerebrovascular insufficiency. Exacerbation of ischemic heart disease with abrupt cessation. May mask hyperthyroidism or hypoglycemia symptoms. Withdrawal before surgery is controversial. May potentiate weakness with myasthenia gravis. Can cause cardiac failure. Caution and consider monitoring renal function in elderly. **Contra:** Active or history of bronchial asthma, severe COPD, sinus bradycardia, 2nd- and 3rd-degree AV block, overt cardiac failure, cardiogenic shock. **P/N:** Category C, not for use in nursing.	Fatigue, headache, nausea, arrhythmia, pruritus, dizziness, dyspnea, asthenia, bradycardia, dizziness.
BETA-BLOCKERS (Selective Beta₁)				
Acebutolol HCl (Sectral)	**Cap:** 200mg, 400mg	**Adults: HTN:** Initial: 400mg/day, given qd-bid. Usual: 200-800mg/day. Max: 1200mg/day. **Ventricular Arrhythmia:** Initial: 200mg bid. Maint: Increase gradually to 600-1200mg/day. **Elderly:** Lower daily doses. Max: 800mg/day. **CrCl <50mL/min:** Decrease daily dose by 50%. **CrCl <25mL/min:** Decrease daily dose by 75%.	**W/P:** Withdrawal before surgery is controversial. Caution with bronchospastic disease, peripheral or mesenteric vascular disease, aortic or mitral valve disease, left ventricular dysfunction, heart failure controlled by digitalis and/or diuretics, hepatic or renal dysfunction. May mask hypoglycemia or hyperthyroidism symptoms. Avoid abrupt discontinuation. May develop antinuclear antibodies (ANA). **Contra:** Persistently severe bradycardia, 2nd- and 3rd-degree heart block, overt cardiac failure, cardiogenic shock. **P/N:** Category B, not for use in nursing.	Fatigue, dizziness, headache, constipation, diarrhea, dyspepsia, flatulence, nausea, dyspnea, urinary frequency, insomnia.
Atenolol (Tenormin)	**Tab:** 25mg, 50mg*, 100mg *scored	**Adults: HTN:** Initial: 50mg qd. Titrate: May increase after 1-2 weeks. Max: 100mg qd. **Angina:** Initial: 50mg qd. Titrate: May increase to 100mg after 1 week. Max: 200mg qd. **AMI:** Initial: 5mg IV over 5 min, repeat 10 min later. If tolerated, give 50mg PO 10 min after the last IV dose, followed by another 50mg PO	**BB:** Avoid abrupt discontinuation of therapy in coronary artery disease. Severe exacerbation of angina and occurrence of MI and ventricular arrhythmias reported in angina patients following abrupt discontinuation of therapy with β-blockers. **W/P:** Withdrawal before surgery is not recommended. Caution with bronchospastic	Bradycardia, hypotension, dizziness, fatigue, nausea, depression, dyspnea.

* Available only in generic form.
BB = black box warning; **W/P** = warnings/precautions; **Contra** = contraindications; **P/N** = pregnancy category rating and nursing considerations.

(Continued)

Prescribing Information for Antihypertensive Agents

GENERIC (BRAND)	FORM/ STRENGTH	DOSAGE	WARNINGS/PRECAUTIONS & CONTRAINDICATIONS	ADVERSE REACTIONS
Atenolol (Tenormin) *(Cont.)*		12 hrs later. Maint: 100mg qd or 50mg bid for 6-9 days. **Renal Impairment/Elderly:** **HTN:** Initial: 25mg qd. **HTN/Angina/AMI:** Max: CrCl 15-35mL/min: 50mg/day. **CrCl <15mL/min:** 25mg/day. **Hemodialysis:** 25-50mg after each dialysis.	disease, conduction abnormalities, left ventricular dysfunction, heart failure controlled by digitalis and/or diuretics, renal or hepatic dysfunction. Can cause heart failure with prolonged use, hyperuricemia, hypercalcemia, hypokalemia, hypophosphatemia. May mask hypoglycemia or hyperthyroidism symptoms. Avoid abrupt discontinuation. Avoid with untreated pheochromocytoma. Possible fetal harm in pregnancy. May aggravate peripheral arterial circulatory disorders. May manifest latent DM. Monitor for fluid or electrolyte imbalance. May develop antinuclear antibodies (ANA). Neonates born to mothers receiving atenolol may be at risk of hypoglycemia and bradycardia. **Contra:** Sinus bradycardia, >1st-degree heart block, cardiogenic shock, overt cardiac failure. **P/N:** Category D, caution in nursing.	
Betaxolol HCl (Kerlone)	**Tab:** 10mg, 20mg	***Adults:*** Initial: 10mg qd. Titrate: May increase to 20mg qd after 7-14 days. Max (usual): 20mg/day. **Severe Renal Impairment/Dialysis:** Initial: 5mg qd. Titrate: May increase by 5mg/day every 2 weeks. Max: 20mg/day. **Elderly:** Initial: 5mg qd.	**W/P:** Caution in CHF controlled by digitalis and diuretics, bronchospastic disease, renal or hepatic dysfunction. Can cause cardiac failure. Avoid abrupt withdrawal. Withdrawal before surgery is controversial. hyperthyroidism symptoms. May decrease IOP and interfere with glaucoma-screening test. Bradycardia may occur more often in elderly. May develop antinuclear antibodies (ANA). **Contra:** Sinus bradycardia, >1st degree heart block, cardiogenic shock, overt cardiac failure. **P/N:** Category C caution in nursing.	Bradycardia, fatigue, dyspnea, lethargy, impotence, dyspepsia, arthralgia, headache, dizziness, insomnia.
Bisoprolol fumarate (Zebeta)	**Tab:** 5mg*, 10mg *scored	***Adults:*** Initial: 2.5-5mg qd. Max: 20mg/day. **Hepatic Dysfunction or CrCl <40mL/min:** Initial: 2.5mg qd; caution with dose titration.	**W/P:** Avoid abrupt withdrawal. May mask hypoglycemia or hyperthyroidism symptoms. Caution with compensated cardiac failure, DM, bronchospastic disease, hepatic/renal impairment, or peripheral vascular disease. May precipitate cardiac failure. Both digitalis glycosides and β-blockers slow atrioventricular conduction and decrease HR. Concomitant use can increase risk of bradycardia. **Contra:** Cardiogenic shock, overt cardiac failure, 2nd- or 3rd-degree AV block, marked sinus bradycardia. **P/N:** Category C, caution in nursing.	Diarrhea, upper respiratory infection, fatigue.
Metoprolol succinate (Toprol-XL)	**Tab, Extended-Release:** 25mg*, 50mg*, 100mg*, 200mg* *scored	***Adults:* HTN:** Initial: 25-100mg qd. Titrate: May increase weekly. Max: 400mg/day. **Angina:** Initial: 100mg qd. Titrate: May increase weekly. Max: 400mg/day. **Heart Failure:** Initial: (NYHA Class II) 25mg qd for 2 weeks. **Severe Heart Failure:** 12.5mg qd for 2 weeks. Titrate: Double dose every 2 weeks as tolerated. Max: 200mg/day. *Pediatrics:* ≥6 yrs: HTN: 1mg/kg qd. Max: 50mg/day. Dose adjust according to BP response. Doses above 2mg/kg have not been studied.	**W/P:** Exacerbation of angina pectoris and MI reported following abrupt withdrawal; taper over 1-2 weeks. Caution with heart failure, bronchospastic disease, DM, hepatic dysfunction, hyperthyroidism, or peripheral vascular disease. May mask symptoms of hyperthyroidism and hypoglycemia. Withdrawal prior to surgery is controversial. **Contra:** Severe bradycardia, >1st degree heart block, cardiogenic shock, sick sinus syndrome (unless a pacemaker is present), decompensated cardiac failure. **P/N:** Category C, caution with nursing.	Bradycardia, shortness of breath, fatigue, dizziness, depression, diarrhea, pruritus, rash, hepatitis, arthralgia.
Metoprolol tartrate (Lopressor)	**Inj:** 1mg/mL; **Tab:** 50mg*, 100mg* *scored	***Adults:* HTN:** Initial: 100mg/day in single or divided doses. Titrate: May increase at weekly (or longer) intervals. Usual: 100-450mg/day. Max: 450mg/day. **Angina:** Initial: 50mg bid. Titrate: May increase weekly. Usual: 100-400mg/day. Max: 400mg/day. **MI (Early Phase):** 5mg IV every 2 min for 3 doses (monitor BP,	**W/P:** Caution with ischemic heart disease, avoid abrupt withdrawal; taper over 1-2 weeks. Withdrawal before surgery is controversial. May mask hyperthyroidism and hypoglycemia symptoms. May exacerbate cardiac failure. Caution with hepatic dysfunction, CHF controlled by digitalis. Avoid in bronchospastic disease.	Bradycardia, shortness of breath, fatigue, dizziness, depression, diarrhea, pruritus, rash, heart block, hypotension.

W/P = warnings/precautions; **Contra** = contraindications; **P/N** = pregnancy category rating and nursing considerations.

Prescribing Information for Antihypertensive Agents

GENERIC (BRAND)	FORM/ STRENGTH	DOSAGE	WARNINGS/PRECAUTIONS & CONTRAINDICATIONS	ADVERSE REACTIONS
BETA-BLOCKERS (Selective Beta₁) *(Cont.)*				
Metoprolol tartrate (Lopressor) *(Cont.)*		HR, and ECG). If tolerated, give 50mg PO q6h for 48 hrs. If not tolerated, give 25-50mg PO q6h. Initiate PO dose 15 min after last IV dose. **MI (Late Phase):** 100mg bid for at least 3 months. Take PO with or immediately following meals.	May decrease sinus HR and/or slow AV conduction. D/C if heart block or hypotension occurs. **Contra:** (HTN, Angina) Sinus bradycardia, >1st degree heart block, cardiogenic shock, overt cardiac failure, sick-sinus syndrome, severe peripheral arterial circulatory disorders, pheochromocytoma. (MI) HR <45 beats/min, 2nd- and 3rd-degree heart block, significant 1st-degree heart block, SBP <100mmHg, moderate to severe cardiac failure. **P/N:** Category C, caution in nursing.	
Nebivolol (Bystolic)	Tab: 2.5mg, 5mg, 10mg	**Adults:** Monotherapy/Combination **Therapy:** Initial: 5mg qd. Titrate: May increase dose if needed at 2-week intervals. Max: 40mg. **Hepatic Impairment/ CrCl <30mL/min:** 2.5mg qd; upward titration may be performed cautiously.	**W/P:** Exacerbation of angina, and occurrence of MI and ventricular arrhythmias reported in patients with CAD following abrupt withdrawal; taper over 1-2 weeks when possible. Avoid with bronchospastic disease. Caution with compensated CHF; consider d/c if heart failure worsens. Caution with PVD, severe renal/moderate hepatic impairment. May mask signs/symptoms of hypoglycemia or hyperthyroidism. Abrupt withdrawal may also exacerbate symptoms of hyperthyroidism or precipitate a thyroid storm. Caution with history of severe anaphylactic reactions. Patients with known/suspected pheochromocytoma should initially receive an α-blocker prior to use of any β-blocker. No studies done in patients with angina pectoris, recent MI, or severe hepatic impairment. **Contra:** Severe bradycardia, heart block >1st degree, cardiogenic shock, decompensated cardiac failure, sick sinus syndrome (unless permanent pacemaker in place), severe hepatic impairment (Child-Pugh >B). **P/N:** Category C, not for use in nursing.	Headache, fatigue, dizziness, diarrhea, nausea.
BETA-BLOCKER COMBINATIONS				
Atenolol/ Chlorthalidone (Tenoretic)	**Tab:** (Atenolol-Chlorthalidone) 50mg-25mg*, 100mg-25mg *scored	**Adults:** Initial: 50mg-25mg tab qd. May increase to 100mg-25mg tab qd. **CrCl 15-35mL/min:** Max: 50mg atenolol/ day. **CrCl <15mL/min:** Max: 25mg qd.	**W/P:** Withdrawal before surgery is not recommended. Caution with bronchospastic disease, conduction abnormalities, left ventricular dysfunction, heart failure controlled by digitalis and/or diuretics, renal dysfunction. Can cause heart failure with prolonged use. May mask hypoglycemia or hyperthyroidism symptoms. Avoid abrupt discontinuation. Avoid with untreated pheochromocytoma. Possible fetal harm in pregnancy. May aggravate peripheral arterial circulatory disorders. Enhanced effects in postsympathectomy patient. Neonates born to mothers receiving atenolol may be at risk of hypoglycemia and bradycardia. **Contra:** Sinus bradycardia, >1st degree heart block, cardiogenic shock, overt cardiac failure, anuria, sulfonamide hypersensitivity. **P/N:** Category D, caution in nursing.	Bradycardia, hypotension, dizziness, fatigue, nausea, depression, dyspnea, blood dyscrasias.
Bisoprolol fumarate/ Hydrochloro-thiazide (Ziac)	**Tab:** (Bisoprolol-HCTZ) 2.5mg-6.25mg, 5mg-6.25mg, 10mg-6.25mg	**Adults:** Initial: 2.5mg-6.25mg tab qd. Maint: May increase every 14 days. Max: 20mg bisoprolol-12.5mg HCTZ/day. **Renal/Hepatic Dysfunction:** Caution in dosing/titrating.	**W/P:** Caution with compensated cardiac failure, DM, bronchospastic disease, hepatic/renal impairment, or peripheral vascular disease. Avoid abrupt withdrawal. Photosensitivity reactions, hypokalemia, hypercalcemia, hypophosphatemia reported. May activate/exacerbate SLE. Enhanced effects in post-sympathectomy patients.	Cough, diarrhea, myalgia, headache, dizziness, fatigue, upper respiratory infection.

W/P = warnings/precautions; **Contra** = contraindications; **P/N** = pregnancy category rating and nursing considerations.

(Continued)

Prescribing Information for Antihypertensive Agents

GENERIC (BRAND)	FORM/ STRENGTH	DOSAGE	WARNINGS/PRECAUTIONS & CONTRAINDICATIONS	ADVERSE REACTIONS
Bisoprolol fumarate/ Hydrochloro-thiazide (Ziac) *(Cont.)*			May mask hyperthyroidism or hypoglycemia symptoms. Monitor for fluid/electrolyte imbalance. May precipitate hyperuricemia, acute gout, cardiac failure. **Contra:** Cardiogenic shock, overt cardiac failure, 2nd- or 3rd-degree AV block, marked sinus bradycardia, anuria, sulfonamide hypersensitivity. **P/N:** Category C, not for use in nursing.	
Metoprolol tartrate/ Hydrochloro-thiazide (Lopressor HCT)	**Tab:** (Metoprolol-HCTZ) 50mg-25mg*, 100-25mg*, 100mg-50mg* *scored	**Adults:** Usual: 100-450mg metoprolol/day and 12.5-50mg HCTZ/day. Max: 50mg HCTZ/day.	**W/P:** Avoid abrupt withdrawal; taper over 1-2 weeks. Withdrawal before surgery is controversial. May mask hyperthyroidism and hypoglycemia symptoms. May cause cardiac failure. Caution with hepatic dysfunction, CHF controlled by digitalis, severe renal disease, allergy or asthma history. Avoid in bronchospastic disease. Monitor for fluid/electrolyte imbalance. May manifest latent DM. Hypokalemia, hyperuricemia, hypercalcemia, hypophosphatemia, and hypomagnesemia may occur. May exacerbate SLE. Enhanced effects in post-sympathectomy patient. **Contra:** Sinus bradycardia, >1st degree heart block, cardiogenic shock, overt cardiac failure, sick-sinus syndrome, severe peripheral arterial circulatory disorders, pheochromocytoma, anuria, sulfonamide hypersensitivity. **P/N:** Category C, not for use in nursing.	Fatigue, dizziness, flu syndrome, drowsiness, hypokalemia, headache, bradycardia.
Nadolol/ Bendroflume-thiazide (Corzide)	**Tab:** (Nadolol-Bendroflumethiazide) 40mg-5mg*, 80mg-5mg* *scored	**Adults:** Initial: 40mg-5mg tab qd. Max: 80mg-5mg tab qd. **CrCl >50mL/min:** Dose q24h. **CrCl 31-50mL/min:** Dose q24-36h. **CrCl 10-30mL/min:** Dose q24-48h. **CrCl <10mL/min:** Dose q40-60h.	**W/P:** Caution in well-compensated cardiac failure, nonallergic bronchospasm, progressive hepatic disease, and renal or hepatic dysfunction. Exacerbation of ischemic heart disease with abrupt withdrawal. Withdrawal before surgery is controversial. May mask hyperthyroidism or hypoglycemia symptoms. Can cause cardiac failure, sensitivity reactions, hypokalemia, hyperuricemia, hypomagnesemia, hypophosphatemia. May activate or exacerbate SLE. Monitor for fluid/electrolyte imbalance. Enhanced effects in postsympathectomy patient. May manifest latent DM. May decrease PBI levels. **Contra:** Bronchial asthma, sinus bradycardia and >1st degree conduction block, cardiogenic shock, overt cardiac failure, anuria, sulfonamide hypersensitivity. **P/N:** Category C, not for use in nursing.	Bradycardia, peripheral vascular insufficiency, dizziness, fatigue, nausea, vomiting, blood dyscrasias, hypersensitivity reactions.
Propranolol HCl/ Hydrochloro-thiazide (Inderide)	**Tab:** (Propranolol-HCTZ) 40mg-25mg*, 80mg-25mg* * scored	**Adults:** Initial: 80-160mg propranolol/day; 25mg-50mg HCTZ/day. Max: (propranolol-HCTZ) 160mg-50mg/day. **Elderly:** Start at low end of dosing range. Do not substitute mg-for-mg of extended-release cap for immediate-release tab plus HCTZ. Dose tab bid and extended-release cap qd.	**W/P:** Caution with well-compensated cardiac failure, nonallergic bronchospasm, Wolff-Parkinson-White Syndrome, hepatic or renal dysfunction. Withdrawal before surgery is controversial. May mask hypoglycemia or hyperthyroidism symptoms. Avoid abrupt discontinuation. May reduce IOP. Can cause cardiac failure, hypokalemia, hyperuricemia, hypercalcemia, hypophosphatemia. May exacerbate or activate SLE. Monitor for fluid/electrolyte imbalance. May manifest latent DM. Enhanced effect in postsympathectomy patient. Concomitant use with alcohol may increase plasma levels of propranolol. **Contra:** Cardiogenic shock, sinus bradycardia and >1st degree block, bronchial asthma, CHF (unless failure is secondary to tachyarrhythmia treatable with propranolol), anuria, sulfonamide	Bradycardia, CHF, hypotension, lightheadedness, mental depression, nausea, vomiting, allergic reactions, blood dyscrasias, pancreatitis.

W/P = warnings/precautions; **Contra** = contraindications; **P/N** = pregnancy category rating and nursing considerations.

Prescribing Information for Antihypertensive Agents

GENERIC (BRAND)	FORM/ STRENGTH	DOSAGE	WARNINGS/PRECAUTIONS & CONTRAINDICATIONS	ADVERSE REACTIONS
BETA-BLOCKER COMBINATIONS *(Cont.)*				
Propranolol HCl/ Hydrochloro- thiazide (Inderide) *(Cont.)*			hypersensitivity. **P/N:** Category C, not for use in nursing. Intrauterine growth retardation, small placenta, and congenital abnormalities have been reported in neonates whose mothers received propra- nolol during pregnancy. Neonates whose mothers received propranolol at parturition have exhibited bradycardia, hypoglycemia, and/or respiratory depression.	
CALCIUM CHANNEL BLOCKERS (Dihydropyridines)				
Amlodipine besylate (Norvasc)	**Tab:** 2.5mg, 5mg, 10mg	**Adults:** HTN: Initial: 5mg qd. Titrate over 7-14 days. Max: 10mg qd. **Small, Fragile, or Elderly/Hepatic Dysfunction/ ConcomitantAntihypertensive:** Initial: 2.5mg qd. **Angina:** 5-10mg qd. **Elderly/Hepatic Dysfunction:** 5mg qd. CAD: 5-10mg qd. **Pediatrics: 6-17 yrs: HTN:** 2.5-5mg qd.	**W/P:** May increase angina or MI with severe obstructive CAD. Caution with severe aortic stenosis, CHF, severe hepatic impairment, and in elderly. **P/N:** Category C, not for use in nursing.	Edema, flushing, palpitation, dizziness, headache, fatigue.
Felodipine (Plendil)	**Tab, Extended-Release:** 2.5mg, 5mg, 10mg	**Adults:** Initial: 5mg qd. Titrate: Adjust at no less than 2 week intervals. Maint: 2.5-10mg qd. **Elderly/Hepatic Dysfunction:** Initial: 2.5mg qd. Take without food or with a light meal. Swallow tab whole.	**W/P:** May cause hypotension and lead to reflex tachycardia with precipitation of angina. Caution with heart failure or ventricular dysfunction, especially with concomitant β-blockers. Monitor dose adjustment with hepatic dysfunction or elderly. Peripheral edema reported. Maintain good dental hygiene; gingival hyperplasia reported. **P/N:** Category C, not for use in nursing.	Peripheral edema, headache, flushing, dizziness.
Isradipine (DynaCirc*)	**Cap:** 2.5mg, 5mg	**Adults:** Initial: 2.5mg bid alone or with a thiazide diuretic. Titrate: May adjust by 5mg/day at 2-4 week intervals. Max: 20mg/day.	**W/P:** May produce symptomatic hypotension. Caution in CHF, especially with concomitant β-blockers. Increased bioavailability in elderly, patients with hepatic functional impairment, and mild renal impairment. **P/N:** Category C, not for use in nursing.	Headache, edema, dizziness, palpitations, chest pain, constipation, fatigue, flushing, abdominal discomfort, tachycardia, rash, pollakiura, weakness, vomiting.
Isradipine (DynaCirc CR)	**Tab, Controlled-Release:** 5mg, 10mg	**Adults:** Initial: 5mg qd alone or with a thiazide diuretic. Titrate: May adjust by 5mg/day at 2-4 week intervals. Max: 20mg/day. Swallow whole.	**W/P:** May produce symptomatic hypotension. Caution in CHF, especially with concomitant β-blockers. Caution with pre-existing severe GI narrowing. Peripheral edema reported. Increased bioavailability in elderly. **P/N:** Category C, not for use in nursing.	Headache, edema, dizziness, constipation, fatigue, flushing, abdominal discomfort.
Nicardipine HCl (Cardene IV)	**Inj:** 2.5mg/mL	**Adults:** IV: Individualized dose; Administer by slow continuous infusion at a concentration of 0.1mg/mL. **Gradual Reduction:** Initial: 50mL/hr (5mg/hr). Titrate: May increase by 25mL/hr (2.5mg/hr) q15 min. Max: 150mL/hr (15mg/hr). **Rapid BP Reduction:** Initial 50mL/hr (5mg/hr). Titrate: 25mL/hr (2.5mg/hr) q5 min. Max 150mL/hr (15mg/hr). Decrease rate to 30mL/hr (3mg/hr) after BP reduction is achieved. **Equiv. PO/IV Dose:** 20mg q8h=0.5mg/hr, 30mg q8h=1.2mg/hr, 40mg q8h=2.2mg/hr.	**W/P:** May induce or exacerbate angina. Caution with CHF, significant left ventricular dysfunction, or pheochromocytoma. Change IV site every 12 hrs to minimize risk of peripheral venous irritation. Monitor BP during administration. Caution in hepatic/renal impairment or reduced hepatic blood flow. **Contra:** Advanced aortic stenosis. **P/N:** Category C, not for use in nursing.	Headache, hypotension, tachycardia, nausea/vomiting.
Nicardipine HCl (Cardene SR)	**Cap, Extended-Release:** 30mg, 45mg, 60mg	**Adults:** Initial: 30mg bid. Usual: 30-60mg bid.	**W/P:** Increased angina reported in patients with angina. Caution with CHF when titrating dose. Caution in hepatic/renal impairment, or reduced hepatic blood flow. May cause symptomatic hypotension. Measure BP 2-4 hrs after 1st dose or dose increase. **Contra:** Advanced aortic stenosis. **P/N:** Category C, not for use in nursing.	Headache, pedal edema, vasodilation, palpitations, nausea, dizziness, asthenia, flushing, increased angina.

* Available only in generic form (brand not available).
W/P = warnings/precautions; **Contra** = contraindications; **P/N** = pregnancy category rating and nursing considerations.

(Continued)

Prescribing Information for Antihypertensive Agents

GENERIC (BRAND)	FORM/ STRENGTH	DOSAGE	WARNINGS/PRECAUTIONS & CONTRAINDICATIONS	ADVERSE REACTIONS
Nifedipine (Adalat CC, Afeditab CR)	Tab, Extended-Release: (Adalat CC, Afeditab CR) 30mg, 60mg, (Adalat CC) 90mg	*Adults:* Initial: 30mg qd. Titrate over 7-14 days. Usual: 30-60mg qd. Max: 90mg/day. Take on empty stomach. Swallow tab whole.	W/P: May cause hypotension; monitor BP initially or with titration. May exacerbate angina from β-blocker withdrawal. CHF risk, especially with aortic stenosis or β-blockers. Peripheral edema reported. May increase angina or MI with severe obstructive CAD. Caution in elderly. P/N: Category C, not for use in nursing.	Headache, flushing, heat sensation, dizziness, peripheral edema, fatigue, asthenia.
Nifedipine (Procardia)	Cap: 10mg, 20mg	*Adults:* Initial: 10mg tid. Titrate over 7-14 days. Usual: 10-20mg tid. Max: 180mg/day. **Elderly:** Start at low end of dosing range.	W/P: May cause hypotension; monitor BP initially or with titration. May exacerbate angina from β-blocker withdrawal. CHF risk, especially with aortic stenosis or β-blockers. Peripheral edema reported. Not for acute reduction of BP or essential HTN. May increase angina or MI with severe obstructive CAD. Avoid with acute coronary syndrome or within 1-2 weeks of MI. Caution in elderly. P/N: Category C, unknown use in nursing.	Dizziness, lightheadedness, giddiness, flushing, muscle cramps, headache, peripheral edema, nervousness/mood changes.
Nifedipine (Procardia XL)	Tab, Extended-Release: 30mg, 60mg, 90mg	*Adults: Angina/HTN:* Initial: 30-60mg qd. Titrate over 7-14 days. Max: 120mg/day. Caution if dose >90mg with angina.	W/P: May cause hypotension; monitor BP initially or with titration. May exacerbate angina from β-blocker withdrawal. CHF risk, especially with aortic stenosis or β-blockers. Peripheral edema reported. May increase angina or MI with severe obstructive CAD. Caution in pre-existing severe GI narrowing. P/N: Category C, unknown use in nursing.	Dizziness, lightheadedness, giddiness, flushing, muscle cramps, headache, weakness, nausea, peripheral edema, nervousness/mood changes.
Nimodipine (Nimotop)	Cap: 30mg	*Adults:* 60mg q 4 hrs for 21 days, 1 hr before or 2 hrs after meals. **Hepatic Cirrhosis:** 30mg q 4 hrs for 21 days. Start therapy within 96 hrs of SAH. If cannot swallow cap, extract contents into syringe and empty into NG tube, then flush with 30mL of 0.9% NaCl.	BB: Do not administer IV or by other parenteral routes. Deaths and serious, life-threatening adverse events have occurred when contents of capsules injected parenterally. W/P: Carefully monitor BP. Monitor BP and HR closely with hepatic dysfunction. Do not administer IV or by other parenteral routes. P/N: Category C, not for use in nursing.	Decreased BP, headache, rash, diarrhea, bradycardia, nausea, abnormal LFTs.
Nisoldipine (Sular)	Tab, Extended-Release: 10mg, 20mg, 30mg, 40mg	*Adults:* Initial: 20mg qd. Titrate: Increase by 10mg weekly or longer. Maint: 20-40mg qd. Max: 60mg/day. **Elderly >65 yrs/Hepatic Dysfunction:** Initial: Do not exceed 10mg/day. Do not chew, divide, or crush tabs.	W/P: May increase angina or MI with severe obstructive CAD. May cause hypotension; monitor BP initially or with titration. Caution with heart failure or compromised ventricular function, especially with concomitant β-blockers. Caution with severe hepatic dysfunction or in elderly. P/N: Category C, not for use in nursing.	Peripheral edema, headache, dizziness, pharyngitis, vasodilation, sinusitis, palpitations.
CALCIUM CHANNEL BLOCKERS (Nondihydropyridines)				
Diltiazem HCl (Cardizem)	Tab: 30mg, 60mg*, 90mg*, 120mg* *scored	*Adults:* Initial: 30mg qid (before meals and qhs). Adjust at 1-2 day intervals. Usual: 180-360mg/day.	W/P: Caution in renal, hepatic, or ventricular dysfunction. Monitor LFTs and renal function with prolonged use. D/C if persistent rash occurs. Symptomatic hypotension may occur. Acute hepatic injury reported. Contra: Sick sinus syndrome and 2nd- or 3rd-degree AV block (except with functioning pacemaker), hypotension (<90mmHg systolic), acute MI, pulmonary congestion. P/N: Category C, not for use in nursing.	Headache, dizziness, asthenia, flushing, 1st-degree AV block, edema, nausea, bradycardia, rash.

BB = black box warning; W/P = warnings/precautions; Contra = contraindications; P/N = pregnancy category rating and nursing considerations.

Prescribing Information for Antihypertensive Agents

GENERIC (BRAND)	FORM/ STRENGTH	DOSAGE	WARNINGS/PRECAUTIONS & CONTRAINDICATIONS	ADVERSE REACTIONS
CALCIUM CHANNEL BLOCKERS (Nondihydropyridines) *(Cont.)*				
Diltiazem HCl (Cardizem CD, Cardizem LA, Cartia XT)	Cap, Extended-Release: (Cardizem CD, Cartia XT) 120mg, 180mg, 240mg, 300mg, (Cardizem CD) 360mg; Tab, Extended-Release: (Cardizem LA) 120mg, 180mg, 240mg, 300mg, 360mg, 420mg	**Adults: HTN:** (CD, Cartia XT) Initial (monotherapy): 180-240mg qd. Titrate: Adjust at 2-week intervals. Usual: 240-360mg qd. Max: 480mg qd. (LA) Initial: 180-240mg qd. Adjust at 2-week intervals. Max: 540mg qd. **Angina:** (CD, Cartia XT) Initial: 120-180mg qd. Adjust at 1-2 week intervals. Max: 480mg/day. (LA) Initial: 180mg qd. Adjust at 1-2 week intervals.	**W/P:** Caution in renal, hepatic, or ventricular dysfunction. Monitor LFTs and renal function with prolonged use. D/C if persistent rash occurs. Symptomatic hypotension may occur. Acute hepatic injury reported. **Contra:** Sick sinus syndrome and 2nd- or 3rd-degree AV block (except with functioning pacemaker), hypotension (<90mmHg systolic), acute MI, pulmonary congestion. **P/N:** Category C, not for use in nursing.	Headache, dizziness, asthenia, flushing, 1st-degree AV block, edema, nausea, bradycardia, rash.
Diltiazem HCl (Dilacor XR, Diltia XT)	Cap, Extended-Release: 120mg, 180mg, 240mg	**Adults: HTN:** Initial: 180-240mg qd. Usual: 180-480mg qd. Max: 540mg qd. **≥60 yrs:** Initial: 120mg qd. **Angina:** Initial: 120mg qd. Titrate: Adjust at 1-2 week intervals. Max: 480mg/day. Swallow whole on an empty stomach in the am.	**W/P:** Caution in renal, hepatic, or ventricular dysfunction. Monitor LFTs and renal function with prolonged use. D/C if persistent rash occurs. Symptomatic hypotension may occur. Acute hepatic injury reported. **Contra:** Sick sinus syndrome, 2nd- or 3rd-degree AV block (except with functioning pacemaker), hypotension (<90mmHg systolic), acute MI, pulmonary congestion. **P/N:** Category C, not for use in nursing.	Rhinitis, pharyngitis, cough, flu syndrome, peripheral edema, myalgia, vomiting, sinusitis, asthenia, nausea, vasodilation, headache, constipation, diarrhea.
Diltiazem HCl (Tiazac, Taztia XT)	Cap, Extended-Release: (Taztia XT, Tiazac) 120mg, 180mg, 240mg, 300mg, 360mg; (Tiazac) 420mg	**Adults: HTN:** Initial: 120-240mg qd. Titrate: Adjust at 2-week intervals. Usual: 120-540mg qd. Max: 540mg qd. **Angina:** Initial: 120-180mg qd Titrate: Increase over 7-14 days. Max: 540mg qd.	**W/P:** Caution in renal, hepatic, or ventricular dysfunction. Monitor LFTs and renal function with prolonged use. D/C if persistent rash occurs. Symptomatic hypotension may occur. Acute hepatic injury reported. **Contra:** Sick sinus syndrome and 2nd- or 3rd-degree AV block (except with functioning pacemaker), severe hypotension (<90mm Hg systolic), acute MI, pulmonary congestion. **P/N:** Category C, not for use in nursing.	Headache, peripheral edema, vasodilation, dizziness, rash, dyspepsia.
Verapamil HCl (Calan)	Tab: 40mg, 80mg*, 120mg* *scored	**Adults: HTN:** Initial: 80mg tid. Usual: 360-480mg/day. **Elderly/Small Stature:** Initial: 40mg tid. **Angina:** Usual: 80-120mg tid. **Elderly/Small Stature:** Initial: 40mg tid. Titrate: Increase daily or weekly. **A-Fib (Digitalized):** Usual: 240-320mg/day given tid-qid. **PSVT Prophylaxis (Non-Digitalized):** 240-480mg/day given tid-qid. Max: 480mg/day. **Severe Hepatic Dysfunction:** Give 30% of normal dose.	**W/P:** Avoid with moderate to severe cardiac failure, and ventricular dysfunction if taking a β-blocker. May cause hypotension, AV block, transient bradycardia, PR interval prolongation. Monitor LFTs periodically; hepatocellular injury reported. Caution with hypertrophic cardiomyopathy, renal or hepatic dysfunction. Decrease dose with decreased neuromuscular transmission. **Contra:** Severe ventricular dysfunction, hypotension, cardiogenic shock, sick sinus syndrome or 2nd- or 3rd-degree AV block (except with functioning ventricular pacemaker), A-Fib/Flutter with an accessory bypass tract. **P/N:** Category C, not for use in nursing.	Constipation, dizziness, nausea, hypotension, headache, edema, CHF, fatigue, elevated liver enzymes, dyspnea, bradycardia, AV block, rash, flushing.
Verapamil HCl (Calan SR)	Tab, Extended-Release: 120mg, 180mg*, 240mg* *scored	**Adults: ≥18 yrs:** Initial: 180mg qam. Titrate: If inadequate response, increase to 240mg qam, then 180mg bid; or 240mg qam plus 120mg qpm, then 240mg q12h. **Elderly/Small Stature:** Initial: 120mg qam. Take with food.	**W/P:** Avoid with moderate to severe cardiac failure, and ventricular dysfunction if taking a β-blocker. May cause hypotension, AV block, transient bradycardia, PR interval, hepatocellular injury reported. Caution with hepatocellular injury reported. Caution with hypertrophic cardiomyopathy, renal or hepatic dysfunction. Decrease dose with decreased neuromuscular transmission. **Contra:** Severe ventricular dysfunction, hypotension, cardiogenic shock, sick sinus syndrome or 2nd- or 3rd-degree AV block (except with functioning ventricular pacemaker), A-Fib/Flutter with an accessory bypass tract. **P/N:** Category C, not for use in nursing.	Constipation, dizziness, nausea, hypotension, headache, edema, CHF, fatigue, elevated liver enzymes, dyspnea, bradycardia, AV block, rash, flushing.

W/P = warnings/precautions; **Contra** = contraindications; **P/N** = pregnancy category rating and nursing considerations.

(Continued)

Prescribing Information for Antihypertensive Agents

GENERIC (BRAND)	FORM/ STRENGTH	DOSAGE	WARNINGS/PRECAUTIONS & CONTRAINDICATIONS	ADVERSE REACTIONS
Verapamil HCl (Covera-HS)	Tab, Extended-Release: 180mg, 240mg	**Adults:** Initial: 180mg qhs. Titrate: May increase to 240mg qhs, then 360mg qhs, then 480mg qhs, if needed. Swallow tab whole. **Elderly:** Start at the low end of the dosing range.	**W/P:** Avoid with moderate to severe cardiac failure, and ventricular dysfunction if taking a β-blocker. May cause hypotension, AV block, transient bradycardia, PR interval prolongation. Monitor LFTs periodically; hepatocellular injury reported. Give 30% of normal dose with severe hepatic dysfunction. Caution with hypertrophic cardiomyopathy, renal or hepatic dysfunction. Decrease dose with decreased neuromuscular transmission. **Contra:** Severe ventricular dysfunction, hypotension, cardiogenic shock, sick sinus syndrome or 2nd- or 3rd-degree AV block (except with functioning ventricular pacemaker), A-Fib/Flutter with an accessory bypass tract. **P/N:** Category C, not for use in nursing.	Constipation, dizziness, nausea, hypotension, headache, edema, CHF, pulmonary edema, fatigue, dyspnea, bradycardia, AV block, rash, flushing.
Verapamil HCl (Isoptin SR)	Tab, Extended-Release: 120mg, 180mg*, 240mg* *scored	**Adults:** Initial: 180mg qam. Titrate: If inadequate response, increase to 240mg qam, then 180mg bid; or 240mg qam plus 120mg qpm, then 240mg q12h. **Elderly/Small Stature:** Initial: 120mg qam. Take with food.	**W/P:** Avoid with moderate to severe cardiac failure, and ventricular dysfunction if taking a β-blocker. May cause hypotension, AV block, transient bradycardia, PR interval prolongation. Monitor LFTs periodically; hepatocellular injury reported. Give 30% of normal dose with severe hepatic dysfunction. Caution with hypertrophic cardiomyopathy, renal or hepatic dysfunction. Decrease dose in those with decreased neuromuscular transmission. **Contra:** Severe ventricular dysfunction, hypotension, cardiogenic shock, sick sinus syndrome or 2nd- or 3rd-degree AV block (except with functioning ventricular pacemaker), A-Fib/Flutter with an accessory bypass tract. **P/N:** Category C, not for use in nursing.	Constipation, dizziness, nausea, hypotension, headache, edema, CHF, pulmonary edema, fatigue, dyspnea, bradycardia, AV block, rash, flushing.
Verapamil HCl (Verelan)	Cap, Extended-Release: 120mg, 180mg, 240mg, 360mg	**Adults:** Usual: 240mg qam. Titrate: May increase by 120mg qam. Max: 480mg qam. **Elderly/Small Stature:** Initial: 120mg qam. Titrate: May increase to 180mg qam, then 240mg qam, then 360mg qam, then 480mg qam. May sprinkle on applesauce; do not crush or chew.	**W/P:** Avoid with moderate to severe cardiac failure, and ventricular dysfunction if taking a β-blocker. May cause hypotension, AV block, transient bradycardia, PR interval prolongation. Monitor LFTs periodically; hepatocellular injury reported. Give 30% of normal dose with severe hepatic dysfunction. Caution with hypertrophic cardiomyopathy, renal or hepatic dysfunction. Decrease dose in those with decreased neuromuscular transmission **Contra:** Severe ventricular dysfunction, hypotension, cardiogenic shock, sick sinus syndrome or 2nd- or 3rd-degree AV block (except with functioning ventricular pacemaker), A-Fib/Flutter with an accessory bypass tract. **P/N:** Category C, not for use in nursing.	Constipation, dizziness, nausea, hypotension, headache, peripheral edema, infection, flu syndrome, fatigue, bradycardia, AV block.
Verapamil HCl (Verelan PM)	Cap, Extended-Release: 100mg, 200mg, 300mg	**Adults:** Usual: 200mg qhs. Titrate: May increase to 300mg qhs, then 400mg qhs. **Renal or Hepatic Dysfunction/Elderly/ Small Stature:** Initial: 100mg qhs. Max: 400mg qhs. May sprinkle on applesauce; do not crush or chew.	**W/P:** Avoid with moderate to severe cardiac failure, and ventricular dysfunction if taking a β-blocker. May cause hypotension, AV block, transient bradycardia, PR interval prolongation. Monitor LFTs periodically; hepatocellular injury reported. Give 30% of normal dose with severe hepatic dysfunction. Caution with hypertrophic cardiomyopathy, renal or hepatic dysfunction. Decrease dose in those with decreased neuromuscular transmission. **Contra:** Severe ventricular dysfunction, hypotension, cardiogenic shock, sick sinus syndrome or 2nd- or	Constipation, dizziness, nausea, hypotension, headache, peripheral edema, infection, flu syndrome, fatigue, bradycardia, AV block.

W/P = warnings/precautions; **Contra** = contraindications; **P/N** = pregnancy category rating and nursing considerations.

Prescribing Information for Antihypertensive Agents

GENERIC (BRAND)	FORM/ STRENGTH	DOSAGE	WARNINGS/PRECAUTIONS & CONTRAINDICATIONS	ADVERSE REACTIONS
CALCIUM CHANNEL BLOCKERS (Nondihydropyridines) *(Cont.)*				
Verapamil HCl (Verelan PM) *(Cont.)*			3rd-degree AV block (except with functioning ventricular pacemaker), A-Fib/Flutter with an accessory bypass tract. **P/N:** Category C, not for use in nursing.	
CALCIUM CHANNEL BLOCKER COMBINATIONS				
Amlodipine besylate/ Atorvastatin calcium (Caduet)	**Tab:** (Amlodipine-Atorvastatin) 2.5mg-10mg, 2.5mg-20mg, 2.5mg-40mg, 5mg-10mg, 5mg-20mg, 5mg-40mg, 5mg-80mg, 10mg-10mg, 10mg-20mg, 10mg-40mg, 10mg-80mg	***Adults:*** Dosing should be individualized and based on the appropriate combination of recommendations for the monotherapies. (Amlodipine): **HTN:** Initial: 5mg qd. Titrate over 7-14 days. Max: 10mg qd. **Small, Fragile, or Elderly/ Hepatic Dysfunction/Concomitant Antihypertensive:** Initial: 2.5mg qd. **Angina:** 5-10mg qd. **Elderly/Hepatic Dysfunction:** 5mg qd. (Atorvastatin): **Hypercholesterolemia/Mixed Dyslipidemia:** Initial: 10-20mg qd (or 40mg qd for LDL-C reduction >45%). Titrate: Adjust dose if needed at 2-4 week intervals. Usual: 10-80mg qd. **Homozygous Familial Hypercholesterolemia:** 10-80mg qd. *Pediatrics:* ≥10 yrs (postmenarchal): (Amlodipine): **HTN:** 2.5-5mg qd. **10-17 yrs (postmenarchal):** (Atorvastatin): **Heterozygous Familial Hypercholesterolemia:** Initial: 10mg/day. Titrate: Adjust dose if needed at intervals of ≥4 weeks. Max: 20mg/day.	**W/P:** May rarely increase angina or MI with severe obstructive CAD. Monitor LFTs prior to therapy, at 12 weeks after initiation, with dose elevation, and periodically thereafter. Reduce dose or withdraw if AST or ALT >3x ULN persist. Caution with heavy alcohol use and/or history of hepatic disease, severe aortic stenosis, CHF. D/C if markedly elevated CPK levels occur, if myopathy is diagnosed or suspected, or if predisposition to renal failure secondary to rhabdomyolysis. Increased risk of hemorrhagic stroke in patients with recent stroke or TIA. **Contra:** Active liver disease, unexplained persistent elevations of serum transaminases, pregnancy, nursing mothers. **P/N:** Category X, not for use in nursing	Headache, edema, palpitation, dizziness, fatigue, constipation, flatulence, dyspepsia, abdominal pain.
Amlodipine besylate/ Benazepril HCl (Lotrel)	**Cap:** (Amlodipine-Benazepril) 2.5mg-10mg, 5mg-10mg, 5mg-20mg, 5mg-40mg, 10mg-20mg, 10mg-40mg	***Adults:*** Usual: 2.5-10mg amlodipine and 10-80mg benazepril per day. **Small/Elderly/Frail/Hepatic Impairment:** Initial: 2.5mg amlodipine.	**BB:** When used in pregnancy, ACE inhibitors can cause injury and even death to the developing fetus. D/C therapy when pregnancy detected. **W/P:** D/C if angioedema, jaundice, or if marked LFT elevation occurs. Risk of hyperkalemia with DM, renal dysfunction. Persistent nonproductive cough reported. Monitor WBCs in collagen vascular disease. Anaphylactoid reactions reported. Fetal/neonatal morbidity and death reported. Monitor for hypotension in high-risk patients (heart failure, surgery/ anesthesia, volume and/or salt depletion, etc). Caution with CHF, severe hepatic or renal dysfunction, and renal artery stenosis. Avoid if CrCl ≤30mL/min. **P/N:** Category C (1st trimester) and D (2nd and 3rd trimesters), not for use in nursing.	Cough, headache, dizziness, edema.
Amlodipine besylate/ Olmesartan medoxomil (Azor)	**Tab:** (Amlodipine-Olmesartan) 5mg-20mg, 10mg-20mg, 5mg-40mg, 10mg-40mg	***Adults:*** **Replacement Therapy:** May substitute for individually titrated components for patients on amlodipine and olmesartan. When substituting for individual components, the dose of 1 or both components may be increased if needed. **Add-On Therapy:** May use as add-on therapy when not adequately controlled on amlodipine or olmesartan. May increase dose after 2 weeks to maximum dose of 10mg-40mg qd.	**BB:** When used in pregnancy during 2nd and 3rd trimesters, drugs that act directly on the renin-angiotensin system can cause injury and even death to developing fetus. When pregnancy is detected, d/c therapy asap. **W/P:** Hypotension, especially in volume- or salt-depleted patients, may occur with treatment initiation; monitor closely. Caution with severe aortic stenosis, heart failure, or severe hepatic impairment. Increased angina or MI with CCBs may occur with dosage initiation or increase. Changes in renal function, oliguria, progressive azotemia, or acute renal failure may occur. **P/N:** Category C (1st trimester) and D (2nd and 3rd trimester), not for use in nursing.	Edema.

BB = black box warning; **W/P** = warnings/precautions; **Contra** = contraindications; **P/N** = pregnancy category rating and nursing considerations.

(Continued)

Prescribing Information for Antihypertensive Agents

GENERIC (BRAND)	FORM/ STRENGTH	DOSAGE	WARNINGS/PRECAUTIONS & CONTRAINDICATIONS	ADVERSE REACTIONS
Amlodipine besylate/ Valsartan (Exforge)	**Tab:** (Amlodipine-Valsartan) 5mg-160mg, 10mg-160mg, 5mg-320mg, 10mg-320mg	***Adults: Combination Therapy from Monotherapy (amlodipine or valsartan):*** Initial: 5mg-10mg amlodipine and 160mg-320mg valsartan qd. Titrate: If inadequate control, may increase after 3-4 weeks of therapy. Max: 10mg-320mg. If receiving amlodipine and valsartan separately, may give same component doses. **Elderly:** Lower initial dose may be required	**BB:** When used in pregnancy, drugs that act directly on the renin-angiotensin system can cause injury and even death to the developing fetus. D/C therapy when pregnancy is detected. **W/P:** May cause excessive hypotension. May increase risk of angina and MI in patients with severe obstructive CAD. Caution with CHF, severe hepatic impairment, renal dysfunction, or renal artery stenosis. **P/N:** Category C (1st trimester) and D (2nd and 3rd trimester), not for use in nursing.	Peripheral edema, vertigo, nasopharyngitis, upper respiratory tract infection, dizziness.
Verapamil HCl/ Trandolapril (Tarka)	**Tab:** (Trandolapril-Verapamil) 2mg-180mg, 1mg-240mg, 2mg-240mg, 4mg-240mg	***Adults: Replacement Therapy:*** 1 tab qd with food. **Severe Hepatic Dysfunction:** Give 30% of normal dose.	**BB:** ACE inhibitors can cause death/injury to developing fetus during 2nd and 3rd trimesters. Stop therapy if pregnancy detected. **W/P:** Monitor for hypotension with surgery or anesthesia. Risk of hyperkalemia with renal insufficiency, DM. D/C if jaundice develops. Avoid with moderate to severe cardiac failure and ventricular dysfunction if taking a β-blocker. May cause angioedema, cough, fetal/ neonatal morbidity, hypotension, AV block, anaphylactoid reactions, transient bradycardia, PR-interval prolongation. Monitor LFTs periodically. Give 30% of normal dose with severe hepatic dysfunction. Caution with CHF, hypertrophic cardiomyopathy, renal or hepatic dysfunction. Decrease dose in those with decreased neuromuscular transmission. Monitor WBC with collagen-vascular disease and/or renal disease. **Contra:** Severe ventricular dysfunction, hypotension, cardiogenic shock, sick sinus syndrome or 2nd- or 3rd-degree AV block (except with functioning ventricular pacemaker), A-Fib/Flutter with an accessory bypass tract, history of ACE inhibitor-associated angioedema. **P/N:** Category C (1st trimester) and D (2nd and 3rd trimesters), not for use in nursing.	AV block, constipation, cough, dizziness, fatigue, headache, increased hepatic enzymes, chest pain, upper respiratory tract infection/congestion.
DIRECT RENIN INHIBITOR & COMBINATION				
Aliskiren (Tekturna)	**Tab:** 150mg, 300mg	***Adults:*** Usual: 150mg qd. Titrate: May increase to 300mg/day if needed. High-fat meals decrease absorption.	**BB:** When used in pregnancy, drugs that act directly on the renin-angiotensin system can cause injury and even death to the developing fetus. D/C therapy when pregnancy is detected. **W/P:** Caution with greater than moderate renal dysfunction (SCr >1.7mg/dL (women) or >2mg/dL (men) and/or GFR <30mL/min), history of dialysis, nephrotic syndrome, or renovascular hypertension. May increase serum K+, especially when used in combination with especially when especially when in diabetics. Angioedema of face, extremities, lips, tongue, glottis, and/or larynx reported; d/c and monitor until complete resolution of signs and symptoms. Hypotension rarely seen. **P/N:** Category C (1st trimester) and D (2nd and 3rd trimesters); not for use in nursing.	Diarrhea, headache, nasopharyngitis, dizziness, fatigue, upper respiratory tract infection, back pain, cough.
Aliskiren/ Hydrochloro-thiazide (Tekturna HCT)	**Tab:** (Aliskiren-HCTZ) 150mg-12.5mg, 150mg-25mg, 300mg-12.5mg, 300mg-25mg	***Adults:*** Initial: Not Controlled on Monotherapy: 150mg/12.5mg qd. Titrate: May increase to 150mg/25mg, 300mg/12.5mg qd if uncontrolled after 2-4 weeks. Max: 300mg/25mg. Avoid with CrCl ≤30mL/min.	**BB:** Drugs that act directly on the renin-angiotensin system can cause injury and even death to the developing fetus. D/C therapy when pregnancy is detected. **W/P:** Angioedema of head and neck may occur; d/c therapy and monitor until	Dizziness, influenza, diarrhea, cough, vertigo, asthenia, arthralgia.

BB = black box warning; **W/P** = warnings/precautions; **Contra** = contraindications; **P/N** = pregnancy category rating and nursing considerations.

Prescribing Information for Antihypertensive Agents

GENERIC (BRAND)	FORM/ STRENGTH	DOSAGE	WARNINGS/PRECAUTIONS & CONTRAINDICATIONS	ADVERSE REACTIONS
DIRECT RENIN INHIBITOR & COMBINATION *(Cont.)*				
Aliskiren/ Hydrochloro-thiazide (Tekturna HCT) *(Cont.)*			signs and symptoms resolve. May cause symptomatic hypotension in volume-and/or salt-depleted patients; correct condition prior to therapy. Avoid with CrCl <30mL/min. Caution with hepatic impairment, or history of allergy or bronchial asthma. May exacerbate or activate SLE. Monitor serum electrolytes periodically to detect possible electrolyte imbalance. **Contra:** Anuria, sulfonamide hypersensitivity. **P/N:** Category D, not for use in nursing.	
DIURETICS (Aldosterone Receptor Blockers)				
Eplerenone (Inspra)	**Tab:** 25mg, 50mg	***Adults:* CHF Post-MI:** Initial: 25mg qd. Titrate: To 50mg qd within 4 weeks. **Maint:** 50mg qd. Adjust dose based on K+ level: See PI. **HTN:** Initial: 50mg qd. May increase to 50mg bid if inadequate effect on BP. Max: 100mg/day. **With Weak CYP3A4 Inhibitors:** Initial: 25mg qd.	**W/P:** Risk of hyperkalemia (>5.5mEq/L); monitor periodically. With CHF post-MI use caution with SCr >2mg/dL (males) or >1.8mg/dL (females), CrCl ≤50mL/min, and in diabetics (also with proteinuria). **Contra:** All: Serum K+ >5.5mgEq/L at initiation, CrCl ≤30mL/min, with potent CYP3A4 inhibitors (eg, ketoconazole, itraconazole, nefazodone, troleandomycin, clarithromycin, ritonavir, nelfinavir). When treating HTN: Type 2 diabetes with microalbuminuria, SCr >2mg/dL (males) or >1.8mg/dL (females), CrCl >50mg/min, with K+ supplements or K+-sparing diuretics (eg, amiloride, spironolactone, triamterene). **P/N:** Category B, not for use in nursing.	Headache, dizziness, hyperkalemia, increased SCr/triglycerides/GGT, angina/MI.
Spironolactone (Aldactone)	**Tab:** 25mg, 50mg*, 100mg* *scored	***Adults:* Hyperaldosteronism:** (Diagnostic) 400mg/day for 3-4 weeks or 400mg/day for 4 days. (Preoperative) 100-400mg/day. Maint: Lowest effective dose. **Edema:** Initial: 100mg/day given qd or in divided doses for at least 5 days. Maint: 25-200mg/day given qd-bid. **HTN:** Initial: 50-100mg/day given qd or in divided doses. Titrate: Adjust at 2-week intervals. **Hypokalemia:** 25-100mg/day.	**BB:** Tumorigenic in chronic toxicity animal studies; avoid unnecessary use. **W/P:** Monitor for fluid/electrolyte imbalance. Caution with renal and hepatic dysfunction. Hyperchloremic metabolic acidosis reported with decompensated hepatic cirrhosis. Mild acidosis, gynecomastia, transient BUN elevation may occur. D/C and monitor ECG if hyperkalemia occurs. Risk of dilutional hyponatremia. **Contra:** Anuria, acute renal insufficiency, significantly impaired renal excretory function, hyperkalemia. **P/N:** Category C, not for use in nursing.	Gastric bleeding, ulceration, gynecomastia, impotence, agranulocytosis, fever, urticaria, confusion, ataxia, renal dysfunction, irregular menses, amenorrhea.
DIURETICS (Loop)				
Bumetanide (Bumex)	**Inj:** 0.25mg/mL; **Tab:** 0.5mg*, 1mg*, 2mg* *scored	***Adults:* ≥18 yrs: PO:** Usual: 0.5-2mg qd. Maint: May give every other day or every 3-4 days. Max: 10mg/day. **IV/IM:** Initial: 0.5-1mg over 1-2 min, may repeat every 2-3 hrs for 2-3 doses. Max: 10mg/day. **Elderly:** Start at low end of dosing range.	**BB:** Can lead to profound water and electrolyte depletion with excessive use. **W/P:** Monitor for volume/electrolyte depletion, hypokalemia, blood dyscrasias, hepatic damage. Elderly are prone to volume/electrolyte depletion. Caution in elderly, hepatic cirrhosis and ascites. Associated with ototoxicity, hypocalcemia, thrombocytopenia, hypomagnesemia, hypokalemia, and hyperuricemia. Hypersensitivity with sulfonamide allergy. D/C if marked increase in BUN or creatinine or if develop oliguria with progressive renal disease. **Contra:** Anuria, hepatic coma, severe electrolyte depletion. **P/N:** Category C, not for use in nursing.	Muscle cramps, dizziness, hypotension, headache, nausea, hyperuricemia, hypokalemia, hyponatremia, hyperglycemia, azotemia, increase serum creatinine.
Ethacrynic acid (Edecrin)	**Tab:** 25mg* *scored	***Adults:*** Initial: 50-100mg qd. Titrate: 25-50mg increments. Usual: 50-200mg/day. After diuresis achieved, give smallest effective dose continuously or intermittently. ***Pediatrics:*** Initial: 25mg. Titrate: Increase by 25mg increments.	**W/P:** Caution in advanced liver cirrhosis. Monitor serum electrolytes, CO_2, BUN early in therapy and periodically during active diuresis. Vigorous diuresis may induce acute hypotensive episode and in elderly cardiac patients, hemoconcentration	Anorexia, malaise, abdominal discomfort, gout, deafness, tinnitus, vertigo, headache, fatigue, rash, chills.

BB = black box warning; **W/P** = warnings/precautions; **Contra** = contraindications; **P/N** = pregnancy category rating and nursing considerations.

(Continued)

Prescribing Information for Antihypertensive Agents

GENERIC (BRAND)	FORM/ STRENGTH	DOSAGE	WARNINGS/PRECAUTIONS & CONTRAINDICATIONS	ADVERSE REACTIONS
Ethacrynic acid (Edecrin) *(Cont.)*		Maint: Reduce dose and frequency once dry weight achieved; may give intermittently.	resulting in thromboembolic disorders. Ototoxicity reported with severe renal dysfunction. Hypomagnesemia and transient increase in serum urea nitrogen may occur. Reduce dose or withdraw if excessive electrolyte loss occurs. Initiate therapy in the hospital for cirrhotic patients with ascites. Liberalize salt intake and supplement with K⁺ if needed. Reduced responsiveness in renal edema with hypoproteinemia; use salt poor albumin. **Contra:** Anuria, infants. D/C if increasing electrolyte imbalance, azotemia, or oliguria develops during treatment of severe, progressive renal disease. D/C if severe, watery diarrhea occurs. **P/N:** Category B, not for use in nursing.	
Furosemide (Lasix)	**Inj:** 10mg/mL; **Sol:** 10mg/mL, 40mg/5mL; **Tab:** 20mg, 40mg*, 80mg *scored	***Adults:* (PO) HTN:** Initial: 40mg bid. **Edema:** Initial: 20-80mg PO. May repeat or increase by 20-40mg after 6-8 hrs. Max: 600mg/day. Alternative Regimen: Dose on 2-4 consecutive days each week. Closely monitor if on >80mg/day. **(Inj) Edema:** Initial: 20-40mg IV/IM. May repeat or increase by 20mg after 2 hrs. **Acute Pulmonary Edema:** Initial: 40mg IV. May increase to 80mg IV after 1 hr. ***Pediatrics:* Edema: (PO)** Initial: 2mg/kg single dose. May increase by 1-2mg/kg after 6-8 hrs. Max: 6mg/kg. **(Inj)** Initial: 1mg/kg IV/IM single dose. May increase by 1mg/kg IV/IM after 2 hrs. Max: 6mg/kg.	**BB:** Can lead to profound water and electrolyte depletion with excessive use. **W/P:** Monitor for fluid/electrolyte imbalance (eg, hypokalemia), renal or hepatic dysfunction. Initiate in hospital with hepatic cirrhosis and ascites. Tinnitus, hearing impairment, hyperglycemia, hyperuricemia reported. May activate SLE. Cross-sensitivity with sulfonamide allergy. Avoid excessive diuresis, especially in elderly. **Contra:** Anuria. **P/N:** Category C, caution in nursing.	Pancreatitis, jaundice, anorexia, paresthesias, ototoxicity, blood dyscrasias, dizziness, rash, urticaria, photosensitivity, fever, thrombophlebitis, restlessness.
Torsemide (Demadex)	**Inj:** 10mg/mL; **Tab:** 5mg*, 10mg*, 20mg*, 100mg* *scored	***Adults:* PO/IV** (bolus over 2 min or continuous): **CHF:** Initial: 10-20mg qd. Max: 200mg single dose. **Chronic Renal Failure:** Initial: 20mg qd. Max: 200mg single dose. **Hepatic Cirrhosis:** Initial: 5-10mg qd with aldosterone antagonist or K+-sparing diuretic. Titrate: Double dose. Max: 40mg single dose. **HTN:** Initial: 5mg qd. Titrate: May increase to 10mg qd in 4-6 weeks, then may add additional antihypertensive agent.	**W/P:** Caution with cirrhosis and ascites in hepatic disease. Tinnitus and hearing loss (usually reversible) reported. Avoid excessive diuresis, especially in elderly. Caution with brisk diuresis, inadequate oral intake of electrolytes, and cardiovascular disease, especially with digitalis glycosides. Monitor for electrolyte/volume depletion. Hyperglycemia, hypokalemia, hypermagnesemia, hypercalcemia, gout reported. May increase cholesterol and TG. **Contra:** Anuria, sulfonamide hypersensitivity. **P/N:** Category B, caution in nursing.	Headache, excessive urination, dizziness, cough, ECG abnormality, asthenia, rhinitis, diarrhea.
DIURETICS (Potassium-Sparing)				
Amiloride HCl*	**Tab:** 5mg	***Adults:*** Initial: 5mg qd. Titrate: Increase to 10mg/day. If hyperkalemia persists, may increase to 15mg/day then to 20mg/day with careful monitoring. Take with food.	**W/P:** Risk of hyperkalemia (≥5.5mEq/L) especially with renal impairment, elderly, DM; monitor levels frequently. D/C if hyperkalemia occurs. Caution in severely ill in whom respiratory or metabolic acidosis may occur; monitor acid-base balance frequently. Hepatic encephalopathy reported with severe hepatic disease. Increased BUN reported. D/C at least 3 days before glucose tolerance test. Monitor electrolytes and renal function in DM. **Contra:** Hyperkalemia, anuria, acute or chronic renal insufficiency, diabetic neuropathy, K⁺-sparing agents (eg, diuretics), and K⁺ supplements, K⁺ salt substitutes, K⁺-rich diet (except with severe hypokalemia). **P/N:** Category B, not for use in nursing.	Headache, nausea, anorexia, vomiting, elevated serum potassium, diarrhea, muscle cramps, impotence.

* Available only in generic form.
BB = black box warning; **W/P** = warnings/precautions; **Contra** = contraindications; **P/N** = pregnancy category rating and nursing considerations.

Prescribing Information for Antihypertensive Agents

GENERIC (BRAND)	FORM/ STRENGTH	DOSAGE	WARNINGS/PRECAUTIONS & CONTRAINDICATIONS	ADVERSE REACTIONS
DIURETICS (Potassium-Sparing) *(Cont.)*				
Triamterene (Dyrenium)	Cap: 50mg, 100mg	*Adults:* Initial: 100mg bid pc. Max: 300mg/day.	**BB:** Abnormal elevation of serum K⁺ levels (≥5.5mEq/L) can occur with all K⁺-sparing agents, including triamterene. Hyperkalemia is more likely to occur with renal impairment and diabetes (even without evidence of renal impairment), and in the elderly, or severely ill. Monitor serum K⁺ at frequent intervals. **W/P:** Check ECG if hyperkalemia occurs. May cause decreased alkali reserve with possibility of metabolic acidosis, mild nitrogen retention. Monitor BUN periodically. May contribute to megaloblastosis in folic acid deficiency. Caution with gouty arthritis; may elevate uric acid levels. May aggravate or cause electrolyte imbalances in CHF, renal disease, or cirrhosis. Caution with history of renal stones. **Contra:** Anuria, severe or progressive kidney disease or dysfunction (except with nephrosis), severe hepatic disease, hyperkalemia, K⁺ supplements, K⁺ salt substitutes, K⁺-sparing agents (eg, diuretics). **P/N:** Category C, not for use in nursing.	Hypersensitivity reactions, hyper- or hypokalemia, azotemia, renal stones, jaundice, nausea, vomiting, diarrhea, weakness, dizziness.
DIURETICS (Thiazide)				
Chlorothiazide (Diuril)	Inj: 0.5g; Sus: 250mg/5mL [237mL]	*Adults:* (PO/IV) Edema: 0.5-1g qd-bid. May give every other day or 3-5 days/week. Substitute IV for oral using same dosage. (PO) HTN: 0.5-1g qd or in divided doses. Max: 2g/day. *Pediatrics:* (PO) Diuresis/HTN: Usual: 10-20mg/kg/day given qd-bid. Max: Infants up to 2 yrs: 375mg/day. 2-12 yrs: 1g/day. <6 months: Up to 15mg/kg bid may be required.	**W/P:** Caution in severe renal disease, liver dysfunction, electrolyte/fluid imbalance. Monitor electrolytes. Hyperuricemia, hyperglycemia, hypokalemia, hyponatremia, hypomagnesemia, hypercalcemia may occur. Increases in cholesterol and triglyceride levels reported. May exacerbate SLE. Sensitivity reactions reported. D/C prior to parathyroid test. Enhanced effects in post-sympathectomy patient. IV use not recommended in infants or children. **Contra:** Anuria, sulfonamide hypersensitivity. **P/N:** Category C, not for use in nursing.	Weakness, hypotension, pancreatitis, jaundice, diarrhea, vomiting, blood dyscrasias, rash, photosensitivity, electrolyte imbalance, impotence.
Chlorthalidone (Thalitone)	Tab: 15mg	*Adults:* HTN: Initial: 15mg qd. Titrate: May increase to 30mg qd, then to 45-50mg qd. Edema: Initial: 30-60mg/day or 60mg every other day, up to 90-120mg/day. Maint: May be lower than initial; adjust to patient. Take in the morning with food.	**W/P:** Caution in severe renal disease, liver dysfunction, allergy history, asthma. May exacerbate or activate SLE. Monitor for fluid and electrolyte imbalance. Hyperuricemia, hypomagnesemia, hypokalemia, hypercalcemia, hypophosphatemia, and hyperglycemia may occur. May manifest latent DM. **Contra:** Anuria, sulfonamide hypersensitivity. **P/N:** Category B, not for use in nursing.	Pancreatitis, jaundice, diarrhea, vomiting, constipation, nausea, blood dyscrasias, rash, photosensitivity, dizziness, headache, electrolyte disturbance, impotence.
Hydrochloro-thiazide*	Tab: 12.5mg, 25mg*, 50mg* *scored	*Adults:* Edema: 25-100mg qd or in divided doses. May give every other day or 3-5 days/week. HTN: Initial: 25mg qd. Titrate: May increase to 50mg/day. *Pediatrics:* Diuresis/HTN: 1-2mg/kg/day given qd-bid. Max: Infants up to 2 yrs: 37.5mg/day. 2-12 yrs: 100mg/day. <6 months: Up to 1.5mg/kg bid may be required.	**W/P:** Caution in severe renal disease, liver dysfunction, electrolyte/fluid imbalance. Monitor electrolytes. Hyperuricemia, hyperglycemia, hypokalemia, hyponatremia, hypomagnesemia, hypercalcemia may occur. Increases in cholesterol and triglyceride levels reported. May exacerbate SLE. Sensitivity reactions reported. D/C prior to parathyroid test. Enhanced effects in post-sympathectomy patients. **Contra:** Anuria, sulfonamide hypersensitivity. **P/N:** Category B, not for use in nursing.	Weakness, hypotension, pancreatitis, jaundice, diarrhea, vomiting, blood dyscrasias, rash, photosensitivity, electrolyte imbalance, impotence.

* Available only in generic form.
BB = black box warning; **W/P** = warnings/precautions; **Contra** = contraindications; **P/N** = pregnancy category rating and nursing considerations.

(Continued)

Prescribing Information for Antihypertensive Agents

GENERIC (BRAND)	FORM/ STRENGTH	DOSAGE	WARNINGS/PRECAUTIONS & CONTRAINDICATIONS	ADVERSE REACTIONS
Hydrochloro-thiazide (Microzide)	**Cap:** 12.5mg	***Adults:*** Initial: 12.5mg qd. Max: 50mg/day.	**W/P:** Caution in severe renal disease, liver dysfunction, electrolyte/fluid imbalance. Monitor electrolytes. Hyperuricemia, hyperglycemia, hypokalemia, hyponatremia, hypomagnesemia, hypercalcemia may occur. Increases in cholesterol and triglyceride levels reported. May exacerbate SLE. Sensitivity reactions reported. D/C prior to parathyroid test. Enhanced effects in post-sympathectomy patient. **Contra:** Anuria, sulfonamide hypersensitivity. **P/N:** Category B, not for use in nursing.	Weakness, hypotension, pancreatitis, jaundice, diarrhea, vomiting, blood dyscrasias, rash, photosensitivity, electrolyte imbalance, impotence.
Indapamide (Lozol)	**Tab:** 1.25mg, 2.5mg	***Adults:* HTN:** 1.25mg qam. Titrate: May increase to 2.5mg qd after 4 weeks, then to 5mg qd after another 4 weeks. Max: 5mg/day. **CHF:** 2.5mg qam. Titrate: May increase to 5mg qd after 1 week. Max: 5mg/day.	**W/P:** Caution in severe renal disease, liver dysfunction. May exacerbate or activate SLE. Monitor for fluid/electrolyte imbalance. Hyperuricemia, hypercalcemia, hypokalemia, hypophosphatemia, and hyperglycemia may occur. Monitor renal function, serum uric acid levels periodically. May precipitate gout. May manifest latent DM. Enhanced effects in post-sympathectomy patient. **Contra:** Anuria, sulfonamide hypersensitivity. **P/N:** Category B, not for use in nursing.	Headache, infection, pain, back pain, dizziness, rhinitis, fatigue, muscle cramps, nervousness, numbness of extremities, electrolyte imbalance, anxiety, agitation.
Methyclothiazide (Enduron)	**Tab:** 5mg* *scored	***Adults:* Edema:** 2.5-10mg qd. Max: 10mg/dose. **HTN:** 2.5-5mg qd.	**W/P:** Caution in severe renal disease, liver dysfunction, electrolyte/fluid imbalance. Monitor electrolytes. Hyperuricemia, hyperglycemia, hypokalemia, hyponatremia, hypomagnesemia, hypercalcemia may occur. Increases in cholesterol and triglyceride levels reported. May exacerbate SLE. Sensitivity reactions reported. D/C prior to parathyroid test. Enhanced effects in post-sympathectomy patient. **Contra:** Anuria, sulfonamide hypersensitivity. **P/N:** Category B, not for use in nursing.	Headache, cramping, weakness, orthostatic hypotension, pancreatitis, hyperglycemia, hyperuricemia, electrolyte imbalance, blood dyscrasias, hypersensitivity reactions.
Metolazone (Zaroxolyn)	**Tab:** 2.5mg, 5mg, 10mg	***Adults:* Edema:** 5-20mg qd. **HTN:** 2.5-5mg qd. **Elderly:** Start at low end of dosing range.	**BB:** Do not interchange rapid and complete bioavailability metolazone formulations for other slow and incomplete bioavailability metolazone formulations; they are not therapeutically equivalent. **W/P:** Risk of hypokalemia, orthostatic hypotension, hypercalcemia, hyperuricemia, azotemia and rapid onset hyponatremia. Cross-allergy with sulfonamide-derived drugs, thiazides, or quinethazone. Sensitivity reactions may occur with 1st dose. Monitor electrolytes. May cause hyperglycemia and glycosuria in diabetics. Caution in elderly or severe renal impairment. May exacerbate or activate SLE. **Contra:** Anuria, hepatic coma or precoma. **P/N:** Category B, not for use in nursing.	Chest pain/discomfort, orthostatic hypotension, syncope, neuropathy, necrotizing angiitis, hepatitis, jaundice, pancreatitis, blood dyscrasias, joint pain.
DIURETIC COMBINATIONS†				
Amiloride HCl/ Hydrochloro-thiazide*	**Tab:** (Amiloride-HCTZ) **Tab:** (Amiloride-HCTZ) 5mg-50mg* *scored	***Adults:*** Initial: 1 tab qd. Titrate: May increase to 2 tabs qd or in divided doses. Max: 2 tabs/day. May give intermittently once diuresis is achieved. Take with food.	**W/P:** Risk of hyperkalemia (≥5.5mEq/L) especially with renal impairment or DM; d/c if hyperkalemia occurs. Monitor for fluid/electrolyte imbalance; hyponatremia and hypochloremia may occur. Caution in severely ill (risk of respiratory or metabolic acidosis). Increases BUN, cholesterol, and TG levels. D/C at least 3 days before glucose tolerance test. May precipitate gout or exacerbate SLE. May precipitate azotemia with renal disease. **Contra:** Hyperkalemia,	Nausea, anorexia, rash, headache, weakness, hyperkalemia, dizziness.

* Available only in generic form. † More combination products are on page 187 (α-Antagonist Combinations), page 192 (ACE Inhibitor Combinations), page 197 (ARBs Combinations), page 202 (Beta-Blocker Combinations), and page 209 (Direct Renin Inhibitor & Combination).
BB = black box warning; **W/P** = warnings/precautions; **Contra** = contraindications; **P/N** = pregnancy category rating and nursing considerations.

Prescribing Information for Antihypertensive Agents

GENERIC (BRAND)	FORM/ STRENGTH	DOSAGE	WARNINGS/PRECAUTIONS & CONTRAINDICATIONS	ADVERSE REACTIONS
DIURETIC COMBINATIONS *(Cont.)*				
Amiloride HCl/ Hydrochloro- thiazide* *(Cont.)*			anuria, sulfonamide hypersensitivity, acute or chronic renal insufficiency, diabetic neuropathy. Concomitant K⁺-sparing agents (eg, spironolactone, triamterene), K⁺ supplements, salt substitutes, K⁺-rich diet (except with severe hypokalemia). **P/N:** Category B, not for use in nursing.	
Chlorthalidone/ Clonidine HCl (Clorpres)	**Tab:** (Clonidine- Chlorthalidone) 0.1mg-15mg*, 0.2mg-15mg*, 0.3mg-15mg* *scored	***Adults:*** Determine dose by individual titration. 0.1mg clonidine-15mg chlorthalidone tab qd-bid; Max: 0.6 mg clonidine-30mg chlorthalidone/day.	**W/P:** Caution with severe renal disease, hepatic dysfunction, asthma, severe coronary insufficiency, recent MI, cerebrovascular disease. May develop allergic reaction to oral clonidine if sensitive to clonidine patch. Avoid abrupt withdrawal. Continue therapy to within 4 hrs of surgery and resume after. Monitor for fluid/electrolyte imbalance. Hyperuricemia, hypokalemia, hyponatremia, hypochloremic alkalosis, and hyperglycemia may occur. **Contra:** Anuria, sulfonamide hypersensitivity. **P/N:** (Clonidine) Category C, caution in nursing. (Chlorthalidone) Category B, not for use in nursing.	Drowsiness, dizziness, constipation, sedation, nausea, vomiting, blood dyscrasias, hypersensitivity reactions, orthostatic symptoms, impotence.
Spironolactone/ Hydrochloro- thiazide (Aldactazide)	**Tab:** (Spironolactone- HCTZ) 25mg-25mg, 50mg-50mg* *scored	***Adults:*** **Edema:** 100mg/day per component qd or in divided doses. Maint: 25-200mg/day per component. **HTN:** 50-100mg/day per component qd or in divided doses.	**BB:** Tumorigenic in chronic toxicity animal studies; avoid unnecessary use. Not for initial therapy. **W/P:** Monitor for fluid/ electrolyte imbalance. Caution with renal and hepatic dysfunction. Hyperchloremic metabolic acidosis reported with decompensated hepatic cirrhosis. Mild acidosis, gynecomastia, transient BUN elevation, hypercalcemia, hyperglycemia, hyperuricemia, hypomagnesemia, and sensitivity reactions may occur. D/C if hyperkalemia occurs. Risk of dilutional hyponatremia. Enhanced effects in post-sympathectomy patient. May increase cholesterol and TG levels. May manifest latent DM. **Contra:** Acute renal impairment, significantly impaired renal excretory function, hyperkalemia, acute or severe hepatic dysfunction, anuria, sulfonamide hypersensitivity. **P/N:** Category C, not for use in nursing.	Gastric bleeding, ulceration, gynecomastia, impotence, agranulocytosis, fever, urticaria, confusion, ataxia, renal dysfunction, blood dyscrasias, electrolyte disturbances, weakness, irregular menses, amenorrhea.
Triamterene/ Hydrochloro- thiazide (Dyazide)	**Cap:** (Triamterene- HCTZ) 37.5mg-25mg	***Adults:*** 1-2 caps qd.	**W/P:** Risk of hyperkalemia (≥5.5mEq/L) especially with renal impairment, elderly, DM or severely ill; monitor levels frequently. Caution in severely ill in whom respiratory or metabolic acidosis may occur; monitor acid-base balance frequently. May manifest DM. Caution with hepatic dysfunction, history of renal stones. Increases uric acid levels, BUN, creatinine. May decrease PBI levels. D/C before parathyroid function tests. May potentiate electrolyte imbalance with heart failure, renal disease, cirrhosis. **Contra:** Hyperkalemia, anuria, acute or chronic renal insufficiency, sulfonamide hypersensitivity, diabetic neuropathy, K⁺-sparing agents (eg, diuretics), K⁺ supplements (except with severe hypokalemia), K⁺ salt substitutes, K⁺-rich diet. **P/N:** Category C, not for use in nursing.	Muscle cramps, GI effects, weakness, blood dyscrasias, arrhythmia, impotence, dry mouth, jaundice, paresthesia, renal stones, hypersensitivity reactions.

* Available only in generic form.
BB = black box warning; **W/P** = warnings/precautions; **Contra** = contraindications; **P/N** = pregnancy category rating and nursing considerations.

(Continued)

Prescribing Information for Antihypertensive Agents

GENERIC (BRAND)	FORM/ STRENGTH	DOSAGE	WARNINGS/PRECAUTIONS & CONTRAINDICATIONS	ADVERSE REACTIONS
Triamterene/ hydrochloro-thiazide (Maxzide/ Maxzide-25)	(Triamterene-HCTZ) **Tab:** (Maxzide) 75mg-50mg*, (Maxzide-25) 37.5mg-25mg* *scored	**Adults:** (37.5mg-25mg tab) 1-2 tabs qd. (75mg-50mg tab) 1 tab qd.	**W/P:** Risk of hyperkalemia (≥5.5mEq/L) especially with renal impairment, elderly, DM or severely ill; monitor levels frequently. Check ECG if hyperkalemia occurs. Caution with history of renal lithiasis, hepatic dysfunction. Monitor BUN and creatinine periodically. D/C if azotemia increases. May contribute to megaloblastosis in folic acid deficiency. Hyperuricemia, hypercalcemia, hypophosphatemia, hypokalemia may occur. May manifest latent DM. May decrease serum PBI levels. Monitor for fluid/electrolyte imbalance. **Contra:** Hyperkalemia, anuria, acute or chronic renal insufficiency, sulfonamide hypersensitivity, diabetic neuropathy, K⁺-sparing agents (eg, diuretics), K⁺ supplements, K⁺ salt substitutes, K⁺-rich diet. **P/N:** Category C, not for use **P/N:** Category C, not for use in nursing.	Jaundice, pancreatitis, nausea, vomiting, taste alteration, drowsiness, dry mouth, depression, anxiety, tachycardia, blood dyscrasias, electrolyte disturbances.
VASODILATORS				
Hydralazine HCl*	**Inj:** 20mg/mL; **Tab:** 10mg, 25mg, 50mg, 100mg	**Adults:** Initial: 10mg qid for 2-4 days. Titrate: Increase to 25mg qid for the rest of the week, then increase to 50mg qid. Maint: Use lowest effective dose. **Resistant Patients:** 300mg/day or titrate to lower dose combined with thiazide diuretic and/or reserpine, or β-blocker. **Pediatrics:** Initial: 0.75mg/kg/day given qid. Titrate: Increase gradually over 3-4 weeks to a max of 7.5mg/kg/day or 200mg/day.	**W/P:** D/C if SLE symptoms occur. May cause angina and ECG changes of MI. Caution with suspected CAD, CVA, advanced renal impairment. May increase pulmonary artery pressure in mitral valvular disease. Postural hypotension reported. Add pyridoxine if peripheral neuritis develops. Monitor CBC and ANA titer before and periodically during therapy. **Contra:** CAD and mitral valvular rheumatic heart disease. **P/N:** Category C, safety in nursing not known.	Headache, anorexia, nausea, vomiting, diarrhea, tachycardia, angina.
Isosorbide dinitrate (Isordil, Isordil titradose)	**Tab:** 5mg*, 10mg*, 20mg*, 30mg*; **Tab, Extended-Release:** 40mg; **Tab, Sublingual:** 2.5mg *scored	**Adults: Prevention:** Initial: 5-20mg bid-tid. Maint: 10-40mg bid-tid. Allow a dose-free interval of at least 14 hrs for both formulations. **Elderly:** Start at low end of dosing range.	**W/P:** Not for use with acute MI or CHF. Severe hypotension may occur. May aggravate angina caused by hypertrophic cardiomyopathy. Caution with volume depletion, hypotension, elderly. Monitor for tolerance. **P/N:** Category C, caution in nursing.	Headache, lightheadedness, hypotension, syncope, rebound HTN.
Isosorbide mononitrate (Imdur)	**Tab, Extended-Release:** 30mg*, 60mg*, 120mg *scored	**Adults:** Initial: 30-60mg qd in am. Titrate: May increase after several days to 120mg/day. Swallow whole with fluids. **Elderly:** Start at lower end of dosing range.	**W/P:** Not for use with acute MI or CHF. Severe hypotension may occur; caution with volume depletion and hypotension. Hypotension may increase angina pectoris. May aggravate angina caused by hypertrophic cardiomyopathy. Monitor for tolerance. May interfere with cholesterol test. **P/N:** Category B, caution with nursing.	Headache, dizziness, hypotension.
Isosorbide mononitrate (Ismo)	**Tab:** 20mg* *scored	**Adults:** 20mg bid; first dose on awakening, then 7 hrs later.	**W/P:** Not for use with acute MI or CHF. Severe hypotension may occur. May aggravate angina caused by hypertrophic cardiomyopathy. Caution with volume depletion, elderly. Monitor for tolerance. **P/N:** Category C, caution in nursing.	Headache, dizziness, nausea, vomiting.
Minoxidil*	**Tab:** 2.5mg*, 10mg* *scored	**Adults:** Initial: 5mg qd. Titrate: Increase by no less than 3 days; may increase every 6 hrs if closely monitored. Usual: 10-40mg/day. Max: 100mg/day. Frequency: Give qd if diastolic BP is reduced to <30mmHg and if reduced to >30mmHg give bid. Give with a diuretic (eg. HCTZ 50mg bid, furosemide 40mg bid) and a β-blocker (equivalent to propranolol 80-160mg/day) or methyldopa (250-750mg bid starting	**BB:** May cause pericardial effusion, occasionally progressing to tamponade, and angina pectoris may be exacerbated. Only for nonresponders to maximum therapeutic doses of two other antihypertensives and a diuretic. Administer under supervision with a β-blocker and diuretic. Monitor in hospital for a decrease in BP in those receiving guanethidine with malignant hypertension. **W/P:** Administer with a	Salt and water retention, pericarditis, pericardial effusion, tamponade, hypertrichosis, nausea, vomiting, rash, ECG changes, hemodilution effects.

* Available only in generic form.
BB = black box warning; **W/P** = warnings/precautions; **Contra** = contraindications; **P/N** = pregnancy category rating and nursing considerations.

	Prescribing Information for Antihypertensive Agents				
GENERIC (BRAND)	**FORM/ STRENGTH**	**DOSAGE**	**WARNINGS/PRECAUTIONS & CONTRAINDICATIONS**	**ADVERSE REACTIONS**
VASODILATORS *(Cont.)*				
Minoxidil* *(Cont.)*		24 hrs before therapy). **Renal Failure/ Dialysis:** Reduce dose. **Pediatrics:** **>12 yrs:** Initial: 5mg qd. Titrate: Increase by no less than 3 days; may increase every 6 hrs if closely monitored. Usual: 10-40mg/day. Max: 100mg/day. Frequency: Give qd if diastolic BP is reduced to <30mmHg and if reduced to >30mmHg give bid. Give with a diuretic (eg, HCTZ 50mg bid, furosemide 40mg bid) and a β-blocker (equivalent to propranolol 80-160mg/day) or methyldopa (250-750mg bid starting 24 hrs before therapy). **<12 yrs:** 0.2mg/kg qd. Titrate: May increase by 50-100% increments. Usual: 0.25-1mg/kg/day. Max: 50mg/day. **Renal Failure/Dialysis:** Reduce dose.	diuretic and β-blocker. Pericarditis, pericardial effusion and tamponade reported. With renal failure or dialysis, reduce dose to prevent renal failure exacerbation and precipitation of cardiac failure. Avoid rapid control with severe HTN. Monitor body weight, fluid and electrolyte balance. Extreme caution with post-MI. Hypersensitivity reactions reported. **Contra:** Pheochromocytoma. **P/N:** Category C, not for use in nursing.	
VASODILATOR COMBINATION				
Hydralazine HCl/ Isosorbide dinitrate (BiDil)	**Tab:** (Hydralazine-Isosorbide) 37.5mg-20mg	**Adults:** Initial: 1 tab tid. Max: 2 tabs tid.	**W/P:** May produce a clinical picture simulating systemic lupus erythematosus including glomerulonephritis. May cause symptomatic hypotension, tachycardia, peripheral neuritis. Caution in patients with acute MI, hemodynamic and clinical monitoring recommended. May aggravate angina associated with hypertrophic cardiomyopathy. **Contra:** Allergies to organic nitrates. **P/N:** Category C, caution in nursing.	Headache, dizziness, chest pain, asthenia, nausea, bronchitis, hypotension, sinusitis, ventricular tachycardia, palpitations, hyperglycemia, rhinitis, paresthesia, vomiting, amblyopia, hyperlipidemia.
MISCELLANEOUS				
Clonidine** (Catapres, Catapres-TTS)	**Patch, Extended-Release** (TTS): 0.1mg/24 hr [4*], 0.2mg/24 hr [4*], 0.3mg/24 hr [4*]; **Tab:** 0.1mg*, 0.2mg*, 0.3mg* *scored	**Adults:** **(Patch)** Apply to hairless, intact area of upper arm or chest weekly. Taper withdrawal of previous antihypertensive. Initial: 0.1mg/24 hr patch weekly. Titrate: May increase after 1-2 weeks. Max: 0.6mg/24 hr. **(Tab)** Initial: 0.1mg bid. Titrate: May increase by 0.1mg weekly. Usual: 0.2-0.6mg/day in divided doses. Max: 2.4mg/day. **(Patch, Tab)** Renal Impairment: Adjust according to degree of impairment.	**W/P:** Avoid abrupt discontinuation. Tabs may cause rash if have allergic reaction to patch. Continue tabs to within 4 hrs of surgery resume and as soon as possible thereafter. Do not remove patch for surgery. Caution with severe coronary insufficiency, conduction disturbances, recent MI, cerebrovascular disease or chronic renal failure. Remove patch before defibrillation or cardioversion due to the potential risk of altered electrical conductivity or MRI due to the occurrence of burns. **P/N:** Category C, caution in nursing.	Dry mouth, drowsiness, dizziness, constipation, sedation, impotence/ sexual dysfunction, nausea, vomiting, alopecia, weakness, orthostatic symptoms, nervousness, localized skin reactions (patch).
Fenoldopam mesylate (Corlopam)	**Inj:** 10mg/mL	**Adults:** Range: Initial: 0.01-0.8 mcg/kg/min IV. Titrate: Increase/decrease by 0.05-0.1mcg/kg/min no more frequently than every 15 min. May use for up to 48 hrs. Refer to PI for detailed dosing info. **Pediatrics:** <1 month-12 years: Initial: 0.2mcg/kg/min. May increase dose every 20-30 min up to 0.3-0.5 mcg/kg/min. Refer to PI for detailed dosing info.	**W/P:** Contains sodium metabisulfite; may cause allergic-type reactions especially in asthmatics. Caution in glaucoma or intraocular HTN. Dose-related tachycardia reported. Symptomatic hypotension may occur; monitor BP. Avoid hypotension with acute cerebral infarction or hemorrhage. Hypokalemia reported; monitor serum electrolytes. **P/N:** Category B, caution in nursing.	Headache, nausea, flushing, extrasystoles, palpitations, bradycardia, heart failure, elevated BUN/glucose/ transaminase, chest pain, leukocytosis, bleeding, dyspnea.
Guanfacine HCl (Tenex)	**Tab:** 1mg, 2mg	**Adults:** 1mg qhs. Titrate: May increase to 2mg qhs after 3-4 weeks. Max: 3mg/day.	**W/P:** Caution with severe coronary insufficiency, recent MI, cerebrovascular disease, chronic renal or hepatic failure. Avoid abrupt discontinuation. Dose-related drowsiness and sedation. **P/N:** Category B, caution with nursing.	Dry mouth, somnolence, asthenia, dizziness, constipation, impotence, headache.

* Available only in generic form.
** Combination information for clonidine/chlorthalidone (Clorpres) is on page 214.
W/P = warnings/precautions; **Contra** = contraindications; **P/N** = pregnancy category rating and nursing considerations.

(Continued)

Prescribing Information for Antihypertensive Agents

GENERIC (BRAND)	FORM/ STRENGTH	DOSAGE	WARNINGS/PRECAUTIONS & CONTRAINDICATIONS	ADVERSE REACTIONS
Mecamylamine HCl (Inversine)	**Tab:** 2.5mg	***Adults:*** Initial: 2.5mg bid after meals. Titrate: Increase by 2.5mg/day at intervals of not less than 2 days. Usual: 25mg/day given tid. Give larger doses at noontime and evening. Reduce dose by 50% with thiazides.	**W/P:** Caution with renal, cerebral, or cardiovascular dysfunction, marked cerebral or coronary insufficiency, prostatic hypertrophy, bladder neck obstruction, urethral stricture. Large doses in cerebral or renal insufficiency may produce CNS effects. Withdraw gradually and add other antihypertensives. May be potentiated by excessive heat, fever, infection, hemorrhage, pregnancy, anesthesia, surgery, vigorous exercise, other antihypertensive drugs, alcohol, salt depletion. D/C if paralytic ileus occurs. **Contra:** Coronary insufficiency, recent MI, uremia, glaucoma, organic pyloric stenosis, uncooperative patients, mild to moderate or labile HTN, with antibiotics or sulfonamides. Administer with great discretion in renal insufficiency. **P/N:** Category C, not for use in nursing.	Ileus, constipation, vomiting, nausea, anorexia, dryness of mouth, syncope, postural hypotension, convulsions, tremor, interstitial pulmonary edema, urinary retention, impotence, blurred vision.
Methyldopa*	**Tab:** 125mg, 250mg, 500mg	***Adults:*** Initial: 250mg bid-tid for 48 hrs. Adjust dose at intervals of not less than 2 days. Maint: 500mg-2g/day given bid-qid. Max: 3g/day. Concomitant **Antihypertensives (other than thiazides):** Initial: Limit to 500mg/day. **Renal Impairment:** May respond to lower doses. ***Pediatrics:*** Initial: 10mg/kg/day given bid-qid. Max: 65mg/kg/day or 3g/day, whichever is less.	**W/P:** Positive Coombs test, hemolytic anemia, and liver disorders may occur. Fever reported within the first 3 weeks of therapy. HTN has recurred after dialysis. Caution with liver disease or dysfunction. D/C if signs of heart failure, or involuntary choreoathetotic movements develop. Edema and weight gain reported. Blood count, Coombs test and LFTs prior to therapy and periodically thereafter. **Contra:** Active hepatic disease, history of methyldopa associated liver disorder, concomitant MAOIs. **P/N:** Category B, caution in nursing.	Sedation, headache, asthenia, edema/weight gain, hepatic disorders, vomiting, diarrhea, nausea, sore or black tongue, blood dyscrasias, BUN increase, gynecomastia, impotence.
Phenoxybenzamine HCl (Dibenzyline)	**Cap:** 10mg	***Adults:*** Initial: 10mg bid. Titrate: Increase every other day to 20-40mg bid-tid, until BP is controlled.	**W/P:** Caution with marked cerebral or coronary arteriosclerosis, or renal damage. May aggravate symptoms of respiratory infections. **Contra:** Conditions where fall in BP may be undesirable. **P/N:** Category C, not for use in nursing.	Postural hypotension, tachycardia, ejaculation inhibition, nasal congestion, miosis, GI irritation, drowsiness, fatigue.
Reserpine*	**Tab:** 0.1mg, 0.25mg	***Adults:*** HTN: Initial: 0.5mg/day for 1-2 weeks. Maint: reduce to 0.1-0.25mg/day. **Psychotic Disorders:** Initial: 0.5mg/day. Range: 0.1-1mg/day.	**W/P:** Caution with renal insufficiency. May cause depression; d/c at 1st sign. Caution with history of peptic ulcer, ulcerative colitis, or gallstones. **Contra:** Active or history of mental depression, active peptic ulcer, ulcerative colitis, current electroconvulsive therapy. **P/N:** Category C, not for use in nursing.	GI effects, dry mouth, hypersecretion, arrhythmia, syncope, edema, dyspnea, muscle aches, dizziness, depression, nervousness, impotence, gynecomastia, rash.

* Available only in generic form.
BB = black box warning; **W/P** = warnings/precautions; **Contra** = contraindications; **P/N** = pregnancy category rating and nursing considerations.

Prescribing Information for Antilipidemic Agents

GENERIC (BRAND)	FORM/ STRENGTH	DOSAGE	WARNINGS/PRECAUTIONS & CONTRAINDICATIONS	ADVERSE REACTIONS
BILE ACID SEQUESTRANTS				
Cholestyramine (Questran, Questran Light)	**Powder:** 4g/pkt [60*, 378g], (**Light**) 4g/scoopful [60*, 268g]	***Adults:*** Initial: 1 pkt or scoopful qd or bid. Maint: 2-4 pkts or scoopfuls/day, given bid. Titrate: Adjust at no less than 4 week intervals. Max: 6 pkts/day or 6 scoopfuls/ day. May also give as 1-6 doses/day. Mix with fluid or highly fluid food. ***Pediatrics:*** Usual: 240mg/kg/day of anhydrous cholestyramine resin in 2-3 divided doses. Max: 8g/day.	**W/P:** May produce hyperchloremic acidosis with prolonged use. Caution in renal insufficiency, volume depletion, and with concomitant spironolactone. Chronic use may produce or worsen constipation. Avoid constipation with symptomatic CAD. May increase bleeding tendency due to vitamin K deficiency. Serum or red cell folate reduced with chronic use. Constipation may aggravate hemorrhoids. Light formulation contains phenylalanine. Measure cholesterol during 1st few months; periodically thereafter. Measure TG periodically. **Contra:** Complete biliary obstruction. **P/N:** Category C, caution in nursing.	Constipation, heartburn, nausea, vomiting, abdominal pain, flatulence, diarrhea, anorexia, osteoporosis, rash, hyperchloremic acidosis (children), vitamin A and D deficiency, steatorrhea, hypoprothrombinemia (vitamin K deficiency).
Colesevelam HCl (Welchol)	**Tab:** 625mg	***Adults: Hyperlipidemia/Type 2 DM:*** 3 tabs bid or 6 tabs qd. Take with liquids and a meal.	**W/P:** Monitor lipids, including TG and non-HDL-cholesterol levels prior to initiation of treatment and periodically thereafter. Caution in TG levels >300mg/dL, dysphagia or swallowing disorders, gastroparesis, GI motility disorders, major GI tract surgery, bowel obstruction, and those susceptible to vitamin K or fat soluble vitamin deficiencies. Coadministered drugs should be given at least 4 hrs prior to treatment; monitor drug levels. Not for use in treatment of type 1 DM or for diabetic ketoacidosis. **Contra:** Bowel obstruction, hypertriglyceridemia-induced pancreatitis, serum TG concentrations >500mg/dL. **P/N:** Category B, caution in nursing.	Asthenia, constipation, dyspepsia, pharyngitis, myalgia, nausea, hypoglycemia, bowel obstruction, dysphagia, esophageal obstruction, fecal impaction, hypertriglyceridemia, pancreatitis, increased transaminases.
Colestipol HCl (Colestid)	**Granules:** 5g/pkt [30* 90*], 5g/ scoopful [300g, 500g]; **Tab:** 1g	***Adults:*** Initial: 2g, 1 pkt or 1 scoopful qd-bid. Titrate: Increase by 2g qd or bid at 1-2 month intervals. Usual: 2-16g/day (tab) or 1-6 pkts or scoopfuls qd or in divided doses. Always mix granules with liquid. Swallow tabs whole with plenty of liquid.	**W/P:** Exclude secondary causes of hypercholesterolemia and perform a lipid profile. May produce hyperchloremic acidosis with prolonged use. Monitor cholesterol and TG based on NCEP guidelines. May cause hypothyroidism. May interfere with normal fat absorption. Chronic use may produce or worsen constipation. Avoid constipation with symptomatic CAD. May increase bleeding tendency due to vitamin K deficiency. **P/N:** Safety in pregnancy not known, caution in nursing.	Constipation, musculoskeletal pain, headache, migraine headache, sinus headache.
CHOLESTEROL ABSORPTION INHIBITOR				
Ezetimibe (Zetia)	**Tab:** 10mg	***Adults:*** 10mg qd. May give with HMG-CoA reductase inhibitor (with primary hypercholesterolemia) or fenofibrate (with mixed hyperlipidemia) for incremental effect. **Concomitant Bile Acid Sequestrant:** Give either ≥2 hrs before or ≥4 hrs after bile acid sequestrant.	**W/P:** Monitor LFTs with concurrent statin therapy. Not recommended with moderate or severe hepatic insufficiency. **Contra:** When used with a statin, refer to the HMG-CoA reductase inhibitor prescribing information. **P/N:** Category C, contraindicated in nursing.	Back pain, arthralgia, diarrhea, sinusitis, abdominal pain, myalgia.
FATTY ACID DERIVATIVE				
Omega-3-acid ethyl esters (Lovaza)	**Cap:** 1g	***Adults:*** 4g qd. Given as single 4-g dose (4 caps) or as two 2-g doses (2 caps bid).	**W/P:** Caution in patients with diabetes, hypothyroidism, hepatic and pancreas problems, known sensitivity or allergy to fish. Lower alcohol use. Lose weight if overweight. Possible increases in alanine aminotransferase levels without a concurrent increase in aspartate aminotransferase levels. Possible increased LDL cholesterol levels. **P/N:** Category C, caution in nursing.	Eructation, infection, flu-syndrome, dyspepsia.

W/P = warnings/precautions; **Contra** = contraindications; **P/N** = pregnancy category rating and nursing considerations.

(Continued)

Prescribing Information for Antilipidemic Agents

GENERIC (BRAND)	FORM/ STRENGTH	DOSAGE	WARNINGS/PRECAUTIONS & CONTRAINDICATIONS	ADVERSE REACTIONS
FIBRATES				
Fenofibrate (Antara)	**Cap:** 43mg, 130mg	***Adults:* Hypercholesterolemia/Mixed Dyslipidemia:** Initial: 130mg qd. **Hypertriglyceridemia:** Initial: 43-130mg/ day. Titrate: Adjust if needed after repeat lipid levels at 4-8 week intervals. Max: 130mg/day. **Renal Dysfunction/ Elderly:** Initial: 43mg/day. Take with meals.	**W/P:** Monitor LFTs regularly; d/c if >3x ULN. May cause cholelithiasis; d/c if gallstones found. D/C if myopathy or marked CPK elevation occurs. Decreased Hgb, Hct, WBCs, thrombocytopenia, and agranulocytosis reported; monitor CBCs during first 12 months of therapy. Acute hypersensitivity reactions (rare) and pancreatitis reported. Rare cases of rhabdomyolysis. Evaluate for myopathy. Monitor lipids periodically initially, d/c if inadequate response after 2 months on 130mg/day. Minimize dose in severe renal impairment. Caution in elderly. **Contra:** Hepatic or severe renal dysfunction (including primary cirrhosis), unexplained persistent hepatic function abnormality, pre-existing gallbladder disease. **P/N:** Category C, not for use in nursing.	Abdominal pain, back pain, headache, abnormal LFTs, respiratory disorder, increased CPK, increased SGPT/SGOT.
Fenofibrate (Lofibra)	**Cap:** 67mg, 134mg, 200mg; **Tab:** 54mg, 160mg	***Adults:* Hypercholesterolemia/Mixed Dyslipidemia:** Initial: **Cap:** 200mg qd. **Hypercholesterolemia/Mixed Hyperlipidemia: Tab:** 160mg qd. **Hypertriglyceridemia:** Initial: **Cap:** 67-200mg/day. **Tab:** 54-160mg qd. Titrate: Adjust if needed after repeat lipid levels at 4-8 week intervals. Max: **Cap:** 200mg/day. **Tab:** 160mg/day. **Renal Dysfunction/Elderly:** Initial: **Cap:** 67mg/ day. **Tab:** 54mg/day. Take with meals.	**W/P:** Monitor LFTs regularly; d/c if >3x ULN. May cause cholelithiasis; d/c if gallstones found. D/C if myopathy or marked CPK elevation occurs. Decreased Hgb, Hct, WBCs, thrombocytopenia, and agranulocytosis reported; monitor CBCs during first 12 months of therapy. Acute hypersensitivity reactions (rare) and pancreatitis reported. Monitor lipids periodically initially, d/c if inadequate response after 2 months on 200mg/day. Minimize dose in severe renal impairment. Caution in elderly. **Contra:** Pre-existing gallbladder disease, unexplained persistent hepatic function abnormality, hepatic or severe renal dysfunction (including primary biliary cirrhosis). **P/N:** Category C, not for use in nursing.	Abdominal pain, back pain, headache, abnormal LFTs, increased CPK, respiratory disorder.
Fenofibrate (Tricor)	**Tab:** 48mg, 145mg	***Adults:* Hypercholesterolemia/Mixed Dyslipidemia:** Initial: 145mg qd. **Hypertriglyceridemia:** Initial: 48-145mg/ day. Titrate: Adjust if needed after repeat lipid levels at 4-8 week intervals. Max: 145mg/day. **Renal Dysfunction/ Elderly:** Initial: 48mg/day. Take without regards to meals.	**W/P:** Monitor LFTs regularly; d/c if >3x ULN. May cause cholelithiasis; d/c if gallstones found. D/C if myopathy or marked CPK elevation occurs. Decreased Hgb, Hct, WBCs, thrombocytopenia, and agranulocytosis reported; monitor CBC during first 12 months of therapy. Acute hypersensitivity reactions (rare) and pancreatitis reported. Monitor lipids periodically initially, d/c if inadequate response after 2 months on 145mg/day. Minimize dose in severe renal impairment. Caution in elderly. **Contra:** Preexisting gallbladder disease, unexplained persistent hepatic function abnormality, hepatic or severe renal dysfunction (including primary biliary cirrhosis). **P/N:** Category C, not for use in nursing.	Abdominal pain, back pain, headache, abnormal LFTs, respiratory disorder, increased CPK.
Fenofibrate (Triglide)	**Tab:** 50mg, 160mg	***Adults:* Hypercholesterolemia/Mixed Hyperlipidemia:** 160mg qd. **Hypertriglyceridemia:** Initial: 50-160mg/ day. Titrate: Adjust if needed after repeat lipid levels at 4-8 week intervals. Max: 160mg/day. **Renal Dysfunction/ Elderly:** Initial: 50mg/day. Take without regards to meals.	**W/P:** Monitor LFTs regularly; d/c if >3x ULN. May cause cholelithiasis; d/c if gallstones found. D/C if myopathy or marked CPK elevation occurs. Decreased Hgb, Hct, WBCs, thrombocytopenia, and agranulocytosis reported; monitor CBCs during first 12 months of therapy. Acute hypersensitivity reactions (rare) and pancreatitis reported. Monitor lipids periodically initially; d/c if inadequate response after 2 months on 160mg/day. Minimize dose in severe renal impairment. Caution in elderly. **Contra:** Severe renal	Abdominal pain, back pain, headache, abnormal LFTs, respiratory disorder, increased CPK, increased SGPT/SGOT.

W/P = warnings/precautions; **Contra** = contraindications; **P/N** = pregnancy category rating and nursing considerations.

Prescribing Information for Antilipidemic Agents

GENERIC (BRAND)	FORM/ STRENGTH	DOSAGE	WARNINGS/PRECAUTIONS & CONTRAINDICATIONS	ADVERSE REACTIONS
Fenofibrate (Triglide) *(Cont.)*			dysfunction, hepatic dysfunction (including primary biliary cirrhosis and unexplained persistent liver function abnormality), pre-existing gallbladder disease. **P/N:** Category C, not for use in nursing.	
Gemfibrozil (Lopid)	**Tab:** 600mg* *scored	**Adults:** 600mg bid. Give 30 min before morning and evening meals.	**W/P:** Abnormal LFTs reported; monitor periodically. Only use if indicated and d/c if significant lipid response not obtained. Associated with myositis. D/C if suspect or diagnose myositis, if abnormal LFTs persist, or gallstones develop. Cholelithiasis reported. Monitor CBC periodically during first 12 months. May worsen renal insufficiency. **Contra:** Hepatic or severe renal dysfunction, including primary biliary cirrhosis; pre-existing gallbladder disease, concomitant cerivastatin. **P/N:** Category C, not for use in nursing.	Dyspepsia, abdominal pain, diarrhea, fatigue, bacterial and viral infections, musculoskeletal symptoms, abnormal LFTs, hematologic changes, hypoesthesia, paresthesia, taste perversion.
HMG-CoA REDUCTASE INHIBITORS (STATINS)				
Atorvastatin calcium (Lipitor)	**Tab:** 10mg, 20mg, 40mg, 80mg	**Adults: Hypercholesterolemia/Mixed Dyslipidemia:** Initial: 10-20mg qd (or 40mg qd for LDL-C reduction >45%). Titrate: Adjust dose if needed at 2-4 week intervals. Usual: 10-80mg qd. **Homozygous Familial Hypercholesterolemia:** 10-80mg qd. **Pediatrics: Heterozygous Familial Hypercholesterolemia: 10-17 yrs** (postmenarchal): Initial: 10mg/day. Titrate: Adjust dose if needed at intervals of ≥4 weeks. Max: 20mg/day.	**W/P:** Monitor LFTs prior to therapy, at 12 weeks or with dose elevation, and periodically thereafter. Reduce dose or withdraw if AST or ALT ≥3x ULN persist. Caution with heavy alcohol use and/or history of hepatic disease. D/C if markedly elevated CPK levels occur, if myopathy is diagnosed or suspected, or if predisposition to renal failure secondary to rhabdomyolysis. Caution in patients with recent stroke or TIA. Rare cases of rhabdomyolysis reported. **Contra:** Active liver disease, unexplained persistent elevations of serum transaminases, pregnancy, nursing mothers. **P/N:** Category X, not for use in nursing.	Constipation, flatulence, dyspepsia, abdominal pain, transaminase and CK elevation in higher doses.
Fluvastatin sodium (Lescol, Lescol XL)	**Cap:** (Lescol) 20mg, 40mg; **Tab, Extended-Release:** (Lescol XL) 80mg	**Adults: ≥18 yrs:** (For LDL-C reduction of ≥25%) Initial: 40mg cap qpm or 80mg XL tab at any time of day or 40mg cap bid. (For LDL-C reduction of <25%) Initial: 20mg cap qpm. Range: 20-80mg/day. **Severe Renal Impairment:** Caution with dose >40mg/day. Take 2 hrs after bile-acid resins qhs. **Pediatrics: Heterozygous Familial Hypercholesterolemia: 10-16 yrs (≥1 yr postmenarche):** Individualize dose: Initial: One 20mg cap. Titrate: Adjust dose at 6-week intervals. Max: 40mg cap bid or 80mg XL tab qd.	**W/P:** Monitor LFTs prior to therapy, at 12 weeks, or with dose elevation. D/C if AST or ALT ≥3x ULN on 2 consecutive occasions. Risk of myopathy and/or rhabdomyolysis reported. D/C if markedly elevated CPK levels occur, if myopathy is diagnosed or suspected, or if predisposition to renal failure secondary to rhabdomyolysis. Less effective with homozygous familial hypercholesterolemia. Caution with heavy alcohol use and/or history of hepatic disease. Evaluate if endocrine dysfunction develops. **Contra:** Active liver disease or unexplained, persistent elevations of serum transaminases, pregnancy, nursing mothers. **P/N:** Category X, not for use in nursing.	Dyspepsia, abdominal pain, headache, nausea, diarrhea, abnormal LFTs, myalgia, flu-like symptoms.
Lovastatin (Altoprev)	**Tab: Extended-Release:** 20mg, 40mg, 60mg	**Adults:** Initial: 20, 40, or 60mg qhs. Consider immediate-release lovastatin in patients requiring smaller reductions. May adjust at intervals of ≥4 weeks. **Concomitant Fibrates/Niacin** (≥1g/day): Try to avoid. Max: 20mg/day. **Concomitant Amiodarone/Verapamil:** Max: 20mg/day. **CrCl <30mL/min:** Consider dose increase of >20mg/day carefully and implement cautiously. Swallow whole; do not chew or crush.	**W/P:** May increase serum transaminases and CPK levels; consider in differential diagnosis of chest pain. D/C if AST or ALT ≥3x ULN persist, if myopathy diagnosed or suspected, and a few days before major surgery. Monitor LFTs prior to therapy, at 6 weeks, 12 weeks, then periodically or with dose elevation. Caution with heavy alcohol use and/or history of hepatic disease. Caution with dose escalation in renal insufficiency. Lovastatin immediate-release found to be less effective with homozygous familial hypercholesterolemia.	Nausea, abdominal pain, insomnia, dyspepsia, headache, asthenia, myalgia.

W/P = warnings/precautions; **Contra** = contraindications; **P/N** = pregnancy category rating and nursing considerations.

(Continued)

Prescribing Information for Antilipidemic Agents

GENERIC (BRAND)	FORM/ STRENGTH	DOSAGE	WARNINGS/PRECAUTIONS & CONTRAINDICATIONS	ADVERSE REACTIONS
Lovastatin (Altoprev) *(Cont.)*			Rhabdomyolysis (rare), myopathy reported. **Contra:** Active liver disease, unexplained persistent elevations of serum transaminases, pregnancy, nursing mothers. **P/N:** Category X, not for use in nursing.	
Lovastatin (Mevacor)	**Tab:** 20mg, 40mg	**Adults:** Initial: 20mg qd at dinner (10mg/ day if need LDL-C reduction <20%). Usual: 10-80mg/day given qd or bid. May adjust every 4 weeks. Max: 80mg/ day. **Concomitant Cyclosporine:** Initial: 10mg/day. Max: 20mg/day. **Fibrates/ Niacin (≥1g/day):** Max: 20mg/day. **Concomitant Amiodarone/Verapamil:** Max: 40mg/day. **CrCl <30mL/min:** Consider dose increase of >20mg/day carefully and implement cautiously. **Pediatrics: Heterozygous Familial Hypercholesterolemia: 10-17 yrs (at least 1-yr postmenarchal):** Initial: If <20% LDL-C Reduction Needed: 10mg qd. If ≥20% **LDL-C Reduction Needed:** 20mg qd. May adjust every 4 weeks. Max: 40mg/day. **Concomitant Cyclosporine:** Initial: 10mg/day. Max: 20mg/day. **Fibrates/Niacin (≥1g/day):** Max: 20mg/day. **Concomitant Amiodarone/Verapamil:** Max: 40mg/day. **CrCl <30mL/min:** Consider dose increase of >20mg/day carefully and implement cautiously.	**W/P:** May increase serum transaminases and CPK levels; consider in differential diagnosis of chest pain. D/C if AST or ALT 3x ULN persist, or if myopathy diagnosed or suspected. Monitor LFTs prior to therapy, at 6 weeks, 12 weeks, then periodically or with dose elevation. Caution with heavy alcohol use and/or history of hepatic disease. Caution with dose escalation in renal insufficiency. Less effective with homozygous familial hypercholesterolemia. Rhabdomyolysis (rare), myopathy reported. D/C a few days before elective major surgery and when any major acute medical or surgical condition supervenes. **Contra:** Active liver disease, unexplained persistent elevations of serum transaminases, pregnancy, nursing mothers. **P/N:** Category X, not for use in nursing.	Headache, constipation, flatulence, dizziness, rash, elevated transaminases or CK levels, GI upset, blurred vision.
Pravastatin sodium (Pravachol)	**Tab:** 10mg, 20mg, 40mg, 80mg	**Adults:** ≥18 yrs: Initial: 40mg qd. Perform lipid tests within 4 weeks and adjust according to response and guidelines. Titrate: May increase to 80mg qd if needed. **Significant Renal/Hepatic Dysfunction:** Initial: 10mg qd. **Concomitant Immunosuppressives** (eg, cyclosporine): Initial:10mg qhs. Max: 20mg/day. **Pediatrics: Heterozygous Familial Hypercholesterolemia: 14-18 yrs:** Initial: 40mg qd. **8-13 yrs:** 20mg qd. **Concomitant Immunosuppressives** (eg, cyclosporine): Initial: 10mg qhs. Max: 20mg/day.	**W/P:** Perform LFTs before therapy, before dose increases, and if clinically indicated. Risk of myopathy, myalgia, and rhabdomyolysis. D/C if AST or ALT ≥3x ULN persists, if elevated CPK levels occur, or if myopathy diagnosed or suspected. Less effective with homozygous familial hypercholesterolemia. Monitor for endocrine dysfunction. Closely monitor with heavy alcohol use, recent history or signs of hepatic disease, or renal dysfunction. **Contra:** Active liver disease, unexplained persistent elevations of LFTs, pregnancy, nursing mothers. **P/N:** Category X, not for use in nursing.	Rash, nausea, vomiting, diarrhea, headache, chest pain, influenza, abdominal pain, increases ALT, AST, CPK levels.
Rosuvastatin calcium (Crestor)	**Tab:** 5mg, 10mg, 20mg, 40mg	**Adults: Hypercholesterolemia/Mixed Dyslipidemia/Hypertriglyceridemia/ Slowing Progression of Atherosclerosis:** Initial: 10mg qd. (20mg qd with LDL-C >190mg/dL). Titrate: Adjust dose if needed at 2-4 week intervals. Range: 5-40mg qd. **Homozygous Familial Hypercholesterolemia:** 20mg qd. Max: 40mg qd. **Asian Patients:** 5mg qd. **Concomitant Cyclosporine:** Max: 5mg qd. **Concomitant Lopinavir/Ritonavir:** Max 10mg qd. **Concomitant Gemfibrozil:** Max: 10mg qd. **Severe Renal Impairment:** **CrCl <30mL/min (not on hemodialysis):** Initial: 5mg qd. Max: 10mg qd.	**W/P:** Increased risk of myopathy with other lipid-lowering therapies, cyclosporine, or lopinavir/ritonavir. Rare cases of rhabdomyolysis with acute renal failure secondary to myoglobinuria reported. Monitor LFTs prior to therapy, at 12 weeks or with dose elevation, and periodically thereafter. Reduce dose or d/c if AST/ALT ≥3x ULN persist. Caution with heavy alcohol use, history of hepatic disease, renal impairment, hypothyroidism, elderly. D/C if markedly elevated CPK levels occur, if myopathy is diagnosed or failure secondary to rhabdomyolysis. Approximately 2-fold elevation in median exposure in Asian subjects. Persistent elevations in hepatic transaminase occurred. Monitor liver enzymes. **Contra:** Rash, pruritus, urticaria, angioedema, active liver disease, unexplained persistent elevations of serum transaminases, pregnancy, nursing mothers. **P/N:** Category X, not for use in nursing.	Headache, myalgia, abdominal pain, asthenia, diarrhea, dyspepsia, nausea, rhabdomyolysis with myoglobinuria and ARF and myopathy, liver enzyme abnormalities.

W/P = warnings/precautions; **Contra** = contraindications; **P/N** = pregnancy category rating and nursing considerations.

Prescribing Information for Antilipidemic Agents

GENERIC (BRAND)	FORM/ STRENGTH	DOSAGE	WARNINGS/PRECAUTIONS & CONTRAINDICATIONS	ADVERSE REACTIONS
Simvastatin (Zocor)	**Tab:** 5mg, 10mg, 20mg, 40mg, 80mg	**Adults:** Initial: 20-40mg qpm. Usual: 5-80mg/day. Titrate: Adjust at ≥4-week intervals. **High Risk for CHD Events:** Initial: 40mg/day. **Homozygous Familial Hypercholesterolemia:** 40mg qpm or 80mg/day given as 20mg bid plus 40mg qpm. **Concomitant Cyclosporine:** Initial: 5mg/day. Max: 10mg/day. **Concomitant Gemfibrozil** (try to avoid): Max: 10mg/day. **Concomitant Amiodarone/Verapamil:** Max: 20mg/day. **Severe Renal Insufficiency:** 5mg/day; monitor closely. **Pediatrics: Heterozygous Familial Hypercholesterolemia: 10-17 yrs (at least 1 yr postmenarchal):** Initial: 10mg qpm. Usual: 10-40mg/day. Titrate: Adjust at ≥4-week intervals. Max: 40mg/day.	**W/P:** Caution with heavy alcohol use, severe renal insufficiency or history of hepatic disease. Monitor LFTs prior to therapy, periodically thereafter for 12 months,or until 12 months after last dose elevation (additional test at 3 months for 80mgdose). D/C if AST or ALT ≥3x ULN persist,if myopathy is suspected or diagnosed, a few days prior to major surgery.Rhabdomyolysis (rare), myopathy reported. **Contra:** Active liver disease, unexplained persistent elevations of serum transaminases, pregnancy, nursing mothers. **P/N:** Category X, not for use in nursing.	Abdominal pain, headache, CK and transaminase elevations, constipation, upper respiratory infection, hepatic failure.
NICOTINIC ACID DERIVATIVE				
Niacin (Niaspan)	**Tab, Extended-Release:** 500mg, 750mg, 1000mg	**Adults:** Take qhs after low-fat snack. Initial: 500mg qhs. Titrate: Increase by 500mg every 4 weeks. Maint: 1-2g qhs. Max: 2g/day. Take ASA or NSAIDs 30 min before to reduce flushing. Do not chew, crush, or break; swallow whole. Women may respond to lower doses than men.	**W/P:** Do not substitute with equivalent doses of immediate-release niacin (severe hepatic toxicity may occur). Associated with abnormal LFTs; monitor LFTs before therapy, every 6-12 weeks during 12 months, then periodically thereafter.D/C if LFTs ≥3x ULN persists or developsigns of hepatotoxicity. Monitor for rhabdomyolysis. Observe closely with history of jaundice, hepatobiliary disease, and peptic ulcer; monitor LFTs and blood glucose frequently. Dose-related rise in glucose tolerance in diabetics. Caution with history of hepatic disease, heavy alcohol use, renal dysfunction, unstable angina, and acute phase of MI. Elevated uric acid levels reported. May reduce platelet and phosphorous levels. **Contra:** Unexplained or significant hepatic dysfunction, active peptic ulcer disease, arterial bleeding. **P/N:** Category C, not for use in nursing.	Flushing episodes (eg, tachycardia, shortness of warmth, redness, itching, tingling), dizziness, breath, sweating, chills, edema, headache, diarrhea.
COMBINATIONS				
Amlodipine/ Atorvastatin (Caduet)	**Tab:** (Amlodipine-Atorvastatin) 2.5mg-10mg, 2.5mg-20mg, 2.5mg-40mg, 5mg-10mg, 5mg-20mg, 5mg-40mg, 5mg-80mg, 10mg-10mg, 10mg-20mg, 10mg-40mg, 10mg-80mg	**Adults:** Dosing should be individualized and based on the appropriate combination of recommendations for the monotherapies. **(Amlodipine): HTN:** Initial: 5mg qd. Titrate over 7-14 days. Max: 10mg qd. **Small, Fragile, or Elderly/ Hepatic Dysfunction/Concomitant Antihypertensive:** Initial: 2.5mg qd. Angina: 5-10mg qd. **Elderly/Hepatic Dysfunction:** 5mg qd. **(Atorvastatin): Hypercholesterolemia/Mixed Dyslipidemia:** Initial: 10-20mg qd (or 40mg qd for LDL-C reduction >45%). Titrate: Adjust dose if needed at 2-4 week intervals. Usual: 10-80mg qd. **Homozygous Familial Hypercholesterolemia:** 10-80mg qd. **Pediatrics:** ≥10 yrs (postmenarchal): **(Amlodipine):** HTN: 2.5-5mg qd. **10-17 yrs (postmenarchal): (Atorvastatin): Heterozygous Familial Hypercholesterolemia:** Initial: 10mg/day. Titrate: Adjust dose if needed at intervals of ≥4 weeks. Max: 20mg/day.	**W/P:** May rarely increase angina or MI with severe obstructive CAD. Monitor LFTs prior to therapy, at 12 weeks after initiation, with dose elevation, and periodically thereafter. Reduce dose or withdraw if AST or ALT >3x ULN persist. Caution with heavy alcohol use and/or history of hepatic disease, severe aortic stenosis, CHF. D/C if markedly elevated CPK levels occur, if myopathy is diagnosed or suspected, or if predisposition to renal failure secondary to rhabdomyolysis. Increased risk of hemorrhagic stroke in patients with recent stroke or TIA. **Contra:** Active liver disease, unexplained persistent elevations of serum transaminases, pregnancy, nursing mothers. **P/N:** Category X, not for use in nursing	Headache, edema, palpitation, dizziness, fatigue, constipation, flatulence, dyspepsia, abdominal pain.

W/P = warnings/precautions; **Contra** = contraindications; **P/N** = pregnancy category rating and nursing considerations.

(Continued)

		Prescribing Information for Antilipidemic Agents		
GENERIC (BRAND)	**FORM/ STRENGTH**	**DOSAGE**	**WARNINGS/PRECAUTIONS & CONTRAINDICATIONS**	**ADVERSE REACTIONS**
Ezetimibe/ Simvastatin (Vytorin)	**Tab:** (ezetimibe-simvastatin) 10mg/ 10mg, 10mg/20mg, 10mg/40mg, 10mg/ 80mg	**Adults:** Take once daily in the evening. Initial: 10mg/20mg qd. **Less Aggressive LDL-C Reductions:** Initial: 10mg/10mg qd. **LDL-C Reduction >55%:** Initial: 10mg/ 40mg qd. Titrate: Adjust at ≥2 weeks. **Homozygous Familial Hypercholesterolemia:** 10mg/40mg or 10mg/80mg qd. **Severe Renal Insufficiency:** Avoid unless tolerant of ≥5mg of simvastatin; monitor closely. **Concomitant Bile Acid Sequestrant:** Take either ≥2 hrs before or ≥4 hrs after bile acid sequestrant. **Concomitant Cyclosporine:** Avoid unless tolerant of ≥5mg of simvastatin. Max: 10mg/10mg/ day. **Concomitant Amiodarone/Verapamil:** Max: 10mg/20mg/day.	**W/P:** Rhabdomyolysis (rare), myopathy reported. D/C therapy if myopathy is suspected or diagnosed, if AST or ALT ≥3x ULN persist, a few days prior to major surgery or when any major medical or surgical condition supervenes. Monitor LFTs prior to therapy and thereafter when clinically indicated. With 10mg/80mg dose, monitor LFTs prior to titration, 3 months after titration and periodically thereafter for 12 months. Caution with heavy alcohol use, severe renal insufficiency, or history of hepatic disease. Avoid use in moderate or severe hepatic insufficiency. **Contra:** Active liver disease, unexplained persistent elevations in serum transaminases, pregnancy, lactation. **P/N:** Category X, not for use in nursing.	Headache, upper respiratory tract infection, myalgia, CK and transaminase elevations, urticaria, arthralgia.
Niacin ER/ Lovastatin (Advicor)	**Tab: Extended-Release** (Niacin-Lovastatin) 500mg-20mg, 750mg-20mg, 1000mg-20mg, 1000mg-40mg	**Adults:** ≥18 yrs: Initial: 500mg-20mg qhs. Titrate: Increase by no more than 500mg of niacin every 4 weeks. Max: 2000mg-40mg. **Concomitant Cyclosporine/Danazol:** Max Lovastatin: 20mg/day. **Concomitant Amiodarone/Verapamil:** Max Lovastatin: 40mg/day. Swallow tab whole. Take with low-fat snack. Pretreat 30 min prior with ASA to reduce flushing.	**W/P:** Do not substitute for equivalent dose of immediate-release niacin. Myopathy, rhabdomyolysis, severe hepatotoxicity reported. Caution with history of liver disease or jaundice, heavy alcohol use, hepatobilliary disease, peptic ulcer, diabetes, unstable angina, acute phase of MI, gout, renal dysfunction. Monitor LFTs prior to therapy, every 6-12 weeks for 1st 6 months, and periodically thereafter. May elevate PT, uric acid levels. D/C if AST or ALT ≥3x ULN persist, if myopathy diagnosed or suspected, and a few days before surgery. May reduce phosphorous levels. May disrupt therapy during a course of treatment with systemic antifungal azole, a macrolide antibiotic or ketolide antibiotic. **Contra:** Active liver disease, unexplained persistent elevations in serum transaminases, active PUD, arterial bleeding, pregnancy, nursing mothers. **P/N:** Category X, not for use in nursing.	Flushing, asthenia, flu syndrome, headache, infection, pain, GI effects, hyperglycemia, myalgia, pruritus, rash.
Niacin ER/ Simvastatin (Simcor)	**Tab, Extended-Release:** (Niacin-Simvastatin) 500mg/ 20mg, 750mg/20mg, 1000mg/20mg	**Adults:** Patients not currently on niacin extended-release or switching from immediate-release niacin: Initial: 500mg/ 20mg qd hs, with a low fat snack. Titrate: Adjust dose at ≥4 weeks. After week 8, titrate to patient response and tolerance. Maint: 1000mg/20mg-2000mg/40mg qd. Max: 2000mg/40mg qd. Doses >2000mg/ 40mg qd are not recommended. Do not break, crush or chew before swallowing.	**W/P:** Do not substitute for equivalent dose of immediate-release niacin. Myopathy and rhabdomyolysis reported; monitor serum creatine kinase (CK) periodically. D/c therapy if myopathy is suspected or diagnosed, if transaminase levels increase ≥3 ULN persist, or a few days prior to major surgery or when any major medical or surgical condition supervenes. Increased risk with higher doses, advanced age (≥65), hypothyroidism, renal impairment. Caution with heavy alcohol use, or history of liver disease; monitor LFTs prior to therapy, every 12 weeks for the first 6 months and periodically thereafter. Severe hepatic toxicity may occur in patients substituting sustained-release niacin for immediate-release niacin at equivalent doses. May increase serum glucose levels in diabetic or potentially diabetic patients, particularly the first few months of therapy; adjust diet and/or hypoglycemic therapy or d/c if necessary. May reduce platelet count. Caution with those predisposed to gout. **Contra:** Active liver disease, unexplained persistent elevations of serum transaminases, active peptic ulcer disease, arterial bleeding, pregnancy, nursing mothers. **P/N:** Category X, not for use in nursing.	Flushing, headache, backpain, diarrhea, nausea, pruritus.

W/P = warnings/precautions; **Contra** = contraindications; **P/N** = pregnancy category rating and nursing considerations.

Index

Page numbers referencing tables are followed by a t, *page numbers referencing figures are followed by an* f.